Canine and Feline

THIRD EDITION

NUTRITION

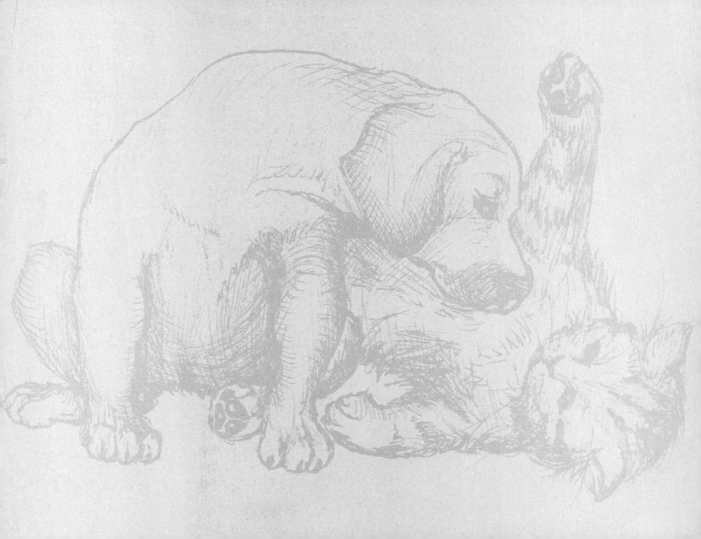

Canine and Feline
NUTRITION

THIRD EDITION

A Resource for Companion Animal Professionals

Linda P. Case, MS
Autumn Gold Consulting
Mahomet, Illinois;
Adjunct Assistant Professor
College of Veterinary Medicine
University of Illinois
Urbana, Illinois

Leighann Daristotle, DVM, PhD
Manager
Scientific Communications
Procter & Gamble Pet Care
Lewisburg, Ohio

Michael G. Hayek, PhD
Associate Director
Research and Development
Procter & Gamble Pet Care
Lewisburg, Ohio

Melody Foess Raasch, DVM
Manager
Scientific Communications
Procter & Gamble Pet Care
Mason, Ohio

with 68 illustrations

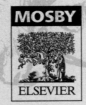

MOSBY

ELSEVIER

MOSBY
ELSEVIER

3251 Riverport Lane
Maryland Heights, Missouri 63043

CANINE AND FELINE NUTRITION, THIRD EDITION   ISBN: 978-0-323-06619-8

Notice

Knowledge and best practice in this field are constantly changing. As new research and experience broaden our understanding, changes in research methods, professional practices, or medical treatment may become necessary.

Practitioners and researchers must always rely on their own experience and knowledge in evaluating and using any information, methods, compounds, or experiments described herein. In using such information or methods they should be mindful of their own safety and the safety of others, including parties for whom they have a professional responsibility.

With respect to any drug or pharmaceutical products identified, readers are advised to check the most current information provided (i) on procedures featured or (ii) by the manufacturer of each product to be administered, to verify the recommended dose or formula, the method and duration of administration, and contraindications. It is the responsibility of practitioners, relying on their own experience and knowledge of their patients, to make diagnoses, to determine dosages and the best treatment for each individual patient, and to take all appropriate safety precautions.

To the fullest extent of the law, neither the Publisher nor the authors, contributors, or editors assume any liability for any injury and/or damage to persons or property as a matter of products liability, negligence or otherwise, or from any use or operation of any methods, products, instructions, or ideas contained in the material herein.

Library of Congress Cataloging-in-Publication Data

Canine and feline nutrition : a resource for companion animal professionals / Linda P. Case ... [et al.]. — 3rd ed.
  p. ; cm.
Includes bibliographical references and index.
ISBN 978-0-323-06619-8 (pbk. : alk. paper)
1. Dogs—Nutrition. 2. Cats—Nutrition. 3. Dogs—Food. 4. Cats—Food. 5. Dogs—Diseases—Nutritional aspects. 6. Cats—Diseases—Nutritional aspects. I. Case, Linda P.
[DNLM: 1. Dogs. 2. Animal Feed. 3. Animal Nutritional Physiological Phenomena. 4. Cats. 5. Nutrition Disorders—veterinary. SF 427.4 C223 2011]
SF427.4.C37 2011
636.7'0852—dc22

                                                    2010001713

Vice President and Publisher: Linda Duncan
Acquisitions Editor: Heidi Pohlman
Publishing Services Manager: Patricia Tannian
Senior Project Manager: Kristine Feeherty
Design Direction: Jessica Williams

Printed in the United States of America

...st digit is the print number: 9   8   7   6   5   4   3   2

To the pet owners who share our appreciation for the infinite ways that dogs and cats enrich our lives and who strive to provide their dogs and cats with the very best care and nutrition, throughout life.

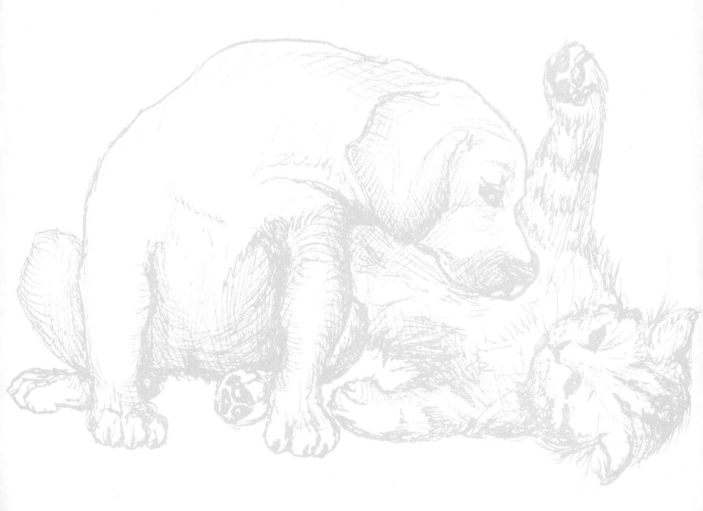

Preface

Humans have a long and very complex history of association with dogs and cats. This relationship has its roots in domestication and has evolved to exist today in a vast variety of forms. Both the dog and the cat originally served a number of functions for humans. While some dogs and cats still fulfill these roles, the primary reason that most people share their lives with dogs and cats today is companionship. In recent years, scientific studies of human-animal interactions have revealed that these relationships are important and enduring components of many pet owners' lives. Pet ownership has also been shown to provide numerous physiological and psychological benefits. Keeping companion animals has become a national pastime, and providing proper care to dogs and cats is of great interest and concern to both pet owners and professionals who work with these animals.

Along with proper health care and medical attention, nutrition is an essential component of pet care. An understanding of basic nutrition and the nutrient requirements of healthy dogs and cats is integral to the understanding of practical feeding practices. Such knowledge enables pet professionals to provide optimal nutritional care throughout life, which contributes to lasting health and longevity. This new edition of *Canine and Feline Nutrition: A Resource for Companion Animal Professionals* provides a thorough examination of the science of companion animal nutrition and practical feeding management for dogs and cats. Information in this book is of value to veterinarians, animal scientists, nutritionists, breeders, exhibitors, judges, trainers, and hobbyists. The book also continues to serve as a textbook for companion animal management and nutrition courses in the fields of animal science and veterinary medicine. It is the authors' intent that this book will complement general animal nutrition textbooks by providing current and comprehensive information about the two most popular companion animal species, the dog and the cat.

This new edition of *Canine and Feline Nutrition* has been reorganized into five sections. These address basic principles of nutrition; nutrient requirements of dogs and cats; pet food production and selection; feeding management throughout the life cycle; and the dietary management of nutritionally responsive disorders. Current research is reviewed, and balanced discussions of different approaches to dietary management are presented. Comparisons between the nutrient requirements and feeding practices of dogs and cats are addressed throughout the book. In order to facilitate use by readers with a wide range of backgrounds and interests, illustrative tables and boxes are included; these present technical material at a level that can be of practical use. The third edition includes more than 30 new tables and figures. Newly structured *Key Points* are located prominently throughout the text to emphasize important learning points in each chapter. References now follow each chapter (rather than sections) to allow easy reference. The third edition also includes two new chapters and numerous added sections within existing chapters.

Section 1 is written as a basic introduction to the science of nutrition, excluding application to specific species. Chapters within this section are organized according to the basic nutrients and the processes of digestion and absorption. In the third edition, new sections regarding taste receptors and their comparative differences between dogs and cats are examined and discussions of small and large intestine microbial populations and their relevance to nutritional health have been expanded. These chapters are of value to students and professionals who require introductory information about the science of nutrition.

Section 2 addresses the specific nutrient requirements of dogs and cats. Chapters in this section examine energy balance in companion animals, comparative nutrient requirements, and the metabolic idiosyncrasies of the cat. New information regarding the cat's metabolic adaptations that reflect its carnivorous history has been added to the new edition. Updated information regarding the energy requirements of dogs and cats living in homes and the effects of various life stage and environmental factors upon energy needs (and estimate equations) is included in the third edition. The essential fatty acid section of Chapter 11 has been expanded to review current understanding of the omega-3 and the omega-6 fatty acid families and their relevance to pet nutrition, as has the section examining taurine nutrition for both dogs and cats in Chapter 12. New information regarding vitamins D and E nutrition for dogs and cats and several of the essential minerals has been added to the final chapter of this section.

Section 3 provides a detailed and updated overview of the formulation, production, and use of commercial and noncommercial pet foods. Chapters include information regarding the history, regulation, and marketing of commercial foods; nutrient content and types of foods; and procedures for evaluating the diets of dogs and cats. New sections examine the roles of all governing agencies, including the Food and Drug Administration, in regulating pet food production and safety. An expanded section reviews the new 2006 National Research Council's *Nutrient Requirements of Dogs and Cats*. Current research and use of functional ingredients in pet foods is another new section in the third edition. Finally, pet foods have been newly classified to reflect the wide variety of pet food forms and types that are available to consumers today. Information regarding organic and natural foods, raw diets, and vegetarian/vegan foods has been added. Practical information about the selection of appropriate pet foods is included and should be of value to both pet owners and companion animal professionals.

Section 4 includes feeding and diet recommendations throughout all life stages for dogs and cats. The third edition includes recent research that has focused on the nutrient needs of neonatal puppies and kittens and the importance of docosahexaenoic acid (DHA), milk production and composition in queens and bitches, and new information regarding the development of gastrointestinal function in puppies and kittens. The

importance of proper feeding management throughout growth, especially for large and giant breeds of dogs, is emphasized. New information regarding the nutritional needs and feeding of geriatric dogs and cats and the feeding of a variety of types of working dogs is included in this newest edition. The importance of both amount and type of dietary fat included in diets for geriatric and for working animals is reviewed. The final chapter in this section examines currently popular nutritional fads and fallacies reported among pet owners and enthusiasts.

Finally, *Section 5* examines the occurrence, treatment, and management of nutritionally responsive disorders in dogs and cats. This section has been extensively revised and expanded in the new edition. The chapters dealing with inherited disorders of metabolism, diabetes mellitus, urolithiasis, nutritionally manageable dermatoses, chronic kidney disease, dental health, cancer, gastrointestinal disease, and feline hepatic lipidosis have all been updated to include reviews of recent research and recommendations for appropriate diets and feeding protocols. Two new chapters have been added in the third edition; these address diet and mobility and the nutritional management of heart disease. The chapters in this section continue to provide an important resource for veterinarians, nutritionists, and breeders who are involved in the treatment or study of these disorders.

In sum, the third edition of *Canine and Feline Nutrition: A Resource for Companion Animal Professionals* continues to provide a comprehensive study of the science of companion animal nutrition. Revisions that include reviews of current research, new chapters and sections, updated figures and tables, user-friendly Key Points, and easily accessible references collectively enhance the book's utility and value as a reference for students, companion animal professionals, and pet owners.

Linda P. Case, MS
Leighann Daristotle, DVM, PhD
Michael G. Hayek, PhD
Melody Foess Raasch, DVM

Acknowledgments

Many colleagues and friends were instrumental in the preparation of the completed manuscript for this book. Nutritionists and veterinarians with acclaimed expertise in the nutrition, feeding management, and therapeutic nutritional care of companion animals have reviewed and edited past and current editions. Collectively, they have provided constructive advice and valuable recommendations. The authors express sincere gratitude to Marcie J. Campion, PhD; Tad B. Coles, DVM; Gary M. Davenport, PhD; Amy Dicke, DVM; Elizabeth Flickinger, PhD; Jocelynn Jacobs, DVM; Russ Kelley, MS; Allan J. Lepine, PhD; Gregory A. Reinhart, PhD; Anna Kate Shoveller, PhD; Gregory D. Sunvold, PhD; Mark A Tetrick, DVM, PhD; and Donna Waltz, PhD. The authors also thank Bruce MacAllister, who created all of the original artwork for the new edition; Susan Yaeger, who provided many of the new graphics; and Sharon Nichols, who helped to compile breed statistics and charts. We thank Jean Gravning and Laurie Geyer, who generously shared photographs of their Nova Scotia Duck Tolling Retrievers, Quincy and Pete. We are also appreciative of the outstanding group of editors and staff at Elsevier, who provided editorial expertise and exceptional attention to detail for all three editions of this book. Special thanks to Anthony J. Winkel, DDS, DVM, who provided the initial encouragement for the third edition, and to our developmental editor, Maureen Slaten, for her unfailing support throughout the research, writing, and production process. Finally, we would like to express our gratitude to two of the book's previous authors, Daniel P. Carey, DVM, and Diane A. Hirakawa, PhD. Their shared vision for increasing our understanding of canine and feline nutrition and for improving the health and quality of life of all companion animals continues to be the most important guiding principle that underlies every chapter of this book.

Linda P. Case, MS
Leighann Daristotle, DVM, PhD
Michael G. Hayek, PhD
Melody Foess Raasch, DVM

Contents

Section 1

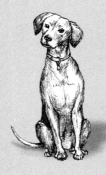

Basics of Nutrition

In recent years, researchers have been able to explain why humans bond so strongly to their pets, and they have also discovered that the relationship between humans and animals is often beneficial to human health. It is not surprising that the strong emotional attachment that people feel for their pets is coupled with an interest in providing them with the best in health care and nutrition. Advances in veterinary medicine have resulted in vaccination programs that protect dogs and cats from many life-threatening diseases and in medical procedures that contribute to lengthened lifespans. Likewise, progress in the field of nutrition has generated an improved understanding of canine and feline dietetics and led to the development of well-balanced pet foods that contribute to long-term health and aid in the prevention and management of chronic disease.

Today's competitive market contains a vast array of foods, snacks, and nutritional supplements for dogs and cats. These products are sold in grocery stores, feed stores, pet shops, and veterinary hospitals. Products vary significantly in nutrient composition, availability, digestibility, palatability, physical form, flavor, and texture. Some foods are formulated to provide adequate nutrition throughout a pet's lifespan, while other foods have been marketed specifically for a particular stage of life or a specific disease state. This large selection of commercial products, combined with the periodic propagation of popular nutritional fads and fallacies, has resulted in much confusion among pet owners and companion animal professionals regarding the nutritional care of dogs and cats.

A basic understanding of the fundamentals of nutrition is a necessary prerequisite for evaluating pet foods and making decisions about a dog's or cat's nutritional status. The term *nutrition* refers to the study of food and the nutrients and other components that it contains. This includes an examination of the actions of specific nutrients, their interactions with each other, and their balance within a diet. In addition, the science of nutrition includes an examination of the way in which an animal ingests, digests, absorbs, and uses nutrients. This section provides an overview of each of the essential nutrients. Energy, water, carbohydrates, fats, proteins, vitamins, and

Basics of Nutrition (continued)

minerals are examined in detail. An examination of the normal digestive and absorptive processes in dogs and cats is also provided. Subsequent sections address the specific nutrient requirements of dogs and cats, the types and compositions of pet foods, feeding management throughout the life cycle, feeding problems, and the management of nutritionally responsive disorders. Information contained in this book will enable pet owners, students, and companion animal professionals to make informed decisions about the diets and nutritional health of dogs and cats throughout all stages of life.

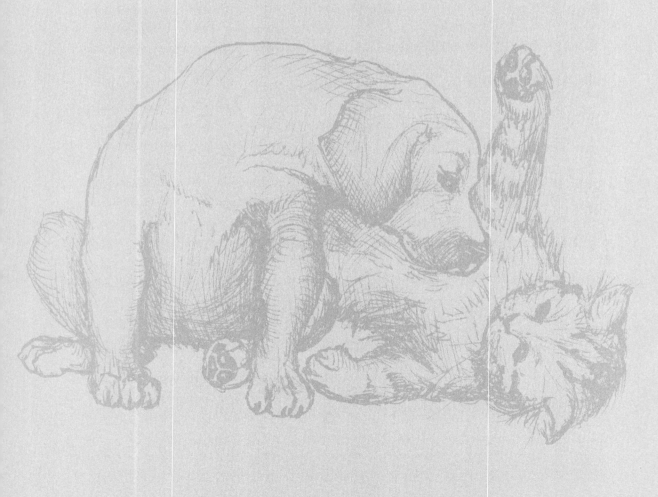

1

Energy and Water

Like all living animals, dogs and cats require a balanced diet to grow normally and maintain health once they are mature. Nutrients are components in the diet that have specific functions within the body and contribute to growth, tissue maintenance, and optimal health. *Essential nutrients* are those components that cannot be synthesized by the body at a rate that is adequate to meet the body's needs. Therefore essential nutrients must be supplied in the diet. *Nonessential nutrients* can be synthesized by the body and obtained either through de novo synthesis or from the diet. Along with a requirement for energy, all animals have a metabolic requirement for six major categories of nutrients. These are water, carbohydrates, proteins, fats, minerals, and vitamins. Energy, although not a nutrient per se, is required by the body for normal growth, maintenance, reproductive performance, and physical work. Approximately 50% to 80% of the dry matter (DM) of a dog's or cat's diet is used for energy.

Nutrition is the study of food, its nutrients, and other components, including an examination of the actions of specific nutrients, their interactions with each other, and their balance within a diet. The six categories of nutrients—water, carbohydrates, proteins, fats, minerals, and vitamins—have specific functions and contribute to growth, body tissue maintenance, and optimal health.

With the exception of water, energy is the most critical component that must be considered in a diet. Like all animals, companion animals require a constant source of dietary energy to survive. Plants obtain energy from solar radiation and convert it to energy-containing nutrients. Animals consume plants and use them either directly for energy or to convert plant nutrients into other energy-containing molecules. The primary form of stored energy in plants is carbohydrate; the main form of stored energy in animals is fat. Energy is necessary for

the performance of the body's metabolic work, which includes maintaining and synthesizing body tissues, engaging in physical work, and regulating normal body temperature. Given its importance, it is not surprising that energy is always the first requirement to be met by an animal's diet. Regardless of a dog's or cat's needs for essential amino acids from dietary protein or essential fatty acids (EFAs) from dietary fat, the energy-yielding nutrients of the diet are first used to satisfy energy needs. Once energy needs are met, nutrients become available for other metabolic functions.

Energy is needed by the body to perform metabolic work, which includes maintaining and synthesizing body tissues, engaging in physical work, and regulating normal body temperature. Energy is always the first requirement met by an animal's diet.

Animals are capable of regulating their energy intake to accurately meet their daily caloric requirements. When allowed free access to a balanced, moderately palatable diet, most dogs and cats will consume enough food to meet, but not exceed, their daily energy needs.[1-3] *Energy density* or *caloric density* refers to the concentration of energy in a given quantity of food (see p. 6). When the energy density of a diet is decreased, animals respond by increasing the quantity of food they consume, which results in a relatively constant energy intake.[3,4] If an animal's food intake is regulated by total energy intake, the composition of all other nutrients in the diet must be balanced with respect to the diet's energy density. This balance should be calculated to ensure that, when a dog or cat consumes a quantity of food adequate to meet his or her caloric needs, all other nutrient requirements will be met in the same volume of food.

Although all dogs and cats have the ability to properly regulate their energy intake, this natural tendency can be overridden by environmental factors. Providing unrestricted access to foods that are both highly palatable and energy-dense can lead to chronic overconsumption in some companion animals. Today's competitive pet food market includes many foods that are high in both palatability and caloric density. Coupled with this fact is a decline in physical activity among many pets in today's society. Many companion animals now lead happy but relatively sedentary lives exclusively as house pets. Cats have moved from the barnyard into the house, where their former working roles as mousers and pest-controllers have been effectively eliminated. Likewise, dogs have evolved from working companions to unemployed house dogs that may lack adequate daily exercise. These two changes have led to an epidemic of obesity among dogs and cats; although reported incidence rates vary, surveys have shown that obesity is a common nutritional problem observed by practicing veterinarians and reported by owners.[5,6] These changes indicate that it may no longer be wise to rely on the inherent abilities of dogs and cats to regulate energy intake. Although companion animals certainly have this ability, many do not self-regulate because of the nature of the food they eat and the type of lifestyle they lead. In most cases, portion-controlled feeding is the best way to control a pet's energy balance, growth rate, and weight status (see Section 4, pp. 194-197).

MEASUREMENT OF ENERGY IN THE DIET

Energy has no measurable mass or dimension, but the chemical energy contained in foods is ultimately transformed by the body into heat, which can be measured. Energy in food is expressed in units of kilocalories (kcal) or kilojoules (kJ). A *calorie* refers to the amount of heat energy necessary to raise the temperature of 1 gram (g) of water from 14.5° Celsius (C) to 15.5° C. Because a calorie is a very small unit, it is not of practical use in the science of animal nutrition. The kcal, which is equal to 1000 calories, is the most commonly used unit of measure. The *kilojoule* is a metric unit and is defined as the amount of mechanical energy required for a force of 1 newton (N) to move a weight of 1 kilogram (kg) by a distance of 1 meter (m). To convert kcal to kJ, the number of kcal is multiplied by 4.184. In the United States, kcal is the most commonly used unit for energy in human and pet foods.

The caloric value of foods can be measured using direct calorimetry. This process involves the complete combustion (oxidation) of a premeasured amount of food in a bomb calorimeter, resulting in the release and measurement of the food's total chemical energy. This energy is called the food's *gross energy* (GE). The three nutrient classes that provide energy in an animal's diet are carbohydrates, fats, and proteins. Animals cannot use all of a food's GE because energy losses occur during digestion and assimilation. *Digestible energy* (DE) signifies the amount of energy available for absorption across the intestinal mucosa. Apparent DE can be calculated by subtracting the indigestible energy excreted in the feces from the GE of the food. Additional energy losses occur as a result of the production of combustible gases and the excretion of urea in the urine. The incomplete oxidation of absorbed dietary protein by the body results in the production of urea. Because the production of combustible gases in dogs and cats is minimal, only urinary losses are typically accounted for. *Metabolizable energy* (ME) is the amount of energy ultimately available to the tissues of the body after losses in the feces and urine have been subtracted from the GE of the food.

ME is the value that is most often used to express the energy content of pet food ingredients and commercial diets. Similarly, the energy requirements of dogs and cats are usually expressed as kcal of ME. ME can be subdivided to calculate net energy (NE) and the energy lost to dietary thermogenesis. *Dietary thermogenesis,* also called the *specific dynamic action of food,* refers to the energy needed by the body to digest, absorb, and assimilate nutrients. *NE* is the energy available to an animal for the maintenance of body tissues and for production needs such as physical work, growth, gestation, and lactation (Figure 1-1). The percent of ME that becomes available as NE is called the *efficiency of utilization.*

The ME of a diet or food ingredient depends on both the nutrient composition of the food and the animal that is consuming it. For example, because of the length and structure of its gastrointestinal tract, a nonruminant herbivore such as a horse can derive a greater amount of energy from grass than can a dog or cat. Therefore the ME value of grass for a horse is higher than the ME value of grass for a companion animal. Several different methods are used to estimate the ME values of a food ingredient or diet for a given species, each with its

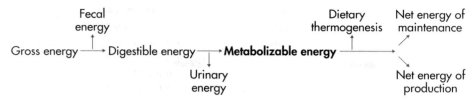

Figure 1-1   Partitioning of dietary energy.

Calculation
Metabolizable energy = (GE$_{food}$) − (GE$_{feces}$ + GE$_{urine}$)

Example
1100 kcal = 3600 (food) − 2500 (feces + urine)

Figure 1-2   Calculation and example of metabolizable energy. *GE,* Gross energy.

own strengths and limitations. These include the direct determination of ME through feeding trials and total collection procedures; calculating an estimate of ME using analyzed levels of protein, carbohydrate, and fat in the diet; and, most recently, predicting ME using regression equations based upon a food's fiber content. New research also suggests that some in vitro methods may provide reliable estimates of the energy content of certain types of commercial pet foods.

Direct Determination in Feeding Trials

The gold standard for determining ME is through data collected in actual feeding trials with the species in question. The diet or food ingredient is fed to a group of test animals, and feces and urine are collected throughout a predesignated time period. Determination of the GE content of the food, feces, and urine allows direct calculation of ME by subtraction (Figure 1-2). Because this approach provides the most accurate estimate of ME, many pet food manufacturers periodically use feeding trials to measure DE or ME of their foods and ingredients. Data that are collected can be used to reflect changes in ME values as new products are developed and to ensure the accuracy of predictive equations that may be used more routinely. When digestibility trials are used, ME values are determined using DE values and a correction factor to account for urinary energy losses from the metabolism of protein. Because cats digest protein calories more efficiently than

dogs, species-specific correction factors have been determined; for cats 0.86 kcal/g digestible protein and for dogs 1.25 kcal/g digestible protein.[7,8]

Calculation Methods

Although direct measurement in the target species is the most accurate method for estimating ME, it is also very time consuming and costly, and requires access to large numbers of representative animals. As a result, routine determinations of ME are conducted with mathematical formulas that estimate ME from analyzed carbohydrate, protein, and fat content, or from fiber content of the food.[9] Recently, although not yet commonly used in industry, experimental methods that utilize in vitro enzymatic assays, measurement of the ratio of total amino acids to non–amino acid nitrogen, or near-infrared spectroscopy have also been reported as accurate predictors of the energy value of dog foods.[10-12]

Pet food manufacturers measure a food's metabolizable energy (ME) either by direct measurement using feeding trials or by calculation from analyzed nutrient levels or standard table values. New in vitro methods of estimating ME include enzymatic assays, measurement of the amino acids and amino acid nitrogen, and near-infrared spectroscopy.

Formulas that have been derived for dog and cat diets include constants that account for fecal and urinary losses of energy. The GE values, which represent total energy content, for mixed carbohydrate, fat, and protein are 4.15, 9.40, and 5.65 kcal/g, respectively.[8] However, as mentioned earlier, animals are incapable of using all of the energy present in food nutrients. Inefficiency in digestion, absorption, and assimilation results in energy losses. In human foods, the *Atwater factors* of 4-9-4 kcal/g are commonly used to estimate ME values for carbohydrate, fat, and protein, respectively. These factors are calculated using estimated digestibility coefficients of 96% for fat and carbohydrate and 91% for protein.[13] A *digestibility coefficient* is the proportion of the consumed nutrient that is actually available for absorption and use by the body. The ME value of protein was further reduced to account for urinary losses of urea.

The Atwater factors work quite well for estimating the ME of homemade dog and cat diets and for commercial products with very high digestibilities such as milk replacers for puppies and kittens and enteral feeding formulas.[8] However, digestibility data collected in dogs and cats fed typical commercial pet foods have shown that Atwater factors tend to overestimate the ME values of most commercial foods. This miscalculation occurs because the digestibility of many pet food ingredients is lower than the digestibility of most foods consumed by humans. Digestibility data collected in dogs from 106 samples of dry, semimoist, and canned commercial dog foods showed that the average digestibility coefficients for crude protein, acid-ether extract (a measure of fat content), and nitrogen-free extract (NFE) (a measure of soluble carbohydrate content) were 81%, 85%, and 79%, respectively.[14] The fact that some pet food ingredients are generally lower in digestibility than the foods consumed by humans causes the Atwater factors to be inaccurate for use in estimating the ME of pet foods. The National Research Council's (NRC's) 1985 recommendations for dogs suggested that digestibility coefficients of 80%, 90%, and 85% be used for the protein, fat, and carbohydrate in commercial dog food, respectively. When GE values were readjusted for digestibility and urinary losses, ME values of 3.5, 8.5, and 3.5 kcal/g were assigned to protein, fat, and carbohydrate, respectively (Table 1-1). These values

are referred to as *modified Atwater factors.* Although these values provide a better estimate of ME values for pet foods than do the Atwater factors, they may still underestimate the ME values of highly digestible foods and overestimate ME values for foods containing high amounts of fiber or poor quality meat sources.[15]

In general, calculation of ME from analyzed levels of carbohydrate, fat, and protein in the diet using modified Atwater factors provides a reasonably accurate estimate of the ME for most pet foods evaluated. This equation is expressed as: $ME_{diet} = (3.5 \times g\ protein) + (8.5 \times g\ fat) + (8.5 \times g\ NFE)$. This is the equation recommended by the Association of American Feed Control Officials (AAFCO) to manufacturers that are reporting ME values on their pet food labels. AAFCO is a regulating group responsible for the standards governing commercially prepared pet foods. Modified equations have been suggested for use with dry cat foods and for weight loss foods that contain high levels of fiber.[15]

ENERGY DENSITY

The *energy density* of a pet food refers to the number of calories provided by the food in a given weight or volume. In the United States, energy density is expressed as kcal of ME per kg or pound (lb) of diet. In most European countries, the unit kJ/kg is used. The importance of energy density in companion animal nutrition cannot be overemphasized. It is the principal factor that determines the quantity of food that is eaten each day and therefore directly affects the amount of all other essential nutrients that an animal ingests. A diet's energy density must be high enough to allow the pet to consume a sufficient amount of the food each day to meet its energy needs. If the energy density is too low, food intake will be restricted by the physical limitations of the gastrointestinal tract, resulting in an energy deficit.

TABLE 1-1   DIGESTIBILITY COEFFICIENTS AND FACTORS

Nutrient	Human food digestibility coefficient	Atwater factor	Pet food digestibility coefficient	Modified Atwater factor
Carbohydrate	96%	4 kcal/g	85%	3.5 kcal/g
Protein	91%	4 kcal/g	80%	3.5 kcal/g
Fat	96%	9 kcal/g	90%	8.5 kcal/g

In other words, the animal would not be physically able to consume enough of the low-energy diet to meet its caloric requirements. Such a diet is said to be "bulk-limited." If levels of the essential nutrients in such a diet are not balanced relative to energy density, multiple nutrient deficiencies could also occur.

When the caloric density of a pet food is high enough for an animal to consume a sufficient quantity to meet its daily energy needs, energy density will be the primary factor that determines the quantity of food that is consumed each day. There is an inverse relationship between energy density and the volume of food that is consumed. As a food's energy density increases, the total volume of food that is consumed decreases. However, feeding a highly palatable pet food can override a pet's tendency to correctly regulate intake. The sale of pet foods that are energy dense and highly palatable has led to recommendations for the use of portion-controlled feeding to manage pets' daily food intake. Maintenance of normal body weight and growth rate are the criteria most often used to determine the appropriate quantity of food. Therefore, even when under the pet owner's control, a dog's or cat's level of energy intake is still the primary factor affecting the quantity of food that is fed.

Because energy intake determines total food intake, it is important that diets are properly balanced, so that requirements for all other nutrients are met when energy needs are satisfied. For this reason, it is more appropriate to express levels of essential nutrients in terms of ME rather than in terms of percentage of the food's weight. Expressing nutrient content as units per 1000 kcal of ME is called *nutrient density*, and provides a standardized format that can be used to compare all types of foods because it accounts for both moisture and energy density differences between products. Actual nutrient intake can be readily determined from a pet's daily energy requirement, and foods of dissimilar energy content can be compared quickly based upon this method of expressing nutrient levels. The energy-contributing nutrients, protein, fat, and carbohydrate, can be expressed either as g per 1000 kcal ME or as a percentage of the total ME of the diet. The latter expression is called the *caloric distribution* of a food and easily allows comparisons between foods with differing moisture or energy contents. Caloric distribution only considers the energy-containing nutrients of the food and does not provide an expression of other essential nutrients in the diet (see Section 3, pp. 145-147).

Energy density (the number of calories provided by a food in a given weight or volume) is the most important factor in determining the quantity of food that a pet eats each day. A food's energy density directly affects the amount of all other essential nutrients that an animal ingests. Therefore, the most accurate way to express levels of essential nutrients in the food is in terms of ME (units per 1000 kcal of ME). This approach also allows comparisons between all types of foods.

Using nutrient density or caloric distribution, values can be compared in any type of food or diet, regardless of water, nutrient, or energy content. For example, a complete and balanced dry dog food contains 27% protein (as a percentage of weight) and supplies 3800 kcal of ME/kg. Modified Atwater factors can be used to estimate the proportion of energy that protein contributes to the food. The calculations in Table 1-2 show that 24.8% of the food's energy is contributed by protein. These figures can be compared with a canned dog food that contains 7% protein on a weight basis and supplies 980 kcal of ME/kg. When expressed as a percentage of calories, the protein in the canned food also supplies approximately 25% of the food's calories (see Table 1-2). If expressed as nutrient density, the

TABLE 1-2	SAMPLE CALCULATION TO CONVERT PERCENTAGE OF WEIGHT TO PERCENTAGE OF ENERGY IN THE DIET					
FOOD TYPE	PROTEIN (%)		MODIFIED ATWATER FACTOR		KCAL/100 G OF FOOD	× 100%
Dry	(27	×	3.5)	÷	380	24.8
Canned	(7	×	3.5)	÷	98	25.0

TABLE 1-3 DETERMINATION OF ENERGY DENSITY FROM GUARANTEED ANALYSIS

Nutrient	Percentage in diet		Modified Atwater factor		Kcal/100 g of food
Protein	26	×	3.5	=	91
Carbohydrate	37	×	3.5	=	129.5
Fat	15	×	8.5	=	127.5
			Total Calories	=	348

348 kcal/100 g × 1000 g/kg = **3480 kcal/kg** (energy density).
3480 kcal/kg × 1 kg/2.2 lb = **1581.8 kcal/lb** food (energy density).

g of protein per 1000 kcal ME are 71 g of protein per 1000 kcal of food.

These two foods appear enormously different when compared in terms of percentage of protein on a weight basis, yet actually contain the same amount of protein when expressed as a percentage of total calories. Differences in the water content and energy density of the two foods account for the large differences in nutrient content when expressed as a percentage of weight. Attempting to compare the two foods when protein is expressed as a percentage of weight can be misleading. Conversion to units of energy allows an accurate comparison of levels of the energy-containing nutrients in different pet foods. Because dogs and cats are fed to meet their caloric requirements, these two foods will supply an equal quantity of protein when fed at the correct level.

Tip: Reading food labels and comparing contents of foods in the store can be very confusing. For example, when the protein content is expressed as a percentage of weight, merely reading the protein content printed on the label of a canned dog food (7% protein) and a dry dog food (27% protein) does not tell the whole story. But when a simple formula is applied to determine the protein as a percentage of calories, one can see that the protein content of the dry and canned foods in this example is almost exactly the same (see Table 1-2).

The energy density of a food must be known in order to estimate the quantity of food necessary to meet a pet's energy requirement. When manufacturers choose to include energy density information on their labels, AAFCO requires that it be expressed in kcal of ME per unit weight or volume. If ME information is not included on a pet food label, it can be estimated using the proximate analysis of the food. If the proximate analysis is not available, the guaranteed analysis provided on the label of all pet foods can be used as a rough estimate of nutrient content. The modified Atwater factors provided earlier are used to calculate the amount of energy contributed by carbohydrate, protein, and fat. For example, the guaranteed analysis on a bag of dry dog food reads as follows:

▸ Crude protein: not less than 26%
▸ Crude fat: not less than 15%
▸ Crude fiber: not more than 5%

An estimate of the mineral content of the food, commonly called *ash,* must then be made. High-quality dry pet foods generally contain between 5% and 8% ash. The food's carbohydrate content can then be estimated by subtraction:

▸ 100% – % protein – % fat – % fiber – % ash – % moisture = % carbohydrate
▸ 100% – 26% – 15% – 5% – 7% – 10% = 37%

The calories provided by each nutrient in 100 g of food can then be estimated (Table 1-3). The total calories obtained from 100 g of food are 348, or 3480 kcal/kg of food. This figure can also be divided by 2.2 to convert to energy density per lb of food. The quantity of food to offer can be estimated by dividing the pet's daily energy requirement by the energy density of the diet. For example, if an adult dog requires 1100 kcal/day and is fed a diet containing 1582 kcal/lb, approximately 11 ounces (oz) of food should be fed each day. An 8-oz cup of dry pet food might weigh 3 oz. Therefore this dog would require a little more than 3½ cups of this food per day (Box 1-1). It is important to be aware that each dog and cat is an individual and that these calculations provide only a guideline or starting point when determining a pet's daily needs. The amount of food should be adjusted to attain optimal growth in young animals and a healthy body weight and condition in adult animals. (Adult pets in optimal condition are well-muscled and lean. Although their ribs cannot be readily seen, they should easily be felt when palpated.)

ENERGY IMBALANCE

Energy imbalance occurs when an animal's daily energy consumption is either greater or less than its daily requirement, leading to changes in growth rate, body weight, and body composition. Excess energy intake is much more common in dogs and cats than is energy deficiency. Overconsumption of energy has been shown to have several detrimental effects on dogs during their growth, especially those of the large and giant breeds. When an excess amount of a balanced, high-energy pet food is fed to growing puppies, maximal growth rate and weight gain can be achieved. However, studies with growing dogs have indicated that maximal growth rate is not compatible with healthy bone growth and development.[16] Feeding growing puppies to attain maximal growth rate appears to be a significant contributing factor in the development of skeletal disorders such as osteochondrosis and hip dysplasia[17,18] (see Section 5, pp. 491-500 for a complete discussion).

A second problem associated with an energy surplus during growth involves fat cell hyperplasia. Studies with laboratory animals have shown that the generation of an excessive number of fat cells in the body, as a result

of overfeeding at a young age, can predispose an animal to obesity later in life.[19,20] Although research on fat cell hyperplasia during growth has not been conducted in the dog or cat, it is possible that these species are affected in a similar manner. In adult dogs and cats, surplus energy intake leads to obesity and its medical complications (see Section 5, pp. 315-321 for a complete discussion).

Inadequate energy intake results in reduced growth rate and compromised development in young dogs and cats and in weight loss and muscle wasting in adult pets. In healthy animals this condition is most commonly seen in hard-working dogs or pregnant or lactating females that are being fed a diet too low in energy density.

WATER

In terms of survivability, water is the single most important nutrient for the body. Although animals can live after losing almost all of their body fat and more than half of their protein, a loss of only 10% of body water results in death.[21] Approximately 70% of lean adult body weight is water, and many tissues in the body are composed of between 70% and 90% water. Intracellular fluid is approximately 40% to 45% of the body's weight, and extracellular fluid accounts for 20% to 25%. The presence of an aqueous medium within cells and in many tissues is essential for the occurrence of most metabolic processes and chemical reactions.

Within the body, water functions as a solvent that facilitates cellular reactions and as a transport medium for nutrients and the end products of cellular metabolism. Because of its high specific heat, water is able to absorb the heat generated by metabolic reactions with a minimal increase in temperature. This property allows the many heat-generating reactions within the body to continue with a minimal change in body temperature. Water further contributes to temperature regulation by transporting heat away from the working organs through the blood and, in some species, by evaporating in the form of sweat on the outer surface of the body. Water is an essential component in normal digestion because it is necessary for hydrolysis (the splitting of large molecules into smaller molecules through the addition of water). The digestive enzymes of the gastrointestinal tract are secreted in solution. This aqueous medium facilitates the interaction of food components with the digestive enzymes. Elimination of waste products from the kidneys also requires a large amount of water, which acts as both a solvent for toxic metabolites and a carrier medium.

Water is the single most important nutrient for the body for survival. Water within the cells is necessary for most metabolic processes and chemical reactions, is important for temperature regulation, and is an essential component of normal digestion. Elimination of waste products from the kidneys also requires a large amount of water.

All animals experience daily water losses. Urinary excretion accounts for the greatest loss of volume in most animals. *Obligatory loss* from the kidneys is the minimum required for the body to rid itself of the daily load of urinary waste products. A certain quantity of water is necessary to act as a solvent for these end products. The remaining portion of urinary water loss, called *facultative loss,* is excreted in response to the normal water reabsorption rate of the kidneys and to mechanisms responsible for maintaining proper water balance in the body. Fecal water accounts for a much smaller portion of water excretion. In healthy animals, the amount of water that actually appears in the feces is very low compared to the amount that is absorbed across the gastrointestinal tract and returned to the body during digestion. Fecal water loss becomes substantial only when aberrations in the intestines' capacity to absorb water occur. A third route of water loss is evaporation from the lungs during respiration. In dogs and cats this water loss is very important for the regulation of normal body temperature during hot weather. Panting substantially increases respiratory water loss and thus heat loss. Because of these mechanisms of temperature regulation, water losses from respiration and evaporation during hot weather can be very high in both dogs and cats.

Daily water consumption must compensate for these continual fluid losses. A pet's total water intake comes from three possible sources: water present in food, metabolic water, and drinking water. The quantity of water present in the food depends on the type of diet. Commercial, dry pet food may contain as little as

7% water, but some canned rations contain up to 84% water. Within limits, increasing the water content of an animal's food increases the diet's acceptability. Many owners are able to increase their pet's consumption of a dry food by adding a small amount of water to it immediately before feeding. Studies have shown that both dogs and cats are able to maintain water balance with no source of drinking water when fed diets containing more than 67% moisture.[22-24] Dogs appear to be able to readily compensate for changes in the amount of water present in food by increasing or decreasing voluntary water intake. Cats also have this ability, but they appear to be less precise in their adjustments and are more likely to underconsume water than are dogs.[25]

Metabolic water is the water produced during oxidation of the energy-containing nutrients in the body. Oxygen combines with the hydrogen atoms contained in carbohydrate, protein, and fat to produce water molecules. The metabolism of fat produces the greatest amount of metabolic water on a weight basis, and protein catabolism produces the smallest amount. For every 100 g of fat, carbohydrate, and protein oxidized by the body, 107, 55, and 41 milliliters (ml) of metabolic water are produced, respectively. The rate of metabolic water production depends on an animal's metabolic rate and the type of diet. But regardless of these factors, metabolic water is fairly insignificant because it accounts for only 5% to 10% of the total daily water intake of most animals.

The last source of water intake is voluntary drinking. Factors affecting a pet's voluntary water consumption include the ambient temperature, type of diet, level of exercise, physiological state, and health. Water intake increases with both increasing environmental temperature and increasing exercise because more evaporative water is lost as a result of the body's cooling mechanisms. The amount of calories consumed also affects voluntary water consumption. As energy intake increases, more metabolic waste products are produced and the heat produced by nutrient metabolism increases. In these circumstances, the body requires more water to excrete waste products in the urine and to contribute to thermoregulation.

Diet type and composition can also dramatically affect voluntary water intake. For example, in a study of dogs that were fed a diet containing 73% moisture, they obtained 38% of their daily water needs from drinking water. When they were abruptly switched to a diet containing only 7% water, voluntary water intake immediately increased to 95% or more of the total daily intake.[25] In the same study, increasing the salt content of the diet caused an increased drinking response in both dogs and cats. When the level of salt in the diet of a group of cats was increased from 1.3% to 4.6%, voluntary water intake nearly doubled. Generally, if fresh, palatable water is available and proper amounts of a well-balanced diet are fed, most healthy pets are able to accurately regulate water balance through voluntary intake of water.

Pets obtain water from food, metabolic water, and drinking water. If the water content of food is increased or decreased, most pets are naturally able to achieve water balance by increasing or decreasing their voluntary intake of drinking water.

References

1. Cowgill GR: The energy factor in relation to food intake: experiments on the dog, *Am J Physiol* 85:45–64, 1928.

2. Durrer JL, Hannon JP: Seasonal variations in caloric intake of dogs living in an arctic environment, *Am J Physiol* 202:375–384, 1962.

3. Romsos DR, Hornshus MJ, Leveille GA: Influence of dietary fat and carbohydrate on food intake, body weight and body fat of adult dogs, *Proc Soc Exp Bio Med* 157:278–281, 1978.

4. Romsos DR, Belo PS, Bennink MR: Effects of dietary carbohydrate, fat and protein on growth, body composition and blood metabolite levels in the dog, *J Nutr* 106:1452–1464, 1976.

5. McGreevy PD, Thomson PC, Pride C, and others: Prevalence of obesity in dogs examined by Australian veterinary practices and the risk factors involved, *Vet Rec* 156:695–707, 2005.

6. Masters AM, McGreevy PD: Dog keeping practices as reported by readers of an Australian dog enthusiast magazine, *Aust Vet J* 86:18–25, 2008.

7. Association of American Feed Control Officials (AAFCO): Official publication, 2008, AAFCO.

8. National Research Council: *Nutrient requirements of dogs*, Washington, DC, 2006, National Academy of Sciences, National Academy Press, pp 28–48.

9. Kienzle E, Biourge V, Schonmeier A: Prediction of energy digestibility in complete dry foods for dogs and cats by total dietary fiber, *J Nutr* 136:2041S–2044S, 2006.

10. Hervera M, Daucells MD, Llanch F, Castrillo C: Prediction of digestible energy content of extruded dog food by in vitro analyses, *Anim Phys Anim Nutr* 91:205–209, 2007.

11. Castrillo C, Baucells M: Vicente F, and others: Energy evaluation of extruded compound foods for dogs by near-infrared spectroscopy, *J Anim Phys Anim Nutr* 89:194–198, 2005.

12. Yamka RM, McLeod KR, Harmon DL, and others: The impact of dietary protein source on observed and predicted metabolizable energy of dry extruded dog foods, *J Anim Sci* 85:204–212, 2007.

13. Harris LE: *Biological energy interrelationships and glossary of energy terms*, Washington, DC, 1966, National Academy of Sciences, National Academy Press.

14. Kendall PT, Burger IH, Smith PM: Methods of estimation of the metabolizable energy content of cat foods, *Feline Pract* 15:38–44, 1985.

15. LaFlamme DP: Determining metabolizable energy content in commercial pet foods, *J Anim Physiol Anim Nutr* 85:222–230, 2001.

16. Kealy RD, Olsson SE, Monti KL, and others: Effects of limited food consumption on the incidence of hip dysplasia in growing dogs, *J Am Vet Med Assoc* 201:857–863, 1992.

17. Richardson DC: The role of nutrition in canine hip dysplasia, *Vet Clin North Am Small Anim Pract* 22:529–540, 1992.

18. Hedhammer A, Wu FM, Krook L, and others: Overnutrition and skeletal disease: an experimental study in growing Great Dane dogs, *Cornell Vet* 64(Suppl 5):1–160, 1974.

19. Bjorntorp P: The role of adipose tissue in human obesity. In Greenwood MRC, editor: *Obesity: contemporary issues in clinical nutrition*, New York, 1983, Churchill Livingstone.

20. Bjorntorp P, Sjostrom L: Number and size of fat cells in relation to metabolism in human obesity, *Metabolism* 20:703–706, 1971.

21. Maynard LA, Loosli JK, Hintz HF, and others: *Animal nutrition*, ed 7, New York, 1979, McGraw-Hill.

22. Caldwell GT: Studies in water metabolism of the cat, *Physiol Zool* 4:324–355, 1931.

23. Danowski TS, Elkinton JR, Winkler AW: The deleterious effect in dogs of a dry protein ration, *J Clin Invest* 23:816–823, 1944.

24. Prentiss PG, Wolf AV, Eddy HE: Hydropenia in cat and dog: ability of the cat to meet its water requirements solely from a diet of fish or meat, *Am J Physiol* 196:625–632, 1959.

25. Anderson RS: Water balance in the dog and cat, *J Small Anim Pract* 23:588–598, 1982.

2

Carbohydrates

Carbohydrates are the major energy-containing constituents of plants, making up between 60% and 90% of dry-matter (DM) weight. This class of nutrients comprises the elements carbon, hydrogen, and oxygen. A structural classification scheme separates carbohydrates into monosaccharides, disaccharides, or polysaccharides. *Monosaccharides,* often referred to as the *simple sugars,* are the simplest form of carbohydrate. A monosaccharide is comprised of a single unit containing between three and seven carbon atoms. The three hexoses (6-carbon monosaccharides) that are nutritionally and metabolically the most important are glucose, fructose, and galactose (Figure 2-1).

Glucose is a moderately sweet, simple sugar found in commercially prepared corn syrup and sweet fruits such as grapes and berries. It is also the chief end product of starch digestion and glycogen hydrolysis in the body. Glucose is the form of carbohydrate found circulating in the bloodstream and is the primary carbohydrate used by the body's cells for energy. Fructose, commonly referred to as *fruit sugar,* is a very sweet sugar found in honey, ripe fruits, and some vegetables. It is also formed from the digestion or acid hydrolysis of the disaccharide sucrose. Galactose is not found in a free form in foods. However, it makes up 50% of the disaccharide lactose, which is present in the milk of all mammalian species. Like fructose, galactose is released during digestion. Within the body, galactose is converted to glucose by the liver and eventually enters the circulation in the form of glucose.

Disaccharides are made up of two monosaccharide units linked together. Lactose, the sugar found in the milk of all mammals, contains a molecule of glucose and a molecule of galactose. It is the only carbohydrate of animal origin that is of any significance in the diet. Sucrose, commonly recognized as table sugar, contains a molecule of glucose linked to a molecule of fructose. It is found in cane, beets, and maple syrup. Maltose is made up of two glucose molecules linked together. This disaccharide is not commonly found in most foods, but it is formed as an intermediate product in the body during the digestion of starch.

Polysaccharides comprise many single monosaccharide units linked together in long and complex chains. Starch, glycogen, dextrins, and dietary fiber are all polysaccharides. Starch is a nonstructural plant storage polysaccharide and is the chief carbohydrate source present in most commercial pet foods. The two major forms of dietary starch are amylose (comprised of linear glucose chains) and amylopectin (comprised

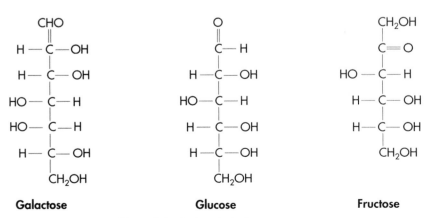

Figure 2-1 Basic carbohydrate structure.

of branched glucose chains). Cereal grains such as corn, wheat, sorghum, barley, and rice are the major ingredients that provide starch. Glycogen is the storage form of carbohydrate in the body. It is found in the liver and muscle, and it functions to help maintain normal glucose homeostasis in the body. Dextrins are polysaccharide compounds that are formed as intermediate products in the breakdown of starch. They are created during normal digestive processes in the body and through the commercial processing of some foods. The monosaccharide units found in starch, glycogen, and dextrin molecules have an alpha-configuration and are linked together by alpha-bonds. This type of bond can be readily hydrolyzed by the endogenous enzymes of the gastrointestinal tract and yields monosaccharide units upon either digestion or chemical hydrolysis.

Although the exact definition of dietary fiber continues to be debated, dietary fiber (also referred to as *nonstarch polysaccharides*) comprises several forms of plant carbohydrate. The major carbohydrate components of dietary fiber include cellulose, hemicellulose, pectin, and the plant gums and mucilages. Lignin, a large phenylpropane polymer, is the only noncarbohydrate component of fiber. Plant fiber differs from starch and glycogen in that its monosaccharide units have a beta-configuration and are linked together by beta-bonds. These bonds resist digestion by the endogenous enzymes of the gastrointestinal tract. As a result, dietary fiber cannot be broken down by enzymes of the intestinal tract to monosaccharide units for absorption in the small intestine.

Although dogs and cats do not directly digest dietary fiber, microbes found in the large intestine (colon) are able to break down certain types of fiber to varying degrees. This bacterial fermentation produces short-chain fatty acids (SCFAs) and other end products. The SCFAs that are produced in greatest abundance are acetate, propionate, and butyrate. The magnitude of bacterial digestion depends on factors such as the species of animal, the type of fiber present in the diet, the gastrointestinal transit time, and the intake of other dietary constituents. Soluble fibers are those that form a viscous solution upon contact with water; it is the physical properties of these fibers that affect gastrointestinal functions such as stomach emptying time and transit time.[1] Most soluble fibers are moderately or

TABLE 2-1 DIETARY FIBER FERMENTATION IN DOGS

FIBER TYPE	SOLUBILITY	FERMENTABILITY
Beet pulp	Low	Moderate
Cellulose	Low	Low
Rice bran	Low	Moderate
Gum arabic	High	Moderate
Pectin	High	High
Carboxymethylcel-lulose	High	Low
Methylcellulose	High	Low
Cabbage fiber	Low	High
Guar gum	High	High
Locust bean gum	High	Low
Xanthan gum	High	Low

From Reinhart GA, Sunvold GD: In vitro fermentation as a predictor of fiber utilization. In *Recent advances in canine and feline nutritional research: proceedings of the 1996 Iams international nutrition symposium,* Wilmington, Ohio, 1996, Orange Frazer Press.

highly fermentable in the large intestine. Conversely, insoluble fibers retain some water within their structural matrix but do not form viscous solutions. These fibers are generally much less fermentable and function to increase fecal mass and decrease intestinal transit time. For example, in dogs and cats, pectin and other soluble fibers are highly fermentable, beet pulp is moderately fermentable, and cellulose is nonfermentable (Table 2-1).

Ruminants and herbivorous animals are able to derive a significant amount of energy from the SCFAs produced by the bacterial fermentation of fiber. However, nonherbivores, such as the dog and the cat, cannot do this because of the relatively short and simple structure of their large intestine. Although SCFAs are produced in these species, there is no mechanism for the absorption of large amounts of SCFAs in the large intestine. Therefore the total energy balance of dogs and cats is not significantly affected by the production of SCFAs from dietary fiber.

However, the SCFAs that are produced from fiber are an important energy source for the epithelial cells lining the gastrointestinal tract in dogs and cats. The enterocytes and colonocytes of the large intestine are active cells that have a high turnover rate and rely on SCFAs as a significant energy source. A series of

TABLE 2-2 EFFECTS OF FIBER SOURCE ON THE CANINE COLON

	CELLULOSE	BEET PULP	PECTIN/GUM ARABIC	INTERPRETATION
Colon weight (g/kg body weight)	6.09	6.52	6.62	More is better
Surface:area ratio	0.146	0.156	0.154	More is better
Cryptitis (number affected of five dogs)	4	1	3	Less is better
DNA content (microgram [μg]/mg)	47.4	40.4	38.4	Less is better

Data from Reinhart GA, Moxley RA, Clemens ET: Dietary fibre source and its effects on colonic microstructure and histopathology of Beagle dogs, *J Nutr* 124:2701S-2703S, 1994.

studies found that dogs fed diets containing moderately fermentable fiber have increased colon weights, mucosal surface area, and mucosal hypertrophy when compared with dogs fed a diet containing a nonfermentable fiber source (Table 2-2).[2] These changes provide a measure of the absorptive capacity of the colon and indicate increased cellular activity and health. Although a highly fermentable fiber source has similar effects on colon weight and morphology, diets containing this type of fiber result in poor stool quality. It appears that the best fiber sources for companion animals are those that are moderately fermentable and provide adequate levels of SCFAs for the intestinal mucosa.[3-5] Fiber in the diets of dogs and cats also functions as an aid in the proper functioning of the gastrointestinal tract and as a dietary diluent that decreases the total energy density of the diet (see Section 2, p. 77, and Section 5, pp. 333-335). Finally, certain fermentable fibers act as prebiotics when included in diets. Prebiotics are food ingredients that provide benefits by stimulating the proliferation of certain desirable bacterial species in the gastrointestinal tract although they are not directly digested by the host animal (see Section 5, pp. 467-472 for a complete discussion).[6]

Moderately fermentable fiber sources (as opposed to highly fermentable and nonfermentable fiber sources), which are a source of bulk and provide adequate levels of short-chain fatty acids (SCFAs) in the large intestine, are good fiber sources for cats and dogs. The SCFAs are an important energy source for the epithelial cells lining the gastrointestinal (GI) tract, and these fiber sources help to maintain GI tract health.

In the body, carbohydrate has several functions. The monosaccharide glucose is an important energy source for many tissues. A constant supply of glucose is necessary for the proper functioning of the central nervous system (CNS), and the glycogen present in the heart muscle is an important emergency source of energy for the heart. Glycogen in the liver and muscle can be hydrolyzed to supply additional carbohydrate fuel to cells when circulating glucose is low. Carbohydrate also supplies carbon skeletons for the formation of nonessential amino acids and is needed for the synthesis of other essential body compounds such as glucuronic acid, heparin, chondroitin sulfate, the immunopolysaccharides, deoxyribonucleic acid (DNA), and ribonucleic acid (RNA). When conjugated with proteins or lipids, some carbohydrates also become important structural components in the body's tissues.

Dietary carbohydrate provides animals with a source of energy and assists in proper gastrointestinal tract functioning. However, only a limited amount of carbohydrate can be stored in the body as glycogen, so when dietary carbohydrate is consumed in excess of the body's energy needs, most is metabolized to body fat for energy storage. Therefore consumption of dietary carbohydrate in excess of an animal's energy needs can lead to increased body fat and obesity. In addition to its function in supplying energy to the body, digestible carbohydrate also has a protein-sparing effect. Just as animals eat to meet their energy needs, the body satisfies its energy requirement before using energy-containing nutrients in the diet for other purposes. If adequate carbohydrate is supplied in the diet, protein will be spared from being used for energy and can then be used for tissue repair and growth. Finally, although dietary fiber does not contribute appreciably to energy balance in dogs and cats, a moderate level in the diet is beneficial. Plant fiber provides SCFAs to cells lining the intestine, helps to stimulate normal peristalsis, provides bulk to intestinal contents, and reduces gastrointestinal transit time (see Section 2, p. 77).

Because carbohydrates are an excellent energy source for the body, optimal levels of digestible carbohydrate in the diet serve to spare dietary protein from being used as an energy source.

References

1. Alvarez E, Sanchez P: Dietary fiber, *Nutr Hosp* 21(Suppl):60–71, 2006.

2. Reinhart GA, Moxley RA, Clemens ET: Dietary fibre source and its effects on colonic microstructure, function and histopathology of Beagle dogs, *J Nutr* 124:2701S–2703S, 1994.

3. Sunvold GD, Fahey GC Jr, Merchen NR, and others: Fermentability of selected fibrous substrates by dog fecal microflora as influenced by diet, *J Nutr* 124:2719S–2720S, 1994.

4. Hallman JE, Moxley RA, Reinhart GA, and others: Cellulose, beet pulp, and pectin/gum arabic effects on canine colonic microstructure and histopathology, *Vet Clin Nutr* 2:137–142, 1995.

5. Sunvold GD, Fahey GC Jr, Merchen NR, and others: Dietary fiber for cats: in vitro fermentation of selected fiber sources by cat fecal inoculum and in vivo utilization of diets containing selected fiber sources and their blends, *J Anim Sci* 73:2329–2339, 1995.

6. Grizard D, Barthomeuf C: Non-digestible oligosaccharides used as probiotic agents: mode of production and beneficial effects on animal and human health, *Reprod Nutr Dev* 39:563–588, 1999.

3

Fats

Dietary fat is part of a heterogeneous group of compounds known as the *lipids*. These compounds are classified together because of their solubility in organic solvents and their insolubility in water. They can be further categorized into simple lipids, compound lipids, and derived lipids. The simple lipids include the triglycerides, which are the most common form of fat present in the diet, and the waxes. Triglycerides are made up of three fatty acids linked to one molecule of glycerol (Figure 3-1), and waxes contain a greater number of fatty acids linked to a long-chain alcohol molecule. Compound lipids are composed of a lipid, such as a fatty acid, linked to a nonlipid molecule. Lipoproteins, which function to carry fat in the bloodstream, are a type of compound lipid. The derived lipids include sterol compounds, such as cholesterol, and fat-soluble vitamins.

Triglyceride is the most important type of fat in the diet; it can be differentiated in foods according to the types of fatty acids that each triglyceride contains. Fatty acids vary in carbon-chain length and may be saturated, monounsaturated, or polyunsaturated. Most food triglycerides contain predominantly long-chain fatty acids that have an even number of carbon atoms ranging between 16 and 26. Two exceptions are butter and coconut oil, which contain appreciable amounts of medium- and short-chain fatty acids (SCFAs). Medium-chain triglycerides (MCTs) refer to triglycerides that primarily contain fatty acids with between 8 and 10 carbon atoms. These fatty acids have been shown to be rapidly hydrolyzed and absorbed in human subjects, reportedly directly entering the portal venous blood system rather than being transported through the lymphatic system.[1] For this reason, MCTs have been identified as a form of dietary fat that may provide benefit to dogs with digestive disorders that affect normal fat digestion and absorption.[2] However, a study that examined the digestion and absorption of MCTs in healthy adult dogs found evidence that these fats were absorbed in the same manner as long-chain fatty acids (via that intestinal lymphatic system) and found no evidence of direct transport via portal venous blood.[3]

In addition, others have reported that the inclusion of high concentrations of MCTs in dog diets can negatively affect diet palatability and cause reduced food intake.[2,4] Therefore additional studies of benefits for this class of fats for pets with gastrointestinal disease are warranted before their use in therapeutic diets can be recommended.

Saturated fatty acids contain no double bonds between carbon atoms and thus are "saturated" with hydrogen atoms. Monounsaturated fatty acids have one double bond, and polyunsaturated fatty acids (PUFAs) contain two or more double bonds (Figure 3-2). The double bonds between carbon atoms in unsaturated fatty acids may exist in either *cis* or *trans* configurations. *Cis* isomers have the hydrogen atoms on each side of the double bond oriented in the same plane, while *trans* isomers have their hydrogen atoms on each side of the bond oriented in opposite planes. Most of the naturally occurring unsaturated fatty acids are *cis* isomers. Conversely, *trans* double bonds are most commonly introduced into fatty acids during the food manufacturing process (both in human and pet foods) or hydrogenation. In humans, the inclusion of *trans* fatty acids in the diet can negatively affect lipoprotein metabolism in the same manner as diets that are rich in saturated fat.[5] However, the impact of these fats upon canine and feline fat metabolism and health has not been studied extensively. In general, the triglycerides in animal fats contain a higher percentage of saturated fatty acids than do those in vegetable fats. Most plant oils, with the exception of palm, olive, and coconut oils, contain between 80% and 90% unsaturated fat; animal fats contain between 50% and 60% unsaturated fat.

Fat has numerous functions within the body. Triglycerides are the body's primary form of stored energy. Major depots of fat accumulation are present under the skin (as subcutaneous fat), around the vital organs, and in the membranes surrounding the intestines. Some of these depots can be readily observed in obese dogs and cats. Fat depots in the body have an extensive blood and nerve supply and are in a constant state of flux,

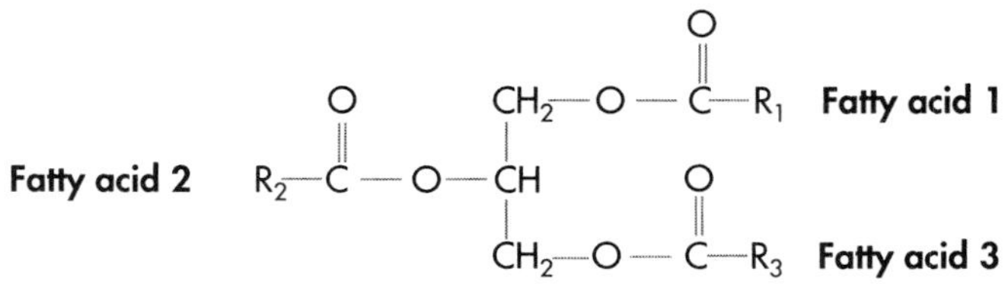

Figure 3-1 Triglyceride structure.

Saturated

Lauric acid

$$CH_3-CH_2-CH_2-CH_2-CH_2-CH_2-CH_2-CH_2-CH_2-CH_2-CH_2-COOH$$

Monounsaturated

Palmitoleic acid

$$CH_3-CH_2-CH_2-CH_2-CH_2-CH_2-CH=CH-CH_2-CH_2-CH_2-CH_2-CH_2-CH_2-CH_2-COOH$$

Polyunsaturated

Linoleic acid

$$CH_3-CH_2-CH_2-CH_2-CH_2-CH=CH-CH_2-CH=CH-CH_2-CH_2-CH_2-CH_2-CH_2-CH_2-CH_2-COOH$$

Alpha-linolenic acid

$$CH_3-CH_2-CH=CH-CH_2-CH=CH-CH_2-CH=CH-CH_2-CH_2-CH_2-CH_2-CH_2-CH_2-CH_2-COOH$$

Arachidonic acid

$$CH_3-CH_2-CH_2-CH_2-CH_2-CH=CH-CH_2-CH=CH-CH_2-CH=CH-CH_2-CH=CH-CH_2-CH_2-CH_2-COOH$$

Figure 3-2 Types of fatty acids.

providing energy in times of need and storage in times of energy surplus. They also serve as insulators, protecting the body from heat loss, and as a protective layer that guards against physical injury to the vital organs. Although animals have a very limited capacity to store carbohydrate in the form of glycogen, they have an almost limitless capacity to store surplus energy in the form of fat.

In addition to providing energy, fat has numerous metabolic and structural functions. Fat insulation surrounds myelinated nerve fibers and aids in the transmission of nerve impulses. Phospholipids and glycolipids serve as structural components for cell membranes and participate in the transport of nutrients and metabolites across these membranes. Lipoproteins provide for the transport of fats through the bloodstream. Cholesterol is used by the body to form the bile salts necessary for proper fat digestion and absorption, and it is also a precursor for the steroid hormones. Along with other lipids, cholesterol forms a protective layer in the skin that prevents excessive water loss and the invasion of foreign substances. The essential fatty acid (EFA) arachidonic acid is the precursor of a group of physiologically and pharmacologically active compounds called *prostacyclins, prostaglandins, leukotrienes,* and *thromboxanes.* These compounds perform extensive hormonelike actions in the body and are involved in processes such as vasodilation and vasoconstriction, muscle contraction, blood pressure homeostasis, gastric acid secretion, regulation of body temperature, regulation of blood clotting mechanisms, and control of inflammation.

In the diet, fat provides the most concentrated form of energy of all the nutrients. Although the gross energy (GE) of protein and carbohydrate is approximately 5.65 and 4.15 kilocalories per gram (kcal/g), respectively, the GE of fat is 9.4 kcal/g. In addition to containing more energy, the digestibility of fat is also usually higher than that of protein and carbohydrate. An early study reported estimates of apparent fat digestibility between 80% and 95% in adult dogs when fed mixtures of plant and animal fat.[6] A second study reported that the apparent digestibility of the fat in several commercially prepared dry-type dog foods varied between 70% and 90%.[7] More recently, a comparison of apparent nutrient digestibilities among six extruded dry dog foods reported that fat digestibility was greater than 90% for all six foods.[8] In each of these studies, within food types, the apparent fat digestibility was consistently higher than either protein or carbohydrate digestibility. Therefore, increasing the percentage of fat in a pet's diet provides a very concentrated, readily digested source of energy that substantially increases the caloric density of the food.

Dietary fat also provides a source of EFAs and acts as a carrier that allows the absorption of the fat-soluble vitamins. The body has a physiological requirement for two distinct families of EFAs: the n-6 and the n-3 series.[9] This terminology denotes the position of the first double bond in the molecule, counting from the terminal (methyl) end of the chain. The most important fatty acid of the n-6 series is linoleic acid (see Figure 3-2). In most animals, gamma-linolenic acid (GLA) and arachidonic acid (AA) can be synthesized from linoleic acid by alternating desaturation and elongation reactions. Therefore, if adequate linoleic acid is provided in the diet, there is not a dietary requirement for GLA or AA. Although the dog is able to synthesize adequate amounts of these fatty acids during all life stages, the cat is one of the few species that does not synthesize adequate amounts of AA during all stages of life, even when adequate linoleic acid is present in the diet.[10] As a result, AA is considered to be conditionally essential for the cat during pregnancy and for normal neonatal development.

In the n-3 family, alpha-linolenic acid (ALA) is also considered to be essential for dogs and cats although exact requirement levels are not well defined.[11] Similar to the n-6 family of fatty acids, the conversion of ALA to physiologically essential long-chain PUFAs such as eicosapentaenoic acid (EPA) and docosahexaenoic acid (DHA) is limited, which may lead to a dietary requirement during periods of reproduction and development (see Section 4, pp. 211 and 228-229 for a complete discussion). Beneficial effects of several of the n-3 fatty acids are reported when these fatty acids are included in the diet at nutritional levels and balanced with n-6 fatty acid content. These effects relate to the fatty acid composition of cell membranes and the production of eicosanoids (see Section 4, pp. 211 and 228-229 and Section 5, Chapters 31, 32, 35, 36, and 37 for complete discussions).

All of the EFAs are polyunsaturated. Linoleic acid and the linolenic acids contain 18 carbon atoms and 2 and 3 double bonds, respectively. AA contains 20 carbon atoms and 4 double bonds (see Figure 3-2). In most animals, the best sources of linoleic acid are vegetable oils such as corn, soybean, and safflower oils. Poultry fat and pork fat also contain appreciable amounts of linoleic acid, while beef tallow and butter fats contain very little. Another form of linoleic acid is called *conjugated linoleic acid* (CLA). CLA is actually a group of compounds, a naturally occurring mixture of linoleic acid isomers that contain modified double bonds. CLAs are naturally produced by rumen bacteria in ruminant animals or through food processing. One particular CLA isomer has been shown to have antiatherogenic properties in laboratory animal models.[12] In dogs and cats, CLA has been reported to provide body composition benefits for overweight animals.[13,14] Additional studies are needed to fully explore the potential dietary benefits of this form of linoleic acid. The final EFA, AA, is found only in animal fats. Some fish oils are rich in this EFA, and pork fat and poultry fat also supply a small amount.

Fat provides the most concentrated form of energy of all the nutrients, is a source of the essential fatty acids, and facilitates absorption of the fat-soluble vitamins. Fat also enhances the palatability and texture of pets' food.

Fat in the diets of companion animals also plays a role in contributing to the palatability and texture of food.[15] This is obviously a critical function because no pet food, regardless of how well-formulated it is, can be nutritious if it is not eaten. A study conducted with cats found that diets containing 25% to 40% fat were preferred to low-fat diets, but increasing the fat content further tended to decrease the diet's acceptability.[16] This effect of dietary fat is complicated by the fact that as the fat content in the diet increases, so does energy density. Animals require decreased quantities of calorie-dense foods to satisfy their energy requirements. However, the increased palatability of foods high in fat can encourage some pets to overconsume. Therefore, although fat does lend increased palatability to a diet, this effect can rapidly lead to overeating as the energy density of the diet rises. For this reason, well-balanced pet foods that are energy-dense and contain moderate to high levels of fat must often be fed on a portion-controlled basis.

As the fat content increases, so does the energy density of the diet. Portion-controlled feeding is usually the best method when feeding a well-balanced, energy-dense pet food containing moderate to high levels of fat.

References

1. Bach AC, Babayan VK: Medium chain triglycerides: an update, *Am J Clin Nutr* 36:950–962, 1982.

2. Remillard RI, Thatcher CD: Dietary and nutritional management of gastrointestinal diseases, *Vet Clin North Am Small Anim Pract* 19:797–817, 1989.

3. Newton JD, McLoughlin MA, Birchard SJ, Reinhart GA: Transport pathways of enterally administered medium-chain triglycerides in dogs. In Reinhart GA, Carey DP, editors: *Recent advances in canine and feline nutrition*, Wilmington, Ohio, 2000, Orange Frazer Press.

4. Van Dongen AM, Stokhof AA, Geelen JH, Beynen AC: The high intake of medium-chain triglycerides elevates plasma cholesterol in dogs (an observation), *Folia Vet* 44:173–174, 2000.

5. Emken EA: Do trans fatty acids have adverse health effects? In Nelson GJ, editor: *Health effects of dietary fatty acids*, Champaign, Ill, 1991, American Oil Chemists' Society, pp 245–263.

6. Orr NWM: The food requirements of Antarctic sledge dogs. In Graham-Jones O, editor: *Canine and feline nutritional requirements*, London, 1965, Pergamon Press.

7. Huber TL, Wilson RC, McGarity SA: Variations in digestibility of dry dog foods with identical label guaranteed analysis, *J Am Anim Hosp Assoc* 22:571–575, 1986.

8. Ahlstrom O, Skrede A: Comparative nutrient digestibility in dogs, blue foxes, mink and rats, *J Nutr* 128:2676S–2677S, 1998.

9. Mead JF: Functions of the n-6 and n-3 polyunsaturated fatty acid acids. In Taylor TG, Jenkins NK, editors: *Proceedings of the XIII International Congress of Nutrition*, London, 1986, John Libbey.

10. Bauer JE: Metabolic basis for the essential nature of fatty acids and the unique dietary fatty acid requirements of cats, *J Am Vet Med Assoc* 229:1729–1732, 2006.

11. Carlson SE: Are n-3 polyunsaturated fatty acids essential for growth and development? In Nelson GJ, editor: *Health effects of dietary fatty acids*, Champaign, Ill, 1991, American Oil Chemists' Society.

12. Nicolosi RJ, Rogers EJ, Kritchevsky D, and others: Dietary conjugated linoleic acid reduces plasma lipoprotein and early atherosclerosis in hypercholesterolemic rabbits, *Artery* 22:266–277, 1997.

13. Bartges JM, Cook M: Influence of feeding conjugated linoleic acid on body composition in healthy adult cats. In *Proc 17th ACVIM*, 1999, p 729.

14. Schoenherr W, Jewell J: Effect of conjugated linoleic acid on body composition of mature obese Beagles, *FASEB J* 13:A262, 1999.

15. Bauer JE: Facilitative and functional fats in diets of cats and dogs, *J Am Vet Med Assoc* 229:680–684, 2006.

16. Kane E, Morris JG, Rogers QR: Acceptability and digestibility by adult cats of diets made with various sources and levels of fat, *J Anim Sci* 53:1516–1523, 1981.

4

Protein and Amino Acids

Proteins are complex molecules that, like carbohydrates and fats, contain carbon, hydrogen, and oxygen. In addition, all proteins contain the element nitrogen, and the majority contain sulfur. All proteins contain approximately 16% nitrogen. This consistency led to the development of the nitrogen balance test, which has been used traditionally to estimate an animal's body protein status. Nitrogen balance tests measure intake and excretion of nitrogen in animals that are fed a test diet. Net loss or gain of nitrogen then indicates increases or decreases in total body protein reserves (see Section 2, p. 89). Amino acids are the basic units of proteins and are held together by peptide linkages to form long protein chains (Figures 4-1 and 4-2). Proteins can range in size from several amino acids to large, complex molecules that consist of several intricately folded peptide chains, and can be classified as either simple or complex forms. Once hydrolysis begins, simple proteins yield only amino acids or their derivatives. Examples include albumin in blood plasma, lactalbumin in milk, zein in corn, and the structural proteins keratin, collagen, and elastin. Complex or conjugated proteins are made up of a simple protein combined with a nonprotein molecule. Examples of complex proteins include the nucleoproteins, glycoproteins, and phosphoproteins.

Proteins in the body have numerous functions. They are the major structural components of hair, feathers, skin, nails, tendons, ligaments, and cartilage. The fibrous protein collagen is the basic material that forms most of the connective tissue throughout the body. Contractile proteins such as myosin and actin are involved in regulating muscle action. All of the enzymes that catalyze the body's essential metabolic reactions and are essential for nutrient digestion and assimilation are also protein molecules. Many hormones that control the homeostatic mechanisms of various systems in the body are composed of protein; for example, insulin and glucagon are two protein hormones involved in the control of normal blood glucose levels. Proteins found in the blood act as important carrier substances. These substances include hemoglobin, which carries oxygen to tissues; transferrin,

which transports iron; and retinol-binding protein, which carries vitamin A. In addition to their transport functions, plasma proteins also contribute to the regulation of acid-base balance. Finally, the body's immune system relies on protein substances; the antibodies that maintain the body's resistance to disease are all composed of large protein molecules.

Proteins are the major structural components of the body. Enzymes essential for nutrient digestion are proteins, as are many hormones, such as insulin and glucagon. Blood proteins act as important carrier substances and contribute to the regulation of acid-base balance. Finally, the body's immune system relies on protein substances; the antibodies that maintain the body's resistance to disease are all composed of large protein molecules.

Protein present in the body is not static; it is in a constant state of flux involving degradation and synthesis. Although tissues vary greatly in their rate of turnover, all protein molecules in the body are eventually catabolized and replaced. During growth and reproduction, additional protein is needed for the accretion of new tissue. A regular influx of protein and nitrogen, supplied by the diet, is necessary to maintain normal metabolic processes and provide for tissue maintenance and growth. The body has the ability to synthesize new proteins from amino acids, provided that all of the necessary amino acids are available to the tissue cells. At the tissue and cellular level it is inconsequential whether the amino acids that are present were synthesized by the body, supplied from the diet as single amino acid units, or supplied from the diet in the form of intact protein. Therefore it is correct to state that the body does not really have a protein requirement per se but rather has a requirement for certain amino acids and a level of nitrogen. This requirement is still addressed as a protein requirement in the diet because most practical diets contain intact protein sources, not individual amino acids.

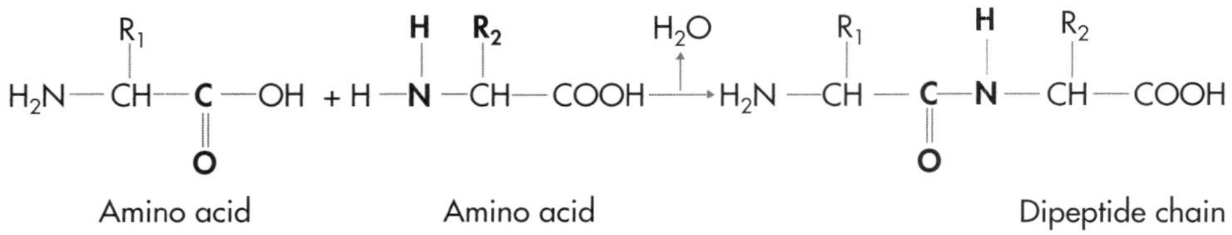

Figure 4-1   Peptide linkage.

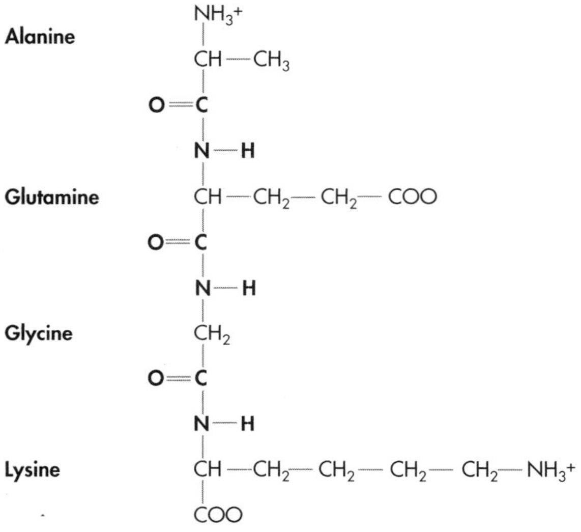

Figure 4-2   Simple protein chain.

BOX 4-1 **ESSENTIAL AND NONESSENTIAL AMINO ACIDS FOR DOGS AND CATS**	
ESSENTIAL AMINO ACIDS	**NONESSENTIAL AMINO ACIDS**
Arginine	Alanine
Histidine	Asparagine
Isoleucine	Aspartate
Leucine	Cysteine
Lysine	Glutamate
Methionine	Glutamine
Phenylalanine	Glycine
Taurine (cats only)	Hydroxylysine
Threonine	Hydroxyproline
Tryptophan	Proline
Valine	Serine
	Tyrosine

There are 22 alpha-amino acids found in protein chains. The term *alpha* denotes the attachment of the amino group (NH_2) to the first (alpha-) carbon in the molecule. Of these 22 alpha-amino acids, if an adequate source of nitrogen is supplied in the diet, dogs and cats are able to synthesize 12 at a sufficient rate to meet the body's needs for growth, performance, and maintenance. These are called the *nonessential,* or *dispensable, amino acids,* and they may be either supplied in the diet or synthesized by the body. The remaining 10 amino acids cannot be synthesized at a rate that is sufficient to meet the body's needs. These are the *essential amino acids,* and they must be supplied in the pet's diet. In addition to these 10, the cat has an additional requirement for taurine, a beta-sulfonic acid (see Section 2, pp. 97-99). The essential and nonessential amino acids are listed in Box 4-1.

Dietary protein serves several important functions. It provides the essential amino acids, which are used for protein synthesis in the growth and repair of tissue, and it is the body's principal source of nitrogen. Nitrogen is essential for the synthesis of the nonessential amino acids and of other nitrogen-containing molecules, such as nucleic acids, purines, pyrimidines, and certain neurotransmitter substances. Amino acids supplied by dietary protein can also be metabolized for energy. The gross energy (GE) of amino acids is 5.65 kilocalories per gram (kcal/g). When fecal and urinary losses are accounted for, the metabolizable energy (ME) of protein in dog and cat diets is approximately 3.5 kcal/g; that is, approximately the same amount of energy supplied by dietary carbohydrate. Animals are unable to store excess amino acids. Surplus amino acids are either used directly for energy or are converted to glycogen or fat for energy storage. An ancillary function of the protein in dog and cat diets is to provide a source of

BOX 4-2 METHODS TO DETERMINE PROTEIN QUALITY

CHEMICAL SCORE

$$\frac{\text{Limiting amino acid in the test protein (\%)}}{\text{Particular amino acid in the reference protein (\%)}}$$

ESSENTIAL AMINO ACID INDEX (EAAI)

$$\left.\frac{\text{Amino acid in the test protein (\%)}}{\text{Same amino acid in the reference protein (\%)}}\right\}\text{Summed for all essential amino acids}$$

TOTAL ESSENTIAL AMINO ACID CONTENT (E/T)

$$\frac{\text{Amount of nitrogen from essential amino acids in the protein source}}{\text{Amount of total nitrogen in the protein source}}$$

PROTEIN EFFICIENCY RATIO (PER)

$$\frac{\text{Weight gained by animals (g)}}{\text{Protein consumed by animals (total g)}}$$

BIOLOGICAL VALUE (BV)

$$\frac{\text{Food nitrogen} - (\text{fecal nitrogen} + \text{urinary nitrogen})}{\text{Food nitrogen} - \text{fecal nitrogen}}$$

NET PROTEIN UTILIZATION (NPU)

$$\text{BV of protein} \times \text{Digestibility of protein}$$

flavor. Different flavors are created when food proteins are cooked in the presence of carbohydrate and fat.[1] In general, as the protein content of a dog or cat diet increases, so does its palatability and acceptability.

Because the protein in the body is in a constant state of flux, a regular intake of dietary protein is necessary to maintain normal metabolic processes and provide for tissue maintenance and growth. Like fat, protein content also contributes to the palatability and acceptability of food.

The degree to which a dog or cat is able to use dietary protein as a source of amino acids and nitrogen is affected by both the digestibility and the quality of the protein included in the diet. Proteins that are highly digestible and contain all of the essential amino acids in their proper proportions relative to the animal's needs are considered high-quality proteins. In contrast, those that are either low in digestibility or limiting in one or more of the essential amino acids are of lower quality. The higher the quality of a protein in a diet, the less quantity will be needed by the animal to meet all of its essential amino acid needs. Various methods for evaluating the protein quality in foods have been developed (Box 4-2). Each of these methods has specific advantages and disadvantages with respect to efficacy of evaluating the overall quality of protein sources included in foods formulated for companion animals.

Several analytical tests predict protein quality based entirely on the protein's essential amino acid composition. A *chemical score* is an index that involves comparing the amino acid composition of a given protein source with the amino acid pattern of a reference protein of very high quality. Egg protein is typically used as the reference protein and is given a chemical score of 100. The essential amino acid that is in greatest deficit in the test protein is called the *limiting amino acid* because it will limit the body's ability to use that protein. The percentage of that amino acid present in the protein relative to the corresponding value in the reference protein determines the chemical score of the test protein. The three amino acids in food proteins that are most often limiting are methionine, tryptophan, and lysine. In some pet foods, arginine and isoleucine have also been reported to be limiting according to analysis by chemical score.[2] Although a chemical score provides useful information concerning the amino acid deficits of a protein source, its value is based entirely on the level of the most limiting amino acid in the protein and does not take into account the proportions of all of the remaining essential amino acids.

A modified version of the chemical score, called the *essential amino acid index* (EAAI), measures the contribution that a protein makes to all of the essential amino acids, rather than only to the one in greatest deficit. A protein's EAAI is calculated as the geometric mean of the ratios of each of the essential amino acids in the test protein to their corresponding values in the reference protein.[3] Finally, the *total essential amino acid content* (E/T) is calculated as the proportion of the total nitrogen in a protein source that is contributed by essential amino acids. Although the chemical score and EAAI both indicate the quality of a protein's amino acid profile, the E/T measures the total quantity of essential amino acids within a particular protein source.

Estimations of protein quality from amino acid composition are helpful in assessing protein quality when combinations of different proteins are used in a food and for assessing protein sources that have been supplemented with purified amino acids. However, these tests are limited by the fact that they provide no information regarding the digestibility of a protein or the availability of its amino acids. For example, the heat used in processing can damage food protein, resulting in a decreased availability of certain amino acids. Simply using an analytical analysis based on amino acid composition would not reveal this change. Two additional in vitro protein quality assays that attempt to provide an estimate of both amino acid composition and availability are the protein solubility index and the immobilized digestive enzyme assay.[4,5] However, these assays have not been tested extensively with protein sources that are typically used in companion animal diets, and a recent study found that they did not produce consistent results.[6]

A thorough assessment of a protein source ultimately requires that feeding trials be conducted in which the protein in question is fed to a predetermined number of test animals. *Protein efficiency ratio* (PER) is one of the simplest and most commonly used feeding tests for measuring protein quality. Weanling male rats or growing chicks are fed an adequate diet containing the test protein for up to 28 days. Changes in weight are measured, and PER is calculated as the grams of weight gained divided by the total grams of protein consumed. The PER value indicates the ability of a protein source to be converted into tissue in a growing animal. One criticism of using PER as a measure of protein quality in dog and cat foods is that this test assumes that weight gain in growing animals is directly related to nitrogen retention. Although this has been proven to be true in rats, this may not be a consistent relationship in growing dogs and cats. In addition, any factor that influences the test animals' rate of growth during the study, regardless of whether it is related to protein quality, will affect the calculated PER value. One method of accounting for these problems is to include a positive and negative control group in the PER study. The positive control group is fed a diet containing a reference protein (egg), and the negative group is fed a protein-free diet. The effects of the nonprotein group are subtracted from the effects in the test protein group when the study is completed.

Biological value (BV) and net protein utilization provide accurate measures of protein quality, but they are more time consuming and labor intensive to conduct than are PER tests. BV is defined as the percentage of absorbed protein that is retained by the body. It is a measure of the ability of the body to convert absorbed amino acids into body tissue. Nitrogen balance studies must be conducted in which nitrogen from food, feces, and urine is collected and measured. Animals are required to be in a state of physiological maintenance, and the diet must contain adequate carbohydrate and fat to ensure that the protein in the diet is not metabolized for energy. True BV can be determined by first accounting for fecal and urinary losses of endogenous nitrogen when the animal is consuming a protein-free diet. One problem with using BV as a measurement of protein quality is that it does not account for protein digestibility. Theoretically, if the small portion of a very indigestible protein that is absorbed is used efficiently by the body, it could still have a very high BV value.

This limitation can be addressed by measuring a protein's *net protein utilization* (NPU). NPU is calculated as the product of a protein's BV and its digestibility. NPU therefore measures the proportion of consumed protein that is retained by the body. A protein that is 100% digestible would have BV and NPU values that were the same. On the other hand, a poorly digested protein would have a much lower NPU value than BV value. Although BV and NPU are considered very important indicators of protein quality, data collected in nitrogen balance experiments can be affected by the level of protein in the diet, the energy intake, and the physiological state of the animal. Overall, in addition to one or more of the tests described earlier, the quality of protein in a pet food is best assessed through in vivo feeding trials in which the food is fed to the animals for which it was developed. Palatability, acceptability, and long-term effects on growth, health, and vitality must also be evaluated to fully determine the quality of a particular protein or mixture of proteins in a food.

Although several laboratory tests are available for evaluating the quality of protein in food, all have their limitations. In addition to these tests, the quality of pet food protein is best assessed by feeding trials in which the food is fed to the animals and life stage for which it was developed. The true quality of a protein or proteins in food must also be evaluated on a long-term basis by assessing the overall health and vitality of the pet.

References

1. Brown RG: Protein in dog foods, *Can Vet J* 30:528–531, 1989.

2. Kronfeld DS: Protein quality and amino acid profiles of commercial dog foods, *J Am Anim Hosp Assoc* 18:679–683, 1982.

3. Oser BL: An integrated essential amino acid index for predicting the biological value of proteins. In Albanese AA, editor: *Protein and amino acid nutrition*, New York, 1959, Academic Press.

4. Araba M, Dale NM: Evaluation of protein solubility as an indicator of over-processing soybean meal, *Poult Sci* 69:76–83, 1990.

5. Schasteen C, Wu J, Schulz M, Parsons CM: An enzyme-based digestibility assay for poultry diets, *Proc Multi-State Poult Feeding and Nutr Conf*, 2002.

6. Dust JM, Grieshop CM, Parsons CM, and others: Chemical composition, protein quality, palatability, and digestibility of alternative protein sources for dogs, *J Anim Sci* 83:2414–2422, 2005.

5

Vitamins

Vitamins are organic molecules that are needed in minute amounts to function as essential enzymes, enzyme precursors, or coenzymes in many of the body's metabolic processes. Although they are organic molecules, vitamins are not classified as carbohydrate, fat, or protein; they are not used as energy sources or structural compounds. With a few exceptions, most vitamins cannot be synthesized by the body and must be supplied in the food.

A general classification scheme for vitamins divides them into two groups: the fat-soluble vitamins and the water-soluble vitamins. The fat-soluble vitamins are A, D, E, and K; the water-soluble group includes vitamin C and members of the B-complex vitamin group. Fat-soluble vitamins are digested and absorbed using the same mechanisms as dietary fat, and their metabolites are excreted primarily in the feces through the bile. In contrast, most of the water-soluble vitamins are absorbed passively in the small intestine and are excreted in the urine. Excesses of fat-soluble vitamins are stored primarily in the liver. With the exception of cobalamin, the body is unable to store significant levels of the water-soluble vitamins. As a result, the fat-soluble vitamins, specifically vitamins A and D, have a much higher potential for toxicity than do the water-soluble vitamins. Similarly, because they can be stored, deficiencies of fat-soluble vitamins develop much more slowly in animals than do deficiencies of the water-soluble vitamins. A summary of food sources and signs of deficiency and excess for the vitamins is given in Table 5-1.

The fat-soluble vitamins are A, D, E, and K; the water-soluble group includes vitamin C and members of the B-complex vitamin group. Fat-soluble vitamins are digested and absorbed using the same mechanisms as dietary fat, and their metabolites are excreted primarily in the feces through the bile. Most of the water-soluble vitamins are absorbed passively in the small intestine and are excreted in the urine.

VITAMIN A

The general term *vitamin A* actually includes several related chemical compounds called *retinol, retinal,* and *retinoic acid.* Of these molecules, retinol is the most biologically active form. In the body, vitamin A has functions involving vision, bone growth, reproduction, and maintenance of epithelial tissue. The role of vitamin A in vision is well established. In the rods of the retina, retinal combines with a protein called *opsin* to form *rhodopsin,* also known as *visual purple.* Rhodopsin is a light-sensitive pigment that enables the eye to adapt to changes in light intensity. When exposed to light, rhodopsin splits into retinal and opsin, and the energy that is released produces nerve transmissions to the optic nerve. In the dark, rhodopsin can then be regenerated by the combination of new retinal and opsin molecules. During periods of vitamin A deficiency, less retinal is available to regenerate rhodopsin; thus the rods of the eye become increasingly sensitive to light changes, which eventually results in night blindness.

Vitamin A is also essential for the formation and maintenance of healthy epithelial tissue. This tissue includes the skin and the mucous membranes lining the respiratory and gastrointestinal tracts. Vitamin A is believed to be necessary for both the proliferation and differentiation of cells and for the production of the mucoproteins found in the mucus produced by some types of epithelial cells.[1] Mucous secretions of epithelial tissue maintain the integrity of the epithelium and provide a barrier against bacterial invasion. In the absence of vitamin A, the differentiation of new epithelial cells beyond the squamous type to mature mucus-secreting cells fails to occur, and normal epithelial cells are replaced by dysfunctional, stratified, keratinized cells.[2] Epithelial tissue that does not function properly leads to lesions in the epithelium and increased susceptibility to infection.

Normal skeletal and tooth development and reproductive performance also depend on vitamin A. The vitamin's role in bone growth appears to involve the

TABLE 5-1 VITAMIN DEFICIENCIES, EXCESSES, AND MAJOR DIETARY SOURCES

VITAMIN	DEFICIENCY	EXCESS	SOURCES
A	Impaired growth, reproductive failure, loss of epithelial integrity, dermatoses	Skeletal abnormalities, hyperesthesia	Fish liver oils, milk, liver, egg yolk
D	Rickets, osteomalacia, nutritional secondary hyperparathyroidism	Hypercalcemia, bone resorption, soft tissue calcification	Liver, some fish, egg yolk, sunlight
E	Reproductive failure, pansteatitis in cats	Nontoxic; may increase vitamin A and D requirements	Wheat germ, corn and soybean oils
K	Increased clotting time, hemorrhage	None recorded	Green leafy plants, liver, some fish meals
Thiamin	CNS dysfunction, anorexia, weight loss	Nontoxic	Meat, wheat germ
Riboflavin	CNS dysfunction, dermatitis	Nontoxic	Milk, organ meats, vegetables
Niacin	Black tongue disease	Nontoxic	Meat, legumes, grains
Pyridoxine	Microcytic hypochromic anemia	None recorded	Organ meats, fish, wheat germ
Pantothenic acid	Anorexia, weight loss	None recorded	Liver, kidney, dairy products, legumes
Biotin	Dermatitis	Nontoxic	Eggs, liver, milk, legumes
Folic acid	Anemia, leukopenia	Nontoxic	Liver, kidney, green leafy vegetables
Cobalamin	Anemia	Nontoxic	Meat, fish, poultry
Choline	Neurological dysfunction, fatty liver	Diarrhea	Egg yolk, organ meats, legumes, dairy products
C	Not required by dogs and cats	Nontoxic	Citrus fruit, dark green vegetables

CNS, Central nervous system.

activity of the osteoclasts and osteoblasts of the epithelial cartilage and may be related to cellular division and the maintenance of cell membranes through glycoprotein synthesis. Experiments with laboratory animals have shown that vitamin A is also essential for spermatogenesis in males and normal estrous cycles in females.[1]

The origin of all vitamin A is the carotenoids, which are synthesized by plant cells. Carotenoids are dark red pigments that provide the deep yellow/orange color of many plants. Vegetables such as carrots and sweet potatoes contain high amounts of these compounds. Deep green vegetables also contain these pigments, but their color is masked by the deep green color of chlorophyll. When animals consume the carotenoids in plants, an enzyme located in the intestinal mucosa, β-carotene 15,15'-dioxygenase, converts these compounds (which are commonly called *provitamin A*) to active vitamin A (Figure 5-1). The active vitamin is then absorbed and stored principally in the liver. Although several different carotenoids are capable of providing vitamin A,

beta-carotene is the most plentiful in foods and has the highest biological activity. Animal products do not contain carotenoids but can provide active vitamin A when included in the diet. Fish liver oils contain the highest amounts, and more common foods such as milk, liver, and egg yolk also contain vitamin A.

Like most animals, dogs are capable of converting carotenoids to active vitamin A; therefore they do not require an animal source of this vitamin in the diet. However, β-carotene 15,15'-dioxygenase is either absent or deficient in the domestic cat. As a result, the cat is unable to convert carotenoid pigments to vitamin A and must receive a source of preformed vitamin A in the diet (see Section 2, pp. 107-108 for a complete discussion). In addition to providing a source of vitamin A, carotenoid pigments also have a role in modulating immune response. Recent studies have shown that both dogs and cats readily absorb beta-carotene and a related carotenoid called *lutein,* and that these pigments may have a function in cell-mediated and humoral immune

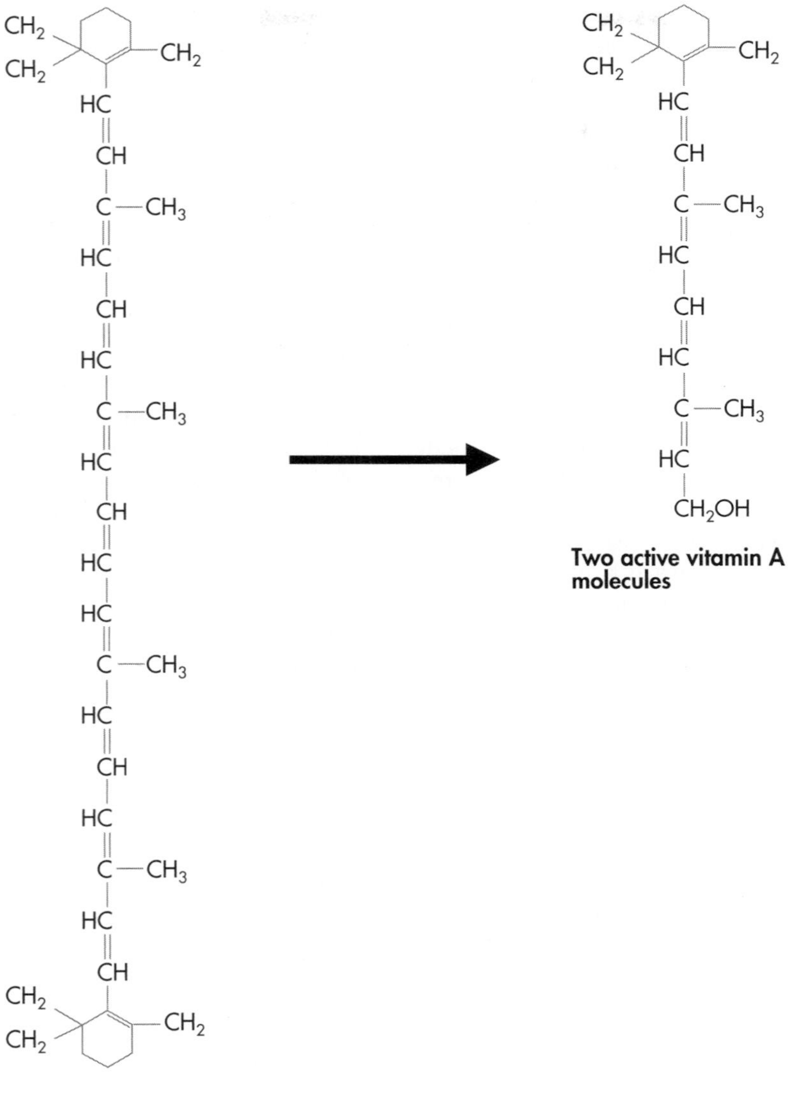

Beta-carotene

Two active vitamin A molecules

Figure 5-1 Conversion of beta-carotene to vitamin A.

response in these species.[3-5] Vitamin A may also have a role in weight maintenance.

VITAMIN D

Vitamin D consists of a group of sterol compounds that regulate calcium and phosphorus metabolism in the body. As with vitamin A, there are provitamin forms of this vitamin. These are vitamin D_2 (ergocalciferol) and vitamin D_3 (cholecalciferol). Vitamin D_2 is formed when the compound ergosterol, which is found in many plants, is exposed to ultraviolet (UV) radiation. This conversion occurs only in harvested or injured plants, not in living plant tissue. Therefore this form of vitamin D is only of significance to ruminants and nonruminant herbivores that are consuming sun-dried or irradiated plant materials. In addition, most species, including cats, use ergocalciferol less efficiently than cholecalciferol.[6] The second form of provitamin D, vitamin D_3, is the form that is of greatest nutritional importance to omnivores and carnivores such as the dog and cat. It is synthesized by the body when 7-dehydrocholesterol, a compound found in the skin of animals, is exposed to UV light from the sun. This form of vitamin D can be obtained either through synthesis in the skin or from the consumption of animal products that contain cholecalciferol. Dogs and cats appear to be dependent upon dietary sources of vitamin D because they have limited ability to convert 7-dehydrocholesterol in the skin to cholecalciferol.[7,8]

Because active vitamin D is synthesized by the body and because of the regulatory functions that it performs within the body, some controversy exists regarding its classification. Although some scientists believe that vitamin D should be considered a hormone, others continue to classify it as a vitamin. Regardless of its categorization, precursors of vitamin D are obtained through the diet, and vitamin D's functions are intricately involved with normal calcium and phosphorus homeostasis in the body. Both ingested and endogenous vitamin D_3 (cholecalciferol) are stored in liver, muscle, and adipose tissue. Cholecalciferol is an inactive storage form of vitamin D. To become active, it must first be transported from the skin or intestines to the liver; there it is hydroxylated to 25-hydroxycholecalciferol. This compound is then transported through the bloodstream to the kidneys, where it is further converted to one of several possible metabolites. Metabolites include 1,25-dihydroxycholecalciferol, also called *calcitriol,* which is the most active form of vitamin D (Figure 5-2). The conversion of 25-hydroxycholecalciferol to calcitriol in the kidneys occurs in response to elevated parathyroid hormone (PTH), which is released from the parathyroid gland in response to decreasing serum calcium. A decrease in serum phosphorus also stimulates the formation of active vitamin D in the kidneys.

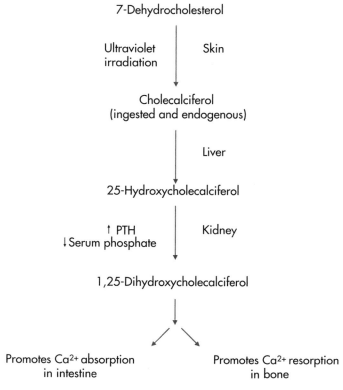

Figure 5-2 Conversion of 7-dehydrocholesterol to active vitamin D. *PTH,* Parathyroid hormone.

Although inactive vitamin D is considered a vitamin, calcitriol is often classified as a hormone because it is produced in the body and because of its mechanism of action in the body.

Active vitamin D functions in normal bone tissue development and maintenance and is an important component in the homeostasis of the body's calcium and phosphorus pools. These effects are mediated through the influence of vitamin D on calcium and phosphorus absorption from the gastrointestinal tract and their deposition in bone tissue. At the site of the intestine, vitamin D stimulates the synthesis of calcium-binding protein, which is necessary for the efficient absorption of dietary calcium and phosphorus. Vitamin D also affects normal bone growth and calcification by acting with PTH to mobilize calcium from bone and by causing an increase in phosphate reabsorption in the kidneys. The net effect of vitamin D's actions in intestines, bones, and kidneys is an increase in plasma calcium and phosphorus to the level that is necessary to allow for the normal mineralization and remodeling of bone. A deficiency of vitamin D causes impaired bone mineralization and results in osteomalacia in adult animals and rickets in growing animals (see Section 2, pp. 108-110).

Dietary sources of vitamin D for dogs and cats are varied. In general, most natural food substances contain very little vitamin D, although egg yolks, liver, and certain types of fish contain moderate amounts. Among the few concentrated food sources of vitamin D are the fish liver oils, particularly cod liver oil. Because natural foods are low in this vitamin, most commercially prepared pet foods are enriched with a purified form of cholecalciferol (vitamin D_3).

VITAMIN E

Vitamin E is the term used to describe a group of chemically related compounds called the *tocopherols* and *tocotrienols,* which have varying levels of biological activity relative to the most potent form, alpha-tocopherol.[9] There are four naturally occurring tocopherols; of these, alpha-tocopherol is the most active form of vitamin E and is the compound most commonly included in pet foods. Several active synthetic forms of vitamin E have also been produced and are used in processed foods. Within the body, vitamin E is found in at least small amounts in almost all tissues and is incorporated into the membrane bilayer of cells. The liver is able to store appreciable amounts of vitamin E.

Vitamin E's chief function in the diet and in the body is as a potent antioxidant. Polyunsaturated fatty acids (PUFAs) that are present in foods and in the lipid membranes of the body's cells are very vulnerable to oxidative damage. Vitamin E interrupts the oxidation of these fats by donating electrons to the free radicals that induce lipid peroxidation (see Section 3, Figure 16-2, p. 156). Peroxidation of the body's lipids can destroy the structural integrity of cell membranes, resulting in impairment of normal cellular functioning. Peroxidation of fats in foods causes rancidity and a loss of the nutritional value of the food's essential fatty acids (EFAs). In addition to its action on PUFAs, vitamin E also protects vitamin A and the sulfur-containing amino acids from oxidative damage. As a direct result of these functions, an animal's requirement for dietary vitamin E depends on the level of PUFAs in its diet and the degree to which dietary fatty acids have undergone peroxidation during processing and storage. Increasing PUFA levels in pet foods causes a concomitant increase in a dog's or cat's vitamin E requirement. A second important interrelationship exists between the trace mineral selenium and vitamin E. Selenium is a cofactor for the enzyme glutathione peroxidase, which functions to reduce the peroxides that are formed during the process of fatty acid oxidation. The inactivation of these peroxides by glutathione peroxidase protects the cell membranes from further oxidative damage. By preventing the oxidation of cell-membrane fatty acids and the formation of peroxides, vitamin E spares selenium. Likewise, selenium creates a similar effect and is able to reduce an animal's vitamin E requirement.

In nature, vitamin E is synthesized by a variety of plants. Food sources that are rich in the tocopherols include wheat germ and the oils of corn, cottonseed, soybean, and sunflower. In general, the vitamin E content of an oil increases according to its linoleic acid concentration. Most animal food sources supply only limited amounts of vitamin E. Egg yolk can contain a moderate amount of vitamin E depending on the diet of the hen, but milk and dairy products are very poor sources. The vitamin E in commercially prepared foods is susceptible to oxidation and destruction along with the fat in the diet. Therefore proper storage of foods is necessary both to prevent oxidative changes to fat and to maintain proper vitamin E levels.

VITAMIN K

Vitamin K comprises a group of compounds called the *quinones*. Vitamin K_1 (phylloquinone) occurs naturally in green plants, and vitamin K_2 (menaquinone) is synthesized by bacteria in the large intestine. Several synthetic analogues have also been prepared. Menadione (vitamin K_3), the most common form of synthetic vitamin K, has a vitamin activity two to three times higher than that of natural K_1. Like all animals, dogs and cats have a metabolic need for vitamin K. However, at least a portion of this requirement can be obtained from bacterial synthesis of the vitamin in the intestine.

The best-known function of vitamin K is its role in the blood clotting mechanism. Specifically, it is required for the liver's synthesis of prothrombin (factor II) and three other clotting factors—factors VII, IX, and X—in the liver. Vitamin K acts as a cofactor for the enzyme that carboxylates glutamic acid residues in a prothrombin-precursor protein to form gamma-carboxyglutamic acid. The conversion of these amino acids facilitates the binding of prothrombin to calcium and phospholipids, a process necessary for the occurrence of normal blood clotting. It appears that vitamin K has a similar role in the activation of other proteins that contain glutamic acid residues in bone and kidney tissue.[10]

Vitamin K is found in green, leafy plants such as spinach, kale, cabbage, and cauliflower. In general, animal sources contain lower amounts of vitamin K; liver, egg, and certain fish meals are fairly good sources. The synthesis of vitamin K by bacteria in the large intestine of dogs and cats can contribute at least a portion, if not all, of the daily requirement in these species. Therefore a dietary supply of this vitamin only becomes significant when bacterial populations in the large intestine are reduced, such as during medical treatment with certain types of antibiotics, or when there is interference with the absorption or use of vitamin K from bacterial sources. Vitamin K is also routinely administered in the treatment of rodenticide poisoning in pets because the active ingredient in many of these poisons is an anticoagulant.

B-COMPLEX VITAMINS

The B-complex vitamins are water-soluble vitamins that were originally grouped together because of similar metabolic functions and occurrence in foods. These nine vitamins act as coenzymes for specific cellular enzymes that are involved in energy metabolism and tissue synthesis. Coenzymes are small organic molecules that must be present with an enzyme for a specific reaction to occur. The vitamins thiamin, riboflavin, niacin, pyridoxine, pantothenic acid, and biotin are all involved in the use of food energy. Folic acid, cobalamin, and choline are important for cell maintenance and growth and/or blood cell synthesis.

Thiamin

Thiamin, also referred to as *vitamin B_1*, is a component of the coenzyme thiamin pyrophosphate, which plays an important role in carbohydrate metabolism. Thiamin pyrophosphate is necessary for the decarboxylation and transketolation reactions that are involved in the use of carbohydrate for energy and conversion to fat and the metabolism of fatty acids, nucleic acids, steroids, and certain amino acids. Because of its importance in carbohydrate metabolism, an animal's thiamin requirement is influenced by the level of carbohydrate present in the diet. A deficiency of thiamin can significantly affect the functioning of the central nervous system (CNS) because of the system's dependency on a constant source of carbohydrate for energy. Natural food sources of thiamin include lean pork, beef, liver, wheat germ, whole grains, and legumes. Although it is present in a large variety of foods, thiamin is a heat-labile vitamin and thus readily destroyed by the high heat involved in the processing of many pet foods. To ensure adequate levels in pet foods, most companies supplement their formulations with this vitamin before processing to ensure that the amount in the finished product is still sufficient. Naturally occurring thiamin deficiency is very rare in dogs and cats and is usually the result of the presence of antithiamin factors in the diet rather than an absolute vitamin deficiency.

Riboflavin

Riboflavin is named for its yellow color (flavin) and because it contains the simple sugar D-ribose. It is relatively stable to heat-processing but is easily destroyed by exposure to light and irradiation. Riboflavin functions in the body as a component of two different coenzymes, flavin mononucleotide and flavin adenine dinucleotide. Both of these coenzymes are required in oxidative enzyme systems that function in the release of energy from carbohydrates, fats, and proteins, as well as in several biosynthetic pathways. Food sources of riboflavin include milk, organ meats, whole grains, and vegetables. In addition, microbial synthesis of riboflavin occurs in the large intestine of most species. The quantity that is synthesized appears to depend on both the species of animal and the level of carbohydrate that is fed. However, the extent to which this source contributes to the daily riboflavin requirement of the dog and cat is unknown.

Niacin

Niacin (nicotinic acid) is closely associated with riboflavin in cellular oxidation-reduction enzyme systems. After absorption, niacin is rapidly converted by the body into nicotinamide, the metabolically active form of the vitamin. Nicotinamide is then incorporated into two different coenzymes, nicotinamide adenine dinucleotide (NAD) and nicotinamide adenine dinucleotide phosphate (NADP). These coenzymes function as hydrogen-transfer agents in several enzymatic pathways involved in the use of fat, carbohydrate, and protein. Meat, legumes, and grains all contain high amounts of niacin. However, a large proportion of the niacin present in many plant sources is in a bound form and unavailable for absorption. The niacin in animal sources is found primarily in an unbound, available form. In addition to consuming niacin in the diet, most animals also synthesize this vitamin as an end product of the metabolism of tryptophan, an essential amino acid. As a result, the level of tryptophan in the diet directly affects an animal's dietary requirement for niacin. Dogs, but not cats, are capable of synthesizing niacin from tryptophan. Although cats possess all of the needed enzymes for this conversion, high activity of a competing enzyme, picolinic carboxylase, converts tryptophan to acetyl coenzyme A, rather than to NAD.[11] Therefore cats must receive their entire niacin requirement from the diet.

Vitamin B₆—Pyridoxine

Pyridoxine, vitamin B_6, comprises three different compounds: pyridoxine, pyridoxal, and pyridoxamine. Pyridoxal, which is a component of the coenzyme pyridoxal 5′-phosphate, is the biologically active form. This coenzyme is necessary for many of the transamination, deamination, and decarboxylation reactions of amino acid metabolism and is active to a lesser extent in the metabolism of glucose and fatty acids. Pyridoxal 5′-phosphate is also required for the synthesis of hemoglobin and the conversion of tryptophan to niacin. In the same manner that the thiamin requirement varies with the carbohydrate level in the diet, the pyridoxine requirement of an animal is influenced by the level of protein in the diet. The three forms of vitamin B_6 are widespread in foods. In animal tissues such as organ meats and fish, the predominant forms are pyridoxal and pyridoxamine. Conversely, plant foods such as wheat germ and whole grains provide this vitamin principally as pyridoxine and pyridoxamine. Naturally occurring dietary deficiencies of this vitamin in dogs and cats have not been reported.

Pantothenic Acid

Pantothenic acid was named after the Greek term *pan,* meaning "all," because this vitamin occurs in all body tissues and in all forms of living tissue. Once absorbed, pantothenic acid is phosphorylated by adenosine triphosphate (ATP) to form coenzyme A. This coenzyme is essential to the process of acetylation, a universal reaction involved in many aspects of carbohydrate, fat, and protein metabolism within the citric acid cycle. Pantothenic acid is found in virtually all foods. As a result, deficiencies of this vitamin are extremely rare. Rich sources of pantothenic acid include organ meats, such as liver and kidney; egg yolk; dairy products; and legumes.

Biotin

The vitamin biotin is a coenzyme required in several carboxylation reactions. It acts as a carbon dioxide carrier in reactions in which carbon chains are lengthened; specifically, biotin is involved in certain steps of fatty acid, nonessential amino acid, and purine synthesis. Biotin is found in many different foods, but its bioavailability varies greatly. Eggs provide a very rich source of biotin, but egg white contains a compound called *avidin,* which binds biotin and makes it unavailable for absorption. Thoroughly cooking eggs destroys avidin and allows the biotin in the yolk to be used. Other food sources of biotin include liver, milk, legumes, and nuts. Intestinal bacteria also synthesize biotin; it is believed that a large proportion, if not all, of an animal's requirement can be met from this source.[12] Deficiencies are not generally a problem; however, the treatment of dogs and cats with antibiotics that decrease the bacterial population of the large intestine can cause an increase in the dietary requirement for biotin.

Folic Acid

Folic acid (folacin) is active in the body as tetrahydrofolic acid. This compound functions as a methyl-transfer agent, transporting single-carbon units in a number of metabolic reactions. An important role of folic acid is its involvement in the synthesis of thymidine, a component of deoxyribonucleic acid (DNA). When folic acid is deficient in the body, the inability to produce adequate DNA leads to decreased cellular growth and maturation. This is manifested clinically as anemia and leukopenia in deficient animals. Food sources of folic acid include green, leafy vegetables and organ meats such as liver and kidney. Like several of the other B vitamins, folic acid is synthesized by the bacteria of the large intestine in dogs and cats. It appears that most, if not all, of the daily requirement of dogs and cats can be met from this source.

Cobalamin

Cobalamin (vitamin B_{12}) contains the mineral cobalt and is unique in that it is the only vitamin that contains a trace element. It is also the only vitamin that is synthesized only by microorganisms. Similar to folic acid, cobalamin is involved in the transfer of single-carbon units during various biochemical reactions. It is also involved in fat and carbohydrate metabolism and is necessary for the synthesis of myelin. As a result, a deficiency of vitamin B_{12} leads to both anemia and impairment of neurological functioning. In most animals, absorption of cobalamin from the diet is facilitated by a group of glycoproteins called *intrinsic factors,* which are produced primarily by the pancreas and secondarily by the gastric mucosa in dogs and cats.[13,14] The absence of this factor can lead to vitamin B_{12} deficiency.

Cobalamin is only found in foods of animal origin. Rich sources of cobalamin include meat, poultry, fish, and dairy products. This vitamin is also unique for a B vitamin because, once absorbed from the diet, excesses can be stored by the body. The liver is the primary storage tissue; muscle, bone, and skin also contain small amounts of cobalamin. Deficiencies of cobalamin are extremely rare as a result of the very small amounts that are needed by the body and the body's ability to store appreciable amounts of the vitamin.

Choline

The last B vitamin, choline, acts as a donor of methyl units for various metabolic reactions in the body. Choline is a precursor for the neurotransmitter substance acetylcholine and is necessary for normal fatty acid transport within cells. Unlike other vitamins, choline is also an integral part of cellular membranes. Choline is a component of two important phospholipids—phosphatidylcholine (lecithin) and sphingomyelin. Lecithin is essential for normal cell-membrane structure and function, and sphingomyelin is found in high concentrations in nervous tissue.

The body is capable of synthesizing choline from the amino acid serine. In this reaction, methionine acts as a methyl donor; folacin and vitamin B_{12} are also necessary. Many animals are capable of synthesizing adequate choline for their needs and so do not require a dietary source. Because choline and methionine both function as methyl donors in the body, diets that are high in methionine can replace some of an animal's choline requirement. Choline is also widespread in food sources. Egg yolk, organ meats, legumes, dairy products, and whole grains all supply high amounts of choline. Because of its synthesis in the body, its presence in many foods, and the ability of methionine to spare choline, naturally occurring dietary deficiencies of choline have not been reported in dogs and cats.

VITAMIN C (ASCORBIC ACID)

Ascorbic acid, commonly known as *vitamin C,* has a chemical structure that is closely related to the monosaccharide sugars. It is synthesized from glucose by plants and most animal species, including dogs and cats. When present in foods, ascorbic acid is easily destroyed by oxidative processes. Exposure to heat, light, alkalies, oxidative enzymes, and the minerals copper and iron all contribute to losses of vitamin C activity. Oxidative loss of vitamin C is inhibited to some extent by an acid environment and by the storage of foods at low temperatures.

The body requires ascorbic acid for the hydroxylation of the amino acids proline and lysine in the formation of collagen and elastin and for the synthesis of acetylcholinesterase. Collagen is the predominant structural protein in animals and is a primary constituent of osteoid, dentine, and connective tissue. It is produced in quantity by osteoblasts during skeletal growth; therefore it is important for normal bone formation. When ascorbic acid is not available, the synthesis of several types of connective tissue within the body is impaired. In animal species that have a dietary requirement for vitamin C, such as humans, nonhuman primates, and guinea pigs, a vitamin C deficiency results in a condition called *scurvy*. Clinical signs of scurvy include impaired wound healing, capillary bleeding, anemia, and faulty bone formation. Bone abnormalities that are associated with scurvy are the result of impaired cartilage synthesis.

With the exception of humans and several other animal species such as guinea pigs, fruit-eating bats, and some other species, all animals are capable of producing adequate levels of endogenous vitamin C and therefore do not have a dietary requirement for this vitamin. Ascorbic acid is produced in the liver from either glucose or galactose through the glucuronate pathway. The adult dog produces approximately 40 milligrams per kilogram (mg/kg) body weight of ascorbate each day.[15]

This is a relatively low amount compared to other mammalian species. However, controlled research studies in the dog have shown that dogs do not require an exogenous source of vitamin C for normal development and maintenance.[16-18] Similarly, no requirement for dietary ascorbic acid has been demonstrated to exist in the cat.[19]

Most vitamins cannot be synthesized by the body and must be supplied in food. Well-balanced pet foods are formulated to provide the necessary supplementation. Vitamin C, however, is one vitamin that can be synthesized from glucose by dogs and cats; in contrast, humans must receive vitamin C from dietary sources.

In recent years a number of breeders, dog show enthusiasts, and pet owners have been routinely administering high levels of supplemental vitamin C to their dogs' diets in the hope of preventing or curing certain developmental skeletal disorders. To date, no controlled research studies have been published that show any efficacy of supplemental ascorbic acid in this role; on the other hand, a substantial amount of evidence exists that directly refutes this claim.[20,21] Currently the use of high amounts of supplemental vitamin C in the diets of healthy dogs and cats is not recommended and may even be contraindicated.

References

1. Goodman DS: Vitamin A and retinoids in health and disease, *N Engl J Med* 310:1023–1031, 1984.

2. Chew BP, Park JS, Wong TS, and others: Importance of beta-carotene nutrition in the dog and cat: uptake and immunity. In Reinhart GA, Carey DP, editors: *Recent advances in canine and feline nutrition, Iams nutrition symposium proceedings,* vol 2, Wilmington, Ohio, 1998, Orange Frazer Press.

3. Schweigert FJ, Raila J, Wichert B, Kienzle E: Cats absorb b-carotene, but it is not converted to vitamin A, *J Nutr* 132:1610S–1612S, 2002.

4. Kim HW, Chew BP, Wong TS, and others: Dietary lutein stimulates immune response in the canine, *Vet Immunol Immunopathol* 74:315–327, 2000.

5. Kim HW, Chew BP, Wong TS, and others: Modulation of humoral and cell-mediated immune responses by dietary lutein in cats, *Vet Immunol Immunopathol* 74:331–341, 2000.

6. Morris JG: Cats discriminate between cholecalciferol and ergocalciferol, *J Anim Physiol Anim Nutr* 86:229–238, 2002.

7. How KL, Hazewinkel AW, Mol JA: Dietary vitamin D dependence of cat and dog due to inadequate cutaneous synthesis of vitamin D, *Gen Comp Endocrinol* 96:12–18, 1994.

8. Morris JF: Ineffective vitamin D synthesis in cats is reversed by an inhibitor of 7-dehydrocholeserol-delta-7-reductase, *J Nutr* 129:903–909, 1999.

9. Chow CK: Vitamin E. In Rucker RB, Suttie JW, McCormick DB, Machlin LJ, editors: *Handbook of vitamins*, New York, 2001, Marcel Dekker, pp 165–197.

10. Gallop PM: Carboxylated calcium–binding proteins and vitamin K, *N Engl J Med* 302:1460–1465, 1980.

11. Ikeda MH, Tsuji H, Nakamura S, and others: Studies on the biosynthesis of nicotinamide adenine dinucleotides. II. Role of picolinic carboxylase in the biosynthesis of NAD from tryptophan in mammals, *J Biol Chem* 240:1395–1401, 1965.

12. Murthy PNA, Mistry SP: Biotin, *Prog Food Nutr Sci* 2:405–455, 1977.

13. Fyfe JC: Feline intrinsic factor (IF) is pancreatic original and mediates ileal cobalamin absorption (abstract), *J Vet Intern Med* 7:133, 1993.

14. Vaillant C, Horadagoda NU, Batt RM: Cellular localization of intrinsic factor in pancreas and stomach of the dog, *Cell Tissue Res* 260:117–122, 1990.

15. Belfield WO, Stone I: Megascorbic prophylaxis and megascorbic therapy: a new orthomolecular modality in veterinary medicine, *J Int Acad Prev Med* 2:10–25, 1975.

16. Innes JRM: Vitamin C requirements in the dog: attempts to produce experimental scurvy. In Innes JRM, editor: *Report of the Cambridge Institute of Animal Pathology*, Cambridge, England, 1931.

17. Naismith DH: Ascorbic acid requirements of the dog, *Proc Nutr Soc* 17:21, 1958.

18. Naismith DH, Pellett PL: The water-soluble vitamin content of blood, serum and milk of the bitch, *Proc Nutr Soc* 19:15, 1960.

19. Carvalho da Silva A, Fajer AB, DeAngelis RC, and others: The domestic cat as a laboratory animal for experimental nutrition studies. II. Comparative growth and hematology on stock and purified rations, *Acta Physiol Latin Am* 1:26–43, 1950.

20. Grondalen J: Metaphyseal osteopathy (hypertrophic osteodystrophy) in growing dogs: a clinical study, *J Small Anim Pract* 17:721–735, 1976.

21. Teare JA, Krook L, Kallfelz FA, and others: Ascorbic acid deficiency and hypertrophic osteodystrophy in the dog: a rebuttal, *Cornell Vet* 69:384–401, 1979.

6

Minerals

Minerals are inorganic elements that are essential for the body's metabolic processes. Only about 4% of an animal's total body weight comprises mineral matter; however, like the vitamins, the presence of these elements is essential for life. A general classification scheme divides minerals into two groups, macrominerals and microminerals. *Macrominerals* are those minerals that occur in appreciable amounts in the body and account for most of the body's mineral content. They include calcium, phosphorus, magnesium, sulfur, iron, and the electrolytes sodium, potassium, and chloride. *Microminerals,* often referred to as the *trace elements,* include a larger number of minerals that are present in the body in very small amounts. These minerals are required in very small quantities in the diet.

Minerals have a variety of functions in the body. They activate enzymatically catalyzed reactions, provide skeletal support, aid in nerve transmission and muscle contractions, serve as components of certain transport proteins and hormones, and function in maintaining water and electrolyte balance. Significant interrelationships exist among many of the mineral elements that can affect mineral absorption, metabolism, and functioning. Specifically, excesses or deficiencies of some minerals can significantly affect the body's ability to use other minerals in the diet. As a result, the level of most minerals in the diet should be considered in relation to other components of the diet, with a goal of achieving an optimal overall dietary balance. Although most of the minerals are discussed separately in this section, the importance of these interrelationships is addressed when they are of practical significance to the nutrition of dogs and cats. A summary of food sources and signs of mineral deficiency and excess is shown in Table 6-1.

Minerals are inorganic elements that make up only about 4% of an animal's total body weight; nonetheless, the essential minerals must be present in the diet to sustain life and maintain health.

CALCIUM AND PHOSPHORUS

Calcium and phosphorus are usually discussed together because their metabolism and the homeostatic mechanisms that control their levels within the body are closely interrelated. Calcium is a principal inorganic component of bone. As much as 99% of the body's calcium is found in the skeleton; the remaining 1% is distributed throughout the extracellular and intracellular fluids. Phosphorus is also an important component of bone. Approximately 85% of the body's phosphorus is found in inorganic combination with calcium as hydroxyapatite in bones and teeth. Most of the remaining portion of this mineral is found (in combination with organic substances) in the soft tissues.

The calcium in bone provides structural integrity to the skeleton and also contributes to the maintenance of proper blood calcium levels through ongoing resorption and deposition. The calcium in bone tissue is not in a static state but is constantly being mobilized and deposited as bone growth and maintenance take place and as the body's needs for plasma calcium fluctuate. The level of circulating plasma calcium is strictly controlled through homeostatic mechanisms and is independent of an animal's dietary intake of calcium. Circulating calcium has essential roles in nerve impulse transmission, muscle contraction, blood coagulation, activation of certain enzyme systems, maintenance of normal cell-membrane permeability and transport, and cardiac function.

Phosphorus that is present in bone is found primarily in combination with calcium in the compound called *hydroxyapatite.* Like calcium, this phosphorus lends structural support to the skeleton and is also released into the bloodstream in response to homeostatic mechanisms. The phosphorus that is found in the soft tissues of the body has a wide range of functions and is involved in almost all of the body's metabolic processes. It is a constituent of cellular deoxyribonucleic acid (DNA) and ribonucleic acid (RNA), several B-vitamin coenzymes, and the cell membrane's phospholipids,

TABLE 6-1 MINERAL DEFICIENCIES, EXCESSES, AND MAJOR DIETARY SOURCES

MINERAL	DEFICIENCY	EXCESS	SOURCES
Calcium	Rickets, osteomalacia, nutritional secondary hyperparathyroidism	Impaired skeletal development; contributes to other mineral deficiencies	Dairy products, poultry and meat meals, bone
Phosphorus	Same as for calcium deficiency	Causes calcium deficiency	Meat, poultry, fish
Magnesium	Soft tissue calcification, enlargement of long bone metaphysis, neuromuscular irritability	Dietary excess unlikely; absorption is regulated according to needs	Soybeans, corn, cereal grains, bone meals
Sulfur	Not reported	Not reported	Meat, poultry, fish
Iron	Hypochromic microcytic anemia	Dietary excess unlikely; absorption is regulated according to needs	Organ meats
Copper	Hypochromic microcytic anemia, impaired skeletal growth	Inherited disorder of copper metabolism causes liver disease	Organ meats
Zinc	Dermatoses, hair depigmentation, growth retardation, reproductive failure	Causes calcium and copper deficiency	Beef liver, dark poultry meat, milk, egg yolks, legumes
Manganese	Dietary deficiency unlikely; impaired skeletal growth, reproductive failure	Dietary excess unlikely	Meat, poultry, fish
Iodine	Dietary deficiency unlikely; goiter, growth retardation, reproductive failure	Dietary excess unlikely; goiter	Fish, beef, liver
Selenium	Dietary deficiency unlikely; skeletal and cardiac myopathies	Dietary excess unlikely; necrotizing myocarditis, toxic hepatitis and nephritis	Grains, meat, poultry
Cobalt	Dietary deficiency unlikely; vitamin B_{12} deficiency, anemia	Not reported	Fish, dairy products

which are important for regulating the transport of solutes into and out of cells. Phosphorus is also necessary for the phosphorylation reactions that are part of many oxidative pathways for the metabolism of the energy-containing nutrients. Phosphorus is a component of the high-energy phosphate bonds of adenosine triphosphate (ATP), adenosine diphosphate, and cyclic adenosine monophosphate.

As mentioned previously, the body has several strictly controlled homeostatic mechanisms that are designed to maintain a constant level of circulating plasma calcium. These mechanisms involve parathyroid hormone (PTH), calcitonin, and active vitamin D (calcitriol). PTH is released into the bloodstream in response to a slight decrease in plasma calcium. This hormone stimulates the synthesis of active vitamin D in the kidneys and increases the resorption of calcium and phosphorus from bone. It also works on the kidney tubules to increase calcium reabsorption and decrease phosphorus reabsorption, resulting in increased retention of calcium in the body and increased losses of urinary phosphate.

In turn, the active vitamin D produced by the kidneys in response to PTH acts at the site of the intestine to increase the absorption of dietary calcium and phosphorus. In conjunction with PTH, vitamin D also enhances the mobilization of calcium from bone by increasing the activity of osteoclasts. Overall, the net action of PTH is to increase the serum concentration of calcium and decrease the serum concentration of phosphorus. The net effect of active vitamin D is to increase levels of both serum calcium and phosphorus (Figure 6-1).

When the blood calcium level is normal, PTH secretion is inhibited through a negative feedback mechanism, and calcitonin, a hormone produced by the parafollicular cells (C cells) of the thyroid gland, is released. Calcitonin functions to reduce blood calcium levels by acting primarily to increase osteoblastic activity and decrease osteoclastic activity in bone tissue. The end result is a decrease in calcium mobilization from the skeleton. Calcitonin is also released in response to hypercalcemia and the release of certain hormones, such as gastrin. Under normal physiological circumstances,

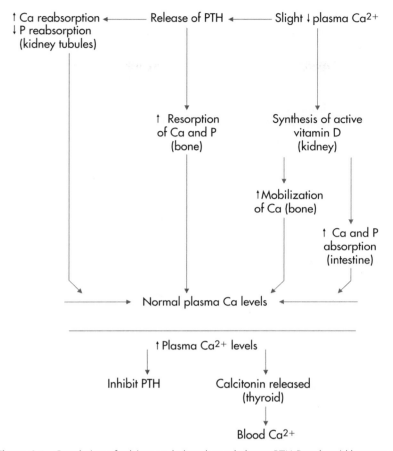

Figure 6-1   Regulation of calcium and phosphorus balance. *PTH,* Parathyroid hormone.

PTH and active vitamin D are the most important regulators of calcium homeostasis, with calcitonin playing a more minor role. However, calcitonin may be of increased importance in the normal homeostatic mechanisms of calcium regulation during growth, pregnancy, and lactation.

In addition to having common homeostatic mechanisms in the body, calcium and phosphorus also have an important relationship to each other within the diet. Once adequate levels of calcium and phosphorus have been included in the diet, it is important to consider the ratio of the amount of calcium to phosphorus. Excess dietary calcium forms an insoluble complex with phosphorus, resulting in decreased phosphorus absorption. Similarly, high levels of phosphorus or phytate in the diet can inhibit calcium absorption. Phytate is a

phosphorus-containing compound found in the outer husks of cereal grains. Although this compound is high in phosphorus, the mineral is poorly available to the body. The recommended ratio of calcium to phosphorus in pet foods is between 1:1 and 2:1.[1] Feeding animals foods that have an improper calcium:phosphorus ratio or supplementing balanced foods with high amounts of either one of these minerals can lead to calcium or phosphorus imbalance. Such problems are usually manifested as skeletal disease in growing and adult animals (see Section 5, pp. 497-499 for a complete discussion).

Foods vary greatly in their calcium content. Dairy products and legumes contain high amounts, but cereal grains, meat, and organ tissues contain very little. The bioavailability of calcium in a food is influenced not only by the source of the mineral, but also by other dietary constituents and the animal's life stage (see Chapter 13, pp. 111-113). Phosphorus, on the other hand, is widely distributed in foods. Foods that contain both phosphorus and calcium include dairy products and legumes. Fish, meats, poultry, and organ meats are also very rich sources of phosphorus. However, these foods are very deficient in calcium, and so their inclusion in the diets of dogs and cats must be balanced by a dietary source of calcium to ensure that an adequate calcium:phosphorus ratio is still maintained.

MAGNESIUM

Although magnesium is a macromineral, its amount in the body is much lower than that of calcium and phosphorus. Approximately 60% to 70% of the magnesium found in the body exists in the form of phosphates and carbonates in bone. Most of the remaining magnesium is found within cells, and a very small portion is present in the extracellular fluid. In addition to its role in providing structure to the skeleton, magnesium functions in a number of metabolic reactions; a magnesium-ATP complex is often the form of ATP that is used as a substrate in many of these processes. As a cation in the intracellular fluid, magnesium is essential for the cellular metabolism of both carbohydrate and protein. Protein synthesis also requires the presence of ionized magnesium. Balanced in the extracellular fluids with calcium, sodium, and potassium, magnesium allows muscle contraction and proper transmission of nerve impulses.

Magnesium is widespread in food sources and is abundant in whole grains, legumes, and dairy products. Naturally occurring magnesium deficiency is not common in dogs and cats. However, excess magnesium in the diets of cats has been implicated as a risk factor for struvite urolithiasis (see Section 5, pp. 362-365 for a complete discussion).

SULFUR

Sulfur is required by the body for the synthesis of a number of sulfur-containing compounds. These include chondroitin sulfate, a mucopolysaccharide found in cartilage; the hormone insulin; and the anticoagulant heparin. As part of the amino acid cysteine, sulfur is found in the regulatory tripeptide glutathione. Glutathione is present in all cells and functions with the enzyme glutathione peroxidase to protect cells against the destructive effects of peroxides. It may also have a role in the transport of amino acids across cell membranes. In addition, sulfur is a constituent of the two B vitamins biotin and thiamin. Within the body, sulfur exists almost entirely as a component of organic compounds. The largest proportion of the body's sulfur is found within proteins as a component of the sulfur-containing amino acids cystine and methionine.

Most dietary sulfur is provided by methionine and cystine. Inorganic sulfates present in the diet are very poorly absorbed by the body and do not contribute an appreciable amount of sulfur. Naturally occurring sulfur deficiency has not been demonstrated in either dogs or cats, and it is believed that diets containing adequate amounts of the sulfur-containing amino acids do provide adequate amounts of sulfur.

IRON

Iron is present in all body cells, but the largest proportion of the body's iron is found as a component of the protein molecules hemoglobin (>65%) and myoglobin (~4%). Hemoglobin is found in red blood cells and transports oxygen from the lungs to the tissues; myoglobin binds oxygen for immediate use by muscle cells. Iron is also a cofactor for several other enzymes and is a component of the cytochrome enzymes, which function in hydrogen ion transport during cellular respiration.

Dietary iron is supplied either as inorganic ions (ferric or ferrous iron) or as organically bound iron, principally as part of the heme molecule. The amount of iron that is absorbed is affected by multiple factors, including the body's need for the mineral, the environment of the intestinal lumen, and the types of foods that are fed.[2,3] Inorganic iron in the ferrous state (+2) is more readily absorbed than iron that is in the ferric state (+3). Therefore an acidic (reducing) environment in the intestine generally enhances iron absorption. Similarly, organic heme iron, which originates from the hemoglobin and myoglobin in animal food sources, is better absorbed than nonheme iron, which is found in plant sources and some animal foods. Low stores of iron in the body and increased metabolic need, such as during periods of growth and gestation, result in increased efficiency of iron absorption.[4] Dietary factors that can inhibit iron absorption include the presence of phytate, phosphates, and oxalates in the diet and the intake of excess dietary zinc or calcium.

Iron is transported in the bloodstream while bound to the transport protein transferrin, and it is stored in tissues while bound to two other proteins, ferritin and hemosiderin. Ferritin and transferrin are also involved in the regulation of iron absorption and transport. Chief storage sites for iron in the body are the liver, spleen, and bone marrow. Most animals are very efficient at conserving iron, so losses of this mineral from the body are minimal. The iron of hemoglobin is recycled and reused when red blood cells are catabolized, and only minute amounts are lost by renal excretion. As a result, the requirement for iron only increases drastically during periods of unusual blood loss, such as in cases of parturition, major surgery, injury, or severe parasitic infection or gastrointestinal disease. Iron deficiency results in a hypochromic, microcytic anemia, which is often manifested clinically by fatigue and depression. Conversely, iron, like most trace elements, is toxic if ingested in excessive amounts.

Organ meats such as liver and kidney are the richest sources of iron; meat, egg yolk, fish, legumes, and whole grains also provide adequate amounts. All of the iron in plants and approximately 60% of the iron in animal foods is in the form of nonheme iron, which is not absorbed as efficiently as heme iron. Common sources of iron that are included in commercial dogs and cat foods include steamed bone meal, dicalcium phosphate, and ferrous sulfate heptahydrate. Anemia as a result of a dietary deficiency of iron is extremely rare in dogs and cats. A chronic blood loss that occurs during severe parasitic infections or hemorrhage is more likely to be the cause of iron deficiency in these species.

COPPER

The metabolism and functions of copper are closely tied to those of iron. Copper is necessary for normal absorption and transport of dietary iron. Along with iron, copper is essential for the normal formation of hemoglobin. Most of the copper found in blood is bound to the plasma protein ceruloplasmin. This protein is a copper-dependent ferroxidase that functions as a carrier of copper and also in the oxidation of plasma iron, which is necessary for binding to transferrin. Ceruloplasmin may also be involved in the mobilization of iron from storage sites in the liver. As a component of several different metalloenzymes, copper is required for the conversion of the amino acid tyrosine to the pigment melanin, for the synthesis of the connective tissues collagen and elastin, and for the production of ATP in the cytochrome oxidase system. Another copper metalloenzyme, superoxide dismutase, functions to protect cells from oxidative damage by superoxide radicals. Copper is also necessary for normal osteoblast activity during skeletal development.

The highest concentration of copper in the body is found in the liver. After absorption from the intestine, copper, complexed with the plasma protein albumin, is transported through the portal vein to the liver. Metallothioneins, small–molecular-weight cytoplasmic proteins, bind copper and are involved in regulating its transport into the liver. Copper is stored in the liver, where it is incorporated into ceruloplasmin and other proteins for use by the body. Excess copper is excreted in the bile.

Sources of copper include liver and the bran and germ portions of grains. In pet foods, supplemental copper is often included in the form of cupric chloride or cupric sulfate. Because of copper's importance in iron metabolism and hemoglobin formation, copper deficiency results in a hypochromic, microcytic anemia similar to that seen with iron deficiency. Other signs of deficiency include depigmentation of colored hair coat and impaired skeletal growth in young animals. Although copper deficiency is not common in dogs and cats, an inherited disorder of copper metabolism that results in copper toxicosis occurs in several different breeds of dogs (see Section 5, pp. 298-299).

ZINC

The trace mineral zinc is widely distributed in many tissues of the body, and its actions influence carbohydrate, lipid, protein, and nucleic acid metabolism. Zinc is a component of many of the metalloenzymes, which include carbonic anhydrase, lactic dehydrogenase, alkaline phosphatase, carboxypeptidase, and aminopeptidase. Zinc also functions as a cofactor in the synthesis of DNA, RNA, and protein and is essential for normal cellular immunity and reproductive functioning. Like iron, the absorption of zinc from the diet is affected by several factors. Metallothioneins have a high affinity for binding to zinc and are involved in the regulation of zinc absorption and metabolism.

The body's efficiency of zinc absorption increases with increasing need for this mineral. Animal sources of zinc, such as meat and eggs, are generally more readily absorbed than are plant sources. Dietary compounds that act to decrease zinc absorption include excess levels of calcium, iron, copper, and fiber, and the presence of phytate.[5]

Because of its role in protein synthesis, zinc deficiency is usually associated with growth retardation in young animals. Other clinical signs include anorexia, testicular atrophy, impaired reproductive performance, immune system dysfunction, conjunctivitis, and the development of skin lesions. In dogs and cats, skin and hair coat changes are usually the first clinical signs of zinc deficiency; these signs have been described as dull, coarse hair coat and skin lesions that show parakeratosis and hyperkeratinization.[6] Although not common, naturally occurring zinc-responsive dermatoses have been identified in companion animals.[7-9] In addition, a genetically influenced abnormality in zinc absorption and metabolism is reported in some dog breeds, resulting in an increased zinc requirement in affected animals (see Section 5, pp. 299-300).[10]

MANGANESE

Like most of the other microminerals, manganese functions as a component of several cell enzymes that catalyze metabolic reactions. A large proportion of manganese is located in the mitochondria of cells where it activates a number of metal-enzyme complexes that regulate nutrient metabolism. These complexes include pyruvate carboxylase and superoxide dismutase. Manganese is also necessary for normal bone development and reproduction. Foods that are good sources of manganese include legumes and whole-grain cereals. Animal-based ingredients are generally poor sources of manganese. Naturally occurring manganese deficiency has not been reported in either dogs or cats. However, manganese deficiency is characterized in other species by decreased growth, impaired reproduction, and disturbances in lipid metabolism.

IODINE

Iodine is required by the body for the synthesis of the hormones thyroxine and triiodothyronine by the thyroid gland. Thyroxine stimulates cellular oxidative processes and regulates basal metabolic rate. The principal sign of iodine deficiency is goiter, an enlargement of the thyroid gland. Cretinism, a syndrome characterized by failure to grow, skin lesions, central nervous system (CNS) dysfunction, and multiple skeletal deformities, can occur in young animals that are fed a severely deficient diet. However, naturally occurring iodine deficiency does not commonly occur in dogs or cats.

SELENIUM

As an essential component of the enzyme glutathione peroxidase, selenium protects cell membranes from oxidative damage. Glutathione peroxidase deactivates lipid peroxides that are formed during oxidation of cell-membrane lipids. In this role, selenium has a close relationship with vitamin E and the sulfur-containing amino acids methionine and cystine. Vitamin E protects the polyunsaturated fatty acids (PUFAs) in cell membranes from oxidative damage, and thus it prevents the release of lipid peroxides. By reducing the number of peroxides that are formed, vitamin E spares the cellular use of selenium. The sulfur-containing amino acids are important in selenium metabolism because they are necessary for the formation of glutathione peroxidase. Sources of selenium include cereal grains, meat, and fish. Because selenium is abundant in foods, naturally occurring deficiencies are not a problem in dogs and cats. However, like other trace elements, the ingestion of excess selenium is toxic.

COBALT

Cobalt is a constituent of vitamin B_{12}. Currently no function for cobalt in the body has been identified. Additional cobalt does not appear to be required by dogs and cats when their diet contains adequate amounts of vitamin B_{12}.

CHROMIUM

Chromium is a component of the organic complex known as *glucose tolerance factor*. This factor functions to enhance the action of the hormone insulin, which is necessary for the normal metabolism of glucose and other nutrients. In humans, chromium deficiency has been shown to be associated with abnormal glucose utilization and insulin resistance.[11] It has also been suggested that a low dietary intake of chromium or an impaired metabolism of chromium may be a factor associated with the development of diabetes (see Section 5, pp. 352-353). A few recent studies with dogs and cats have examined the effects of supplemental chromium (usually supplied as chromium tripicolinate) on glucose metabolism, insulin sensitivity, and immune responsiveness (see Section 5, pp. 352-353 for a complete discussion).[12-14]

OTHER MICROMINERALS

There are several trace elements that have been shown to be required by other species of mammals, but they have not yet been demonstrated to be essential for dogs and cats. These include molybdenum, tin, fluorine, nickel, silicon, vanadium, and arsenic. It is highly likely that dogs and cats also require these elements, even though minimum requirements have not yet been established. These minerals are widespread in food ingredients and are required by the body in very minute amounts. Conversely, all have been shown to be highly toxic when fed in large doses.

ELECTROLYTES

Potassium

Potassium is the main cation in the intracellular fluid. Approximately one third of a cell's potassium is bound to protein; the rest is found in the ionized form. Ionized potassium within cells provides the osmotic force that maintains proper fluid volume. Cellular potassium is also required for numerous enzymatic reactions. The small concentration of potassium present in the extracellular fluid aids in the transmission of nerve impulses and the contraction of muscle fibers. The maintenance of potassium balance is especially important for the normal functioning of heart muscle. Many foods contain potassium. Meats, poultry, and fish are all rich sources, and whole-grain cereals and most vegetables also contain high amounts. Because of the abundance of potassium in most foods, potassium deficiency of a dietary origin is highly unusual in dogs and cats.

Sodium

Ionized sodium is the major cation found in the extracellular fluid. Sodium in this compartment provides the primary osmotic force that maintains the aqueous environment of the extracellular fluid. It functions in conjunction with other ions to maintain the normal irritability of nerve cells and the contractibility of muscle fibers. Sodium is also necessary for the maintenance of the permeability of cell membranes. The sodium "pump" controls the electrolyte balance between the intracellular and extracellular fluid compartments. The chief source of sodium in the diet is table salt (sodium chloride), which is used for food preservation in most commercially prepared foods. In addition to processed products, foods that have naturally high sodium content include dairy products, meat, poultry, fish, and egg white. Because of this mineral's abundance in foods, sodium deficiency is not a problem in dogs and cats. Conversely, excess sodium intake has been implicated as a possible causal factor in hypertension in some human populations.[15] These observations, coupled with the high sodium content of some commercial pet foods, led investigators to examine the effects of high sodium intake in dogs. Results indicate that hypertension is not a common problem in this species. Moreover, dogs and cats appear to be physiologically capable of adapting to wide variations in sodium intake.[16-19]

Chloride

Chloride ions account for about two thirds of the total anions present in the extracellular fluid. They are necessary for the regulation of normal osmotic pressure, water balance, and acid-base balance in the body. Chloride is also necessary for the formation of hydrochloric acid (HCl) in the stomach. HCl is required for the activation of several gastric enzymes and for the initiation of digestion in the stomach. Because most of the chloride that animals consume is associated with sodium, the daily amount consumed generally parallels sodium intake. Like potassium and sodium, dietary chloride deficiency has not been found to be a common problem in dogs and cats.

References

1. Association of American Feed Control Officials (AAFCO): Official publication, 2008, AAFCO.

2. Fernandez R, Phillips S: Components of fiber impair iron absorption in the dog, *Am J Clin Nutr* 35:107–112, 1982.

3. Hill EC, Burrows C, Ellison G, Bauer J: The effect of texturized vegetable protein from soy on nutrient digestibility compared to beef in cannulated dogs, *J Anim Sci* 79:2162–2171, 2001.

4. Meyer H: Mineral metabolism and requirements in bitches and suckling pups. In Anderson R, editor: *Nutrition and behaviour in dogs and cats*, Oxford, UK, 1985, Pergamon Press, pp 13–24.

5. Hunt JR, Johnson PE, Swan PB: Dietary conditions influencing relative zinc availability from foods to the rat and correlations with in vitro measurements, *J Nutr* 117:1913–1923, 1987.

6. Sanecki RK, Corbin JE, Forbes RM: Tissue changes in dogs fed a zinc-deficient ration, *Am J Vet Res* 43:1642–1646, 1983.

7. Sousa CA, Stannard AA, Ihrke PH: Dermatosis associated with feeding generic dog food: 13 cases (1981-1982), *J Am Vet Med Assoc* 192:767–680, 1988.

8. Ohlen B, Scott D: Zinc-responsive dermatosis in puppies, *Canine Pract* 13:6–10, 1986.

9. Huber TD, Laflamme D, Medleau L, and others: Comparison of procedures for assessing adequacy of dog foods, *J Am Vet Med Assoc* 199:731–734, 1991.

10. Colombini S, Dunstan R: Zinc-responsive dermatosis in northern-breed dogs: 17 cases (1990-1996), *J Am Vet Med Assoc* 211:451–453, 1997.

11. Anderson RA: Chromium, glucose tolerance and diabetes, *Biol Trace Element Res* 32:19–24, 1992.

12. Appleton DJ, Rand JS, Sunvold GD, Priest J: Effect of chromium supplementation on glucose tolerance and insulin sensitivity in normal cats. In *Proceedings XXIV WSAVA Congress*, Lyon, France, 1999.

13. Spears J, Brown T Jr, Hayek M, Sunvold G: Effect of dietary chromium on the canine immune response. In Reinhart GA, Carey DP, editors: *Recent advances in canine and feline nutrition: Iams nutrition symposium proceedings,* vol 2, Wilmington, Ohio, 1998, Orange Frazer Press, pp 555–564.

14. Spears J, Brown T, Sunvold G, Hayek M: Influence of chromium on glucose metabolism and insulin sensitivity. In Reinhart GA, Carey DP, editors: *Recent advances in canine and feline nutrition: Iams nutrition symposium proceedings,* vol 2, Wilmington, Ohio, 1998, Orange Frazer Press, pp 103–112.

15. Houston MC: Sodium and hypertension, *Arch Intern Med* 146:179–185, 1986.

16. Wilhelmj CM, Waldmann EB, McGuire TF: Effect of prolonged high sodium chloride ingestion and withdrawal upon blood pressure of dogs, *Proc Soc Exp Bio Med* 77:379–382, 1951.

17. National Research Council: *Nutrient requirements of dogs and cats*, Washington, DC, 2006, National Academy Press.

18. Kirk CA, Jewell DE, Lowry SR: Effects of sodium chloride on selected parameters in cats, *Vet Ther* 7:333–346, 2006.

19. Luckschander N, Iven C, Hosgood G, and others: Dietary NaCl does not affect blood pressure in health cats, *J Vet Intern Med* 18:463–467, 2004.

7

Digestion and Absorption

The process of digestion breaks down the large, complex molecules of many nutrients into their simplest, most soluble forms so that absorption and use by the body can take place (Table 7-1). The two basic types of action involved in this process are mechanical digestion and chemical (or enzymatic) digestion. Mechanical digestion involves the physical mastication (chewing), mixing, and movement of food through the gastrointestinal tract. Chemical digestion involves splitting the chemical bonds of complex nutrients through enzymatically catalyzed hydrolysis. The three major types of foods that require digestion are fats, carbohydrates, and proteins. Before absorption takes place, most of the fat in food is hydrolyzed to glycerol, free fatty acids (FFAs), and some monoglycerides and diglycerides. Complex carbohydrates are broken down to the simple sugars—glucose, galactose, and fructose. Protein molecules are hydrolyzed to single amino acid units and some dipeptides. As dietary nutrients are digested, they are transported through the digestive tract by a series of contractions of the muscular walls of the gastrointestinal tract. The process of digestion and absorption begins when food first enters the mouth and ends with the excretion of waste products and undigested food particles in the feces (Figures 7-1 and 7-2).

Digestion and absorption begin in the mouth, with the mastication (chewing) of food and its mixture with saliva. Digestion continues throughout the gastrointestinal system and ends with the excretion of waste products and undigested food particles in the feces.

MOUTH

In all species, the mouth functions to bring food into the body, initiate physical mastication, and mix the food with saliva. Saliva is secreted in response to the sight and smell of food. It acts as a lubricant to facilitate both chewing and swallowing and also serves to solubilize the dietary components that stimulate the taste buds and impart flavor to food. In addition to its function in digestion, saliva is also important to the dog (and less so in cats) for evaporative cooling. Compared to many ruminant and herbivorous species that thoroughly masticate their food, dogs and cats often swallow large boluses of food with little or no chewing. However, there are also important differences between dogs and cats. Although domesticated dogs and cats have the same number of incisor and canine teeth (six incisors and two canines on both the top and bottom jaws), the dog's mouth contains more premolars and molars than does the cat's mouth. These teeth are associated with an increased capacity to chew and crush food, which is indicative of

TABLE 7-1 DIGESTIVE END PRODUCTS OF CARBOHYDRATE, PROTEIN, AND FAT

NUTRIENT	ENZYMES	END PRODUCTS
Carbohydrate	Amylase	Glucose
	Lactase	Galactose
	Sucrase	Fructose
	Maltase	
Protein	Dipeptidase	Dipeptides
	Amino peptidase	Single amino
	Pepsinogen	acids
	Pepsin	
	Nucleotidase	
	Nucleosidase	
	Trypsin	
	Chymotrypsin	
	Carboxypeptidase	
	Nuclease	
Fat	Intestinal lipase	Glycerol
	Pancreatic lipase	Free fatty acids
		Monoglycerides, diglycerides

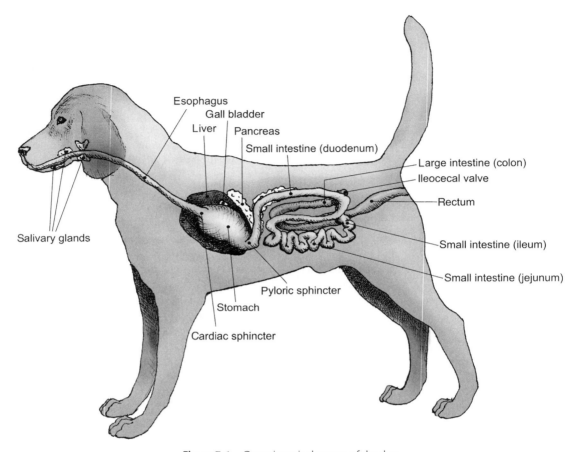

Figure 7-1 Gastrointestinal system of the dog.

a diet containing a larger proportion of plant material. Thus the dentition of dogs is suggestive of a more omnivorous diet than is the dentition of cats, which is more typical of the pattern seen in most obligate carnivores.[1] Although both dogs and cats are considered to be "meat-eaters," the dog has evolved to consume a diet that is more omnivorous in nature than that of the cat.

Another important role of the mouth is its importance in taste perception (gustation). *Taste* refers to the sensation that arises from stimulation of the taste buds, spherical or ovoid clusters of papillae that are located on the surface of the tongue. Taste receptor cells are located at the tip of each taste bud and are classified into five general receptor types: sweet (sugars), sour (acids), salty, bitter (alkaloids, peptides), and umami (monosodium glutamate, disodium guanylate, "meaty" flavors). Dogs and cats possess taste systems that are consistent with the general pattern seen in other carnivorous species. Early studies classified the cat's taste system into four general types of units (I, II, IIA, and IIB).[2] A similar and closely corresponding set of units has been identified in the domestic dog.[3] In general, both dogs and cats are highly sensitive to the tastes of amino acids and to various types of organic acids and nucleotides. All of these are substances found in abundance in animal tissues.[4] Another similarity between dogs and cats is that neither species exhibits a strong preference for salt solutions.[5] Although there is evidence that salty flavors may enhance the attractiveness of some foods for dogs and that cats show a slight preference for salt at relatively high concentrations, these species do not demonstrate

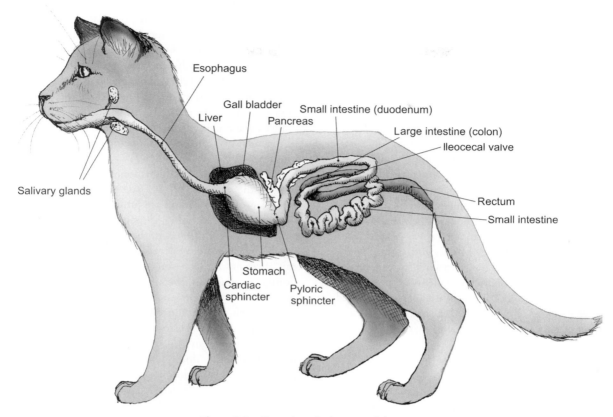

Figure 7-2   Gastrointestinal system of the cat.

the "salt appetite" that is reported in other omnivores and herbivorous species.

Dogs and cats also have several interesting differences in taste receptors. One of the most dramatic is in their sensitivity to the taste of sweet. Dogs, but not cats, are sensitive to and show preferences for sweet foods.[6,7] (This is one of the reasons that theobromine toxicity, as a result of chocolate ingestion, is a significant risk to pet dogs but not to pet cats.) Recent studies have shown that one of two receptor genes known to encode for the sweet-taste receptors in taste buds is not expressed in cats.[8] This defect may be responsible for the lack of response to sweet flavors observed in the domestic cat and in several other felid species. In lieu of these receptors, cats possess a receptor that is highly sensitive to quinine, tannic acid, and alkaloids—flavors that are thought to be perceived as bitter.[9] In contrast,

dogs are typically repelled by most bitter flavors. There is speculation that these differences between dog and cat taste systems reflect the cat's evolutionary adherence to a more strictly carnivorous feeding pattern, leading to taste preferences for foods derived from only animal tissue, and a loss of the ability to perceive flavors that are more typically found in fruits and vegetables. In contrast, the dog evolved from a canid species that, although also a predator, was more omnivorous in nature. Further, the process of domestication selected for a more varied omnivorous diet in dogs, as scavenging gradually replaced cooperative hunting as a primary feeding behavior.[10] The impact that taste and other special sense perceptions such as odors and food textures have upon food selection and preferences in dogs and cats are discussed in detail in Chapter 19 (see pp. 191-193).

Dogs show a preference for sweet foods, while cats do not. Conversely, cats (but not dogs) are attracted to flavors that are typically perceived as bitter. These differences may reflect the cat's evolutionary adherence to a more strictly carnivorous feeding pattern and the dog's historically more omnivorous diet.

ESOPHAGUS

Food passes from the mouth to the stomach through the esophagus. The cells of the mucosal lining of the esophagus secrete mucus in response to the presence of food, which further aids in lubricating food as it passes to the stomach. As the food reaches the end of the esophagus, the cardiac sphincter, a ring of muscle at the junction between the esophagus and stomach, relaxes to allow food to enter the stomach. This ring relaxes in response to the peristaltic movements of the esophagus. It then immediately constricts after food has passed to prevent reflux of the stomach contents back into the lower esophagus.

STOMACH

The stomach acts as a reservoir for the body, allowing food to be ingested as a meal rather than continuously throughout the day. The proximal section of the stomach is capable of expansion to allow storage of large meals, a function that is assumed to be of greater importance for dogs, who tend to eat large meals at a given time, than for cats, who prefer to eat multiple small meals per day (see Chapter 19, pp. 192-193). In addition to its storage function, the stomach also initiates the chemical digestion of protein (and possibly of fat, in the dog), mixes food with gastric secretions, and regulates the entry of food into the small intestine. The gastric glands, which are located in the mucosal lining of the corpus portion of the stomach, secrete mucus, hydrochloric acid (HCl), and the proteolytic enzyme pepsinogen. In dogs, gastric lipase is secreted throughout the stomach, but appears to be much less important for fat digestion than pancreatic lipase.[11] For this reason, it is believed that the majority of fat digestion still takes place in the small intestine. Mucous secretions protect the gastric mucosa and also lubricate the ingested food. HCl is necessary to maintain a proper pH for the occurrence of enzymatic

action. It functions to slightly alter the composition of ingested fat and protein in preparation for further action by digestive enzymes in the small intestine. Along with previously formed pepsin, HCl also converts pepsinogen to the enzyme pepsin. This enzyme initiates hydrolysis of protein molecules to smaller polypeptide units in the stomach. The activity of pepsin is highest in the acidic environment of the stomach and is reduced and eventually inactivated when food leaves the stomach and is exposed to the neutral pH of the small intestine.[12]

Both neurological and hormonal stimuli are important for the secretion of HCl and mucus by the stomach. Neurological stimuli are produced in response to the anticipation of eating, the sight and smell of food, and the presence of food in the stomach. In addition, psychological stimuli such as fear, stress, and anxiety can affect gastric secretions and gastrointestinal functioning in animals. The hormone gastrin is released in response to the presence of food and distention of the stomach. It is produced by mucosal glands in the antrum portion of the stomach. Gastrin stimulates the secretion of HCl and mucus and also increases gastric motility. Another local hormone, enterogastrone, is produced by glands located in the duodenal mucosa. Enterogastrone is secreted in response to the presence of fat entering the duodenum and counteracts the activity of gastrin by inhibiting acid production and gastric motility.

Peristaltic movements of the stomach slowly mix the ingested food with gastric secretions, preparing it for entry into the small intestine. The mucosal cells located in the antral portion of the stomach secrete mucus that has a more alkaline pH and is low in digestive enzymes. Thorough mixing in this portion results in the production of a semifluid mass of food called *chyme*. Chyme must pass through the pyloric sphincter to enter the small intestine for further digestion. Like the cardiac sphincter, the pyloric sphincter is a ring of muscle that is usually in a constricted state. This ring relaxes in response to the strong peristaltic contractions that originate in the stomach and travel toward the intestine. While open, the sphincter allows small amounts of chyme to enter the duodenum. The pyloric sphincter controls the rate of passage of food from the stomach into the small intestine. The rate of gastric emptying is affected by a number of factors, including the osmotic pressure, particle size, and viscosity of the chyme, as well as the degree of gastric acidity and volume. In general, large meals have a slower rate of emptying than small meals, liquids leave the stomach faster than solids, and very high-fat meals may cause a decrease in stomach-emptying rate. Diets that contain soluble fiber as a fiber source cause a decreased rate of stomach emptying when compared with diets that contain insoluble dietary fiber (see Chapter 2, p. 14, Table 2-1). In addition, there is evidence in cats that dry cat foods leave the stomach at a slower rate than canned foods, except when very small meals are consumed.[13] The shape of the kibble in dry cat food can also influence the rate of gastric emptying, with triangular-shaped pieces leaving the stomach at a slower rate than round pieces.[14]

SMALL INTESTINE

Before reaching the small intestine, most of the digestive processes that occur in dogs and cats are mechanical in nature. The chyme that is delivered through the pyloric sphincter to the duodenum is a semifluid mass made up of food particles mixed with gastric secretions. Carbohydrates and fats are almost unchanged in composition, but the protein in the food has been partially hydrolyzed to smaller polypeptides. Even this digestion is not crucial, however, because the enzymes of the small intestine are capable of completely digesting intact dietary protein. Therefore the major task of chemical digestion and the subsequent absorption of nutrients occur in the small intestine.

Further mechanical digestion also occurs in the small intestine through the coordinated contractions of its muscle layers. These movements thoroughly mix the food mass with intestinal secretions, increase the exposure of digested food particles to the mucosal surface, and slowly propel the food mass through the intestinal tract. Constant sweeping motions of the intestinal villi that line the surface of the mucosa mix the chyme that is in contact with the intestinal wall and increase the efficiency of absorption of digested particles. After food has entered the small intestine, large quantities of mucus are secreted by the Brunner's glands, which are located immediately inside the duodenum. This mucus protects the intestinal mucosa from irritation and erosion by the gastric acids that are entering from the stomach and further lubricates the food mass.

Nutrient Digestion

The pancreas and the glands located in the duodenal mucosa secrete enzymes into the intestinal lumen that chemically digest fat, carbohydrate, and protein. Enzymes secreted by the intestinal cells include intestinal lipase, amino peptidase, dipeptidase, nucleotidase, nucleosidase, and enterokinase. Intestinal lipase converts fat to monoglycerides, diglycerides, glycerol, and FFAs. Amino peptidase breaks the peptide bond located at the N-terminal of the protein molecule, slowly releasing single amino acids from the protein chain. Dipeptidase breaks the peptide bond of dipeptides to release two single amino acid units. Both nucleosidase and nucleotidase hydrolyze nucleoproteins to their constituent bases and pentose sugars. Lastly, enterokinase converts inactive trypsinogen, a proenzyme secreted by the pancreas, to its active form (trypsin).

The final digestion of carbohydrate takes place at the brush border of the small intestine. The cells of the brush border secrete the enzymes maltase, lactase, and sucrase, which respectively convert the disaccharides maltose, lactose, and sucrose to their constituent monosaccharides; glucose, fructose, and galactose. Protease enzymes secreted by the pancreas include trypsin, chymotrypsin, carboxypeptidase, and nuclease. Several of these are secreted in an inactive form and are activated by other components in the small intestine after release. In addition, pancreatic lipase and amylase are released into the intestinal lumen and respectively function to hydrolyze dietary fat and starch into smaller units. Cholesterol esterase secreted by the pancreas catalyzes the formation of cholesterol esters. Free cholesterol must be esterified to fatty acids to facilitate its absorption into the body. The pancreas also secretes a large volume of bicarbonate salts into the small intestine. These salts function to neutralize the acidic chyme and provide the proper pH for the digestive enzymes to function.

Bile is another important component of nutrient digestion in the small intestine. It is produced by the liver and stored in the gallbladder. Bile's primary function in the small intestine is the emulsification of dietary fat and the activation of certain lipases. These two processes result in the formation of very small, water-soluble globules called *micelles*. The formation of micelles results in an increased surface area for the action of lipase and also arranges lipid molecules into water-miscible forms that are able to gain access to the aqueous layer covering the microvilli, ultimately facilitating absorption of fat into the body.

Hormonal control of digestion in the small intestine involves several components. Secretin is produced by the mucosa of the upper portion of the duodenum in response to the entry of acidic chyme into the duodenum. It stimulates the release of bicarbonate from the pancreas and controls the rate of bile flow from the gallbladder. Cholecystokinin is also released from this portion of the intestinal mucosa in response to the presence of fat in the food mass. This hormone stimulates contraction of the gallbladder, resulting in a release of bile into the intestinal lumen. Cholecystokinin also stimulates secretion of the pancreatic enzymes.

Most of the important tasks of chemical digestion and the subsequent absorption of nutrients occur in the small intestine.

Small Intestinal Microflora

Although of greater significance in the large intestine, the small intestines of healthy dogs and cats also contain resident microbial populations. In dogs, bacterial numbers in the duodenum and ileum are relatively low, rarely exceeding 10^4 colony forming units (CFUs) per milliliter (ml).[15] These numbers increase to approximately 10^6 CFU per ml in the distal portion of the ileum as it approaches the ileal-cecal junction. Species that are typically found in the dog's small intestine include primarily streptococci, lactobacilli, and *Bifidobacterium* spp. in the duodenum and jejunum and several species of anaerobic bacteria and *Escherichia coli* in the ileum. Compared with dogs, healthy cats have significantly higher concentrations of microbes present in their small intestine, having duodenal counts as high as 10^8 CFUs.[16] Also, species differences are found when comparing typical bacteria present in the small intestines of cats and dogs. The primary microbes found in the duodenum of cats include the aerobe *Pasteurella* and the anaerobes *Bacteroides, Eubacteria,* and *Fusobacteria.*

Microflora present in the small intestine function to prevent colonization of pathogenic microbes by competing for available nutrients, maintaining an appropriate lumen environment, and producing inhibitory compounds. In both dogs and cats, small intestinal bacteria have also been found to produce short-chain fatty acids (SCFAs), which may further influence the lumen environment and intestinal health.[17,18] In addition, certain nutrients and dietary components may influence small intestinal microbial populations. For example, fructooligosaccharides (FOS), a type of naturally occurring fiber that is fermented by certain intestinal bacteria, have been found to enhance the growth of beneficial bacteria and reduce the numbers of potentially pathogenic bacteria in the small intestine of dogs and cats.[19,20] A similar fiber, mannanoligosaccharides (MOS) can also beneficially alter small intestinal bacterial populations, albeit via a different mechanism[21] (see Chapter 35, pp. 467-470 for a complete discussion).

Nutrient Absorption

In dogs and cats, the chemical digestion of food is completed in the small intestine. Digestible protein, carbohydrate, and fat are hydrolyzed to amino acids, dipeptides, monosaccharides, glycerol, FFAs, and monoglycerides and diglycerides. As these small units are produced, they are absorbed by the body along with dietary vitamins and minerals. Absorption involves the transfer of digested nutrients from the intestinal lumen into the blood or lymphatic system for delivery to tissues throughout the body. Like digestion, the greatest part of absorption takes place in the small intestine.

The structure of the inner wall of the small intestine is designed to provide a high amount of surface area for the absorption of nutrients. The mucosal folds, villi, and microvilli of the mucosa produce an absorptive inner surface area that is approximately 600 times that of the outer serosal layer of the intestine. Villi are finger-like projections that cover the convoluted folds of the mucosa. Each individual villus contains a vascular network of venous and arterial capillaries and a lymph vessel called a *lacteal*. These function to transport absorbed nutrients to either the portal or lymphatic circulations. The surface of each villus is covered with numerous, minute projections called *microvilli*. These are often collectively referred to as the *brush border* of the small intestine. The cells lining the luminal surface of the villi are highly specialized absorptive cells called *enterocytes*. These cells have a lifespan of only 2 to 3 days, during which they absorb nutrients from the lumen of the small intestine. Old cells are continually sloughed off and excreted in the feces, giving these cells one of the highest turnover rates of any tissue in the body.

Nutrient absorption is accomplished in the small intestine through several processes. Some small molecules are absorbed by passive diffusion according to the osmotic gradient; for example, electrolytes and water molecules both flow across the mucosa in response to osmotic pressure. Facilitated diffusion involves the transport of large molecules across the cellular membrane in concurrence with the pressure gradient. Carrier proteins located in the membranes of the enterocytes facilitate transport of these nutrients into the cells. In contrast, active transport involves the transport of nutrient molecules across the intestinal epithelial membrane against a concentration gradient. This transport mechanism differs from passive diffusion in that more energy is required to transport materials against a concentration gradient. For example, the most common type of active transport mechanism involves a membrane protein carrier coupled with the active transport of sodium (the sodium pump).

Although some passive diffusion is believed to occur, most simple carbohydrates are absorbed by the body through an active process that is linked to sodium transport and uses a specific carrier protein. Single amino acids and some dipeptides and tripeptides are also absorbed in this manner. Small peptides that are absorbed into the cell are immediately hydrolyzed to single amino acid units before being released into the portal circulation. Sugars and amino acids are absorbed into the villus capillaries and from there enter the portal vein, which transports these nutrients to the liver. Absorption of fat involves the interaction of the fat-containing micelles with the aqueous layer surrounding the brush border. Micelles contain bile acids, monoglycerides, diglycerides, and long-chain fatty acids. Because they are water-miscible, the micelles are able to travel to the brush border, where they are disrupted and their component fat particles are absorbed into the cell. The bile remains in the lumen and eventually moves down the intestine to be reabsorbed and circulated back to the liver. Within the enterocyte, most of the fatty acids and glycerol are resynthesized into triglycerides, combined with cholesterol, phospholipid, and protein, and released into the central lacteal as either chylomicrons or very–low-density lipoprotein (VLDL) transport

particles. The central lacteal drains into the major lymph vessels, and the particles eventually enter the blood circulation near the heart.

The liver functions to further process the absorbed monosaccharides and amino acids that arrive through the portal circulation. Some monosaccharides are converted to the storage carbohydrate form glycogen, and a certain quantity of glucose is secreted directly into the circulation. Some amino acids are released into the bloodstream, where they circulate to tissues for absorption into cells. Excess amino acids are either converted to other nonessential amino acids or metabolized by the liver for energy.

Most minerals are absorbed by the body in an ionized form. The water-soluble vitamins are transported by passive diffusion, but some may be absorbed by an active process when the diet contains low levels. Vitamin B_{12} is unique in its requirement for an intrinsic factor for proper absorption (see Chapter 5, p. 34). Fat-soluble vitamins are made soluble by combination with bile salts and are then absorbed by passive diffusion through the lipid phase of the mucosal cell membrane. In general, when there is normal fat absorption, there is normal fat-soluble vitamin absorption.

LARGE INTESTINE (COLON)

The contents of the small intestine enter the large intestine through the ileocecal valve. The cecum is an intestinal pocket located next to the junction of the colon and the small intestine. This portion of the intestine varies in size and functional capacity among species of mammals. The cecum of nonruminant herbivores such as the horse and rabbit is relatively large and has a highly enhanced digestive capacity. Likewise, both the cecum and large intestine of the omnivorous pig are enlarged when compared with those of the carnivorous species. Microbial digestion of dietary fiber in the cecum and colon of nonruminant herbivores contributes significantly to the nutrient intake and balance of these animals. In comparison, carnivorous species such as the cat and mink have a vestigial cecum, and the length of their large intestine is relatively short. Relative to body size, the dog's cecum is not as large as the pig's, but it is somewhat larger than the cat's. This observation is consistent with the fact that the dog has adapted to consuming a diet that is more omnivorous in nature than that of the cat. The extent to which bacterial digestion of dietary fiber in the cecum and colon contributes to energy balance in these species is small compared to the contribution for nonruminant herbivore species. However, SCFAs produced by bacterial fermentation of fiber are an important energy source for colonocytes and contribute to intestinal health.[22,23] In addition, adherent bacteria in the large intestine influence function of the intestinal mucosa and help to regulate the enteric immune system[22] (see Section 5, pp. 465-467 for a complete discussion of the role of colonic bacteria in intestinal health).

A chief function of the large intestine in dogs and cats is the absorption of water and certain electrolytes. Unlike the small intestine, the large intestine has no villi and therefore has a lower capacity for absorption. Although it is able to efficiently absorb water and electrolytes, it has no mechanisms for active transport. Along with a large volume of water, sodium is absorbed into the body from the large intestine. As mentioned previously, the bacterial colonies of the colon are capable of digesting some of the indigestible fiber and other nutrients in the diet that have escaped digestion in the small intestine. The products of this bacterial digestion contribute to the characteristic smell and color of canine and feline feces. Undigested food residues, sloughed cells, bacteria, and unabsorbed endogenous secretions make up the fecal matter that eventually reaches the rectum and is excreted from the body.

Fecal characteristics in dogs and cats can be significantly affected by the quantity and type of indigestible matter that is present in the animal's diet. Bacterial digestion of these materials produces various gases, SCFAs, and other byproducts. When protein reaches the large intestine in an undigested state, bacterial degradation results in the production of the amines indole and skatole. In addition, hydrogen sulfide gas is produced from the sulfur-containing amino acids of undigested or poorly digested protein. Hydrogen sulfide gas, indole, and skatole impart strong odors to fecal matter and intestinal gas. Certain types of carbohydrates found in legumes such as soybeans are resistant to digestion by the endogenous enzymes of the small intestine. These carbohydrates reach the colon and are metabolized by bacteria, with a resultant production of intestinal gas (flatulence). Hydrogen, carbon dioxide, and methane gases are produced from the bacterial digestion of carbohydrates. A similar effect occurs with certain types of fiber. While nonfermentable fibers resist digestion in the small intestine and fermentation in the large intestine, fermentable fibers are used as an energy source by intestinal bacteria, resulting in the production of gases and SCFAs. The degree to which flatulence and strong fecal odors occur in dogs and cats that are fed poorly digestible materials varies with the amounts and types of materials fed and the intestinal flora present in the colons of individual animals.

In contrast to the small intestine, a primary function of the large intestine (colon) in dogs and cats is the absorption of water and certain electrolytes, especially sodium.

References

1. Morris JG, Rogers QR: Comparative dog and cat nutrition. In Burger IH, Rivers JPW, editors: *Nutrition of the dog and cat*, Cambridge, England, 1989, Cambridge University Press.

2. Boudreau JC, Alev N: Classification chemoresponsive tongue units of the cat geniculate ganglion, *Brain Res* 54:157–175, 1973.

3. Boudreau J, White T: Flavor chemistry of carnivore taste systems. In Bullard RW, editor: *Flavor chemistry of animal foods, American Chemical Society symposium series 67*, Washington DC, 1978, ACS, pp 102–108.

4. Kumazawa T, Nakamura M, Kurihara K: Canine taste nerve response to umami substances, *Physiol Behav* 49:875–881, 1991.

5. Yu S, Rogers QR, Morris JG: Absence of salt (NaCl) preference of appetite in sodium-replete or depleted kittens, *Appetite* 29:1–10, 1997.

6. Ferrell F: Preference for sugars and nonnutritive sweeteners in young Beagles, *Neurosci Biobehav Rev* 8:199–203, 1984.

7. Houpt KA, Coren B, Hintz HF, Hilderbrant JE: Effect of sex and reproductive status on sucrose preference, food intake, and body weight of dogs, *J Am Vet Med Assoc* 174:1083–1085, 1979.

8. Li X, Li W, Wang H, and others: Cats lack a sweet taste receptor, *J Nutr* 136:1932S–1934S, 2006.

9. Bradshaw JWS: The evolutionary basis for the feeding behavior of domestic dogs (*Canis familiaris*) and cats (*Felis catus*), *J Nutr* 136:1927S–1931S, 2006.

10. Macdonald DW, Carr GM: Variation in dog society: between resource dispersion and social flux. In Serpell J, editor: *The domestic dog: its evolution, behaviour and interactions with people*, Cambridge, England, 1995, Cambridge University Press, pp 199–216.

11. Carriere F, Laugier R, Barrowman JA, and others: Gastric and pancreatic lipase levels during a test meal in dogs, *Scand J Gastroenterol* 28:443–454, 1993.

12. Smeets-Peeters M, Watson T, Minekus M, Havenaar R: A review of the physiology of the canine digestive tract related to the development of in vitro systems, *Nutr Res Rev* 11:45–69, 1998.

13. Goggin JM, Hoskinson JJ, Butine MD, and others: Scintigraphic assessment of gastric emptying of canned and dry diets in healthy cats, *Am J Vet Res* 59:388–392, 1998.

14. Armbrust LJ, Hoskinson JJ, Lora-Michiels NM, Milliken GA: Gastric emptying in cats using foods varying in fiber content and kibble shapes, *Vet Radiol Ultrasound* 44:339–343, 2003.

15. Kearns RJ, Hayek MG, Sunvold GD: Microbial changes in aged dogs. In Reinhart GA, Carey DP, editors: *Recent advances in canine and feline nutritional research: Iams nutrition symposium proceedings*, vol 2, Wilmington, Ohio, 1998, Orange Frazer Press, pp 337–351.

16. Johnston K, Lamport A, Batt RM: An unexpected bacterial flora in the proximal small intestine of normal cats, *Vet Rec* 132:362–363, 1993.

17. Brosley BP, Hill RC, Scott KC: Gastrointestinal volatile fatty acid concentrations and pH in cats, *Am J Vet Res* 61:359–361, 2000.

18. Strickling JA, Harmon DL, Dawson KA, Gross KL: Evaluation of oligosaccharide addition to dog diets: influences on nutrient digestion and microbial populations, *Anim Feed Sci Technol* 86:205–219, 2000.

19. Sparkes AH, Papasouliotis K, Sunvold G, and others: Bacterial flora in the duodenum of healthy cats and effect of dietary supplementation with fructo-oligosaccharides, *Am J Vet Res* 59:431–435, 1998.

20. Willard MD: Effects of dietary supplementation of fructo-oligosaccharides on small intestinal bacterial overgrowth in dogs, *Am J Vet Res* 55:654–659, 1992.

21. Ofek I, Beachey EH: Mannose binding and epithelial cell adherence of *Escherichia coli*, *Infect Immunol* 22:247–254, 1978.

22. Buddington RK, Buddington KK, Sunvold GD: The use of fermentable fibers to manage the gastrointestinal tract. In Reinhart GA, Carey DP, editors: *Recent advances in canine and feline nutritional research: Iams nutrition symposium proceedings*, vol 3, Wilmington, Ohio, 2000, Orange Frazer Press, pp 169–179.

23. Drackley JK, Beaulieu AD, Sunvold GD: Energetic substrates for intestinal cells. In Reinhart GA, Carey DP, editors: *Recent advances in canine and feline nutritional research, Iams nutrition symposium proceedings*, vol 2 Wilmington, Ohio, 1998, Orange Frazer Press, pp 463–472.

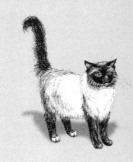

Nutrient Requirements of Dogs and Cats

Dogs and cats must be fed a proper diet that supplies all of the essential nutrients in their correct quantities and proportions to maintain health throughout all stages of life. The primary goals of feeding companion animals include maintaining optimal health, promoting a normal (but not excessive) growth rate, supporting gestation and lactation, and, in some cases, contributing to high-quality performance. Proper feeding throughout the pet's life also contributes to long-term health, vitality, and longevity.

As a result of the advances that have been made in companion animal nutrition during the past 40 years, frank nutrient deficiencies are rare in dogs and cats today. Rather, changes in nutrient status occur more often as a result of overfeeding, excessive supplementation, or exposure to inhibitory substances. It is important to recognize that individual nutrients do not function in isolation; interactions among essential nutrients are necessary for normal cellular metabolism. These relationships affect nutrient absorption, use, and excretion. Pet food companies use information about nutrient requirements and interactions to formulate balanced and complete pet foods for various stages of companion animals' lives. Because of the intricate interactions between dietary components, the balance of nutrients within the diet and the absolute quantity of each individual nutrient must always be considered.

All dogs and cats require an adequate intake of nutrients each day to maintain optimal health. Requirements for energy and certain nutrients can vary significantly during the lifetime of an individual pet. Increased demands occur during growth, reproduction, and physical work. A decreased requirement for energy and some nutrients occurs as animals attain adulthood, after neutering, and as they age. In addition to changing needs within the life cycle, the nutrient requirements of individual animals also vary considerably. For example, the energy needs for an adult Pug that spends a lot of time dozing on the couch will be significantly lower than the energy requirement of an adult Cairn Terrier that weighs the same amount but has an inherently higher activity level.

Standards of nutrient requirements for dogs and cats are necessary to provide general guidelines for commercial pet food companies to use when

Nutrient Requirements of Dogs and Cats (continued)

formulating diets. Ideally these standards should include current information concerning minimum and maximum levels of nutrients, nutrient requirements for different stages of life and activity levels, and estimates of the bioavailability of nutrients in commonly used pet food ingredients. Currently there are two sets of published standards that provide nutrient requirement information for dogs and cats. The first is produced by the National Research Council (NRC) and is titled *Nutrient Requirements of Dogs and Cats*. The recommendations of the current (2006) NRC were compiled by an ad hoc committee of companion animal nutritionists, convened in the year 2000. Previously, two separate publications, the *Nutrient Requirements of Dogs* and the *Nutrient Requirements of Cats*, were issued in 1985 and 1986, respectively. These publications were revised and combined into a single volume in 2006. The current NRC publication provides an overview of the digestive physiology and feeding behavior of dogs and cats, and concentrates on providing nutrient requirement estimates for dogs and cats. Unlike earlier editions, the 2006 NRC edition includes information on the influence of age, physiological state, and living environment on nutrient needs as well as sections addressing diet formulation and nutrient availability in processed foods.

The second group is the Association of American Feed Control Officials (AAFCO). The AAFCO has developed a set of practical standards, called Nutrient Profiles, for dog and cat foods. These profiles were first published in the early 1990s and provide recommendations for minimum and maximum levels of nutrients that are included in commercial pet foods. The levels of nutrients listed in these reports are intended for processed foods at the time of feeding. Minimum nutrient levels are reported for two different categories: growth and reproduction, and adult maintenance. Maximum nutrient levels are reported for nutrients with a potential for overuse or toxicosis. Both the canine and feline profiles are updated periodically as new information becomes available. All pet food companies are required to use these profiles when formulating dog and cat foods to meet established nutrient levels and to adhere to AAFCO guidelines.

8

Nutritional Idiosyncrasies of the Cat

Although the dog and cat have about equal status as companion animals in our society, it is important to recognize that they belong to two separate species. This truth is evidenced by well-defined physiological, behavioral, and dietary differences. In the following chapters, differences between the cat's and the dog's requirements for a number of nutrients are discussed in detail. These differences include the cat's unique energy and glucose metabolism, higher protein requirement, a requirement for dietary taurine, sensitivity to a deficiency of the amino acid arginine, inability to convert beta-carotene to active vitamin A, and inability to convert the amino acid tryptophan to niacin.

An examination of the phylogeny and evolutionary relationship of the domestic dog and cat offers some clues to their inherent dietary dissimilarities. Although both species are of the class Mammalia and the order Carnivora, the dog belongs to the modern-day Canoidea superfamily, and the cat belongs to the Feloidea superfamily.[1] Included with the dog in the Canoidea superfamily are several families with very diverse dietary habits. For example, the Ursid (bear) and the Procyonid (raccoon) families are both omnivorous, but species of the Ailurid (panda) family are strictly herbivorous. The only carnivorous species included with dogs are the Mustelids (weasels). The Feloidea superfamily, on the other hand, includes three families: the Viverrids (genet), the Hyaenids (hyena), and the Felids (cat) (Figure 8-1). All of the species in these families, including the cat, have evolved as strict carnivores. Therefore, the evolutionary history of the dog suggests a predilection for a diet that is more omnivorous in nature while the history of the cat indicates that this species has consumed a purely carnivorous diet throughout its evolutionary development.

Although equally popular as pets, dogs and cats have diverse nutritional needs. Dogs are omnivores, while cats have remained carnivores throughout their evolution. Cats cannot obtain all necessary nutrients from plants and plant products and must consume some animal tissues to meet their needs for high protein levels, taurine, arachidonic acid, and preformed vitamin A.

The adherence of the cat to a highly specialized diet has resulted in specific metabolic adaptations that manifest themselves as peculiarities in nutritional requirements. The consequence of these changes is an animal that cannot obtain all necessary nutrients solely from plants and plant products and therefore requires the consumption of animal tissues to meet certain nutrient requirements. These specific nutritional idiosyncrasies are exhibited in the domestic cat (*Felis catus*) but not in its frequent housemate, the domestic dog (*Canis familiaris*). This fact is of practical significance in light of the prevailing belief among some pet owners that cats may be fed as if they were small dogs.

The nutritional idiosyncrasies of the cat result in more stringent dietary requirements than those of a more omnivorous species, such as the dog. While all of these nutritional peculiarities are of metabolic significance, some are of greater practical importance than others when considering the optimal nutrition and proper feeding practices for pet cats (Box 8-1). The domestic cat's high protein requirement, along with its need for taurine, arachidonic acid, and preformed vitamin A, imposes a requirement for the inclusion of animal tissues in the diet of this species. Although it is possible to develop a cereal-based ration for cats (i.e., vegetarian or vegan diets), such a formulation requires close attention to nutrient levels and the appropriate supplementation with purified forms of taurine, arachidonic acid, and preformed vitamin A.[2,3]

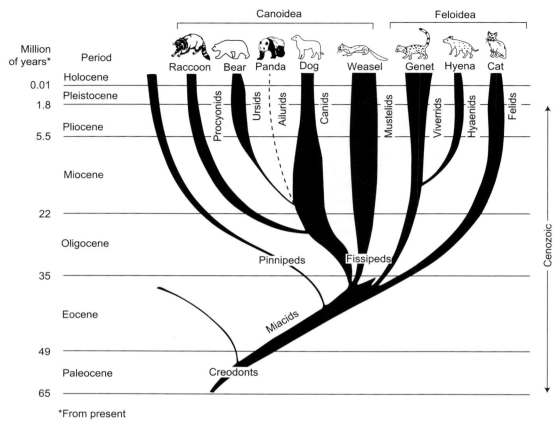

Figure 8-1   Phylogenic tree of the dog and cat.
(From Morris J, Rogers Q. In Burger IH, Rivers JPW, editors: *Nutrition of the dog and cat,* Cambridge, England, 1989, Cambridge University Press.)

BOX 8-1   NUTRITIONAL IDIOSYNCRASIES OF THE CAT

IDIOSYNCRASIES OF PRACTICAL IMPORTANCE	IDIOSYNCRASIES OF ACADEMIC INTEREST
High protein requirement	Unique energy and glucose metabolism
Taurine requirement	Sensitivity to arginine deficiency
Arachidonic acid requirement	Inability to convert tryptophan to niacin
Preformed vitamin A requirement	

References

1. Colbert EH: *Evolution of the vertebrates,* ed 3, New York, 1980, John Wiley & Sons.

2. Gray CM, Sellon RK, Freeman LM: Nutritional adequacy of two vegan diets for cats, *J Am Vet Med Assoc* 225:1670–1675, 2004.

3. Morris JG: Idiosyncratic nutrient requirements of cats appear to be diet-induced evolutionary adaptations, *Nutr Res Rev* 15:153–168, 2002.

9

Energy Balance

All animals must meet their bodies' energy needs. Energy balance is achieved when energy expenditure is equal to energy intake, resulting in minimal changes in the body's store of energy. Positive energy balance occurs when caloric intake exceeds energy expenditure. In growing and pregnant animals, a positive energy balance is needed for the synthesis of new tissue and fetal development, respectively. In adult, nonreproducing animals, positive energy balance results primarily in an increase in the quantity of fat stored by the body. Negative energy balance occurs when caloric intake is lower than energy expenditure. Weight loss and decreases in both fat and stores of lean body tissue occur during negative energy balance. The daily energy requirement for dogs and cats depends on the amount of energy that the body expends each day. Many factors can influence the energy requirement of a pet, and these factors must all be considered when determining the number of calories and the quantity of food required by a particular companion animal.

ENERGY EXPENDITURE

The body's energy expenditure can be partitioned into three major components: basal metabolic rate, voluntary muscular activity, and dietary thermogenesis.[1] A fourth component, called *adaptive* or *nonshivering thermogenesis,* represents energy that is expended in response to environmental conditions and yields heat but no useful work. Nonshivering thermogenesis was first demonstrated in small, warm-blooded animals and is essential for cold adaptation in many species, including dogs.[2,3]

> *There are three major components of energy expenditure: (1) the energy expended during rest (resting metabolic rate), (2) the energy expended during voluntary muscle activity, and (3) the energy/heat produced by thermogenesis.*

Basal Metabolic Rate and Resting Fed Metabolic Rate

Basal metabolic rate (BMR) contributes the greatest portion of an animal's total energy expenditure. It is defined as the amount of energy expended while an animal is resting in a thermoneutral environment and in a postabsorptive state (i.e., after an overnight fast). BMR represents the energy cost of maintaining homeostasis in all of the integrated systems of the body during periods of rest, when the body is not digesting food. Homeostasis refers to a state of internal stability within the body. A related value is the *resting fed metabolic rate* (RFMR), which is measured when the animal is not in a postabsorptive state and so includes the heat produced when food is consumed (dietary thermogenesis). The RFMR accounts for approximately 60% to 75% of an animal's total daily energy expenditure. Factors influencing RFMR include sex and reproductive status, thyroid gland and autonomic nervous system function, body composition, body surface area, and nutritional state.[1]

Research has shown that BMR and RFMR are positively correlated with the total amount of respiring cell mass present in the body. Fat-free mass or lean body mass is the closest approximation available of the total respiring cell mass. The amount of fat-free mass or lean body tissue is the strongest predictor of an animal's metabolic rate, followed by body surface area and body weight (BW).[4,5] As a pet's lean body mass and body surface area increase, BMR and RFMR increase proportionately. Similarly, when an animal becomes overweight and experiences an increase in body fat and a decrease in the proportion of lean tissue to total BW, energy expenditure per unit BW decreases.[6]

Voluntary Muscular Activity

Voluntary muscular activity is the most variable component of energy expenditure. Muscular activity contributes approximately 30% of the body's total energy expenditure in moderately active individuals.

The metabolic efficiency of performing physical work is invariable, but the total amount of energy expended is affected by both the duration and the intensity of the activity. In addition, the energy cost of any type of weight-bearing activity, such as walking or running, rises as BW increases. This effect is a direct result of the added energy necessary to move a greater body mass. Therefore the energy expenditure of a pet with a high activity level depends on the duration and intensity of the exercise and the size and weight of the animal.

Dietary Thermogenesis

Dietary thermogenesis, also called the *specific dynamic effect of food* or *meal-induced thermogenesis,* refers to the heat produced in response to and following the consumption of a meal. The ingestion of nutrients causes an obligatory increase in heat production by the body as a result of the metabolic costs of digestion, absorption, metabolism, and storage of nutrients. This heat is not useful to an animal that is living in a thermal neutral environment, but will contribute to the maintenance of body temperature when an animal is exposed to a cold environment. A series of studies showed that dietary thermogenesis occurs in two phases in dogs. The first is a rise in metabolic rate that occurs in response to the presence of food, called the *cephalic phase;* the second, postprandial phase, occurs for up to six hours after the consumption of a meal.[7,8] Together, the two phases of dietary thermogenesis represent approximately 10% of daily energy expenditure for dogs. However, the magnitude of this heat production is influenced by the caloric and nutrient composition of the diet and by the nutritional state of the animal. The number of meals fed each day also affects dietary thermogenesis, with an increase in the number of meals causing an increase in the total amount of heat produced each day (see p. 65). Because cats generally consume diets that are higher in protein than dogs and tend to consume multiple meals per day, dietary thermogenesis may account for slightly more than 10% of metabolizable energy (ME) in the cat.[9]

Another type of heat production is called *adaptive thermogenesis.* This is an additional energy expenditure that is not accounted for by the obligatory and short-term thermogenesis of meal ingestion. Adaptive thermogenesis is manifested primarily as a change in the BMR in response to environmental stresses. These stresses include changes in ambient temperature, alterations in food intake, and emotional stress. For example, cold adaptation in small mammals has been shown to rely on increased heat production that is disassociated from any productive work and is separate from shivering thermogenesis.[10] This heat loss, referred to as *nonshivering thermogenesis,* also occurs in dogs that are exposed to cold environments.[11]

Overconsumption affects thermogenesis in some animals. When energy intake increases above daily needs in rats, dietary thermogenesis increases above the normal levels necessary for the metabolism of food and maintenance of body temperature.[12] This increased energy loss is a result of less efficient use of food calories. In the long term, the amount of weight gained during the period of overeating is less than that normally expected from the increased caloric intake. This process may represent the body's tendency to protect the status quo of energy balance during periods of overconsumption. However, although this process has been shown to occur in laboratory animals and some human subjects, dogs do not appear to show a similar increase in dietary thermogenesis in response to overeating.[13] Dietary thermogenesis during periods of overconsumption has not been studied in cats.

Factors Affecting Energy Expenditure

Various factors influence a pet's total daily energy expenditure (Table 9-1). An individual animal's BMR is affected by body composition, age, caloric intake,

TABLE 9-1 FACTORS AFFECTING COMPONENTS OF ENERGY EXPENDITURE

COMPONENT	FACTORS
Basal metabolic rate	Gender, reproductive status, hormonal status, autonomic nervous system function, body composition, body surface area, nutritional stage, age
Voluntary muscular activity	Weight-bearing activity, duration of exercise, intensity of exercise, size and weight of animal
Meal-induced thermogenesis	Caloric and nutrient composition of meal, nutritional state
Adaptive thermogenesis	Ambient temperature, alterations in food intake, emotional stress

and hormonal status. The BMR component of energy expenditure naturally decreases as a pet ages, primarily as a result of a gradual loss of lean body tissue. Changes in BMR can also occur as a result of food restriction. When caloric intake is decreased, an initial decrease in BMR occurs because of hormonal influences. If caloric restriction continues, the loss of lean body tissue due to weight loss causes a persistent reduction in BMR. This decrease will not be corrected until normal levels of lean body tissue have been restored. Similarly, persistent overeating can lead to an increase in total energy expenditure. Part of this increase results from the increase in lean body tissue with weight gain and increased dietary thermogenesis. A pet's reproductive status also affects resting metabolic rate (RMR). A study with cats reported that gonadectomized (neutered) male and female cats have lower estimated RMR values than those for intact cats of the same age.[14] These differences may be a factor in overweight conditions in pets (see Section 5, pp. 316-318).

Changes in voluntary activity and exercise level can significantly affect energy expenditure in dogs and cats. Just like people, companion animals tend to become more sedentary as they age. This change is usually first observed when the pet reaches maturity. In many breeds and individuals, play behaviors do not persist strongly into adulthood, and the onset of maturity is accompanied by a decline in physical activity. Later in life, voluntary activity may decline further because of chronic disease, the onset of arthritis, or a decreased tolerance for exercise. These changes will be reflected in a decline in the pet's total energy requirement. It follows that increasing a pet's daily exercise will increase the energy requirement. A portion of the higher energy expenditure occurs because of the direct calorie-consuming benefit of exercise. However, just as important, the long-term, cumulative effects of exercise cause changes in BW and condition. Regular exercise results in a higher proportion of lean tissue to fat tissue in the pet's body. The amount of exercise necessary to decrease body fat and maintain or increase lean body tissue is related to the duration and intensity of the physical activity. As discussed previously, an increase in lean body tissue increases BMR. Therefore voluntary activity not only directly burns energy; it also contributes to a higher percentage of lean body tissue and a higher BMR over the long term.

As pets age, regular exercise is important to maintain adequate energy expenditure and to help to maintain the body's lean mass. Voluntary activity burns energy, increases lean body tissue, and results in a higher basal metabolic rate.

FOOD AND ENERGY INTAKE

The other half of the energy balance equation is energy intake. Food intake is regulated in all animals by a complex system involving both internal physiological controls and external cues. The internal signals and external stimuli that affect appetite, hunger, and satiety are presented in Box 9-1. A growing number of studies have investigated the internal signals that govern food intake in dogs and cats. Although much of the scientific knowledge regarding these signals has been collected primarily in laboratory animals, it can be used to provide insight into mechanisms that may be operating in other species.

Internal Controls of Food Intake

In all mammals, the natural state for the body is one of hunger. This state is held in check by the presence of food in the gastrointestinal tract; the digestion, absorption, and metabolism of nutrients; and the amount of nutrients stored in the body at any one time. The systems controlling food intake are complex, and include feedback to the brain from adipose and the gastrointestinal tract via hormonal and nervous system signals.

BOX 9-1 FACTORS AFFECTING ENERGY INTAKE	
INTERNAL SIGNALS	**EXTERNAL STIMULI**
Gastric distention	Food availability
Physiological response to sight, sound, and smell of food	Timing and size of meals
Changes in plasma concentrations of specific nutrients, hormones, and peptides	Food composition and texture
	Diet palatability

During a meal, food causes stomach distension and the immediate release of gastrointestinal hormones such as cholecystokinin (CCK) and glucagon-like peptide 1 (GLP-1), which signal fullness in the short term.[15] Physical distention of the stomach and the distal small intestine stimulates the vagus nerve and relays satiety information to the brain.[16] However, the presence of food in the stomach alone will not inhibit food intake until significant gastric distention occurs, so the relative importance of this mechanism in influencing meal size and meal termination, especially when consuming an energy-dense diet, is fairly minor. A second physiological control of food intake is the ileal brake. Under normal physiological conditions, undigested nutrients can reach the terminal small intestine and cause delayed gastric emptying and reduced intestinal tract motility, making the ileal brake a relatively important mechanism in food intake control.[17] Activation of the ileal brake reduces hunger and food intake in addition to influencing gastrointestinal motility and secretions.

In the stomach, gastric cells release one of the few known orexigenic hormones, ghrelin. Blood ghrelin peaks prior to meal initiation and the administration of ghrelin stimulates appetite and increases gastric emptying rate in dogs and cats.[18-20] In the proximal small intestine, I-cells in the duodenum and jejunum release CCK in response to the presence of fat and protein. CCK mediates gastric acid secretion, gastric emptying, gall bladder contraction, and pancreatic enzyme secretion in multiple species, including the dog and cat, where it also acts as a potent anorectic agent.[18,21] In dogs and cats, GLP-1 and peptide YY (PYY) both are released from L-cells in the ileum and colon and influence satiety in response to the presence of unabsorbed carbohydrates and fats.[22,23] GLP-1 increases insulin secretion and reduces pancreatic enzyme secretion. It also reduces gastric acid secretion, slows gastric emptying rate, and functions to stimulate the ileal brake, exerting an endocrine distal-to-proximal feedback in the gastrointestinal tract.[24] In contrast, PYY acts as a paracrine or neurocrine agent, as plasma levels do not reflect the local activity of PYY.[25]

Other hormones influence the sensation of satiation and hunger over longer periods of time. These include leptin and insulin. Leptin is a product of the *ob* gene and is synthesized primarily by adipose tissue. Leptin signals the availability of energy stores to the hypothalamus and, when it is increased, reduces food intake and BW. Blood leptin concentrations do not change in response to meals, but are proportional to total body fat stores in dogs and cats.[26,27] Increased leptin concentrations also are associated with the diminished insulin sensitivity seen in overweight cats.[28]

Insulin may be an important internal control signal for both appetite and satiety. The exogenous administration of this hormone stimulates hunger and increases food intake in human subjects. The mechanisms involved appear to be an insulin-induced decrease in the use of cellular glucose (glucoprivation) and severe hypoglycemia. Insulin may also act directly on the hypothalamus to mediate this effect. Studies with rats have shown that both insulin and the adrenal glucocorticoid corticosterone function synergistically with central neurotransmitter substances to stimulate eating. In human subjects, feelings of hunger are positively correlated with low levels of blood glucose.[29] Excess plasma glucose, however, does not depress food intake.

Insulin may also be involved in signaling satiety and the cessation of eating. It has been theorized that the size of the fat deposit in an animal's body may be regulated by the concentration of insulin in the cerebrospinal fluid. The insulin levels in the cerebrospinal fluid increase and decrease proportionately as fat cells increase and decrease in size. These changes happen without the daily fluctuations that occur in plasma insulin levels. The insulin receptors of the cerebrospinal fluid, which are not accessible to the plasma insulin pool, appear to be involved in the regulation of food intake and total body adiposity. A study with rats demonstrated that when insulin was infused into the cerebrospinal fluid over a period of several weeks, food intake and BW decreased significantly.[30] On the other hand, when the spinal pool of insulin was experimentally decreased by the injection of insulin antibodies, food intake and BW both increased. These changes occurred independently of changes in plasma insulin concentration. Insulin levels in cerebrospinal fluid may modulate the brain's response to other internal satiety signals, such as the release of gut peptides, and may be important in the long-term control of body fat stores.

The complex actions of the myriad of orexigenic and anorexic hormones are received and coordinated by the brain. Specifically, the hypothalamus is known to be involved in mediating both quantitative and qualitative changes in food intake. The arcuate nucleus in the hypothalamus plays a central role in mediating signals of energy storage and needs. The arcuate nucleus stimulates food intake through neuropeptide Y (NPY)-containing neurons and signals satiety through pro-opiomelanocortin (POMC) neurons.[31] Insulin and leptin inhibit NPY-containing neurons and stimulate POMC-containing neurons. PYY also inhibits NPY release in the brain.[16] In addition, several different neurotransmitter substances are believed to be involved in this process.[31] Stimulatory neurotransmitters include catecholamine, norepinephrine, and three classes of neuropeptides (opioids, pancreatic polypeptides, and galanin). Direct injections of these compounds into the hypothalamus of rats potentiate eating in both hungry and satiated animals. In addition, obesity as a result of overeating can be induced in laboratory animals by the chronic administration of norepinephrine. Although multiple sites of the brain and nervous system respond, the medial paraventricular nucleus is the area of the hypothalamus most sensitive to these neurotransmitters. Interestingly, there is evidence suggesting that these compounds affect specific nutrient selection by animals, rather than simply increasing total caloric intake.[31] Norepinephrine injection causes an increase in the consumption of carbohydrates, and the administration of opioids and galanin results in increased fat consumption.

Aberrations in any of the internal control systems for appetite, hunger, and satiety can result in pathological changes in food intake. For example, lesions involving the ventromedial center of the hypothalamus lead to overeating, but lesions of the lateral nucleus result in an inhibition of food intake. Endocrine imbalances such as insulinoma, hypopituitarism, hyperadrenocorticism, and possibly hypothyroidism may affect food intake. Any metabolic dysfunction that affects neurotransmitter substances or the gut peptides could also potentially result in changes in food intake.

Interestingly, the condition of obesity can further perturb appetite, hunger, and satiety signaling. Excess weight gain can elicit insulin resistance in cats and dogs.[27,28,32] Relative to normal-weight controls, obese humans have faster gastric emptying rates and lower postprandial PYY and GLP-1 responses. These abnormalities were ameliorated with weight loss and suggest weaker satiety signaling in obese individuals.[16] In addition, other physiological conditions, such as spaying and neutering, may impact internal controls of food intake. In a survey of dogs in the United Kingdom, neutered females and males were approximately twice as likely to be obese as their intact counterparts.[33] Neutering has been demonstrated to increase food intake, BW, and body fat in male and female cats, which can be mitigated almost entirely by the administration of estradiol.[34,35] Furthermore, intact female rats and ovariectomized female rats and male rats administered estrogen, were much more sensitive to the anorectic effects of leptin in the brain compared to male rats and ovariectomized female rats not supplemented with estrogen.[36] This suggests that sex hormones play a central role in regulating internal satiety signals.

External Controls of Food Intake

External controls of food intake include stimuli such as diet palatability, food composition and texture, and the timing and environment of meals. Exposure to highly palatable foods is considered an important environmental factor contributing to food overconsumption in humans, laboratory animals, and companion animals.[37] Studies with human subjects have demonstrated that the quantity of food consumed varies directly with its palatability, and palatability does not appear to increase with levels of food deprivation. In other words, if food is perceived to be very appealing, an individual tends to consume more of it, regardless of the initial level of hunger. Similarly, when rats are offered a highly palatable diet, they overeat and become obese.[38] This effect has been observed with high-fat diets, calorically dense diets, and "cafeteria" diets that provide a large variety of palatable food items.[39,40] It appears that the novelty of being presented with several different types of palatable foods can override normal satiety signals.[41] A similar practice that is not uncommon with companion animals is the feeding of a variety of table scraps and calorically dense treats. The persistent feeding of highly desirable and appealing foods to some dogs and cats may override the body's natural tendency to balance energy intake and lead to the overconsumption of energy.

Dogs and cats have preferences for certain flavors and types of pet foods, and these preferences are influenced by a number of factors. For example, an early study reported that beef was a preferred type of meat for dogs, and that cooking the meat enhanced its attractiveness.[42] It was theorized that early experience with cooked meat, such as that present in commercial pet foods, was the cause of the development of a preference for cooked products. Dogs also have a strong preference for sucrose, while cats do not show a strong attraction to sucrose-sweetened foods or fluids.[43,44] Both dogs and cats prefer warm food to cold food, and palatability generally increases along with the fat content of the diet (although this increase in acceptance may be related to texture as well as taste). Many of the taste preferences of dogs and cats can be explained by the type of taste buds or "units" found on their tongues (see Chapter 7, pp. 46-47).[45] For example, both dogs and cats have a high proportion of taste buds that are sensitive to amino acid flavors. It is postulated that these provide them with the ability to distinguish among the different types of meats that may be found in a carnivorous diet.

Not surprisingly, most dogs prefer canned and semimoist pet food rather than dry; cooked rather than uncooked meat; beef over other meats; and warm food rather than cold. To a degree, palatability increases along with the fat content of the diet.

Palatability is an important diet characteristic that is heavily promoted in the marketing of commercial pet foods. In addition to the pet's preferences, many pet owners select a pet food based on their own perceptions of the food's appeal (see Section 3, pp. 177-180 for a complete discussion of palatability of commercial pet foods).

The timing and social setting of meals also influence eating behavior. Dogs and cats rapidly become conditioned to receiving their meals at a particular time of day. This conditioning manifests itself both behaviorally and physiologically. Pets generally become more active at mealtime, and gastric secretions and gastric motility increase in anticipation of eating. In addition, dogs tend to increase food intake when consuming food in the presence of other dogs in their social group (conspecifics). This process is called *social facilitation*. For example, some pet owners find that a dog fed

free-choice without difficulty begins to overconsume and gain weight when another dog is added to the household. In most dogs, social facilitation causes a moderate increase in the dog's interest in food and an increased rate of eating. However, for some, the increase in food intake that occurs in response to another animal's presence can be extreme enough to singularly cause excessive food intake. In some situations, however, the addition of a new dog or cat to the home can inhibit food consumption in other pets. This can occur when agonistic relationships develop or when one pet is fearful of another.

There is also evidence that food choice in dogs can be influenced by the experience of conspecifics and by the behavior of their owner. For example, in a small pilot study, 12 pairs of dogs were matched according to body size and then randomly assigned to be either a demonstrator or an observer dog.[46] Demonstrator dogs were taken to another room and were offered a serving of dry dog food flavored with either dried basil or dried thyme. After the demonstrator had consumed at least 20 grams (g) of the food, the two dogs were reunited and allowed to socialize for 10 minutes. The observer dog was then removed and offered an equal amount of both of the flavored foods. Although all of the observer dogs sampled both foods, dogs showed a significant preference for the flavor that had been previously consumed by their paired demonstrator dog. Because all of the observer dogs sniffed the mouths and heads of their demonstrators, it was theorized that olfactory cues may be important for the social transmission of food preferences. Interestingly, another set of studies demonstrated that dogs were capable of performing correctly in quantity discrimination tasks and consistently selected a large quantity over a small quantity of palatable food.[47,48]

Recently, another form of social learning affecting food choice has also been described in dogs. An owner's food preferences can influence the food choices that their dog makes. In one study, a group of 50 dogs was first tested for quantity discrimination and showed a significant preference for the larger quantities of food (1 piece vs. 8 pieces of kibble).[49] However, when the owner of the dog demonstrated a preference for the smaller quantity of food before allowing the dog to choose, dogs switched and began to choose the smaller quantity of food more frequently. In addition, when dogs were presented with two bowls containing identical quantities of food, and the owner showed an interest in one of the bowls, their dogs chose the preferred bowl 82% of the time. These results illustrate the importance of the dog's social environment, and specifically the influence of an owner's preferences, upon feeding behavior in dogs. Similar studies are needed that examine the influence of owner behavior and food choice on food preferences in cats.

> *A dog's social environment can influence feeding behavior and food selection. For example, dogs often respond to the presence of other dogs by increasing their rate of eating and are also capable of learning food preferences from other dogs. Similarly, the owner's behavior can influence a dog's food choices!*

The frequency with which meals are provided is another external factor that can affect food intake and energy needs of dogs and cats. Metabolically, increasing the number of meals per day while keeping total energy intake constant results in increased energy loss from dietary thermogenesis. In a study with adult dogs, a group that was fed four times per day increased oxygen consumption 30%, but a second group that was fed the same amount of food in just one meal daily exhibited only a 15% increase in oxygen consumption.[50] In contrast, the presence of food, particularly palatable food, is a potent external cue for meal ingestion and offering increased number of meals per day may lead to excess consumption in individuals that are highly sensitive to external cues. A study was conducted to compare the effects of free-choice feeding with portion-controlled feeding on the growth and development of growing puppies.[51] Puppies that had access to food throughout the day gained weight more rapidly and were heavier than puppies fed using the portion-controlled regimen. However, the two groups exhibited similar amounts of skeletal growth as measured by forelimb and body length. These results indicate that both groups were developing maximally, but the free-choice fed group was depositing more body fat than was the portion-controlled group. In addition to affecting growth, multiple feedings of a highly palatable food may lead to overconsumption and excess weight gain in adult dogs and cats. This tendency to overconsume may more than compensate for the increased energy loss from dietary thermogenesis.

A final external factor that may contribute to energy intake is the nutrient composition of the diet. Nutrient composition affects both the efficiency of nutrient metabolism and the amount of food that is voluntarily consumed. Dietary fat, protein, and fiber are the nutrients of greatest interest. Although most animals decrease their intake of a high-fat diet in an attempt to balance energy needs, the greater caloric density of the diet and its increased palatability can still cause increased energy consumption in some individuals. In addition, dietary fat has a weaker effect on satiety than either carbohydrate or protein.[52] Additionally, the metabolic efficiency of converting dietary fat to body fat for storage is higher than the efficiency of converting dietary carbohydrate or protein to body fat. Only 3% of the energy content of fat is lost when it is stored as body fat. This loss can be compared with a loss of 23% of the energy content of dietary carbohydrate and protein when these nutrients are converted to body fat.[37] Therefore, if an animal is consuming more than its caloric requirement of a particular diet and if the excess calories are provided by fat, more weight will be gained than if the excess calories are coming from either carbohydrate or protein.

This phenomenon was illustrated in an early study with companion animals; puppies that consumed a high-fat diet had similar growth in lean body mass when compared with puppies fed diets lower in fat, but the former accumulated significantly more body fat.[53] Similarly, when adult dogs were fed either a high-fat or a high-carbohydrate diet, the dogs fed the high-fat diet consumed only 13% more energy than those fed the high-carbohydrate diet, but they retained 117% more energy.[54] Even though a portion of this increased weight gain was attributed to the small difference in energy intake, there appeared to be increased efficiency of fat deposition in the dogs consuming the high-fat diet. Finally, the protein content of a diet may also influence energy intake; this effect may be related to palatability as well as the effects of dietary protein upon satiety.[55] A recent study reported that dogs preferentially avoided a protein-free diet and tended to select foods that contain between 25% and 30% of their calories from protein.[56] In contrast, an earlier study reported that cats did not demonstrate a clear preference for high vs. low levels of protein when offered diets containing varying concentrations of soy protein or casein[57] (see Chapters 18 and 19 for complete discussions of food selection and factors affecting satiety).

DETERMINATION OF ENERGY REQUIREMENTS OF DOGS AND CATS

The total daily energy requirement of an animal is the sum of the energy that is needed for the BMR, dietary thermogenesis, voluntary muscular activity, and maintenance of normal body temperature when exposed to adverse weather conditions. Adult animals in a state of maintenance only require enough energy to support activity and maintain the body's normal metabolic processes and tissue stores. On the other hand, dogs and cats that are growing, reproducing, or working have increased energy needs.

Dogs

Formulating an exact equation to estimate the energy requirements of dogs is a difficult task because of the wide variety of body sizes and weights in this species. The amount of energy that is used by the body is correlated with total body surface area. Body surface area per unit of weight decreases as animals increase in size. As a result, the energy requirements of animals with widely differing weights are not well correlated with BW; they are more closely related to BW raised to a specified power. This unit of BW is called *metabolic body weight*. Representing weight as metabolic body weight helps to account for differences in body surface area between animals of varying sizes. Historically, coefficient values used with dogs have ranged between 0.67 and 0.88.[58]

An allometric equation for ME requirement is represented as ME = K (representing a constant) × weight (W) kilograms (kg)$^{0.75}$. This provides a reasonable starting point when estimating the daily energy requirements for different sizes of adult dogs at maintenance. The National Research Council (NRC) guidelines provide a series of K values that are used to adjust for different activity levels and living situations (Box 9-2).[9]

However, an important consideration (and limitation) when using an allometric equation lies in the selection of an appropriate K value. For example, a value of 95 is recommended for inactive pet dogs living in home environments, while a value of 130 is suggested for active pet dogs that have ample opportunities to exercise. Using these values, a 50-pound (lb) (22.7-kg)

BOX 9-2 CALCULATION OF ESTIMATED ENERGY REQUIREMENTS OF ADULT DOGS AT MAINTENANCE

INACTIVE ADULT DOGS*

ME requirement = $95 \times W_{kg}^{0.75}$

Examples:

ME requirement of a 10-kg (22-lb) dog = $95 \times (10 \text{ kg})^{0.75}$ = **534 kcal ME/day**

ME requirement of a 22.7-kg (50-lb) dog = $95 \times (22.7 \text{ kg})^{0.75}$ = **988 kcal ME/day**

ACTIVE ADULT DOGS*

ME requirement = $130 \times W_{kg}^{0.75}$

Examples:

ME requirement of a 10-kg (22-lb) dog = $130 \times (10 \text{ kg})^{0.75}$ = **731 kcal of ME/day**

ME requirement of a 22.7-kg (50-lb) dog = $130 \times (22.7 \text{ kg})^{0.75}$ = **1352 kcal ME/day**

ME, Metabolizable energy.
*NOTE: Estimates use equations provided by the National Research Council: *Nutrient requirements of dogs and cats*, Washington, DC, 2006, National Academy Press. (Other energy equations are available and may also be used.)

---

inactive adult dog has an estimated daily caloric requirement of approximately 988 kcal (see Box 9-2). The same dog, if considered active, would have an estimated caloric requirement of 1352 kilocalories (kcal), a difference of more than 360 kcal per day. Therefore, once a K value has been selected for use, the resulting caloric estimate must be considered to be just a starting point to determine the daily energy requirement of a particular animal. Variability among individual dogs and the environmental conditions under which dogs are kept can result in a requirement that is substantially more or less than this initial estimate.

The initial amount of food that is estimated should be adjusted according to the dog's long-term response to feeding. For example, using the previous example, an inactive adult dog weighing 50 pounds (22.7 kg) would require approximately 988 kcal of ME per day. If a food containing 3800 kcal/kg (1727 kcal/lb) was fed, the dog would require 0.260 kg (260 g) of food. This is equal to 9.1 ounces (oz). One 8-oz cup of dry dog food typically contains 3 to 4 oz of food. Therefore

TABLE 9-2 CALCULATION OF THE AMOUNT OF FOOD TO FEED DOGS AND CATS

	ENERGY REQUIREMENT (KCAL OF ME/DAY)		ENERGY DENSITY (KCAL/KG)		QUANTITY (KG)				POUNDS		OUNCES		CUPS PER DAY
Dog (22.7 kg)	988	÷	3800	=	0.26	×	2.2	=	0.572	=	9.2	=	2.6
Cat (4 kg)	253	÷	4200	=	0.060	×	2.2	=	0.132	=	2.12	=	0.60
Puppy (10 kg)	1462	÷	3800	=	0.385	×	2.2	=	0.846	=	13.5	=	3.86
Kitten (1 kg)	250	÷	4200	=	0.059	×	2.2	=	0.129	=	2.06	=	0.58

ME, Metabolizable energy.

the initial feeding level of this dog should be a little more than 2½ cups of food per day (Table 9-2). Alternatively, if this dog was considered to be somewhat active, with a requirement of 1352 kcal per day, feeding approximately 3½ cups of the same food would meet this requirement. Therefore, if the owner is uncertain about their dog's actual activity level, an initial feeding amount of 3 cups might be appropriate, which can then be adjusted up or down in response to the dog's body condition and weight.

The energy requirements predicted by allometric equations are calculated for dogs at adult maintenance. Stages of life that result in increased energy needs include growth, gestation, lactation, periods of strenuous physical work, and exposure to extreme environmental conditions (Table 9-3). The body type and conformation of particular breeds can also affect an individual dog's maintenance energy requirement.[59] For example, adult Newfoundland dogs have lower energy requirements than adult Great Danes of similar weight. This difference may be a reflection of variation in proportions of lean body tissue in the two breeds and may also be influenced by differences in activity levels. More research into energy differences in different breeds is necessary because such information may be helpful in explaining the predisposition to obesity seen in certain breeds and breed types.

After weaning, growing puppies require approximately twice the energy intake per unit of BW as adult dogs of the same weight. For example, an active puppy that weighs 22 lb (10 kg) would require 2 × 731 kcal, or 1462 kcal, per day. This would correspond to a little less than 4 cups of food per day when a food containing

TABLE 9-3 ENERGY REQUIREMENTS FOR DIFFERENT STAGES OF LIFE

STAGE	ENERGY REQUIREMENT
Dogs	
Postweaned	2 × adult maintenance ME*
40% adult body weight	1.6 × adult maintenance ME
80% adult body weight	1.2 × adult maintenance ME
Late gestation	1.25 to 1.5 × adult maintenance ME
Lactation†	3 × adult maintenance ME
Prolonged physical work	2 to 4 × adult maintenance ME
Decreased environmental temperature	1.2 to 1.8 × adult maintenance ME
Cats	
Postweaned	250 kcal ME/kg body weight
20 weeks	130 kcal ME/kg body weight
30 weeks	100 kcal ME/kg body weight
Late gestation	1.25 × adult maintenance ME
Lactation	3 to 4 × adult maintenance ME

ME, Metabolizable energy.
*Adult maintenance for a dog of comparable weight.
†Equation based upon number of puppies and week of lactation:
ME = adult maintenance + [BW (kg) × (24n + 12m) × L]. (BW = body weight; n = number of puppies up to 4; m = number of puppies between 5 and 8; L = week of lactation.)

3800 kcal/kg is fed (see Table 9-2). If a more energy-dense food was fed, a smaller volume would be estimated. When puppies reach about 40% to 50% of their adult weight, this level of food should be reduced to 1.6 times maintenance levels; it should be further reduced to 1.2 times maintenance levels when 80% of adult weight is achieved (see Table 9-3).[9] The age at which a puppy will attain these proportions of adult weight will vary with the adult size of the dog. In general, large breeds of dogs mature more slowly than do small breeds. With the exception of the giant breeds, most puppies achieve 40% of their adult weight between 3 and 4 months of age and 80% of adult weight between 4½ and 8 months. Large breeds of dogs do not attain full adult size until they are more than 10 months of age; small breeds reach adult size at a slightly earlier age.[60] It is also important to recognize that attaining adult size is not synonymous with physical maturity in terms of skeletal maturation and muscle development (see Chapter 22, pp. 221-226). Although there is limited information published regarding breed differences in energy needs during growth, activity differences among breeds and temperament types can affect energy requirements during development, especially during the latter half of the growth period.[61]

Energy needs increase substantially for female dogs during gestation and lactation. During the first 3 to 4 weeks of the 9-week gestation, energy needs remain the same as for maintenance. After the fourth week of pregnancy, energy requirements increase gradually to provide for rapid fetal growth. The energy needs of a pregnant female will increase to approximately 1.25 to 1.5 times the normal maintenance requirement by the end of the gestation period. Alternatively, increased needs during the latter half of gestation (after 4 weeks until parturition) can be estimated using the equation ME (kcal) = maintenance energy + (26 kcal × BW kg).[62]

Lactation is one of the most energy-demanding stages of life for an animal. Depending on the size of the litter, the energy needs of a bitch during lactation can increase to as much as three times the normal maintenance requirement. Using the previous example, a female with a normal weight of 22.7 kg and maintenance energy needs of 988 kcal may require up to 3 × 988 kcal, or 2964 kcal, during peak lactation. This is equal to almost 8 cups of food per day. The ability of a bitch to consume this large volume of food may be limited by the size of her stomach. Therefore it is important to feed a food that is highly digestible and nutrient dense during this stage of life and if necessary, to increase the number of meals that are offered (see Section 4, pp. 204-205 for a complete discussion). When a more precise estimate is needed, energy requirements of lactating females can be calculated using an equation that accounts for both the number of puppies in the litter and for the week of lactation (see Table 9-3).[9,63]

Both physical work and environmental stresses can cause increased energy needs in dogs. Short bouts of intense physical exercise may cause only a slight increase in energy requirement, but a regular program of prolonged exercise may increase energy needs up to two to four times maintenance requirements. In addition, exposure to cold and hot weather conditions can also increase a dog's energy requirement. Dogs must expend additional energy to support normal body temperature in cold conditions and for the body's cooling mechanisms in warm conditions. Depending on the severity, living in cold weather conditions can increase energy requirements by 1.2 to 1.8 times maintenance.[64]

The energy requirements of cats and dogs are higher during growth, reproduction, physical activity, and exposure to cold environmental conditions. During lactation, the energy needs of dogs and cats can increase as much as three times normal, depending on litter size. Table 9-3 provides methods of calculating energy requirements and the amounts to feed.

Cats

The mature BW of most domestic cats varies between about 2 and 7 kg (4 and 15 lb). Because cats do not show the extreme variability in body size and weight that dogs do, their energy needs have been traditionally expressed as a linear relationship with BW. However, this approach tended to overestimate the energy needs of larger cats. Recent studies of the maintenance energy requirements of cats of different sizes and ages have found that using metabolic BW provides a more accurate energy estimate for cats, just as it does for dogs.[65,66] An exponent of 0.67 has been suggested for cats with optimal or lean body condition, and an exponent of 0.40 is suggested for cats that are overweight or obese.[9] Maintenance energy needs for lean cats are estimated using the equation $ME = 100 \times BW_{kg}^{0.67}$, and for overweight cats with the equation $ME = 130 \times BW_{kg}^{0.40}$. Although these two equations account for different body sizes and body conditions in cats, an individual animal's activity level and age will also influence the maintenance energy requirement. In a recent study, indirect calorimetry was used to measure daily energy expenditure of young adult cats of both sexes.[67] The results provided an estimate of approximately 60 kcal/kg BW for young adults, regardless of sex. Another study provided similar values for young adults and also showed that the energy needs of middle-aged cats generally decreased to approximately 45 kcal/kg BW.[68] Similar to dogs, these age-related changes in energy needs have been attributed to the additive effects of reduced activity and changes in body composition.[69,70]

As with dogs, energy equations for cats provide a rough estimate to use as a starting point when determining an optimal amount of food for an individual. An example using these equations is provided in Box 9-3. Using the NRC equations, an adult 4.0-kg (8.8-lb) cat in optimal body condition would require approximately 253 kcal of ME per day. The alternative equation (60 kcal/BW_{kg}) provides an estimate of 240 kcal. If the cat was a senior, the estimate is reduced to approximately 180 kcal. Finally, the estimated energy need of an overweight adult cat weighing 8 kg (17.6 lb) is approximately 299 kcal per day. See Table 9-2 for feeding estimates for an adult cat in optimal body condition.

The energy requirements of cats increase during growth, reproduction, physical activity, and extreme environmental conditions (see Table 9-3). The energy and nutrient requirements of growing kittens are highest per unit of BW at about 5 weeks of age. Young, rapidly growing kittens require approximately 200 to 250 kcal of ME per kg of BW. This requirement declines to 130 kcal/kg by 20 weeks of age, and to 100 kcal/kg by 30 weeks of age. For example, a 3-month-old kitten weighing 1 kg (2.2 lb) requires up to 250 kcal/day. If a dry kitten food containing 4200 kcal/kg is fed, the kitten should be given 59 g or approximately 2 oz of food. This is equal to a little more than ½ cup of food per day. A more complex equation that accounts for differences in expected adult size and that is calculated specifically for a post-weaned kitten's current BW is provided by the NRC.[9] However, this equation relies upon an estimate of adult weight—information that may not be available to many owners. The estimates provided by this equation

---

BOX 9-3   CALCULATION OF ENERGY REQUIREMENTS OF ADULT CATS AT MAINTENANCE

LEAN ADULT CATS (NRC FORMULA)*
$ME = 100 \times W_{kg}^{0.67}$

Examples:

ME requirement of a 4-kg (8.8-lb) cat = $100 \times (4 \text{ kg})^{0.67}$ = 253 kcal of ME/day

ME requirement of a 6-kg (13.2-lb) cat = $100 \times (6 \text{ kg})^{0.67}$ = 332 kcal of ME/day

ALTERNATE FORMULA (YOUNG ADULT CATS)†
$ME = 60 \times W_{kg}$

Examples:

ME requirement of a 4-kg (8.8-lb) cat = 60×4 kg = 240 kcal of ME/day

ME requirement of a 6-kg (13.2-lb) cat = 60×6 kg = 360 kcal of ME/day

OVERWEIGHT CATS (NRC FORMULA)*
$ME = 130 \times W_{kg}^{0.40}$

Examples:

ME requirement of a 6-kg (13.2-lb) cat = $130 \times (6 \text{ kg})^{0.40}$ = 266 kcal of ME/day

ME requirement of a 8-kg (17.6-lb) cat = $130 \times (8 \text{ kg})^{0.40}$ = 299 kcal of ME/day

OLDER ADULT CATS‡
$ME = 45 \times W_{kg}$

Examples:

ME requirement of a 4-kg cat = 45×4 kg = 180 kcal of ME/day

ME requirement of a 6-kg cat = 45×6 kg = 270 kcal of ME/day

ME, Metabolizable energy; *NRC,* National Research Council.
*National Research Council: *Nutrient requirements of dogs and cats,* Washington, DC, 2006, National Academy Press. (Other energy equations are available and may also be used.)
†Wichert B, Muller L, Gebert S, and others: Additional data on energy requirements of young adult cats measured by indirect calorimetry, *J Anim Phys Anim Nutr* 91:278–281, 2007.
‡Laflamme DP, Ballam JM: Effect of age on maintenance energy requirements of adult cats. In *Proc Purina Nutr Forum,* St Louis, 2001.

are usually similar to estimates provided by the more general recommendations.

Studies with reproducing queens have indicated that energy requirements of cats increase throughout gestation, rather than only during the last 4 to 5 weeks.[71] By the end of the 9-week gestation, an increase of about 25% above normal maintenance energy needs is usually required. The accretion of excess maternal body tissues during gestation allows the queen to prepare adequately for the intense energy demands of lactation. The queen then uses these maternal stores and additional dietary energy to meet her increased energy needs during lactation. Depending on the size of the litter, a queen's dietary energy requirement during peak lactation may be as high as 2.5 times her maintenance requirement (see Chapter 20, pp. 200-205 for a complete discussion).

During all physiological stages, the energy requirement of a particular cat is influenced by the cat's activity level, body condition, and length and thickness of the cat's coat and by the environmental conditions in which the cat is living. Therefore these estimates should be used only as a starting point when determining the exact needs of an individual animal. Evaluation of the cat's BW and condition can then be used to adjust the initial energy requirement estimate.

WATER

The daily drinking water requirement of a dog or cat depends on several factors. Voluntary water intake will increase in response to any change that causes an increase in water losses from the body, such as increased physical activity, increased body or environmental temperature, changes in the kidneys' ability to concentrate urine, or the onset of lactation. An animal's water needs increase dramatically during periods of intense or prolonged exercise, when exposed to high environmental temperature or humidity, and in females, during the weeks of peak lactation. In addition, the amount of water present in the pet's food significantly affects voluntary water intake. If the water content of the food is very high, both dogs and cats are able to maintain normal water balance with no additional drinking water.[72,73]

Several approaches are used to estimate dog and cats' maintenance water needs. Fluid therapy estimates are based upon BW and use an estimate

of 50 to 60 ml/BW_{kg}.[74] Using this formula, a 23-kg (50-lb) dog would require 1150 to 1380 ml of water per day. Another formula estimates dogs' exogenous water requirement in a thermoneutral environment as two to three times the dry-matter (DM) intake of food, expressed in grams. Using the previous example, an inactive adult dog weighing 23 kg requires approximately 1000 kcal/day. If the dog is fed a dry food that has an energy density of 3500 kcal/kg, the dog should receive 285 g of food per day. Dry pet foods contain approximately 8% moisture. Therefore the dog will be consuming 262 g of dry matter (DM). Multiplying this number by 3 gives an estimated water requirement of 785 ml of water per day, which is somewhat lower than the previous estimate. Finally, other recommendations suggest that dogs require an amount of drinking water that is roughly equal to the number of kcal consumed per day (i.e., a 1:1 ratio). In this case, the requirement would be equal to 1000 ml/day, which is similar to the estimate provided by the first equation. In general, water requirements of cats are thought to be somewhat lower than those for dogs. For example, the relationship between water intake needed to maintain balance and caloric intake in cats is reported to be 0.6 to 1, lower than recommendation for dogs.[75] Therefore, while the formulas that are used for dogs can also be used for cats, they may generally overestimate maintenance needs for cats.

The best method of ensuring adequate water intake in both dogs and cats is to provide fresh, clean water at all times, regardless of the animal's physiological state, caloric needs, or DM intake. Dogs typically consume more water per unit BW than do cats and respond more rapidly to mild dehydration by voluntarily increasing their water consumption.[76] In contrast, cats are less sensitive to dehydration than dogs and take longer to restore water balance through spontaneous drinking. Cats are also capable of producing more concentrated urine than dogs, an adaptation that helps to conserve water loss. The cat's relatively weak thirst drive and tendency to consume smaller volumes of water are attributed to its evolution from a desert-dwelling species. However, the cat's drinking behaviors and production of a concentrated urine are also risk factors for urolith formation in susceptible cats (see Chapter 30, pp. 365-366 for a complete discussion).

References

1. Blaxter K: *Energy metabolism in animals and man*, Cambridge, UK, 1989, Cambridge University Press.

2. Sellers EA, Reichman S, Thomas N, and others: Acclimatization to cold in rats: metabolic rates, *Am J Physiol* 167:651–655, 1951.

3. Davis TR: Contribution of skeletal muscle to nonshivering thermogenesis in the dog, *Am J Physiol* 213:1423–1426, 1967.

4. Ravussin E, Burnand B, Schutz Y, and others: Twenty-four hour energy expenditure and resting metabolic rate in obese, moderately obese and control subjects, *Am J Clin Nutr* 35:566–573, 1982.

5. Forbes GB, Welle SL: Lean body mass in obesity, *Int J Obes* 7:99–107, 1983.

6. Pouteau ES, Mariot L, Martin H, and others: Effect of weight variations (fattening and slimming) on energy expenditure in dogs (abstract), *J Vet Intern Med* 14:390, 2000.

7. Diamond P, Brondel L, Leblanc L: Palatability and postprandial thermogenesis in dogs, *Am J Physiol* 248:E75–E79, 1985.

8. LeBlanc J: Nutritional implications of cephalic phase responses, *Appetite* 34:214–216, 2000.

9. National Research Council: *Nutrient requirements of dogs and cats*, Washington, DC, 2006, National Academy Press.

10. Rothwell N, Stock MJ: Luxuskonsumption, diet-induced thermogenesis and brown fat: the case in favor, *Clin Sci* 64:19–23, 1983.

11. Davis TR: Contribution of skeletal muscle to nonshivering thermogenesis in the dog, *Am J Physiol* 213:1423–1426, 1967.

12. Sims EAH: Experimental obesity, dietary-induced thermogenesis, and their clinical implications, *Clin Endocrinol Metabol* 5:377–395, 1976.

13. Crist KA, Romsos DR: Evidence for cold-induced but not for diet-induced thermogenesis in adult dogs, *J Nutr* 117:1280–1286, 1987.

14. Root MV: Early spay-neuter in the cat: effect on development of obesity and metabolic rate, *Vet Clin Nutr* 2:132–134, 1995.

15. Graaf CD, Blom WAM, Smeets PAM, and others: Biomarkers of satiation and satiety, *Am J Clin Nutr* 79:946–961, 2004.

16. Näslund E, Grybäck P, Backman L, and others: Distal small bowel hormones: correlation with fasting antroduodenal motility and gastric emptying, *Dig Dis Sci* 43:945–952, 1998.

17. Maljaars PWJ, Peters HPF, Mela DJ, Masclee AAM: Ileal brake: a sensible food target for appetite control. A review, *Physiol Behav* 95:271–281, 2008.

18. Maljaars J, Peters HPF, Masclee AM: Review article: the gastrointestinal tract: neuroendocrine regulation of satiety and food intake, *Aliment Pharmacol Ther* 26(Suppl 2):241–250, 2007.

19. Bhatti SF, Hofland LJ, van Koetsveld PM, and others: Effects of food intake and food withholding on plasma ghrelin concentrations in healthy dogs, *Am J Vet Res* 67:1557–1563, 2006.

20. Ida T, Miyazato M, Naganobu K, and others: Purification and characterization of feline ghrelin and its possible role, *Domest Anim Endocrinol* 32:93–105, 2007.

21. Inui A, Okita M, Inoue T, and others: Mechanism of actions of cholecystokinin octapeptide on food intake and insulin and pancreatic polypeptide release in the dog, *Peptides* 9:1093–1100, 1998.

22. Wen J, Phillips SF, Sarr MG, and others: PYY and GLP-1 contribute to feedback inhibition from the canine ileum and colon, *Am J Physiol* 269:G945–G952, 1995.

23. Bado A, Cloarec D, Moizo L, and others: Neurotensin and oxyntomodulin-(30-37) potentiate PYY regulation of gastric acid and somatostatin secretions, *Am J Physiol* 265:G113–G117, 1993.

24. Schirra J, Goke B: The physiological role of GLP-1 in human: incretin, ileal brake or more? *Regul Pept* 128:109–115, 2008.

25. Koda S, Date Y, Murakami N, and others: The role of the vagal nerve in peripheral PYY3-36-induced feeding reduction in rats, *Endocrinology* 146:2369–2375, 2005.

26. Jeusette IC, Lhoest ET, Istasse LP, Diez MO: Influence of obesity on plasma lipid and lipoprotein concentrations in dogs, *Am J Vet Res*. 66:81–86, 2005.

27. Hoenig M, Thomaseth K, Waldron M, Ferguson DC: Insulin sensitivity, fat distribution, and adipocytokine response to different diets in lean and obese cats before and after weight loss, *Am J Physiol Regul Integr Comp Physiol* 292:R227–R234, 2007.

28. Appleton DJ, Rand JS, Sunvold GD: Plasma leptin concentrations are independently associated with insulin sensitivity in lean and overweight cats, *J Feline Med Surg* 4:83–93, 2002.

29. Silverstone T, Besser M: Insulin, blood sugar and hunger, *Postgrad Med J* 47:427–429, 1971.

30. Woods SC, Porte D Jr, Bobbioni E: Insulin: its relationship to the central nervous system and to the control of food intake and body weight, *Am J Clin Nutr* 42:1063–1071, 1985.

31. Leibowitz SF, Hoebel BG: Behavioral neuroscience and obesity. In Bray G, Bouchard C, editors: *Handbook of obesity, etiology and pathophysiology*, ed 2, New York, 2004, Marcel Dekker, pp 301–371.

32. Rocchini AP, Yang JQ, Gokee A: Hypertension and insulin resistance are not directly related in obese dogs, *Hypertension* 43:1011–1016, 2004.

33. Edney AT, Smith PM: Study of obesity in dogs visiting veterinary practices in the United Kingdom, *Vet Rec* 118:391–396, 1986.

34. Martin L, Siliart B, Dumon H, and others: Leptin, body fat content and energy expenditure in intact and gonadectomized adult cats: a preliminary study, *J Anim Physiol Anim Nutr* 85:195–199, 2001.

35. Cave NJ, Backus RC, Marks SL, Klasing KC: Oestradiol, but not genistein, inhibits the rise in food intake following gonadectomy in cats, but genistein is associated with an increase in lean body mass, *J Anim Physiol Anim Nutr* 91:400–410, 2007.

36. Clegg DL, Brown LM, Woods SC, Benoit SC: Gonadal hormones determine sensitivity to central leptin and insulin, *Diabetes* 55:978–987, 2006.

37. Blundell J, Stubbs J: Diet composition and the control of food intake in humans. In Bray G, Bouchard C, editors: *Handbook of obesity, etiology and pathophysiology*, ed 2, New York, 2004, Marcel Dekker, pp 427–460.

38. Scalafani A, Springer O: Dietary obesity in adult rats: similarities to hypothalamic and human obesity syndromes, *Physiol Behav* 17:461–471, 1976.

39. Slattery JM, Potter RM: Hyperphagia: a necessary precondition to obesity? *Appetite* 6:133–142, 1985.

40. Rogers PJ, Blundell JE: Meal patterns and food selection during the development of obesity in rats fed a cafeteria diet, *Neurosci Biobehav Rev* 8:441–453, 1984.

41. Rolls BJ, Rowe EA, Turner RC: Persistent obesity in rats following a period of consumption of a mixed energy diet, *J Physiol (Lond)* 298:415–427, 1980.

42. Lohse CL: Preferences of dogs for various meats, *J Am Anim Hosp Assoc* 10:187–192, 1974.

43. Castonguay TW, Giles TC, Harrison JE, Rogers QR: Variations in sucrose concentration and its effect on food intake in the domestic cat, *Soc Neurosci Abst* 13:464, 1987.

44. Houpt KA, Smith SL: Taste preferences and their relation to obesity in dogs and cats, *Can Vet J* 22:77–81, 1981.

45. Thorne CJ: Understanding pet response: behavioral aspects of palatability. In *Proceedings of the petfood forum*, Chicago, 1997, Watts Publishing.

46. Lupfer-Johnson G, Ross J: Dogs acquire food preferences from interacting with recently fed conspecifics, *Behav Proc* 74:104–106, 2007.

47. Ward C, Smuts B: Quantity-based judgments in the domestic dog (*Canis lupus familiaris*), *Anim Cogn* 10:71–80, 2006.

48. West RE, Young RJ: Do domestic dogs show any evidence of being able to count? *Anim Cogn* 5:183–186, 2002.

49. Prato-Previde E, Marshall-Pescini S, Valsecchi P: Is your choice my choice? The owners' effect on pet dogs' (*Canis lupus familiaris*) performance in a food choice task, *Anim Cogn* 11:167–174, 2008.

50. Leblanc J, Diamond P: The effect of meal frequency on postprandial thermogenesis in the dog (abstract), *Fed Proc* 44:1678, 1985.

51. Alexander JE, Wood LLH: Growth studies in Labrador Retrievers fed a calorie-dense diet: time-restricted versus free choice feeding, *Canine Pract* 14:41–47, 1987.

52. Backus R: Management of satiety, *Waltham Focus* 16:27–32, 2006.

53. Romsos DR, Belo PS, Bennink MR, and others: Effects of dietary carbohydrate, fat and protein on growth, body composition and blood metabolite levels in the dog, *J Nutr* 106:1452–1464, 1976.

54. Romsos DR, Hornshus MJ, Leveille GA: Influence of dietary fat and carbohydrate on food intake, body weight and body fat of adult dogs, *Proc Soc Exp Biol Med* 157:278–281, 1978.

55. Gerstein D, Woodward-Lappel G: Clarifying concepts about macronutrients' effects on satiation and satiety, *J Am Diet Assoc* 104:1151–1153, 2004.

56. Torres CL, Hickenbottom SJ, Rogers QR: Palatability affects the percentage of metabolizable energy as protein selected by adult Beagles, *J Nutr* 133:3516–3522, 2003.

57. Cook N, Kane E: Self-selection of dietary casein and soy protein by the cat, *Physiol Behav* 34:583–594, 1985.

58. Kienzle E, Rainbird A: Maintenance energy requirement of dogs: what is the correct value for the calculation of metabolic body weight in dogs? *Am J Clin Nutr* 121:S39–S40, 1991.

59. Earle KE: Calculations of energy requirements of dogs, cats and small psittacine birds, *J Small Anim Pract* 34:163–173, 1993.

60. Allard RL, Douglass GM, Kerr WW: The effects of breed and sex on dog growth, *Compan Anim Pract* 2:15–19, 1988.

61. Rainbird A, Kienzle E: Investigations on energy requirements of dogs in relation to breed and age, *Kleintierpraxis* 35:145–158, 1990.

62. Meyer H, Zentek J: Body composition of newborn puppies and nutrient requirements of pregnant bitches, *Adv Anim Physiol Anim Nutr* 16:7–25, 1985.

63. Scantlebury M, Butterwick R, Speakman JR: Energetics of lactation in the domestic dog (*Canis familiaris*) breeds of two sizes, *Compar Biochem Physiol-Part A* 125:197–210, 2000.

64. Blaza SE: Energy requirements of dogs in cold conditions, *Canine Pract* 9:10–15, 1982.

65. Earle KE, Smith PM: Digestible energy requirements of adult cats at maintenance, *J Nutr* 121:S45–S46, 1991.

66. Nguyen PH, Dumon R, Frenais B, and others: Energy expenditure and requirement assessed using three different methods in adult cats, *Compend Contin Educ Pract Vet* 23(9A):86, 2001.

67. Wichert B, Muller L, Gebert S, and others: Additional data on energy requirements of young adult cats measured by indirect calorimetry, *J Anim Phys Anim Nutr* 91:278–281, 2007.

68. Laflamme DP, Ballam JM: Effect of age on maintenance energy requirements of adult cats. In *Proc Purina Nutr Forum*, St Louis, 2001.

69. Taylor EJ, Adams C, Neville R: Some nutritional aspects of ageing in dogs and cats, *Proc Nutr Soc* 54:645–656, 1995.

70. Martin L, Siliart B, Bumon H, and others: Leptin, body fat content and energy expenditure in intact and gonadectomized adult cats: a preliminary study, *J Anim Physiol Anim Nutr* 85:195–199, 2001.

71. Loveridge GG, Rivers JPW: Body weight changes and energy intakes of cats during pregnancy and lactation. In Burger IH, Rivers JPW, editors: *Nutrition of the dog and cat*, New York, 1989, Cambridge University Press.

72. Danowski TS, Elkinton JR, Winkler AW: The deleterious effect in dogs of a dry protein ration, *J Clin Invest* 23:816–823, 1944.

73. Prentiss PG, Wolf AV, Eddy HE: Hydropenia in the cat and dog: ability of the cat to meet its water requirements solely from a diet of fish or meat, *Am J Physiol* 196:625–632, 1959.

74. Schaer M: General principles of fluid therapy in small animal medicine, *Vet Clin North Am Small Anim Pract* 19:203–213, 1989.

75. Seefeldt SL, Chapman TE: Body water content and turnover in cats fed dry and canned rations, *Am J Vet Res* 40:183–185, 1979.

76. Anderson RS: Water balance in the dog and cat, *J Small Anim Pract* 23:588–598, 1982.

10

Carbohydrate Metabolism

All animals have a metabolic requirement for glucose. This requirement can be supplied either through endogenous synthesis or from dietary sources of carbohydrate. Gluconeogenic pathways in the liver and kidneys use propionic acid, lactic acid, glycerol, and certain amino acids to produce glucose, which is then released into the bloodstream to be carried to the body's tissues.

DIETARY REQUIREMENT FOR CARBOHYDRATE

The dog is capable of meeting its metabolic requirement for glucose from gluconeogenic pathways throughout growth and adult maintenance, provided that sufficient fat and protein are included in the diet.[1] However, the need for an exogenous source of carbohydrate during the metabolically stressful periods of gestation and lactation has been debated. During gestation the female dog's needs increase because glucose provides a major energy source for fetal development. Similarly, during lactation, additional glucose is needed for the synthesis of lactose, the disaccharide present in milk. It is assumed that the female cat's glucose requirement also increases during these physiological periods.

An early study with dogs examined the degree of reproductive success in females that were fed diets with varying levels of carbohydrates.[2] The data indicated that pregnant dogs did require a source of carbohydrate to whelp and rear healthy puppies. Dogs that had been fed a carbohydrate-free diet throughout gestation became hypoglycemic and ketotic near the end of their pregnancies, and also showed reduced blood concentrations of the amino acid alanine. Only 63% of their puppies were alive at birth, and puppy mortality was high shortly after birth. However, these results were subsequently refuted by data from a second study that also examined the effects of feeding a carbohydrate-free diet to female dogs throughout gestation and lactation.[3] These data indicated that a carbohydrate-free diet did not affect duration of gestation, litter size, litter weight,

or puppy viability. Ultimately, the difference in the results of the two experiments was attributed to differences in the protein levels of the diets that were fed. The diet in the first study contained only 26% protein, compared with 51% and 45% protein diets in the second set of experiments. Feeding a higher protein diet provides sufficient amounts of gluconeogenic amino acids to allow the maintenance of plasma glucose levels despite the heavy demands of gestation and lactation. Alanine, glycine, and serine appear to be the principal gluconeogenic amino acids in dogs.[4] The reduced blood levels of alanine exhibited by the dogs in the first study suggest that insufficient alanine was available to allow adequate gluconeogenesis. The hypoglycemia observed in these dogs was probably a result of the lack of gluconeogenic precursors rather than an innate inability to synthesize sufficient glucose during gestation and lactation.

These results were further supported by a study that examined the ability of varying levels of dietary protein to ameliorate the effects of carbohydrate-free diets on gestation and lactation.[5] These data confirmed that feeding carbohydrate-free diets to pregnant and lactating dogs can cause adverse effects. However, performance was not impaired when the protein level in the diet was sufficiently high. The investigators estimated that if carbohydrate is provided in the diet, female dogs require about 7 grams (g) of digestible crude protein per unit of metabolic body weight. However, if no carbohydrate is supplied in the diet, this protein requirement must be increased to approximately 12 g of protein. Lactating females appear to require between 13 and 18 g of protein per unit of metabolic weight when fed a diet containing carbohydrate and 30 g when fed a carbohydrate-free diet. This information indicates that although glucose is a metabolically essential nutrient for the dog, carbohydrates are not an indispensable component of the diet, even during the metabolically demanding stages of gestation and lactation. Although specific studies have not been conducted during pregnancy and lactation in the cat, this species' unique pattern of gluconeogenesis, coupled with its carnivorous nature, suggests that it too can survive all stages of life while consuming a carbohydrate-free diet.

> *Although glucose is a metabolically essential nutrient for the dog and the cat, digestible carbohydrates are not an indispensable component of the diet. Dogs, and probably cats, can synthesize adequate glucose from gluconeogenic pathways to meet their metabolic needs throughout life, provided that sufficient protein is included in the diet to supply gluconeogenic amino acids.*

CARBOHYDRATE METABOLISM IN CATS

Compared with the dog and other omnivorous species, the cat has several unique mechanisms for metabolizing dietary carbohydrate. The cat's ability to maintain normal blood glucose levels and health when fed a carbohydrate-free diet is partly related to its unique pattern of gluconeogenesis. In most animals, maximal gluconeogenesis for the maintenance of blood glucose levels occurs during the postabsorptive state, when dietary soluble carbohydrate is no longer available. However, carnivorous species are similar to ruminant species in that they maintain a constant state of gluconeogenesis with a slightly increased rate immediately after feeding.[6] Because the body is limited in its ability to conserve amino acids, and a carnivorous diet typically contains little soluble carbohydrate, the immediate use of gluconeogenic amino acids for the maintenance of blood glucose levels is an adaptive advantage.

The enzyme activity values in the cat's liver indicate that gluconeogenic amino acids in the diet are deaminated and converted to glucose, rather than being directly oxidized for energy.[7] Liver phosphoenolpyruvate carboxykinase (PEPCK), a major gluconeogenic enzyme, does not change in activity level when cats that were previously fed high-protein diets are subjected to fasting.[8] In addition, no significant changes in hepatic PEPCK activity occur when cats are switched from a low-protein diet (17.5%) to a high-protein diet (70%).[9]

These data support the supposition that the hepatic gluconeogenic enzymes in cats always have a high rate of activity, necessitating the rapid conversion of excess dietary amino acids to glucose. This lack of enzymatic adaptation to change in dietary protein concentration is also seen in other carnivorous species, including trout, vultures, and barn owls.[10-12]

There are also differences between cats and omnivores in the relative importance of various gluconeogenic and carbohydrate-metabolizing pathways. Compared with omnivorous species, the cat has a high hepatic activity of the enzyme serine-pyruvate aminotransferase and low activity of the enzyme serine dehydratase.[9,13] It appears that the cat is able to convert the amino acid serine to glucose by a route that does not involve either pyruvate or serine dehydratase. An alternative pathway has been proposed for the conversion of serine to glucose.[14] It has been observed that a high activity of the first enzyme in this alternative pathway, serine-pyruvate aminotransferase, appears to be associated with carnivorous dietary habits in mammals.

After glucose is absorbed into the body, it must be phosphorylated to glucose-6-phosphate before it can be metabolized. The liver of most omnivorous animals, including the domestic dog, has two primary enzymes that catalyze this reaction: glucokinase and hexokinase. Hexokinase is active when low levels of glucose are delivered to the liver, and glucokinase operates whenever the liver receives a large load of glucose from the portal vein. The cat's liver has active hexokinase but has minimally active glucokinase.[15] The hepatic glucokinase that is present functions at a very low rate, and its activity cannot be up-regulated in response to a large intake of carbohydrate. Interestingly, recent studies show that, compared with dogs, the activity of feline hepatic hexokinase and two other glycolytic enzymes, phosphofructokinase and pyruvate kinase, are relatively high.[16] It is possible that the high activity rates of these enzymes compensate for the low activity of glucokinase in the cat's liver. Cats also show minimal activity of hepatic glycogen synthetase, an enzyme essential for converting glucose to glycogen for storage in the liver.[17] Together these metabolic patterns may limit the cat's ability to rapidly minimize the hyperglycemia that occurs after a large dietary glucose load. Conversely, the cat's carbohydrate-metabolizing enzyme patterns support an ability to maintain normal blood glucose levels through the consistent delivery of glucose via gluconeogenic catabolism of amino acids.

As obligate carnivores, cats possess several unique metabolic adaptations that allow them to maintain normal blood glucose concentrations through the consistent delivery of glucose via the gluconeogenic catabolism of amino acids.

UTILIZATION OF DIETARY CARBOHYDRATE

The fact that dogs and cats do not require carbohydrate in their diets is usually immaterial because most commercial foods include at least a moderate level of this nutrient. In general, dry pet foods contain the highest amount of carbohydrate. Commercial dry foods may include up to 60% carbohydrate, and canned foods contain anywhere between 0% and 30% (as-fed basis). The largest proportion of carbohydrate in pet foods is provided by starch (nonstructural polysaccharides). Pancreatic amylases are the major enzymes involved in the digestion of amylase, amylopectin, and maltodextrins. Although the activity of pancreatic amylase is higher in dogs than in cats, both dogs and cats efficiently digest cooked starch.[18-20] Dietary starch provides an economical and digestible energy source, and it is also essential for the extrusion process used in the preparation of most dry pet foods. The digestibility and utilization of dietary starch by dogs and cats is affected by several factors, including the type of starch, degree of heat treatment, and size of the starch granules. Heating greatly increases digestibility, and finely ground starch is more digestible than coarsely ground granules.[18,21]

Although cooked starch provides an excellent energy source, certain individual disaccharides, such as sucrose and lactose, are not well tolerated by pets. An animal's ability to digest and use these sugars is governed by the levels and activities of sucrase (beta-fructofuranosidase) and lactase (beta-galactosidase) found in the cells of the intestinal lumen. As in most species, the activity of lactase in dogs and cats is high early in life and decreases with age.[18] Queen's milk contains approximately 3% to

5% lactose, which provides about 20% of its metabolizable energy (ME).[22] Although kittens can digest this high level of lactose, some adult cats develop diarrhea when consuming high levels of lactose. As a result of a loss of lactase activity with age, feeding adult companion animals large amounts of milk or other dairy products often results in maldigestion. Small quantities of these foods can be digested by most pets, but large quantities cause diarrhea because of the osmotic effect of the sugar that escapes digestion and the volatile fatty acids that are produced by bacterial fermentation of the sugar in the large intestine. In addition, adult cats have low intestinal activity of sucrase, suggesting limited capacity to digest sucrose (table sugar).[23] Although it has not been demonstrated in puppies and kittens, data from other species indicate that very young animals have low levels of sucrase activity during the first few weeks of life. For this reason, sucrose solutions should not be used as energy sources for very young or orphaned puppies and kittens.

As dogs and cats reach maturity, their ability to digest milk and other dairy products decreases because of decreased lactase activity in the intestinal mucosa. Similarly, it is thought that very young animals have low levels of sucrase, which indicates that oral sucrose solutions are not recommended for very young or orphaned puppies and kittens.

Fiber is the other carbohydrate component commonly present in pet foods. Although dietary fiber is not a required nutrient per se, the inclusion of optimal amounts of fiber in the diets of companion animals is necessary for normal functioning and health of the gastrointestinal tract. Nonfermentable fiber functions to increase the bulk of the diet, contributes to satiety, and maintains normal intestinal transit time and gastrointestinal tract motility. Fermentable fibers have varying effects upon gastric emptying, and their fermentation by colonic bacteria produces short-chain fatty acids (SCFAs) that are important energy sources for colonocytes, the mucosal cells of the colon (see Section 5, pp. 465-467 for a complete discussion). Common sources of dietary fiber in pet foods include tomato, citrus, and grape pomace; beet pulp; powdered cellulose, pea fiber, and the hulls of soybeans and peanuts. Corn, rice, wheat, oats, and barley all contribute digestible carbohydrates and supply small amounts of dietary fiber, as do various types of vegetables that are used with increasing frequency in commercial pet foods. In addition, protein sources in cereal-based pet foods add varying amounts of dietary fiber to the ration. The amount of fiber in pet foods varies with the type of food and the ingredients that are included (see Chapter 16).

References

1. Romsos DR, Belo PS, Bennink MR, and others: Effects of dietary carbohydrate, fat and protein on growth, body composition and blood metabolite levels in the dog, *J Nutr* 106:1452–1464, 1976.

2. Romsos DR, Palmer HJ, Muiruri KL, and others: Influence of a low carbohydrate diet on performance of pregnant and lactating dogs, *J Nutr* 111:678–689, 1981.

3. Blaza SE, Booles D, Burger IH: Is carbohydrate essential for pregnancy and lactation in dogs? In Burger IH, Rivers JPW, editors: *Nutrition of the cat and dog*, New York, 1989, Cambridge University Press.

4. Brady LJ, Armstrong MK, Muriuri KL, and others: Influence of prolonged fasting in the dog on glucose turnover and blood metabolites, *J Nutr* 107:1053–1061, 1977.

5. Kienzle E, Meyer H: The effects of carbohydrate-free diets containing different levels of protein on reproduction in the bitch. In Burger IH, Rivers JPW, editors: *Nutrition of the dog and cat*, New York, 1989, Cambridge University Press.

6. Morris JG, Rogers QR: Nutritionally related metabolic adaptations of carnivores and ruminants. In *International symposium on plant, animal and microbial adaptations to terrestrial environments, man and the biosphere*, Halkidiki, Greece, 1982.

7. Beliveau GP, Freedland RA: Metabolism of serine, glycine and threonine in isolated cat hepatocytes (*Felis domestica*), *Comp Biochem Physiol* 71B:13–18, 1982.

8. Kettlehut IC, Foss MC, Migliorini RH: Glucose homeostasis in a carnivorous animal (cat) and in rats fed a high-protein diet, *Am J Physiol* 239:R115–R121, 1978.

9. Rogers QR, Morris JG, Freedland RA: Lack of hepatic enzymatic adaptation to low and high levels of dietary protein in the adult cat, *Enzyme* 22:348–356, 1977.

10. Cowey CB, Cooke DJ, Maty AJ, Adron JW: Effects of quantity and quality of dietary protein on certain enzyme activities of rainbow trout, *J Nutr* 111:336–345, 1981.

11. Migliorini RH, Linder C, Moura JL, and others: Gluconeogenesis in a carnivorous bird (black vulture), *Am J Physiol* 225:1389–1392, 1973.

12. Myers MR, Klasing KC: Low glucokinase activity and high rates of gluconeogenesis contribute to hyperglycemia in barn owls (*Tyto alba*) after a glucose challenge, *J Nutr* 129:1896–1904, 1999.

13. Rowsell EV, Carnie JA, Wahbi SD, and others: L-serine dehydratase and L-serine-pyruvate aminotransferase activities in different animal species, *Comp Biochem Physiol* 63:543–555, 1979.

14. Morris JG, Rogers QR: Metabolic basis for some of the nutritional peculiarities of the cat, *J Small Anim Pract* 23:599–613, 1982.

15. Ballard FJ: Glucose utilization in mammalian liver, *Comp Biochem Physiol* 14:437–443, 1965.

16. Washizu T, Tanaka A, Sako T, and others: Comparison of the activities of enzymes related to glycolysis and gluconeogenesis in the liver of dogs and cats, *Res Vet Sci* 67:203–204, 1999.

17. Zoran DL: The carnivore connection to nutrition in cats, *J Am Vet Med Assoc* 221:1559–1567, 2002.

18. Morris JG, Trudell J, Pencovic T: Carbohydrate digestion by the domestic cat (*Felis catus*), *Br J Nutr* 37:365–373, 1977.

19. Kienzle E: Carbohydrate metabolism in the cat. 1. Activity of amylase in the gastrointestinal tract of the cat, *J Anim Physiol Anim Nutr* 69:92–101, 1994.

20. Kienzle E: Carbohydrate metabolism in the cat. 2. Digestion of starch, *J Anim Physiol Anim Nutr* 69:102–114, 1994.

21. De Wilde RO, Jansen T: The use of different sources of raw and heated starch in the ration of weaned kittens. In Burger IH, Rivers JPW, editors: *Nutrition of the cat and dog*, New York, 1989, Cambridge University Press.

22. Keen CL, Lonnerdal B, Clegg MS, and others: Developmental changes in composition of cats' milk: trace elements, minerals, protein, carbohydrate and fat, *J Nutr* 112:1763–1769, 1982.

23. Meyer H, Kienzle E: Dietary protein and carbohydrates: relationship to clinical disease. In *Proceedings of the Purina international nutrition symposium*, Orlando, Fla, 1991.

11

Fat Requirements

FAT AS AN ENERGY SOURCE

The dietary fat requirement of dogs and cats depends on the animal's need for energy (calories) and for essential fatty acids (EFAs). Dietary fat contributes more than twice the amount of metabolizable energy (ME) per unit weight than does protein or carbohydrate and is also a highly digestible nutrient. The apparent digestibility of most fats included in pet foods is typically 90% or higher.[1-3] Because of its high energy content and digestibility, increasing the level of fat in a pet's diet appreciably increases energy density. Both dogs and cats are able to maintain health when consuming diets that contain wide ranges of fat content, provided that other nutrients are adjusted to account for the changes in energy density. Because animals normally eat or are fed to meet their energy needs, consumption of a more energy-dense ration will result in decreased consumption of the total volume of food. Therefore, if nutrients are not adjusted in relation to fat, nutrient deficiencies can result.

Dietary fat provides a concentrated source of energy that is highly digestible. Dogs and cats can thrive on foods containing a wide range of fat content, provided that other nutrients are adjusted to account for the changes in energy density.

Periods of high energy demand in dogs and cats occur during growth, gestation, lactation, and prolonged periods of physical exercise. Feeding an energy-dense, high-fat diet during these periods can allow an animal to consume adequate calories without having to ingest excessive amounts of dry matter (DM). In addition, feeding a diet containing a sufficient concentration of dietary fat during strenuous physical work may have metabolic benefits. Fatty acids are the primary source of energy used by the body during prolonged physical exertion. Studies of dogs engaging in endurance events

such as long-distance sled races have found that the consumption of a high-fat diet enhances dogs' ability to use fatty acids for energy, which can ultimately contribute to improved performance[4,5] (see Chapter 24, pp. 245-248 for a complete discussion).

However, most adult pets today live relatively sedentary lifestyles and do not need foods containing high concentrations of fat. Although high-fat pet foods are capable of providing good nutrition and supporting optimal health, sedentary animals may be inclined to overconsume these diets because of their high palatability and energy density. If adult pets are fed performance diets, strict portion-controlled feeding should be used to prevent excessive energy consumption and weight gain. Likewise, feeding high-fat, energy-dense foods during periods of rapid growth must be strictly monitored. This is especially important for large and giant breeds of dog because high-fat (energy-dense) foods that are balanced for all essential nutrients are capable of supporting a high rate of growth if they are fed *ad libitum*. Maximal growth rate has been shown to be incompatible with proper skeletal development in dogs and is a risk factor for the development of several skeletal disorders. Portion-controlled feeding should therefore be used to control a growing pet's weight gain, rate of growth, and body condition (see Section 4, pp. 231-233, and Section 5, pp. 496-497).

FAT AS A SOURCE OF ESSENTIAL FATTY ACIDS

In addition to providing energy, fat is necessary in the diet of dogs and cats as a source of the EFAs. Two families of fatty acid are essential: the omega-6 (n-6) and the omega-3 (n-3) fatty acids. The n-6 fatty acids have their first carbon double bond located at the sixth position on the carbon chain from the methyl end and the n-3 fatty acids have the first double bond located at the third carbon position (see Chapter 3, p. 19). The parental forms of the n-6 and n-3 families are linoleic acid and alpha-linolenic acid, respectively. Linoleic acid is comprised of an 18-carbon chain and has two double bonds (18:2n-6), and alpha-linolenic acid is the same length, but contains three double bonds (18:3n-3). Both of these fatty acids can be converted in the body to other long-chain polyunsaturated fatty acids (LCP-UFA) through elongation and desaturation reactions.

The LCPUFAs of greatest physiological importance are arachidonic acid (AA), synthesized from linoleic acid, and eicosapentaenoic acid (EPA) and docosahexaenoic acid (DHA), produced from alpha-linolenic acid (see Chapter 31, Figure 31-3, p. 388). During metabolism, the n-6 and n-3 families compete for the same enzymes and metabolic pathways, although their end products differ. Because of the basic difference in the location of the first double bond, interconversion between the two families of fatty acids is not possible. Therefore dietary requirements for linoleic acid (n-6) and alpha-linolenic acid (n-3) and their respective derivative LCPUFAs must be addressed distinctly, and the competitive relationship between the two families of fatty acids must always be considered when examining dietary effects of EFAs.

Two key liver enzymes involved in the production of LCPUFAs are delta-6-desaturase and delta-5-desaturase. In dogs, as in humans, the rate of conversion of the parent fatty acid to other LCPUFAs is regulated by delta-6-desaturase. This enzyme functions at a high enough rate to provide dogs with adequate quantities of AA to meet needs when dietary linoleic acid is present.[6] In addition, adult dogs are capable of converting alpha-linolenic to both EPA and to a precursor of DHA, docosapentaenoic acid (DPA), although at relatively low rates of conversion.[7] There is evidence that the DPA that is produced in the liver of dogs and cats from alpha-linolenic acid is transported to target tissues such as the retina, where it is converted to DHA.[8,9] As a result, the adult dog does not have a dietary maintenance requirement for AA and probably does not require EPA or DHA, provided that adequate levels of linoleic acid and alpha-linolenic acid are provided in the diet. Conversely, there is evidence that adequate EPA and DHA may be necessary for healthy reproductive performance in dogs (see below).

In contrast, cats are rather unusual in that the rate of delta-6-desaturase activity in the feline liver is limited, leading to reduced production of LCPUFAs from parent fatty acids.[10,11] This imposes a greater dependency on dietary sources of AA (and possibly also upon EPA and DHA) upon the cat. Early studies reported that when linoleic acid but not AA was included in the diet, cats developed impaired platelet aggregation and thrombocytopenia, and queens failed to deliver viable kittens.[12,13] However, the male cat's reproductive performance was not impaired by a lack of dietary AA. This difference was attributed to the testes' ability to produce adequate AA from linoleic acid for its own use. More recent studies confirmed that adult male cats do not demonstrate a dietary requirement for AA, and further examined the needs of reproducing females.[14] These results suggest that like males, female cats do not typically require a dietary source of AA for initial reproductive success. However, a dietary source of AA may be needed for healthy litters in queens that experience multiple pregnancies. These studies suggest that while adult cats have less capacity for producing AA than do adult dogs, they are still able to synthesize adequate amounts to meet their needs during normal adult maintenance. The degree to which adult cats are capable of converting alpha-linolenic acid to its derivative LCPUFAs has not been studied in detail. However, one study of the effects of dietary fatty acids on skin and plasma fatty acid profiles provided evidence that suggested negligible conversion of alpha-linolenic acid to EPA or DHA in cats.[15]

Finally, it is known that EFA status of the body is negatively influenced by the physiological stress of pregnancy and lactation.[16] Recent studies with dogs have shown that reproducing female dogs develop reduced EFA status and these changes are exacerbated with increasing number of litters.[17] Specifically, increased EFAs are needed during gestation and lactation to supply fetal tissues with EFAs through the placenta and after birth through the milk. Of particular importance to reproducing females and their developing fetuses is DHA, which is needed for normal neurological and retinal development in puppies and kittens (see Chapter 22, pp. 228-229 for a complete discussion).[18] Because females have limited ability to enrich their milk with DHA and EPA from dietary alpha-linolenic acid, the best way to supply developing fetuses and neonates with needed LCPUFAs is through dietary enrichment of the mother's diet with these fatty acids during pregnancy and lactation.[19,20] In addition, recent evidence shows that, similar to humans and other species, newborn puppies can convert milk alpha-linolenic acid to DHA early in life, but they lose this ability after the neonatal stage of life.[21,22] The minimum amount of alpha-linolenic acid that is needed to supply adequate DHA for the neonate is not known and requires further study. Therefore, while dietary n-6 and n-3 LCPUFAs are probably not required by either dogs or cats during adult maintenance, increased demands occur during early development, growth, gestation, and lactation to make these LCPUFAs conditionally essential.[23]

Increased essential fatty acids (EFAs) are needed during gestation and lactation to supply fetal tissues with EFAs through the placenta and after birth through the milk. Of particular importance to reproducing females and fetuses is docosahexaenoic acid, which is needed for normal neurological and retinal development in puppies and kittens. The best way to supply the needed long-chain polyunsaturated fatty acids is through dietary enrichment of the mother's diet with these fatty acids during pregnancy and lactation.

FUNCTIONS OF ESSENTIAL FATTY ACIDS FOR DOGS AND CATS

Most mammals, including dogs and cats, are capable of synthesizing the nonessential 16- and 18-carbon fatty acids from glucose or amino acids. These fatty acids belong to two families, the n-7 and n-9 fatty acids, and are produced in highest quantities when an animal is fed a low-fat diet. Alternatively, when fed a diet containing adequate fat, animals preferentially use the fatty acids provided by the diet to meet their needs. The two 18-carbon EFAs, linoleic acid (n-6) and alpha-linolenic acid (n-3) are synthesized by terrestrial plants, while marine plants are capable of inserting further double bonds and elongating these carbon chains to produce the n-3 LCPUFAs. However, no plants are capable of producing AA from linoleic acid. As a result, AA is found only in animal tissues. Each of the EFAs and those that are classified as conditionally essential have important roles in cell membranes, the immune system,

and the circulatory system. Because of the competition between linoleic acid and alpha-linolenic acid for the same metabolic pathways, the effects of these fatty acids will be influenced by both their absolute quantities in the diet and by their relative levels to each other.

Linoleic Acid and Arachidonic Acid

Linoleic acid has essential functions in maintaining the epidermal water barrier of the skin. It is incorporated into a fraction of cellular phospholipids in the epidermal keratinocytes called *ceramides*. Ceramides are extruded from keratinocytes into the intercellular spaces as lamellar granules and function to enhance cell cohesion and create an effective water barrier.[24] Linoleic acid's important role in skin health is reflected in the changes to skin and coat that are seen during EFA deficiency. Linoleic acid is also important as a precursor of the LCPUFAs that are incorporated into cell membranes in the form of phospholipids and other lipid components. These function to maintain normal membrane fluidity, structure, and function. The type of fatty acids that predominate in a cell membrane differs among cell types and is also influenced by the fatty acid composition of the diet. The n-6 fatty acids that are derived from linoleic acid are found as storage fatty acids in adipose tissue, and in liver, kidney, and muscle cells. Linoleic acid–derived fatty acids found in cell membranes also have interactive roles with regulatory proteins that are important for cell metabolism and signaling.

The most important LCPUFA produced from linoleic acid is AA, which is a major cell membrane fatty acid and a precursor of certain types of eicosanoids. The eicosanoids are a diverse group of 20-carbon substances that are produced and released from cell membranes in response to physical or chemical trauma and that have local effects upon immune and inflammatory responses. The four primary types of eicosanoids are the prostaglandins, prostacyclins, thromboxanes, and leukotrienes. AA, which generally comprises more than 20% of the total fatty acids in cell membrane phospholipids in the skin, is converted to prostaglandins of the 2 series (prostaglandin E_2) and leukotrienes of the 4 series (leukotriene B_4). These eicosanoids are proinflammatory and are important mediators of inflammatory and allergic responses (see Chapter 31, pp. 386-395 for a complete discussion).

Arachidonic acid, produced from linoleic acid, is a major cell membrane fatty acid and a precursor of certain types of eicosanoids. The eicosanoids are 20-carbon substances that are released from cell membranes in response to physical or chemical trauma and have local effects on immune and inflammatory responses. The four primary types of eicosanoids are the prostaglandins, prostacyclins, thromboxanes, and leukotrienes.

Alpha-Linolenic Acid, EPA, and DHA

Alpha-linolenic acid does not appear to have direct functions itself, although there is evidence that it may contribute to a healthy transepidermal water barrier.[25,26] This effect is attributed to alpha-linolenic acid providing a sparing effect for linoleic acid as a source of LCPUFAs, which allows increased accumulation of linoleic acid in ceramide fractions of the skin. The primary role of alpha-linolenic acid is as the parent fatty acid for the synthesis of EPA and DHA. EPA is incorporated into cell membranes and, like AA, serves as a precursor for the eicosanoids. Important eicosanoids produced from EPA are prostaglandins of the 3 series (prostaglandin E_3) and leukotrienes of the 5 series (leukotriene B_5). These eicosanoids are less potent mediators of inflammation than those produced from AA and can effectively reduce inflammatory and allergic responses when they replace AA. This is the basis for the use of n-3 fatty acids in the management of certain inflammatory skin diseases and other inflammatory disorders (see Section 5, pp. 386-396 for complete discussions).

DHA is found in large amounts in the cell membranes of neurological tissues and is one of the most abundant fatty acids found in the retina. It is essential for normal neurological and visual development during fetal and neonatal life. Alpha-linolenic acid can be converted to DHA in very young animals and less efficiently in adults. There is also evidence that adult dogs are capable of converting dietary alpha-linolenic acid to an intermediate fatty acid, DPA, which is found in circulating plasma phospholipids.[22] The canine retina is capable of converting DPA to DHA, and it is theorized that circulating DPA produced in the liver provides the substrate for this conversion. Similarly, adult cats are able to convert small amounts of alpha-linolenic acid to EPA and DPA in the liver and feline neurological tissue appears to be able to convert DPA to DHA.[27] Therefore, dietary alpha-linolenic acid may provide a source of retinal and nerve tissue DHA, although it is not known if amounts that are converted can meet physiological needs throughout life. Providing at least small amounts of dietary DHA may be a more effective way of meeting requirements, at least during fetal growth and early in life.

DIETARY FAT AND ESSENTIAL FATTY ACID REQUIREMENTS

Dogs

Although there is not an absolute requirement for dietary fat per se, fat is needed in the diet to provide EFAs and energy and to enhance diet palatability. A minimum amount of dietary fat is also needed as a carrier for the fat-soluble vitamins. Most dry dog foods that are marketed for adult maintenance contain between 5% and 13% fat (DM basis). In comparison, the fat content of dry dog foods that are formulated for gestation, lactation, or performance may be 20% or greater. The current Association of American Feed Control Officials' (AAFCO's) *Nutrient Profiles* minimum fat recommendations are 5% for adult maintenance and 8% for growth and reproduction (DM basis) provided in a food containing 3500 kcal/kg.[28] An adult dog maintenance food should also provide a minimum of 1% of the food's dry weight as linoleic acid.

Although a requirement for alpha-linolenic acid has not been established for dogs, a minimum requirement of approximately 0.044% DM (or 0.09% ME) in foods containing approximately 1% linoleic acid is suggested.[23] Because the n-3 and n-6 fatty acids compete for metabolic pathways, the amount of alpha-linolenic acid in the food must always be determined relative to the level of linoleic acid. If the linoleic acid content of the food is higher than 1%, alpha-linolenic acid should also be increased to maintain an appropriate balance between the two families of fatty acids. The current

National Research Council (NRC) recommends that a ratio of linoleic acid to alpha-linolenic acid of between 2.6 and 26 should be maintained in all foods. Although EPA and DHA are considered to be conditionally essential during certain stages of life for dogs, a minimum dietary requirement for these LCPUFAs has not been established for dogs. The current NRC provides an adequate intake (AI) estimate of 0.11 g of EPA and DHA combined per 1000 kcal of diet.[23]

Cats

A minimum level of fat is needed in the cat's diet for the same purposes as with dogs. Also similar to dogs, cats are capable of thriving on a relatively wide range of dietary fat, provided the diet includes proper levels of all essential nutrients. In general, cat foods contain slightly higher amounts of dietary fat than do most dog foods. For example, dry maintenance cat foods contain between 8% and 13% fat (DM basis). The current AAFCO's *Nutrient Profiles* minimum fat recommendation for cats during all life stages is 9% in a food containing 4000 kcal/kg.[28]

Exact estimates for the EFA requirement in cats are difficult to make because adequate levels of linoleic acid in the diet decrease the cat's requirement for AA, and high levels of AA can meet some of the needs for linoleic acid.[29] In addition, recent evidence suggests that most adult cats do not have a dietary requirement for AA and are capable of synthesizing adequate levels from dietary linoleic acid. The AAFCO's Nutrient Profiles for cat foods recommends 0.5% linoleic acid and 0.02% AA in diets containing 4000 kcal of ME/kg. The current NRC provides similar estimates along with the caveat that the AA recommendation is a presumed adequate intake rather than a minimum requirement for adult maintenance.[23] Similar to dogs, requirements have not been established for alpha-linolenic acid or for any of its LCPUFA derivatives for the cat. The NRC provides an AI estimate of 0.1 g of EPA and DHA combined per 1000 g diet in a food containing 4000 kcal/g.[23]

DEFICIENCIES AND EXCESSES

Low amounts of fat in the diet can lead to deficiencies in both total energy and EFAs. In addition, the palatability of dog and cat diets is strongly affected by fat content. To a limit, increasing fat results in enhanced palatability. Similarly, decreasing fat below a certain level causes decreased acceptability of the diet. This effect is believed to be the result of both the texture and the flavor that fat contributes to a pet food. Because low-fat diets may not be readily accepted by pets, their potential for causing an energy or EFA deficiency is exacerbated by their causing a decrease in food intake.

Because linoleic acid is important for the maintenance of the epidermal water barrier, and because skin cells have a high rate of turnover, the skin is particularly vulnerable to EFA deficiencies. In dogs, linoleic acid deficiency results in a dry, dull coat; hair loss; skin lesions; and poor wound healing. Over time, the skin becomes pruritic, greasy, and susceptible to infection. A change in the surface lipids in the skin alters the normal bacterial flora and can predispose the animal to secondary bacterial infections.[30] Epidermal peeling, interdigital exudation, and otitis externa have also been reported in EFA-deficient dogs.[31] Linoleic acid deficiency in cats results in similar dermatological signs. In addition, kittens will fail to grow normally, and may develop fatty degeneration of the liver and fat deposition in the kidneys.[32,33]

Although not reported in dogs and cats, deficiency signs of n-3 fatty acids in other species include nervous system abnormalities, decreased visual acuity, retinal abnormalities, and reductions in learning and memory.[34,35] These signs reflect the high concentrations of n-3 LCPUFAs found in the brain and retinal rod cells of most species and the importance of these fatty acids during early development. Although signs of n-3 EFA deficiency have not been reported in dogs and cats, the high concentrations of DHA in nervous and retinal tissues and high demands during reproduction and early development suggest that deficiencies in dogs and cats would produce similar signs.

Today, overt EFA deficiencies are not common in dogs and cats. When they do occur, deficiencies are usually associated with the consumption of diets that are either poorly formulated or have been stored improperly. Most well-formulated diets contain sufficient amounts of EFAs. However, exposure to high environmental temperatures and humidity for long periods can promote oxidation of the unsaturated fatty acids in the food. This process is commonly referred to as *rancidity*. If insufficient antioxidants are present, EFA activity is destroyed. As the unsaturated fats are destroyed by oxidation, not only is EFA activity lost, but so are the vitamins D, E, and biotin. EFA deficiency in dogs and cats can also occur as a complication of other diseases, such as pancreatitis, biliary disease, hepatic disease, and malabsorption.

Although uncommon, essential fatty acid (EFA) deficiency results in a dry, dull coat; hair loss; skin lesions; and poor wound healing. Over time, the skin becomes pruritic, greasy, and susceptible to infection. A change in the surface lipids in the skin alters the normal bacterial flora and can predispose the animal to secondary bacterial infections. EFA deficiency can result from feeding poorly formulated or rancid foods, but it can occur secondary to pancreatitis, biliary disease, hepatic disease, or malabsorption.

Although commercially prepared foods will not normally cause fat or EFA deficiency, many pet owners believe that supplementing their pet's diet with corn oil or some other type of fat will improve coat quality. This will only be effective if the pet is truly suffering from an EFA or fat deficiency. If that is the case, completely changing the diet to a well-formulated pet food that supplies all of the essential nutrients in their correct proportions, including fat and EFAs, is recommended. Simply adding a source of fat or EFAs to a deficient diet without assessing levels of both n-3 and n-6 fatty acids in the diet may or may not solve the EFA deficit and has the potential to further imbalance a food that is already inadequate. Conversely, fatty acid supplementation or altering the fatty acid levels or ratios in the diet can be effective in treating certain inflammatory and hyperproliferative skin diseases in companion animals. Recent research indicates that modifying the fatty acid profile of the diet can promote the formation of fewer inflammatory agents, resulting in a reduction in clinical signs (see Section 5, pp. 386-395 for a complete discussion).

Excess fat intake can also be detrimental to a pet's health. As stated previously, dogs and cats are able to digest and assimilate diets containing high levels of fat. However, providing more fat than the gastrointestinal tract can effectively digest and absorb results in fatty stools (steatorrhea) and diarrhea. This problem is most commonly observed when pet owners provide their dog or cat with table scraps composed predominantly of fatty foods. The long-term consumption of diets that are very high in fat may lead to weight gain and obesity because of the high palatability and energy density of the diet. Feeding diets that are very high in fat and do not have all other nutrients balanced relative to energy density may result in the development of deficiencies in other essential nutrients.

Lastly, excessive levels of LCPUFAs in the diet cause an increase in an animal's vitamin E requirement. Vitamin E functions as an antioxidant in the body, protecting cellular membrane lipids from peroxidation. The vitamin is preferentially oxidized before the unsaturated fatty acids, thus protecting the fatty acids from rancidity; however, vitamin E is destroyed in this process. Therefore as the level of unsaturated fatty acids in an animal's diet increases, so does the animal's requirement for vitamin E. If a pet food contains very high levels of LCPUFAs or if an owner is supplementing a balanced diet with high amounts of corn or vegetable oil, vitamin E in the diet must concomitantly be increased. For example, when hunting dogs were fed high amounts of high fat food scraps as their primary diet, they developed clinical signs of vitamin E deficiency.[36] Similarly, a condition called *pansteatitis,* or "yellow fat disease," occurs in cats when their diets are high in unsaturated fatty acids and marginal or low in vitamin E (see Section 4, p. 279).

References

1. Peachey SE, Dawson JM, Harper EJ: The effect of ageing on nutrient digestibility by cats fed beef tallow, sunflower oil, or olive oil-enriched diets, *Growth Dev Aging* 63:49–58, 1999.

2. Kane E, Morris JG, Rogers QR: Acceptability and digestibility by adult cats of diets made with various sources and levels of fat, *J Anim Sci* 53:1516–1523, 1981.

3. Meyer H, Zentek J, Freudenthal U: Digestibility of beef tallow in dogs, *Wien Tierarzt Monat* 79:202, 1992.

4. Downey RL, Kronfeld DS, Banta CA: Diet of Beagles affects stamina, *J Am Anim Hosp Assoc* 16:273–277, 1980.

5. Reynolds AJ, Taylor CR, Hoppeler H, and others: The effect of diet on sled dog performance, oxidative capacity, skeletal muscle microstructure, and muscle glycogen metabolism. In Carey DP, Norton SA, Bolser SM, editors: *Recent advances in canine and feline nutritional research, Proceedings of the 1996 Iams International Nutrition Symposium*, Wilmington, Ohio, 1996, Orange Frazer Press, pp 181–198.

6. Dunbar BL, Bauer JE: Conversion of essential fatty acids by delta-6-desaturase in dog live microsomes, *J Nutr* 132:1701S–1703S, 2002.

7. Bauer JE, Dunbar BL, Bigley KE: Dietary flaxseed in dogs results in differential transport and metabolism of (n-3) polyunsaturated fatty acids, *J Nutr* 128:2641S–2644S, 1998.

8. Alvarez RA, Aguirre GD, Acland GM: Docosapentaenoic acid is converted to docosahexaenoic acid in the retinas of normal and prcd-affected Miniature Poodle dogs, *Invest Sci* 35:402–408, 1994.

9. Pawlowsky R, Barnes A, Salem N Jr: Essential fatty acid metabolism in the feline: relationship between liver and brain production of long-chain polyunsaturated fatty acids, *J Lipid Res* 35:2032–2040, 1994.

10. Rivers JPW, Sinclair AJ, Crawford MA: Inability of the cat to desaturate essential fatty acids, *Nature (Lond)* 258:171–173, 1975.

11. Hassam AG, Rivers JPW, Crawford MA: The failure of the cat to desaturate linoleic acid: its nutritional implications, *Nutr Metabol* 21:321–328, 1977.

12. MacDonald ML, Anderson BC, Rogers QR, and others: Essential fatty acid requirements of cats: pathology of essential fatty acid deficiency, *Am J Vet Res* 45:1310–1317, 1984.

13. MacDonald ML, Rogers QR, Morris JG: Effects of linoleate and arachidonate deficiencies on reproduction and spermatogenesis in the cat, *J Nutr* 114:719–726, 1984.

14. Morris JG: Do cats need AA in the diet for reproduction? *Proc Symp Compar Nutr Soc* 4:65–69, 2002.

15. Chew BP, Park JS, Wong TS, and others: Role of omega-3 fatty acids on immunity and inflammation in cats. In Carey DP, Norton SA, Bolser SM, editors: *Recent advances in canine and feline nutritional research: proceedings of the 2000 Iams international nutrition symposium*, Wilmington, Ohio, 2000, Orange Frazer Press, pp 55–67.

16. Holman RT, Johnson SB, Osburn PL: Deficiency of essential fatty acids and membrane fluidity during pregnancy and lactation, *Proc Natl Acad Sci U S A* 88:4835–4839, 1991.

17. Kelley R, Lepine AJ: Improving puppy trainability through nutrition. In *Proc North Am Vet Conf*, 2005, pp 21–26.

18. Lauritzen L, Hansen HS, Jorgensen MH, Michaelson KE: The essentiality of long-chain n-3 fatty acids in relation to development and function of the brain and retina, *Prog Lipid Res* 40:1–94, 2001.

19. Bauer JE, Heinemann KM, Bigley KE, and others: Maternal diet alpha-linolenic acid during gestation and lactation does not increase canine milk docosahexaenoic acid, *J Nutr* 134:2035S–2038S, 2004.

20. Heinemann M, Waldron MK, Bigley KE: Long-chain (n-3) polyunsaturated fatty acids are more efficient than alpha-linolenic acid in improving electroretinogram responses of puppies exposed during gestation, lactation, and weaning, *J Nutr* 135:1960–1966, 2005.

21. Bauer JE, Heinemann KM, Lees GE, Waldron MK: Docosahexaenoic acid accumulates in plasma of canine puppies raised on alpha-linolenic acid-rich milk during suckling but not when fed alpha-linolenic acid-rich diets after weaning, *J Nutr* 136:2087S–2089S, 2006.

22. Bauer JE, Dunbar BL, Bigley KE: Dietary flaxseed in dogs results in differential transport and metabolism of n-3 polyunsaturated fatty acids, *J Nutr* 136:1991S–1994S, 2006.

23. National Research Council: *Nutrient requirements of dogs and cats*, Washington, DC, 2006, National Academy Press.

24. Kirby NA, Hester SL, Bauer JE: Dietary fats and the skin and coat of dogs, *J Am Vet Med Assoc* 230:1641–1644, 2007.

25. Rees CA, Bauer JE, Burkholder WJ: Effects of dietary flaxseed and sunflower seed supplementation on normal canine serum polyunsaturated fatty acids and skin and hair coat condition scores, *Vet Dermatol* 12:111–117, 2001.

26. Campbell KL, Roudebust P: Effects of four diets on serum and cutaneous fatty acids, transepidermal water losses, skin surface lipids, hydration and condition of the skin and hair coat of dogs. In *Proc Ann Am Assoc Vet Derm*, 1995, pp 80–81.

27. Pawlosky RJ, Denkins Y, Ward G: Retinal and brain accretion of long-chain polyunsaturated fatty acids in developing felines: the effects of corn-based maternal diets, *Am J Clin Nutr* 65:465–472, 1997.

28. Association of American Feed Control Officials (AAFCO): Official publication, 2008, AAFCO.

29. MacDonald ML, Rogers QR, Morris JG: Nutrition of the domestic cat, a mammalian carnivore, *Ann Rev Nutr* 4:521–562, 1984.

30. Codner EC, Thatcher CD: The role of nutrition in the management of dermatoses, *Semin Vet Med Surg (Small Anim)* 5:167–177, 1990.

31. Hansen AE, Wiese HF: Fat in the diet in relation to nutrition of the dog. I. Characteristic appearance and changes of animals fed diets with and without fat, *Tex Rep Biol Med* 9:491–515, 1951.

32. Sinclair AJ, McLean JG, Monger EA: Metabolism of linoleic acid in the cat, *Lipids* 14:932–936, 1979.

33. Rivers JPW: Essential fatty acids in cats, *J Small Anim Pract* 23:563–576, 1982.

34. Neuringer M, Anderson GJ, Conner WE: The essentiality of the n-3 fatty acids for the development and function of the retina and brain, *Ann Rev Nutr* 8:517–541, 1988.

35. Conner WE, Neuringer M, Reisbeck S: Essential fatty acids: the importance of n-3 fatty acids in the retina and brain, *Nutr Rev* 50:2129–2134, 1996.

36. Davidson MG, Geoly FJ, Gilger BC, and others: Retinal degeneration associated with vitamin E deficiency in hunting dogs, *J Am Vet Med Assoc* 213:645–651, 1998.

12

Protein Requirements

A requirement for dietary protein actually represents the need for essential amino acids and adequate nonessential amino acids to maintain body protein and to supply nitrogen for the synthesis of nonessential amino acids and other essential nitrogen-containing compounds (see Section 1, p. 21). This requirement is commonly expressed as a protein requirement because amino acids and nitrogen-containing compounds are most typically supplied in the diet in the form of intact protein. Adult animals require dietary protein to maintain whole-body protein turnover.[1] This turnover represents the synthesis and breakdown of proteins in all tissues of the body, including skin, hair, skeletal muscle, digestive enzymes, hormones, serum transport proteins, and mucosal cells. It is the sum of the losses of all of the body's individual proteins and nitrogen-containing compounds that ultimately determines an individual's daily protein (amino acid) requirement. Young animals have the same maintenance requirements as adult animals, plus an added requirement for the deposition or growth of new tissue.

> *Protein in the diets of adult dogs, adult cats, puppies, and kittens is necessary for the replacement of protein losses in the skin, hair, digestive enzymes, and mucosal cells, as well as amino acid losses from normal cellular protein catabolism. Puppies and kittens also require protein for growth.*

DETERMINING PROTEIN REQUIREMENTS

Historically, the response criteria that have been used to determine protein requirements in dogs and cats are nitrogen balance and growth rate. Nitrogen balance studies are based upon the fact that protein, on the average, contains 16% nitrogen. The nitrogen contents of food, feces, and urine are commonly measured using analytical tests, the *Kjeldahl method* and the *Leco Nitrogen Protein Analyzer.*[2] Measuring nitrogen intake and excretion provides a rough estimate of the body's protein status. Nitrogen balance is calculated as:

Nitrogen balance = Nitrogen intake from food - Nitrogen excretion through urine and feces

The nitrogen in the feces is comprised of unabsorbed dietary protein and nitrogen from endogenous sources, such as intestinal cells and gut microflora. Urinary nitrogen is composed primarily of urea, which is the end product of amino acid catabolism. Further nitrogen losses occur from desquamated cells of the skin surface, hair, and nails. However, these losses are very difficult to measure and are usually not considered when measuring nitrogen balance in experimental studies.

Requirement studies with growing animals use maximum positive nitrogen balance and growth rate as response variables to indicate an adequate level of protein in the diet. Studies of adult companion animals at maintenance use zero nitrogen balance to indicate dietary protein adequacy. Zero nitrogen balance provides an indirect measure of whole-body protein turnover and suggests that the body's daily loss of protein is replaced by intake, without a net gain or loss in total body protein. Although the majority of requirement studies have used zero nitrogen balance to assess the protein requirement of adult animals during maintenance, it is important to recognize that there are certain limitations to the use of the nitrogen balance technique. First, nitrogen balance does not provide information regarding the adequacy of (or requirement for) individual amino acids. Therefore amino acid requirement studies have been conducted independently of protein requirement studies (see pp. 95-101). Second, the minimum level of protein needed to maintain zero nitrogen balance may not be adequate to promote optimal performance and health. For example, in an early study, when adult dogs were fed diets containing just enough protein to attain zero nitrogen balance, they

TABLE 12-1 STATES OF NITROGEN BALANCE

State	Balance	Physiological stage
Zero	N intake = N excretion	Maintenance
Positive	N intake > N excretion	Growth, gestation, recovery from illness
Negative	N intake < N excretion	Inadequate nutrition, severe illness or injury, urinary N loss during renal failure, gastrointestinal tract loss during certain diseases

N, Nitrogen.

were found to be more susceptible to the toxicity of certain drugs.[3] In addition, higher levels of protein in the diet may be needed to obtain adequate individual amino acid intakes to maintain lean body mass and protein reserves. (Although protein is not stored in the body as is fat and, to a lesser degree, carbohydrate, the term *reserves* refers to the ability of the body to mobilize protein from prioritized body tissues during periods of stress.) For example, many diseases cause a loss of muscle mass, which is generally considered the largest protein depot. Therefore it is prudent to consider that estimates obtained using zero nitrogen balance may represent a minimum protein requirement for adult animals. Adequate intake (AI) estimates for dogs and cats are expected to be slightly higher than this minimum amount for healthy adults, especially during periods of physiological stress. AI estimates also account for variations in the population of interest.

Nitrogen equilibrium (zero balance) is the normal state for healthy adult animals during maintenance. An animal is described as being in a state of positive nitrogen balance when protein intake exceeds excretion. Positive nitrogen balance occurs when new tissue is being synthesized by the body, such as during the physiological stages of growth and gestation or the recovery phase following a prolonged illness. Positive nitrogen balance cannot occur when there is insufficient protein intake or a significant imbalance of the essential amino acids. Negative nitrogen balance results when protein excretion exceeds intake. An animal that exhibits negative balance is losing nitrogen from tissues more rapidly than it is being replaced. This loss of nitrogen may occur for several reasons. If the animal is consuming an insufficient amount of energy or is anorectic, body tissues must be catabolized to provide energy to the body. If inadequate levels of available protein and/or amino acids or an inappropriate ratio of amino acids are fed, tissue replacement cannot occur. Severe or prolonged

illness or injury results in a catabolic state in animals that is evidenced by excessive breakdown of the body's tissues and negative nitrogen balance. Excess losses of nitrogen from the urine during renal failure or from the gastrointestinal tract during some types of gastrointestinal disease can also cause negative nitrogen balance to occur (Table 12-1).

FACTORS AFFECTING PROTEIN REQUIREMENT

The determination of the exact protein requirements for dogs and cats is a difficult task because many factors affect an individual animal's need for protein. Dietary factors that affect protein turnover (nitrogen balance) include protein quality and amino acid composition, protein digestibility, and the energy density of the diet. In addition, an animal's activity level, physiological state, and prior nutritional status can all influence protein requirement as determined by nitrogen balance, whole-body protein turnover, or growth rate (Box 12-1).

An animal's protein requirement varies inversely with the protein source's digestibility and with its ability to provide all of the essential amino acids in their correct quantities and ratios. As protein digestibility and quality increase, the level of protein that must be included in the diet to meet the animal's needs decreases. Early protein requirement studies with dogs and cats used either purified or semipurified diets; the protein and amino acids in these types of diets are highly digestible and available. In contrast, most of the protein sources used in commercial pet foods have comparatively lower digestibility coefficients. For example, protein digestibility in a semipurified diet approaches 95%, but that of high-quality, commercial diets range between 80% and 90%. On the other hand, low-quality, commercial pet foods can have protein digestibilities of less than

FACTORS AFFECTING PROTEIN REQUIREMENT

Protein quality: As protein quality increases, protein requirement decreases.

Amino acid composition: As amino acid composition improves, protein requirement decreases.

Protein digestibility: As protein digestibility increases, protein requirement decreases.

Energy density: As energy density increases, protein requirement as a percentage of the diet increases.

75%. Because of these differences, requirement studies with purified or semipurified diets generally underestimated the protein requirements of animals consuming mixed protein diets that contained less available or inappropriate ratios of the essential amino acids.

Protein quality also influences an animal's protein requirement. The higher the biological value of a protein, the less the amount that is needed to meet all of an animal's essential amino acid needs (see Section 1, pp. 23-25). Therefore, as the quality of the protein in the test diet increases, the estimated requirement decreases. Again, the diets that were used in early amino acid and protein requirement studies had amino acid contents that were adjusted to carefully fit the needs of the experiment. Few, if any, naturally occurring protein sources have amino acid compositions that specifically fit the requirements of the animal consuming it. Most practical sources of dietary protein contain excesses of some amino acids and slight or severe deficiencies of others relative to an animal's requirement. Commercial pet foods correct for these inadequacies by using mixtures of protein sources that have complimentary profiles of essential amino acids and individual amino acids.

The caloric density of the diet used in a requirement study significantly affects the estimated protein requirement. This effect occurs because the presence of nonprotein calories has a protein-sparing effect. A diet must first meet an animal's energy needs before the energy-containing nutrients can be used for other purposes. Therefore, adequate nonprotein calories in the form of carbohydrate or fat spare the protein in the diet from being metabolized for energy. If sufficient nonprotein calories are not provided, at least a portion

of the dietary protein will be metabolized as an energy source. At caloric intakes that are less than the animal's energy requirement, protein will not be available for the building or replacing of body tissues because it will all be used for energy. Therefore, when a diet is limiting in both energy and protein, weight loss and a loss of lean body tissue result. Nitrogen balance studies have shown that when the dietary protein level is held constant, nitrogen retention increases as caloric intake increases and approaches the animal's energy requirement.[4]

A second aspect of the relationship between protein and energy must also be examined. Assuming that adequate nonprotein energy is present in the diet, as the energy density of the diet increases, a higher proportion of protein is required for maximal nitrogen retention; however, the protein-to-energy ratio remains the same. The most important factors that affect the energy density of commercial pet foods are dietary fat concentration and diet digestibility. The relationship between energy density and protein content is illustrated by the results of one of the first requirement studies of growing dogs.[5] When a diet containing 25% crude protein and 20% fat was fed, maximal growth rate resulted. However, when the fat content of the diet was increased to 30%, 29% crude protein was necessary to support maximal growth. The reason for this change relates to an animal's tendency to eat to satisfy its energy needs. Provided that these controls are in place, an animal will naturally consume less of a more energy-dense ration. Pet owners who use portion-controlled feeding regimens usually adjust quantity according to their pet's body weight and/or growth rate. Therefore portion-controlled feeding schedules are still regulated according to a pet's energy requirements. When lower quantities of food are fed because of greater energy density, protein must contribute a higher proportion of the diet so that the animal is still able to meet its total protein needs. Although protein is the most commonly used example, this relationship with energy also applies to all other essential nutrients.

Finally, protein requirement studies must take into account an animal's prior nutritional status and physiological state. The amount of absorbed protein needed to produce nitrogen equilibrium depends on the degree of protein depletion. Although it seems paradoxical, dogs with depleted body protein reserves require lower levels of nitrogen to achieve nitrogen balance than do dogs with normal reserves.[6] This effect may be the result of an increased efficiency of absorption and use of dietary protein when in a depleted state, and to the metabolic down-regulation of protein catabolism. Ensuring that all dogs are in nitrogen balance and have adequate body protein reserves by feeding a high-protein diet before the onset of a requirement study can help to eliminate this discrepancy. Conversely, correcting for lean body mass (a measure of protein reserves) can also at least partially account for differences in protein requirements. However, nitrogen balance studies still cannot provide information regarding the presence or degree of change in protein synthesis, breakdown, and oxidation that can occur in response to differing levels of protein or essential amino acids in the diet. In recent years the use of ^{13}C-labeled leucine infusion as a measure of whole-body protein metabolism has been used to further elucidate these changes.[7,8] Physiological state also directly affects the body's need for protein and will therefore affect the outcome of requirement studies that use nitrogen balance. For example, in growing puppies and kittens, the rate of growth and, subsequently, the protein requirement decrease slightly with age.[9-12]

PROTEIN REQUIREMENTS

Dogs

Numerous studies have been conducted on the minimum protein requirement of the adult dog. However, differences in the protein sources, energy densities, and amino acid ratios of the experimental diets have led to a great deal of confusion regarding this requirement. Early studies showed that when diets containing very high-quality protein sources are fed, adult dogs require between 4% and 7% of their metabolizable energy (ME) calories to be supplied as protein.[13-15] The current National Research Council (NRC) recommends a minimum protein requirement of 80 g of crude protein per kg diet in foods with an energy density of 4.0 kilocalories (kcal) ME/g, when proteins that are of high quality (both bioavailable and with the correct amounts of the essential amino acids) are fed.[16] This is equivalent to just 7% of the diet's ME. The NRC's recommended allowance is slightly higher (8.75% of ME), presumably to account for lower digestibility coefficients of protein sources used in practical diets. It is important

to consider that when lower-quality protein sources are fed, protein requirement estimates will increase significantly, typically as high as 20% of the ME calories.[17] For this reason, the current American Association of Feed Control Officials' (AAFCO's) *Nutrient Profiles* for dogs recommends that adult maintenance dog foods contain at least 18% of ME calories as protein (see below).[18]

The protein requirement of growing puppies is significantly higher than that of adult dogs. Early studies using mixed protein sources reported minimum protein requirements of between 17% and 22% of ME for growing dogs.[5,19,20] These experiments used maximum weight gain as an indicator of minimum protein needs. More recent studies, which also used weight gain as the major response criterion, reported minimum requirement estimates for recently weaned puppies of approximately 180 g crude protein/kg diet in a food containing 4.0 kcal/g.[17,21,22] This is equivalent to just 16% of ME. However, the protein sources used in all of these studies were either highly digestible protein or supplied as free amino acids. Interestingly, weight gain in growing dogs is maximized at lower protein intakes than is nitrogen retention. For example, nitrogen balance data with young puppies fed a highly digestible protein source provided a slightly higher protein requirement estimate of 20% of ME.[21] The current NRC recommends that a minimum of 16% of a diet's calories should be supplied as high-quality protein to maximize nitrogen retention in newly weaned puppies between the ages of 8 and 14 weeks.[16] After 14 weeks, the minimum requirement decreases to about 12.25% of ME. However, just as with adult maintenance diets, these estimates increase substantially when feeding practical diets that contain less available protein sources. The NRC recognizes this and recommends minimum levels of 21% (250 grams/kilogram [g/kg]) for puppies less than 14 weeks of age and 17.5% for puppies over 14 weeks of age when fed practical diets.[16] The current AAFCO *Nutrient Profiles* recommend a minimum level of 22% protein ME for growth and reproduction and do not distinguish between newly weaned and adolescent puppies (Table 12-2).

Cats

Early studies of the cat's nutrient requirements showed that it has a protein requirement substantially higher than that of other mammals, including the dog.[23,24]

TABLE 12-2   SUGGESTED MINIMUM LEVELS OF PROTEIN IN THE DIETS OF DOGS AND CATS AS A PERCENTAGE OF METABOLIZABLE ENERGY (ME)

	NRC*	AAFCO†
Dogs		
Adult maintenance	8.75% of ME	18% of ME
Growth and reproduction	21% of ME (Puppies ≤ 14 weeks)	22% of ME
	17.5% of ME (Puppies > 14 weeks)	
Cats		
Adult maintenance	17.5% of ME	22.75% of ME
Growth and reproduction	~20% of ME	26.25% of ME

AAFCO, Association of American Feed Control Officials; *NRC*, National Research Council.
*National Research Council: *Nutrient requirements of dogs and cats*, Washington, DC, 2006, National Academy Press.
†Association of American Feed Control Officials (AAFCO): Official publication, 2008, AAFCO.

When growing kittens were fed varying levels of dietary protein, supplied as minced herring and minced liver, growth was reported to be satisfactory only when protein exceeded 30% of the dry weight of the diet.[24] In comparison, growing puppies fed mixed diets required only 20% protein for adequate growth and development. One of the first studies of the protein requirement of the adult cat reported that 21% dietary protein was necessary to maintain nitrogen balance when cats were fed a mixed diet containing liver and whitefish as the primary protein sources.[25]

Subsequent experimentation using crystalline amino acids and protein isolates allowed more precise definition of the minimum protein requirements of growing kittens and adult cats. One study reported a protein requirement of 18% to 20% (by weight) in growing kittens fed either crystalline amino acid diets or casein diets supplemented with methionine.[26] Another study reported requirements as low as 16% of ME calories when growing kittens were fed a purified diet containing all of the essential amino acids in their assumed correct concentrations and ratios.[27] Using a similar semipurified diet, the protein requirement of adult cats was determined to be 12.5% of ME.[28] The profound effect that protein digestibility, amino acid balance, and amino acid availability have on determining an animal's dietary protein requirement is illustrated by the substantially lower values that were obtained when semipurified and purified diets were used to determine requirements. However, the comparison of these figures with the ideal minimum protein requirements of other mammals still demonstrates that the cat, together with

other obligate carnivores such as the fox and the mink, has a higher requirement for dietary protein (see pp. 94-95 for a complete discussion). For example, although the cat requires 20% of a 100%-available, well-balanced protein for growth and 12% for maintenance, the dog requires only 12% and 4%, respectively. It should be noted that these values are substantially lower than the protein requirement of a cat fed a practical diet containing protein sources that are not balanced for individual amino acids or highly bioavailable.

The current NRC recommendations use nitrogen balance data from a study reporting on a group of 18 adult cats to provide a recommended minimum requirement of protein for adult cats of 160 g crude protein/kg food in a diet containing 4 kcal/kg.[16,29] This is equivalent to a minimum requirement of 14% of ME. Adding a safety allowance to this minimum provides an estimate of 200 g/kg food (17.5% of ME) as a recommended allowance (RA) (see Table 12-2). The NRC's minimum requirement for kittens after weaning is 180 g/kg, equivalent to 15.75% of ME and the RA is 225 g/kg (~20% of ME). Once again, it is important to recognize that all of these values assume highly available and well-balanced protein sources that contain all of the necessary amino acids.[30,31] Conversely, the AAFCO *Nutrient Profiles* provide nutrient estimates for use in the actual formulation of pet foods. Therefore, it is not surprising that the AAFCO *Nutrient Profiles* for cat foods, as with dog foods, suggest a higher level of protein for inclusion in commercially prepared foods.[18] A level of 30% of the diet (dry matter [DM]) is suggested for growth and reproduction in foods containing 4 kcal of ME/g of food. This value is equivalent to 26.25% of ME calories. A level of 26% of the diet, equivalent to 22.75% ME, is suggested for adult maintenance (see Table 12-2).

THE CAT'S HIGH PROTEIN REQUIREMENT

The cat's comparatively high dietary requirement for protein is the result of increased needs for the maintenance of whole-body protein turnover, rather than increased needs for growth. Approximately 60% of the growing kitten's protein requirement is used for the maintenance of body tissues; only 40% is used for growth. The opposite is true in most of the other species that have been studied. For example, the growing rat requires only 35% of its dietary protein for maintenance and 65% for growth; similarly, the growing dog uses only 33% of its protein requirement for maintenance and 66% for growth.[32] The higher growth rate of puppies compared with kittens causes this increased need for dietary protein during growth; when compared during adult maintenance, cats have almost twice the requirement for bioavailable protein compared with dogs.[16]

The elevated protein requirement for maintenance results from the inability of the amino acid and amino acid nitrogen catabolic enzymes in the cat's liver to effectively down-regulate in response to reduced dietary protein intake. When most mammals are fed diets high in protein, the enzymes involved in amino acid catabolism, nitrogen disposal, and gluconeogenesis increase in activity to use the carbon backbone of surplus amino acids and convert excess nitrogen to urea for excretion. Conversely, when low-protein diets are fed, the activity of these enzymes declines (i.e., is down-regulated), which allows for the conservation of amino acids for whole-body protein synthesis and results in lower amounts of nitrogen to be produced via the urea cycle.[33,34] This adaptive mechanism is a distinct advantage because it allows animals to conserve amino acids while consuming low-protein diets. The ability to up- and down-regulate these catabolic enzymes provides a mechanism by which potentially toxic amino acids can be catabolized when animals are consuming high-protein diets. For example, an early study fed adult cats either high-protein (70%) or low-protein (17.5%) diets for 1 month.[35] The activities of three urea cycle enzymes

and seven nitrogen catabolic enzymes in the liver were then measured. With the exception of one transaminase enzyme, no significant differences in enzyme activity were found between the cats fed the low-protein diet and the cats fed the high-protein diet. Several gluconeogenic and lipogenic enzymes were also measured, none of which exhibited any change in activity in response to the changes in dietary protein level. On the other hand, similar rat hepatic enzymes decrease in activity from 2.75-fold to 13-fold after rats are changed from a high-protein diet to a low-protein diet.[34]

In addition to the inability of the cat's protein-catabolizing enzymes to down-regulate in response to reduced dietary protein, the enzymes involved in nitrogen catabolism function at relatively high rates of activity. This metabolic state causes the cat to catabolize a substantial amount of amino acids after each meal, regardless of its protein content. Thus the cat does not have the capability to conserve nitrogen from the body's general nitrogen pool and has a higher urinary obligatory nitrogen loss when fed low-protein (or protein-free) diets.[36] This difference is of important significance when considering the nutritional care of cats that are ill or anorectic, as long-term food deprivation causes a much higher loss of urinary nitrogen in cats compared with other species (see Chapter 33, pp. 432-434 for a complete discussion).[37] The only alternative that ensures adequate conservation of body protein stores is the consistent consumption of a diet containing high levels of protein. Recent studies have shown that although cats do not adapt to low-protein diets, they do efficiently adapt to medium- and high-protein diets.[38,39] This appears to occur via increased liver mass, increased delivery of substrate to urea cycle enzymes, and to allosteric regulation of rate-controlling enzyme activities. It can be theorized that because of the cat's strict adherence to a carnivorous diet, it experienced little selective pressure throughout its evolutionary history to develop metabolic adaptations to low-protein diets. Additionally, a high rate of gluconeogenesis from amino acid catabolism would provide endogenous glucose to an animal that evolved to ingest a low-carbohydrate diet, thus having selective advantage.[40]

Another factor that contributes to an animal's dietary protein requirement is its need for essential amino acids. When the protein nutrition of the cat was first studied, it was postulated that its high dietary protein requirement might be the result of an unusually high requirement for one or more of the essential amino acids. However, results of several experimental studies have shown that with the exception of slightly higher requirements for leucine, threonine, methionine, and arginine, as well as a unique dietary requirement for taurine (see below), the cat's requirements for specific essential amino acids are not significantly higher than those of other species such as the rat, dog, or pig.[41] More recently, studies have shown that the growing kitten appears to be less sensitive to the amino acid imbalances that are seen in omnivores and herbivores when one or more amino acid is limiting and total protein level of the diet is increased.[42,43] In other animals, but not in cats, increasing dietary crude protein causes a concomitant increase in essential amino acid requirements.

The protein requirement of the cat is higher than that of the dog as a result of the cat's greater need for the maintenance of normal body tissues rather than from increased need for growth. This is because of the inability of certain catabolic enzymes in the cat's liver to down-regulate in response to changes in dietary protein intake.

ESSENTIAL AMINO ACIDS IN DOG AND CAT NUTRITION

The following 10 amino acids have been identified as being essential for growing puppies and kittens: arginine, histidine, isoleucine, leucine, lysine, methionine, phenylalanine, threonine, tryptophan, and valine. Although both the dog and the cat have a dietary requirement for arginine, the cat is unusual in its immediate and severe reaction to the consumption of an arginine-free meal. The other amino acids that are of special concern in the feeding of dogs and cats are lysine, the sulfur amino acids (SAAs) methionine and cysteine (and the production of felinine), and the amino-sulfonic acid, taurine. Of less practical concern, but of academic interest, is the cat's inability to convert the amino acid tryptophan to the B vitamin niacin.

Arginine

The amino acid arginine is not considered a dietary essential for many adult animals because most species can synthesize adequate amounts to meet their metabolic needs. However, arginine has been shown to be essential for both dogs and cats throughout life.[44-46] Arginine is needed by the body for normal protein synthesis and as an essential component of the urea cycle. Arginine functions in the urea cycle as an ornithine and urea precursor. In this capacity arginine allows the large amounts of nitrogen generated from amino acid catabolism to be converted to urea for excretion from the body. If nitrogen cannot be liberated through the urea cycle by the presence of arginine, then both free urea and ammonia will begin to rise in the blood. A lack of arginine in the diet causes an immediate and severe deficiency response in the cat. Cats will develop hyperammonemia within several hours of consuming a single arginine-free meal.[47] Clinical signs include emesis (vomiting), muscle spasms, ataxia, hyperesthesia (sensitivity to touch), and tetanic spasms. These signs can eventually lead to coma and death. Dogs show similar, but less severe, clinical signs of arginine deficiency following consumption of an arginine-free meal, suggesting a low level of endogenous arginine production.[48]

The metabolic basis for the cat's extreme sensitivity to arginine deficiency is related to an inability to synthesize *de novo* ornithine. In most animals, the amino acids glutamate and proline act as precursors for ornithine synthesis in the intestinal mucosa. However, the cat's intestinal mucosal cells have extremely low levels of active pyrroline-5-carboxylate synthase, an essential enzyme in this pathway.[49] The cat also has low activity of a second essential enzyme, ornithine aminotransferase.[50] In addition to being unable to synthesize ornithine, the cat is also unable to synthesize citrulline from ornithine for use by extrahepatic tissues, even if dietary ornithine is provided. Studies in the rat demonstrated that the normal route of arginine synthesis for use by extrahepatic tissues involves both the liver and the kidneys. Arginine cannot leave the liver to provide for extrahepatic tissues because high activity of liver arginase prevents its accumulation to a concentration above that of the bloodstream. However, citrulline, which is produced from ornithine either in the intestinal mucosa or in a urea cycle intermediate in the liver, can travel to the kidneys where it is then converted to arginine. This arginine provides the kidneys and other tissues of the body with their needs for normal growth and tissue maintenance in most animals. In the cat, however, citrulline is not produced in the intestinal mucosa (because of the inability to produce ornithine), and the citrulline produced in the liver appears to be unable to leave the hepatocyte to be converted to arginine by the kidneys. As a direct result of these metabolic deficiencies, arginine becomes an essential amino acid for both urea cycle function and for normal growth and maintenance in the cat (Table 12-3). The importance of arginine for normal functioning of the urea cycle, coupled with the cat's high and inflexible rate of protein catabolism, causes the cat to be extremely sensitive to arginine deficiency. Like the cat, the growing dog also has a dietary requirement for arginine. However, the response of the growing dog to an arginine-deficient diet is not as severe as that observed in the immature cat.[48]

Arginine deficiency in the cat has immediate and devastating effects. Severe hyperammonemia, emesis, muscle spasms, ataxia, hyperesthesia, and tetanic spasms can lead to coma and death. Taurine deficiency can lead to retinal degeneration and dilated cardiomyopathy.

Lysine

The growing dog's dietary requirement for lysine appears to increase as the level of total protein in the diet increases.[51] This effect has been demonstrated in other species and may be the result of amino acid imbalances and antagonisms with lysine at higher levels of protein intake. Although this effect has been demonstrated with other essential amino acids, it is especially important with lysine because lysine is often the first limiting amino acid in cereal-based dog foods.[52] In addition, the lysine that is present in the diet is susceptible to certain types

of processing damage that can occur in commercially prepared pet foods. The exposure of protein to excessive heat induces cross-linking between amino acids, resulting in decreased digestibility of the food's total protein. Even mild heat treatment can result in a reaction between the epsilon-amino group of lysine and the amino groups of free amino acids with reducing sugars. The resultant Maillard products are resistant to digestion and result in a reduction in the amount of available lysine that can be supplied by the food. The limiting amino acids in cereal proteins are lysine and tryptophan. Conversely, meat products contain adequate amounts of these amino acids. The inclusion of meat proteins in a pet food, coupled with properly controlled processing methods, ensures that the ration contains an adequate level of available lysine. In a completely cereal-based dog food, either supplemental lysine or a meat source of lysine must be added (see Section 3, pp. 150-151).

Methionine and Cysteine

The SAA methionine is essential for dogs and cats, but cysteine is dispensable. Cysteine may become indispensable if there is not enough methionine to provide for the total sulfur (methionine + cysteine) requirement. Because methionine is used by the body to synthesize cysteine, approximately half of the methionine requirement can be met by dietary cysteine.[53,54] Therefore it is preferable to address a total SAA requirement rather than a specific methionine requirement for animals. Interestingly, cats have a higher need for SAA (methionine and cysteine) when compared with most other mammals. For example, while growing dogs require a minimum of 1.40 g/1000 kcal of ME, the minimum requirement of growing cats is approximately 25% higher than this (1.75 g/1000 kcal).[16]

The cat's greater need for SAA appears to be the result of several metabolic factors. First, the cat, along with other members of the Felidae family, uses methionine and cysteine to produce a unique sulfur amino acid called *felinine*.[55] Felinine is synthesized in the liver and is excreted in the urine of all cats, but is found in highest concentration in the urine of adult, intact males.[56] The urine of intact tom cats contains felinine concentrations that are up to sixfold greater than those found in castrated males and intact females. Conversely, castrated males and intact females excrete proportionally

TABLE 12-3   ARGININE SYNTHESIS

Reaction	Most Mammals	Cats
Glutamate + proline → ornithine (intestine)	Normal	Low
Ornithine → citrulline (intestine)	Normal	Little activity
Citrulline travels to the kidney	Does occur	Does not occur
Citrulline → arginine (kidney)	Does occur	Does not occur

higher amounts of a felinine metabolite, called *N-acetyl-felinine,* which may drive a higher sulfur amino acid requirement for these cats.[57] When both felinine and *N*-acetyl-felinine are combined, intact male cats still have 1.7 to 2.3 times greater excretion than castrated males and intact females. This suggests that male intact cats may have a greater requirement for the SAAs than sterilized female and male cats. Although it has not been exclusively proven, it is believed that felinine, or more likely, a breakdown product of felinine, acts as a urinary pheromone for territorial marking in male cats and is at least partly responsible for the pungent odor of sprayed urine.[58] Other potential causes for the cat's high SAA requirement are its needs for the maintenance of a thick hair coat and for the increased methylation reactions necessary for the synthesis of phospholipids. Increased phospholipid synthesis is believed to be necessary for the absorption and transport of the high level of fat that is normally included in a cat's diet. Lastly, the cat's requirement for dietary taurine further adds to the cat's total requirement for SAAs in the diet.

Methionine is usually the first limiting amino acid in most commercial pet foods that contain animal tissues and plant protein sources. This fact, coupled with the high SAA requirement for cats and the need for methionine as a precursor for taurine (see below), results in methionine being an important consideration for pet food companies during the formulation of nutritionally balanced cat and dog foods.

Taurine

Taurine is a unique beta–amino-sulfonic acid that is not incorporated into large proteins but is found as a free amino acid in tissues or as a constituent of small peptides. It is synthesized by most mammals from methionine and cysteine during normal sulfur amino acid metabolism (Figure 12-1). The myocardium and retina contain high concentrations of free taurine, and these two tissues are able to concentrate taurine to levels that are 100-fold to 400-fold greater than those found in plasma.[59] Taurine is conjugated with a number of compounds and is involved in many aspects of metabolism. Its most important roles are in bile acid conjugation, retinal function, and normal functioning of the myocardium. Taurine also appears to be necessary for healthy reproductive performance in dogs and cats.[60,61]

CATS   Cats are able to synthesize only small amounts of taurine and so require a dietary source of taurine to meet daily needs.[62] This inability is partially the result of the cat's low activity of two enzymes that are essential

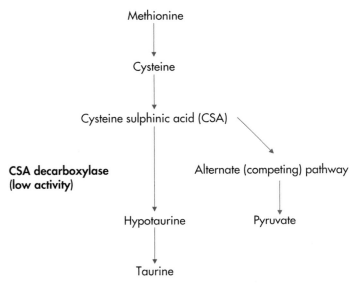

Figure 12-1   Taurine synthesis and metabolism in the cat.

for taurine synthesis: cysteine dioxygenase and cysteine sulfinic acid decarboxylase. In addition, the competing pathway of cysteine catabolism, which produces pyruvate and sulfite rather than taurine from methionine and cysteine, is very responsive to increased cysteine concentrations (see Figure 12-1).[63] The cat is not unique in its limited capacity for taurine synthesis. Low levels of *de novo* synthesis have also been reported in humans, Old World monkeys, rabbits, and guinea pigs. However, the cat requires dietary taurine because of an unusually high metabolic demand. The domestic cat uses only taurine for bile-salt formation and, in contrast to other animals, cannot convert to conjugation of bile acids with glycine when the taurine supply is limited.[64] For example, although humans and Old World monkeys also have only a limited capacity for taurine synthesis and prefer to conjugate bile acids with taurine, they will switch to glycine conjugation when dietary taurine is low. Conversely, the cat has a continual requirement for taurine to replace fecal losses that occur from incomplete recovery of bile salts by the enterohepatic circulation. The dog also uses only taurine to conjugate bile acids, but provided that the diet contains adequate protein and SAA, dogs are capable of synthesizing adequate taurine to meet their metabolic needs (see pp. 99-100).

Feline central retinal degeneration (FCRD) was the first clinical deficiency syndrome recognized as caused by taurine deficiency in the cat. Taurine's primary role in the proper functioning of the retina involves the photoreceptor cells, where it regulates the flux of calcium and potassium ions across the photoreceptor pigment–epithelial cell barrier.[65] When taurine is absent, the photoreceptor cell membranes become disrupted and dysfunctional, which eventually leads to cellular death and the loss of cells. A concomitant degeneration of the underlying tapetum lucidum can also occur. Although abnormalities in electroretinograms can be observed in as few as 6 weeks of consuming a taurine-free diet, visual impairment is only observed clinically when cats are in the later stages of retinal degeneration.[66-68] At this point, irreversible blindness occurs in most cats.[69]

Taurine is also necessary for normal functioning of the myocardium. Although it is not the only underlying cause in cats, a deficiency of taurine results in the development of dilated cardiomyopathy (DCM).[70] This degenerative disease has been reported in several species and causes decreased myocardial contractility, which eventually leads to cardiac failure. Along with the retina, the myocardium is one of the tissues in the body that is able to concentrate taurine to levels much greater than those found in the plasma. The classic study by Pion et al.[70] reported data from 21 clinical cases of DCM in pet cats. All of the cats were found to have significantly lower plasma taurine concentrations when compared with clinically normal cats. When the affected cats were supplemented with taurine (0.5 g twice daily), all the cats clinically improved within 2 weeks. At 3 to 4 weeks, the cats showed improved echocardiographs that eventually resulted in complete normalization of left ventricular function. At the time of publication, all surviving cats were clinically and echocardiographically normal. In addition, two experimental cats that had been fed a purified diet containing marginally low levels of taurine for 4 years developed DCM. These cats also exhibited full recovery as a result of taurine supplementation. The authors proposed that low levels of taurine in plasma and myocardial tissue are a major cause of the development of DCM in cats. Although the exact biochemical defect of taurine-induced DCM is not fully understood, taurine appears to confer a calcium- and potassium-stabilizing effect on heart tissue and may thereby ensure cationic stability and membrane integrity.

Finally, taurine is needed for normal reproductive success in queens. Gestating cats that are taurine-depleted are more likely to resorb or abort fetuses, have fewer live births, and produce kittens with lower birth weights and growth rates.[71,72] The effects of taurine deficiency on reproduction appear to be related to fetal development rather than to an effect on the queen's estrus cycle or ability to ovulate.[73] In addition, queens that are fed taurine-deficient diets have significantly lower concentrations of taurine in their milk, without any other changes in nutrient content.[71]

An exact dietary taurine requirement for cats is impossible to define because the need for dietary taurine is affected by the type and composition of the diet that is fed. The most important factors are the level and type of dietary protein and fiber, and the degree of heat treatment that is used during processing. There are two primary mechanisms through which diet characteristics influence taurine status in cats. First, certain fibers and peptides in food can bind with taurocholic acid in the small intestine, making it unavailable for enterohepatic reutilization.[74,75] Rice bran has been implicated as a cause of decreased plasma and whole-blood taurine levels in both cats and dogs, and it is theorized that either the fiber, fat, or protein found in rice bran forms nonabsorbable complexes with bile acids (see p. 100).[75,76] These conjugates are then excreted in the feces, leading to increased daily loss of taurine (i.e., increased taurine turnover). Second, thermal processing of certain types of protein results in the production of Maillard products, which can contribute to taurine depletion.[77] Maillard products are complexes of reducing sugars and amino acids that are formed during heat treatment. Because these products are less digestible than untreated protein, they provide an intestinal environment that favors increased numbers of taurine-degrading bacteria. Increased bacterial populations include species that are capable of cleaving taurocholic acid and oxidizing free taurine for energy, reducing the enterohepatic reutilization of bile acids. Maillard products may also affect taurine status by indirectly influencing the release of the hormone cholecystokinin (CCK), which in turn stimulates the release of additional bile acids into the intestinal lumen during digestion.[78] In all of these situations, a substantial proportion of the taurine requirement of adult cats is required to replace taurine lost in the feces or oxidized by microbes. Therefore any factor that can bind taurocholic acid or increases the microbial degradation of taurine will lead to an increased dietary requirement.

Because of the effects of protein level, fiber, and heat processing upon the availability of taurine, the current NRC provides several different recommendations.[16] The NRC's AI for all life stages when a food containing a highly available and digestible protein source is fed just a 400-mg taurine/kg diet (in a food containing 4000 kcal/kg). However, this estimate is not generally practical, and recommendations of 1000 mg taurine/kg dry diet and 1700 mg taurine/kg wet (canned) diet are provided for commercial foods. The current AAFCO *Nutrient Profiles* for cat foods provide the same minimum for dry foods and a slightly higher minimum for canned (1000 mg/kg and 2000 mg/kg, respectively).[18] Higher nutrient intake recommendations are provided for canned foods compared with dry foods to account for the high heat treatment, water content, and generally higher protein levels in canned foods, factors which lead to greater taurine losses during production and during feeding.[62,79]

Taurine is present primarily in animal tissues, with greatest concentrations found in muscle tissue. Seafoods provide the most concentrated source ($\geq$1000 mg/kg of dry weight), and poultry also contains high levels.[80] Although a carnivorous diet ensures the cat an adequate taurine intake, the consumption of a diet containing high amounts of plant products and cereal grains may not provide sufficient taurine. Of special concern are cereal-based dog foods that contain lower levels of protein and taurine. Therefore, while these diets are adequate for dogs, the practice of feeding dog foods to cats may result in taurine deficiency and the development of FCRD, and so should be strongly discouraged.

Feeding cereal-based dog foods to cats can be harmful; such foods have lower protein and taurine levels and can cause protein and taurine deficiency.

DOGS Unlike the cat, dogs that are fed diets containing adequate levels of protein and SAA are capable of synthesizing enough taurine to meet their needs. As a result, a need for dietary taurine has not been generally recognized in dogs. However, in recent years, the high prevalence of DCM in certain breeds and families of dogs, along with evidence of low plasma and whole-blood taurine levels in some of these dogs has led researchers to examine taurine status as a potential underlying cause of DCM.[80-82] The presence of increased incidence of DCM in American Cocker Spaniels and Newfoundlands may reflect a genetic anomaly in taurine homeostasis that makes certain breeds more susceptible to taurine-responsive DCM.[83,84] Although not related to a specific breed, a familial component to DCM (and potentially to taurine homeostasis) has also been reported in cats.[85]

Dietary factors that are important considerations for taurine status in dogs include low dietary protein, feeding a primary protein source that contains low or less available SAAs, and the use of rice bran. For example, although anecdotal, researchers reported taurine deficiency and DCM in two unrelated dogs that were fed a vegetarian diet containing soybean curd as its primary protein source. Soybean protein is low in SAAs and the formation of bile acid complexes may further contribute to fecal loss of taurine.[86] A controlled study reported that feeding a diet containing marginally low protein (10% DM) to healthy adult dogs for 4 years caused significant reductions in plasma taurine concentrations even though the diet met AAFCO guidelines for protein and individual amino acids.[82] Another study identified lamb meal as a consistent dietary ingredient of commercial dog foods that were associated with reduced plasma and whole-blood taurine concentrations in healthy dogs.[76] This finding was corroborated by a study that measured taurine status in a group of 19 adult Newfoundlands that were fed commercial dry diets.[84] However, neither of these studies was controlled and both included dogs fed a variety of commercial foods. It was theorized that the association between lamb meal and taurine status could be due to low levels of available amino acids present in the lamb meal, to excessive heat damage of the protein, or to the confounding factor of the inclusion of rice bran in many lamb meal–containing foods.[87] Similar to cats, rice bran may function to increase gastrointestinal tract loss of taurine through the formation of bile acid conjugates.

Most recently, there is evidence that breed size and maintenance energy requirements of dogs influences rate of endogenous taurine synthesis and, ultimately, the need for dietary taurine.[88,89] It is theorized that increased body size in dogs is associated with enhanced risk for developing taurine deficiency and that this risk may be exacerbated by genetic predispositions in some breeds of dogs.[90] Newfoundlands have been shown to have a significantly lower rate of *de novo* taurine synthesis when compared with Beagles on a metabolic body weight and liver weight basis. It appears that this difference may be attributed to lower total intake of food (and thus of taurine precursors, methionine and cystine) relative to metabolic body weight, leading to reduced taurine balance and resulting in taurine depletion. These results were supported by a controlled study that compared taurine synthesis rates in large dogs compared with Beagles and found that the large dogs had lower *de novo* synthesis of taurine compared with small dogs when fed diets containing marginally low levels of SAAs.[89] Together, these studies suggest that certain dogs may possess a genetic predisposition to taurine depletion and development of DCM and this susceptibility may be related to breed size and metabolic rate. Dogs with increased susceptibility to taurine depletion

may require a dietary source of taurine under certain environmental or physiological conditions or when fed foods containing certain types of protein or dietary fiber. Simply increasing dietary protein might achieve taurine homeostasis, provided the protein source was of high quality and not excessively heat processed. Increasing the protein concentration of poor-quality proteins, or in diets that are excessively heat-treated, may be counterproductive as these diets can result in increased microbially mediated fecal loss of taurine.[91]

Cats' Inability to Convert Tryptophan to Niacin

The requirement for the B vitamin niacin is met in most animals through both the consumption of dietary nicotinamide and through the conversion of the essential amino acid tryptophan to nicotinic acid (Figure 12-2). The efficiency of conversion of tryptophan to niacin

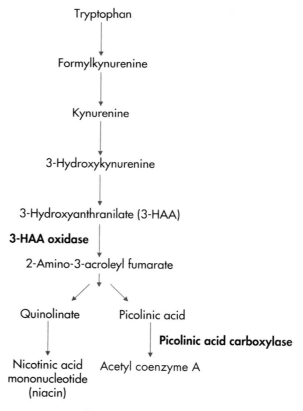

Figure 12-2 Niacin synthesis.

varies among species but is generally quite low (3%).[92] This is a result of the existence of more dominant competing pathways of tryptophan metabolism. A branch point in the pathway involved in tryptophan catabolism results in the synthesis of either quinolinic acid or picolinic acid. Quinolinic acid is further metabolized to form niacin; picolinic acid is converted to glutarate. Although most species have high levels of picolinate carboxylase activity that result in a higher production of picolinic acid, a substantial amount of niacin is still produced from the quinolinic acid branch. The activity of picolinate carboxylase in cats is 30 to 50 times higher than its activity in rats, resulting in negligible niacin synthesis from tryptophan in the cat.

Animal tissues are well supplied with nicotinamide. The regular consumption of a carnivorous diet throughout evolutionary history would probably not result in selective pressure for the cat to synthesize niacin from precursor substances. However, it has been postulated that the high-protein diet of the cat would exert pressure toward a high rate of tryptophan catabolism (i.e., the picolinic acid branch of the pathway). The rapid metabolism of tryptophan would prevent the accumulation of the amino acid and its intermediates, such as serotonin, to toxic levels. Animal proteins contain significantly higher levels of tryptophan than do plant proteins. Thus the high activity of picolinic carboxylase in the cat may prevent the accumulation of tryptophan and its byproducts in the bloodstream following the consumption of a meal containing high amounts of animal protein.

The inability of the cat to convert tryptophan to niacin is of little practical significance to the feeding management of pet cats because nicotinamide is widely distributed in feed ingredients. Sources of this vitamin in commercial pet foods include animal and fish byproducts, distillers' grains and yeast, and certain oil meals. Therefore the chance of inducing a niacin deficiency through improper feeding practices is slim, regardless of the cat's inability to convert tryptophan to niacin for use by the body.

PROTEIN DEFICIENCY IN DOGS AND CATS

Signs of protein deficiency include retarded growth in young animals and weight loss, reduced lean body mass, and impaired reproductive and work performance in adults. When protein deficiency occurs with adequate energy intake, concentrations of plasma amino acids decrease in the short term and serum albumin concentration decreases in the long term. Reduction in plasma protein levels can eventually lead to edema or ascites. A deficiency of protein commonly occurs with energy deficiency; this state is referred to as *protein/calorie malnutrition* (PCM). When PCM occurs, the animal exhibits lethargy, reduced digestive efficiency, compromised immune function, and reduced resistance to infectious disease. There is also some evidence that general undernutrition and protein deficiency during development can affect brain development and learning capabilities later in life.

Protein deficiency is rare in companion animals that are fed balanced commercial pet foods. This is probably because the majority of commercial foods contain more protein than is needed to meet the minimum requirement.[93] When protein deficiency does occur, it is usually because owners are attempting to economize by feeding low-quality, poorly formulated rations during periods of high nutrient need, such as pregnancy or lactation. Additionally, cats that are fed cereal-based dog foods that contain marginally adequate levels of protein are at risk for the development of protein and/or taurine deficiency.

PROTEIN EXCESS IN DOGS AND CATS

As discussed previously, there is some evidence suggesting that it may be beneficial to feed animals levels of protein that are higher than the minimum level necessary to maintain nitrogen equilibrium, and that whole-body protein turnover provides a better estimate of an animal's maintenance protein needs. When protein in excess of needs is consumed, there are two possible uses for the additional protein (amino acids). If the animal is in negative energy balance, the excess protein will be used as an energy source. Conversely, if the animal is in zero or positive energy balance (i.e., consuming adequate or excess energy than it is expending, respectively), the excess protein will be deposited as fat and the nitrogen will be excreted in the urine. Unlike fat and carbohydrate, excess amino acids are not stored by the body for future use.

All companion animals have the ability to metabolize excess protein. This process results in the production of urea and its excretion in the urine. Historically, protein intake that was greater than an animal's requirement was theorized to have detrimental effects on kidney function, especially in aging animals. This was based on the theory that the catabolism of excess protein and subsequent urinary excretion of urea and other nitrogenous waste products was responsible for the progression of renal dysfunction.[94] However, while the control of dietary protein is used to reduce uremia and its associated clinical signs in animals with chronic renal disease, there is no evidence showing that protein intake initiates or contributes to the progression of kidney dysfunction (see Section 5, pp. 412-414 for a complete discussion).[95]

As animals age, they experience reduced renal weight and a gradual decline in kidney function. These are normal occurrences and have been extensively studied in humans and rats.[96,97] However, these changes should not be extrapolated to suggest a need to reduce dietary protein.[98] A study with dogs evaluated clinical changes in renal function in a colony of Beagles for a period of 13 years. The data from this study indicate that normal kidney aging can lead to a nephron loss of up to 75% before clinical or biochemical signs occur.[99] Animals with less than a 75% loss are usually clinically normal, but they may be more susceptible to renal insult than are younger animals still possessing renal reserve capacity. This knowledge led to the untested practice of systematically reducing the protein content in the diets of elderly animals in an attempt to prevent or minimize progression of kidney dysfunction. However, recent studies have shown that geriatric dogs actually benefit from slightly higher levels of high-quality protein and this increased dietary protein can help to ameliorate the age-associated loss of muscle mass.[100] Therefore there is no evidence indicating a need to systematically reduce protein levels in the diets of healthy older pets. It is recommended that protein in the diets of geriatric pets should not be restricted simply because of advancing age (see Section 4, pp. 268-270 for a complete discussion).

> *Contrary to popular belief, there is no research-based, conclusive evidence that protein ingestion contributes to the development of kidney dysfunction in healthy dogs and cats. Moreover, there is no evidence that the protein intake of geriatric pets should be restricted just because of old age.*

References

1. Shoveller AK, Atkinson JL, Davenport GM: Protein and amino acids for adult dogs: recommendations. In *Iams Nutr Symp, OVC Proc*, 2006, pp 11–17.

2. Bradstreet RB: *The Kjeldahl method for organic nitrogen*, New York, 1965, Academic Press.

3. Allison JB, Wannemacher RW, Migliarese JF: Diet and the metabolism of 2-aminofluorene, *J Nutr* 52:415–425, 1954.

4. Allison JB: Optimal nutrition correlated with nitrogen retention, *Am J Clin Nutr* 4:662–672, 1956.

5. Ontko JA, Wuthier RE, Phillips PH: The effect of increased dietary fat upon the protein requirement of the growing dog, *J Nutr* 62:163–169, 1957.

6. Allison JB, Seeley RD, Brown JH, and others: The evaluation of proteins in hypoproteinemic dogs, *J Nutr* 31:237–242, 1946.

7. Humbert B, Bleis P, Martin L, and others: Effects of dietary protein restriction and amino acids deficiency on protein metabolism in dogs, *J Anim Physiol Anim Nutr* 85:255–262, 2001.

8. Humbert G, Martin L, Dumon H, and others: Dietary protein level affects protein metabolism during the postabsorptive state in dogs, *J Nutr* 132:1676S–1678S, 2002.

9. Case LP, Czarnecki-Maulden GL: Protein requirements of growing pups fed practical dry-type diets containing mixed-protein sources, *Am J Vet Res* 51:808–812, 1990.

10. Payne PR: Assessment of the protein values of diets in relation to the requirements of the growing dog. In Graham-Jones O, editor: *Canine and feline nutritional requirements*, London, 1965, Pergamon Press.

11. Dickinson CD, Scott PP: Nutrition of the cat. II. Protein requirements for growth of weanling kittens and young cats maintained on a mixed diet, *Br J Nutr* 10:311–316, 1956.

12. Anderson PA, Baker DH, Sherry PA, and others: Nitrogen requirement of the kitten, *Am J Vet Res* 41:1646–1649, 1980.

13. Arnold A, Schad JS: Nitrogen balance studies with dogs on casein or methionine-supplemented casein, *J Nutr* 53:265–273, 1954.

14. Kade CF Jr, Phillips JH, Phillips WA: The determination of the minimum requirement of the adult dog for maintenance of nitrogen balance, *J Nutr* 36:109–121, 1948.

15. Melnick D, Cowgill GR: The protein minima for nitrogen equilibrium with different proteins, *J Nutr* 13:401–424, 1937.

16. National Research Council: *Nutrient requirements of dogs and cats*, Washington, DC, 2006, National Academy Press.

17. Schaeffer MC, Rogers QR, Morris JG: Protein in the nutrition of dogs and cats. In Burger IH, Rivers JPW, editors: *Nutrition of the dog and cat*, New York, 1989, Cambridge University Press.

18. Association of American Feed Control Officials (AAFCO): Official publication, 2008, AAFCO.

19. Heiman V: The protein requirements of growing puppies, *J Am Anim Hosp Assoc* 111:304–308, 1947.

20. Gessert CG, Phillips PH: Protein in the nutrition of the growing dog, *J Nutr* 58:415–421, 1956.

21. Burns RA, LaFaivre MH, Milner JA: Effects of dietary protein quantity and quality on the growth of dogs and rats, *J Nutr* 112:1843–1853, 1982.

22. Delaney SJ, Hill AS, Backus RC, and others: Dietary crude protein concentration does not affect the leucine requirement of growing dogs, *J Anim Physiol Anim Nutr* 85:88–100, 2001.

23. Jansen GR, Deuth MA, Ward GM, and others: Protein quality studies in growing kittens, *Nutr Rep Int* 11:525–536, 1975.

24. Dickinson CD, Scott PP: Nutrition of the cat. II. Protein requirements for growth of weanling kittens and young cats maintained on a mixed diet, *Br J Nutr* 10:311–316, 1956.

25. Greaves JP, Scott PP: Nutrition of the cat. III. Protein requirements for nitrogen equilibrium in adult cats maintained on a mixed diet, *Br J Nutr* 14:361–369, 1960.

26. Smalley KA, Rogers QR, Morris JG: The nitrogen requirement of the kitten using crystalline amino acid diets or casein diets. In *Proceedings of the twelfth international congress on nutrition*, San Diego, 96:538, August 16-21, 1981 (abstract).

27. Anderson PA, Baker DH, Sherry PA, and others: Nitrogen requirement of the kitten, *Am J Vet Res* 41:1646–1649, 1980.

28. Burger IH, Blaza SE, Kendall PT: The protein requirement of adult cats, *Proc Nutr Soc* 40:102a, 1981.

29. Burger IH, Blaze SE, Kendall PT, Smith PM: The protein requirement of adult cats at maintenance, *Feline Pract* 14:8–14, 1984.

30. Taylor TP, Morris JG, Willits NH, Rogers QR: Optimizing the pattern of essential amino acids as the sole source of dietary nitrogen supports near-maximal growth in kittens, *J Nutr* 126:2243–2252, 1996.

31. Rogers QR, Morris JG: Some highlights in elucidating the peculiar nutritional needs of cats, *Compend Cont Educ Vet* 30(Suppl):9–16, 2008.

32. Russell K, Lobley GE, Millward DK: Whole-body protein turnover of a carnivore, *Felis silvestris catus*, *Br J Nutr* 89:29–37, 2003.

33. Schimke RT: Adaptive characteristics of urea cycle enzymes in the rat, *J Biol Chem* 237:459–467, 1962.

34. Szepesi B, Freedland RA: Alterations in the activities of several rat liver enzymes at various times after initiation of a high protein regimen, *J Nutr* 93:301–310, 1967.

35. Rogers QR, Morris JG, Freedland RA: Lack of hepatic enzymatic adaptation to low and high levels of dietary protein in the adult cat, *Enzyme* 22:348–356, 1977.

36. Hendriks WH, Moughan P, Tarttelin MF: Urinary excretion of endogenous nitrogen metabolites in adult domestic cats using a protein-free diet and the regression technique, *J Nutr* 127:623–629, 1997.

37. Biourge V, Groff JM, Fisher C: Nitrogen balance, plasma free amino acid concentrations and urinary orotic acid excretion during long term fasting in cats, *J Nutr* 124:1094–1103, 1994.

38. Rogers QR, Morris JG: Up-regulation of nitrogen catabolic enzymes is not required to readily oxidize excess protein in cats, *J Nutr* 132:2819–2820, 2002.

39. Russell K, Murgatroyd PR, Batt RM: Net protein oxidation is adapted to dietary protein intake in domestic cats (*Felis silvestris catus*), *J Nutr* 132:456–460, 2002.

40. Backus RC: Advances in knowledge about feline metabolism, *Compend Cont Educ Vet* 30(Suppl):17–24, 2008.

41. Rogers JG, Morris QR: Essentiality of amino acids for the growing kitten, *J Nutr* 109:718–723, 1979.

42. Strieker MJ, Morris JG, Rogers QR: Increasing dietary crude protein does not increase the essential amino acid requirements of kittens, *J Anim Physiol Anim Nutr* 90:344–353, 2006.

43. Strieker MJ, Morris JG, Rogers QR: Increasing dietary crude protein does not increase the methionine requirement of kittens, *J Anim Physiol Anim Nutr* 91:465–474, 2007.

44. Burns RA, Milner JA, Corbin JE: Arginine: an indispensable amino acid for mature dogs, *J Nutr* 111:1020–1024, 1981.

45. Ha YH, Milner JA, Corbin JE: Arginine requirements in immature dogs, *J Nutr* 108:203–210, 1978.

46. Morris JG, Rogers QR: Arginine: an essential amino acid for the cat, *J Nutr* 108:1944–1953, 1978.

47. Morris JG, Rogers QR: Ammonia intoxication in the near-adult cat as a result of a dietary deficiency of arginine, *Science* 199(4327):431–432, 1978.

48. Czarnecki GL, Baker DH: Urea-cycle metabolism in the dog with emphasis on the role of arginine, *J Nutr* 114:581–586, 1984.

49. Rogers QR, Phang JM: Deficiency of pyrroline-5-carboxylate synthetase in the intestinal mucosa of the cat, *J Nutr* 115:146–150, 1985.

50. Morris JG: Nutritional and metabolic responses to arginine in carnivores, *J Nutr* 115:524–531, 1985.

51. Milner JA: Lysine requirements of the immature dog, *J Nutr* 111:40–45, 1981.

52. Brown RG: Protein in dog foods, *Can Vet J* 30:528–531, 1989.

53. Teeter RG, Baker DH, Corbin JE: Methionine and cystine requirements of the cat, *J Nutr* 108:291–297, 1978.

54. Burns RA, Milner JA: Sulfur amino acid requirements of the immature Beagle dog, *J Nutr* 111:2117–2122, 1981.

55. Hendriks WH, Rutherford SM, Rutherford KJ: Importance of sulfate, cysteine and methionine as precursors to felinine synthesis by domestic cats (*Felis catus*), *Comp Biochem Physiol C* 129:211–216, 2001.

56. Hendriks WH, Tarttelin MF, Moughan PJ: Twenty-four hours felinine excretion patterns in intact and castrated cats, *Physiol Behav* 58:467–469, 1995.

57. Rutherford-Marwick KJ, McGrath MC, Weidgraaf K, Hendriks WH: Gamma-glutamylfelinylglycine metabolite excretion in the urine of the domestic cat (*Felis catus*), *J Nutr* 136:2075S–2077S, 2006.

58. Rutherford SM, Kitson TM, Woolhouse AD, and others: Felinine stability in the presence of selected urine compounds, *Amino Acids* 32:235–242, 2007.

59. Huxtable RJ: The physiological actions of taurine, *Physiol Rev* 72:101–163, 1992.

60. Backus RC, Ko KS, Fascetti AJ, and others: Low plasma taurine concentration in Newfoundland dogs is associated with low plasma methionine and cyst(e)ine concentration and low taurine synthesis, *J Nutr* 136:2525–2533, 2006.

61. Sturma JA, Lu P: Role of feline maternal taurine nutrition in fetal cerebellar development: an immunohistochemical study, *Amino Acids* 13:369–377, 1997.

62. Morris JG, Rogers QR: The metabolic basis for the taurine requirement of cats. Taurine: nutritional value and mechanisms of action, *Adv Exp Med Biol* 315:33–44, 1992.

63. Morris JG, Rogers QR: Why is the nutrition of cats different from that of dogs? *Tijdschr Diergeneesk* 1:64S–67S, 1991.

64. Rabin AR, Nicolosi RJ, Hayes KC: Dietary influence of bile acid conjugation in the cat, *J Nutr* 106:1241–1246, 1976.

65. Hayes KC, Carey RE, Schmidt SY: Retinal degeneration associated with taurine deficiency in the cat, *Science* 188:949–951, 1975.

66. Hayes KC, Rabin AR, Berson EL: An ultrastructural study of nutritionally induced and reversed retinal degeneration in cats, *Am J Pathol* 78:505–524, 1978.

67. Wen GY, Sturman JA, Wisniewski HM, and others: Tapetum disorganization in taurine-depleted cats, *Invest Ophthalmol Vis Sci* 18:1201–1206, 1979.

68. Leon A, Levick WR, Sarossy WR: Lesion topography and new histological features in feline taurine deficiency retinopathy, *Exp Eye Res* 61:731–741, 1995.

69. Barnett KC, Burger IH: Taurine deficiency retinopathy in the cat, *J Small Anim Pract* 21:521–526, 1980.

70. Pion PD, Kittleson MD, Rogers QR, and others: Myocardial failure in cats associated with low plasma taurine: a reversible cardiomyopathy, *Science* 237:764–768, 1987.

71. Sturman JA, Gargano AD, Messing JM, Imaki H: Feline maternal taurine deficiency: effect on mother and offspring, *J Nutr* 116:655–667, 1986.

72. Sturman JA, Messing JM: Dietary taurine content and feline reproduction and outcome, *J Nutr* 121:1195–1203, 1991.

73. Dieter JA, Stewart DR, Haggarty MA, and others: Pregnancy failure in cats associated with long-term dietary taurine insufficiency, *J Reprod Fertil Suppl* 47:457–463, 1993.

74. Hickman MA, Morris JG, Rogers QR: Intestinal taurine and the enterohepatic circulation of taurocholic acid in the cat, *Adv Exp Med Biol* 315:45–54, 1992.

75. Stratton-Phelps MR, Cackus RC, Rogers QR, Fascetti AJ: Dietary rice bran decreases plasma and whole-blood taurine in cats, *J Nutr* 132:1745S–1747S, 2002.

76. Delaney SJ, Kass PH, Rogers QR, Fascetti AJ: Plasma and whole blood taurine in normal dogs of varying size fed commercially prepared food, *J Anim Physiol Anim Nutr* 87:236–244, 2003.

77. Kim SW, Rogers QR, Morris JG: Maillard reaction products in purified diets induce taurine depletion in cats which is reversed by antibiotics, *J Nutr* 126:195–201, 1996.

78. Morris JG, Rogers QR, Seungwook WK, and others: Dietary taurine requirement of cats is determined by microbial degradation of taurine in the gut, *Vet Clin Nutr* 1:118–127, 1994.

79. Douglass GM, Fern EB, Brown RC: Feline plasma and whole blood taurine levels as influenced by commercial dry and canned diets, *J Nutr* 121:S179–S180, 1991.

80. Spitze AR, Wong DL, Rogers QR, Fascetti AJ: Taurine concentrations in animal feed ingredients; cooking influences taurine content, *J Anim Physiol Anim Nutr* 87:251–262, 2003.

81. Freeman LM, Michel KE, Brown DJ: Idiopathic dilated cardiomyopathy in Dalmatians: nine cases (1990-1995), *J Am Vet Med Assoc* 209:1592–1596, 1996.

82. Sanderson SL, Gross KL, Ogburn PN: Effects of dietary fat and L-carnitine on plasma and whole blood taurine concentrations and cardiac function in health dogs fed protein-restricted diets, *Am J Vet Res* 62:1616–1623, 2001.

83. Kittleson ME, Keene B, Pion PD: Results of the Multicenter Spaniel Trial (MUST): taurine- and carnitine-responsive dilated cardiomyopathy in American Cocker Spaniels with decreased plasma taurine concentration, *J Vet Intern Med* 11:204–211, 1997.

84. Backus RC, Cohen G, Pion PD, and others: Taurine deficiency in Newfoundlands fed commercially available complete and balanced diets, *J Am Vet Med Assoc* 223:1130–1136, 2003.

85. Lawler DF, Templeton AJ, Monti KL: Evidence for genetic involvement in feline dilated cardiomyopathy, *J Vet Intern Med* 7:383–387, 1993.

86. Kim SW, Morris JG, Rogers QR: Dietary soybean protein decreases plasma taurine in cats, *J Nutr* 125:2831–2837, 1995.

87. Johnson ML, Parsons CM, Fahey CG Jr: Effects of species raw material source, ash content, and processing temperature on amino acid digestibility of animal by-product meals by cecectomized roosters and ileally cannulated dogs, *J Anim Sci* 76:1112–1122, 1998.

88. Backus RC, Ko KS, Fascetti AJ, and others: Low plasma taurine concentration in Newfoundland dogs is associated with low plasma methionine and cyst(e)ine concentrations and low taurine synthesis, *J Nutr* 136:2525–2533, 2006.

89. Ko KS, Backus RC, Berg JR, and others: Differences in taurine synthesis rate among dogs relate to differences in their maintenance energy requirement, *J Nutr* 137:1171–1175, 2007.

90. Torres CL, Backus RC, Rascetti AJ, Rogers QR: Taurine status in normal dogs fed a commercial diet associated with taurine deficiency and dilated cardiomyopathy, *J Anim Physiol Anim Nutr* 87:359–372, 2003.

91. Backus RC, Morris JG, Kim SW, and others: Dietary taurine needs of cats varies with dietary protein quality and concentration, *Vet Clin Nutr* 5:18–22, 1998.

92. Ikeda M, Tsuji H, Nakamura S, and others: Studies on the biosynthesis of nicotinamide adenine dinucleotide. II. A role of picolinic carboxylase in the biosynthesis of nicotinamide adenine dinucleotide from tryptophan in mammals, *J Biol Chem* 240:1395–1401, 1965.

93. Kallfelz FA: Evaluation and use of pet foods: general considerations in using pet foods for adult maintenance, *Vet Clin North Am Small Anim Pract* 19:387–403, 1989.

94. Murphy DH: Too much of a good thing: protein and a dog's diet, *Int J Study Anim Prob* 4:101–107, 1983.

95. Finco DR, Brown SA, Crowell WA, and others: Effects of aging and dietary protein intake on uninephrectomized geriatric dogs, *Am J Vet Res* 55:1282–1290, 1994.

96. Lowenstein LM: The rat as a model for aging in the kidney. In Gibson DC, Adelman RC, Finch C, editors: *Development of the rodent as a model system of aging*, Washington, DC, 1978, US Department of Health, Education, and Welfare.

97. Goldman R: Aging of the excretory system: kidney and bladder. In Finch EE, Hayflick L, editors: *Handbook of the biology of aging*, New York, 1977, Van Nostrand Reinhold.

98. Milward DJ, Fereday A, Gibson N, Pacy PJ: Aging, protein requirements, and protein turnover, *Am J Clin Nutr* 66:774–786, 1997.

99. Cowgill LD, Spangler WL: Renal insufficiency in geriatric dogs, *Vet Clin North Am Small Anim Pract* 11:727–749, 1981.

100. Davenport G, Gaasch S, Hayek MG, Cummins KA: Effect of dietary protein on body composition and metabolic responses of geriatric and young-adult dogs, *J Vet Intern Med* 15:306, 2001.

13

Vitamin and Mineral Requirements

FAT-SOLUBLE VITAMINS

Vitamins are organic dietary constituents that are necessary for growth and the maintenance of life, but they are not used by the body as an energy source or incorporated as part of tissue structure (see Section 1, pp. 27-36). The fat-soluble vitamins include vitamins A, D, E, and K. These vitamins are absorbed from the small intestine in much the same way as dietary fat and are stored primarily in the liver.

Vitamin A

All animals have a physiological requirement for active vitamin A (retinol). However, most mammals, including the dog but with the exception of the cat, have the ability to convert vitamin A precursors to active vitamin A (see Section 1, pp. 27-29). Carotenoid pigments, of which beta-carotene is the most important, are cleaved by a dioxygenase enzyme in the intestinal mucosa to yield vitamin A aldehyde (retinal). Retinal is then reduced by a second enzyme to form active vitamin A (retinol). Retinol is esterified to fatty acids and absorbed into the body along with dietary fat.[1,2] The dioxygenase enzyme that is essential for the splitting of the beta-carotene molecule is either absent or grossly deficient in the domestic cat. Studies have shown that neither dietary nor intravenous beta-carotene can prevent the development of vitamin A deficiency in the domestic cat.[3] As a result, the cat must have a source of preformed vitamin A present in the diet.

> All animals have a physiological requirement for vitamin A, but most mammals, including the dog, are able to convert vitamin A precursors such as the carotenoid pigments to active vitamin A. The cat, however, cannot convert carotenoids to retinol and so must have a source of dietary preformed vitamin A.

The most common forms of preformed vitamin A in foods are derivatives of retinol, such as retinyl palmitate and retinyl acetate. The largest quantities of these compounds are found in fish liver oils and animal livers. Nutrient requirements for vitamin A and its content in pet foods are expressed either as international units (IUs) or retinol equivalents (RE). One IU of vitamin A is equal to 0.3 micrograms (μg) of retinol or 0.3 RE. The 2006 National Research Council (NRC) recommendations suggest an adequate intake (AI) for dogs, during all life stages, of 303 RE/1000 kilocalories (kcal) of diet and a recommended allowance of 379 RE/1000 kcal.[4] These values are equivalent to 1060 RE/kilogram (kg) and 1326 RE/kg in a food containing 3.5 kcal/gram (g). The 2008 Association of American Feed Control Officials (AAFCO) *Nutrient Profiles* for dog foods recommends that dog foods containing an energy density of 3.5 kcal/kg should include a minimum of 5000 IU/kg for growth, reproduction, and adult maintenance.[5] This value is equivalent to 1500 RE/kg diet.

Because cats cannot convert carotenoid pigments to active vitamin A, the requirement is expressed in units of retinol for cats. The NRC's recommendations for cats suggests an AI of 200 μg retinol/1000 kcal of food for growing kittens and adult maintenance, and 400 μg/1000 kcal during pregnancy and lactation.[4] The recommended allowances are 250 μg and 500 μg, respectively. These recommended allowances are equivalent to 1000 μg/kg and 2000 μg/kg in a food with an ME of 4.0 kcal/g of dry matter (DM) (Table 13-1). The AAFCO *Nutrient Profiles* recommend a minimum of 5000 IU/kg of diet on a dry-matter basis (DMB) for adult maintenance and 9000 IU/kg for growth and reproduction in foods containing 4.0 kcal/kg.[5] These values are equivalent to 1500 μg and 2700 μg, respectively.

Vitamin A deficiency is rarely observed in dogs and cats because commercial pet foods contain adequate amounts and because dogs are able to convert the carotenoids found in plant matter into active vitamin A. Experimental vitamin A deficiency results in abnormal bone growth and neurological disorders in young animals. Stenosis of the neural foramina causes pinching of

TABLE 13-1 RECOMMENDED FAT-SOLUBLE VITAMIN LEVELS (ADULT MAINTENANCE)

	VITAMIN A	VITAMIN D	VITAMIN E	VITAMIN K
Dog*				
NRC (Recommended allowance)	1326 RE	483 IU	26.25 IU	1.40 mg
AAFCO	1500 RE	500 IU	50 IU	—†
Cat‡				
NRC (Recommended allowance)	1000 µg	280 IU	38 IU	1.0 mg
AAFCO	1500 µg	500 IU	30 IU§	0.1 mg‖

AAFCO, Association of American Feed Control Officials; *IU,* international units; *NRC,* National Research Council; *RE,* retinol equivalents.
*Estimates are per kg of diet containing 3500 kcal/kg.
†No requirement established.
‡Estimates are per kg of diet containing 4000 kcal/kg.
§Additional vitamin E is needed in diets containing high amounts of fish oils.
‖A dietary source of vitamin K is not needed except in food containing 25% or more fish (dry-matter basis).

cranial and spinal nerves as they pass through the abnormally shaped bone. If the deficiency persists, shortening and thickening of the long bones occur, along with abnormal development of the bones of the skull.[6] Vitamin A deficiency in adult animals affects reproduction, vision, and functioning of the epithelium. Clinical signs include anorexia, xerophthalmia and conjunctivitis, corneal opacity and ulceration, skin lesions, and multiple disorders of the epithelial layers in the body.[7]

Vitamin A toxicity is not common in the animal kingdom because the precursor for vitamin A, beta-carotene, is not a toxic substance. The intestinal mucosa regulates the hydrolysis of beta-carotene and the subsequent absorption of retinol into the body. In addition, the dog appears to have a relatively high tolerance for preformed vitamin A.[8,9] The cat differs from the dog because it cannot use carotenoids and must consume all of its vitamin A as preformed retinyl palmitate or free retinol from animal tissues. The absorption of preformed vitamin A is not regulated by the intestinal mucosa, and high amounts of this vitamin are readily absorbed by the body. If cats are fed foods having a concentrated source of vitamin A, they are unable to protect themselves from absorbing toxic levels. These foods include organ meats, such as liver and kidney, and various fish oils. Vitamin A toxicosis in cats results in a disorder called *deforming cervical spondylosis*. The effects of excess vitamin A on bone growth and remodeling cause the development of bony exostoses (outgrowths) on the cervical vertebrae. These changes eventually cause pain, difficult movement, lameness, and crippling in severe cases (see Section 4, pp. 280-282 for a complete discussion).

Vitamin D

Vitamin D is essential for normal calcium and phosphorus metabolism and homeostasis. The actions of vitamin D on the intestine, skeleton, and kidneys result in increased plasma levels of calcium and phosphorus. This facilitates normal mineralization and remodeling of bone and cartilage and maintains the concentration of calcium in the extracellular fluid that is necessary for normal muscle contraction and nervous tissue excitability. Many animals have the ability to synthesize vitamin D_3 (cholecalciferol) from 7-dehydrocholesterol when the skin is exposed to ultraviolet (UV) radiation. However, dogs and cats have limited ability to convert 7-dehydrocholesterol in the skin to vitamin D_3 and therefore are dependent upon a dietary source of this essential vitamin.[10] Studies with cats have found that this inability is caused by a high activity of the enzyme 7-dehydrocholesterol-delta-7-reductase, which catalyzes the conversion of 7-dehydrocholesterol to cholesterol.[11] Because cats rapidly convert 7-dehydrocholesterol to cholesterol, they have limited capacity for synthesizing cholecalciferol and, ultimately, active vitamin D (see Section 1, pp. 29-31).

The level of dietary vitamin D that is needed by a dog or cat depends upon the calcium and phosphorus levels in the diet and the age of the animal. Recent studies with dogs also suggest that differences may occur in vitamin D_3 metabolism and calcium homeostasis between large and small-breed dogs during periods of growth.[12,13] Specifically, the well-documented increased susceptibility of large-breed dogs to developmental skeletal disease may be related to relationships between elevated concentrations of circulating growth hormone, insulin-like growth factor, and active vitamin D_3 during growth (see Section 5, pp 496-497 for a complete discussion). Regardless of breed-size differences, all growing animals experience a high rate of skeletal calcification and so are more sensitive to dietary deficiency than are adult animals. The interrelationship between vitamin D, calcium, and phosphorus has been demonstrated by studies that have produced experimental vitamin D deficiencies in dogs and cats by limiting or imbalancing calcium and phosphorus levels.[14,15] For example, studies with kittens found that clinical signs of vitamin D deficiency did not occur when the level of calcium in a vitamin D–deficient diet was increased from 7 g/kg to 12 g/kg.[16] However, plasma levels of 25-hydroxycholecalciferol were less than normal in these kittens and increased significantly when the kittens were switched to a diet containing 124 IUs of vitamin D/kg. Normal plasma levels of 25-hydroxycholecalciferol were maintained when the diet's vitamin D content was further increased to 250 IU/kg. The current AAFCO *Nutrient Profiles* advise that dog foods and adult maintenance cat foods contain a minimum of 500 IU/kg of vitamin D. The recommendation for kitten diets is 750 IU/kg.

Unlike many animals, dogs and cats have limited ability to convert 7-dehydrocholesterol in the skin to vitamin D_3 and therefore must have a source of vitamin D_3 in their diets. The level that is needed depends on the animal's age and stage of development, as well as the concentrations of calcium and phosphorus in the food. In dogs, breed size may also influence an individual animal's vitamin D requirement.

As in other species, experimental induction of vitamin D deficiency in growing dogs and cats results in the development of rickets.[17,18] Rickets is characterized by bone malformation caused by insufficient deposition of calcium and phosphorus. The long bones are affected, resulting in bowing of the legs and thickening of the joints. When the deficient diet is replaced with a food containing vitamin D, signs resolve, normal bone mineralization can occur, and circulating levels of vitamin D metabolites increase to normal values. Vitamin D deficiency has also been produced in kittens that were fed a diet containing no vitamin D and 1% calcium and phosphorus.[19] Deficiency signs were exacerbated when the diet's phosphorus level was decreased to 0.65% and calcium was increased to 2%. Because practical ingredients that are included in commercially produced pet foods naturally contain vitamin D_3, deficiency is rare in companion animals, and when observed is usually associated with either a strict vegetarian diet, the presence of disease, or an inborn error of metabolism.

Vitamin D deficiency in adult animals leads to osteomalacia. This disorder is caused by decalcification of bone and results in an increased tendency of the long bones to fracture. Cats with vitamin D deficiency become reluctant to move and show decreased inclination to groom themselves. A progressive posterior paralysis develops, eventually leading to quadriparesis in advanced cases. These neurological changes are associated with degeneration of the spinal cord caused by abnormal growth and remodeling of cervical vertebrae. In most animals, vitamin D deficiency develops concomitantly with deficiencies or imbalances in dietary calcium and phosphorus. Low levels or imbalances of these minerals exacerbate vitamin D deficiency and may precipitate the signs of rickets in growing animals or osteomalacia in adults.

Hypervitaminosis D caused by excess levels of dietary vitamin D is well documented and results in hypercalcemia and calcification of soft tissues. The most common cause in pet dogs and cats is not dietary, but rather occurs as a result of accidental cholecalciferol rodenticide poisoning.[20-22] In addition, several cases of hypervitaminosis D were reported to occur in dogs in the United Kingdom and cats in Japan; these animals were fed commercial foods that mistakenly contained excessive levels of vitamin D.[23,24] In both these cases, the commercial foods contained excessively high concentrations of vitamin D because of a manufacturing error that subsequently led to product recalls. A survey of commercial cat foods marketed in the United States found that none of the foods was deficient in vitamin D content, based upon an arbitrary minimum requirement of 250 IU/kg, but some did contain less than the AAFCO minimum of 500 IU/kg.[19] Conversely, 20 of the 49 foods sampled contained more than 7500 IU/kg, and 15 contained more than 10,000 IU/kg, levels that are well above the AAFCO's maximum allowance of 5000 IU/kg. The sources of high vitamin D levels are generally ingredients such as fish meals and fish oils that contain naturally high concentrations of the vitamin, rather than supplemental vitamin D. Regardless of these findings, no reports of clinical vitamin D toxicity in cats have been reported in the United States, although there is some evidence of a connection between feline oral resorptive lesions and high dietary vitamin D (see Chapter 34, p. 447). The lack of toxicity reports may be in part due to evidence that cats appear to be relatively resistant to cholecalciferol toxicosis, when compared with other species.[25]

Vitamin E

Vitamin E functions as a biological, chain-breaking antioxidant that neutralizes free radicals and prevents the peroxidation of lipids within cellular membranes. An animal's requirement for vitamin E depends on dietary levels of polyunsaturated fatty acids (PUFAs) and selenium, a trace mineral. Vitamin E and selenium function synergistically. Although vitamin E protects cell membrane fatty acids by quenching the free radicals formed during oxidation, selenium (as a component of the enzyme glutathione peroxidase) reduces peroxide formation. This process further protects membrane fatty acids from oxidative damage (see Section 1, p. 31). Increasing the level of unsaturated fat in the diet causes an increase in an animal's vitamin E requirement. In commercial pet foods, vitamin E also protects unsaturated dietary fats from destructive oxidation. The vitamin is preferentially oxidized before the unsaturated fatty acids, thus protecting them from rancidity. However, in this process, vitamin E is destroyed. Therefore, as the level of unsaturated fatty acids in a food increases, its concentration of vitamin E should also increase.

A naturally occurring deficiency of vitamin E is not common in dogs and cats. However, the ingestion of poorly prepared or poorly stored foods or supplementation with large amounts of PUFAs can precipitate a relative deficiency of this vitamin.[26,27] Experimentally induced vitamin E deficiency in dogs results in skeletal muscle degeneration, decreased reproductive performance, retinal degeneration, and impaired immunological response.[28,29] Supplementation with large amounts of vitamin E has been theorized to be beneficial in the treatment of some types of skin disorders in dogs, such as discoid lupus erythematosus, demodicosis, and acanthosis nigricans,

with varying levels of success reported (see Section 5, p. 384).[30,31] However, these responses are believed to reflect a pharmacological response to high doses of vitamin E, rather than a response to a dietary deficiency state. Although study results have been conflicting, it has also been theorized that dogs engaging in prolonged or strenuous activity that results in oxidative stress may benefit from supplemental vitamin E, and that vitamin E may help to enhance the immune response (see Section 4, pp. 255-256 for a complete discussion).[32]

A condition called *pansteatitis,* or "yellow fat disease," occurs in cats that are fed diets containing marginal or low levels of vitamin E and high amounts of unsaturated fatty acids. Signs of pansteatitis include anorexia, depression, pyrexia (fever), hyperesthesia of the thorax and abdomen, a reluctance to move, and the presence of "swollen fat."[33,34] A diet that contains high levels of fish oil may cause a threefold to fourfold increase in a cat's daily requirement for vitamin E. Early cases of pansteatitis occurred almost exclusively in cats that were fed a canned, commercial, fish-based cat food, of which red tuna was the principal type of fish. Later cases of the disease occurred in cats that were fed diets consisting wholly or largely of canned red tuna, fish scraps, and, in two cases, an imbalanced homemade diet comprised almost completely of whole pig's brain.[35] Red tuna packed in oil contains high levels of PUFAs and low levels of vitamin E. The addition of large amounts of fish products to a cat's diet appears to be the most common cause of this disease (see Section 4, p. 279).

Vitamin K

Vitamin K includes a class of compounds known as *quinones*. This vitamin is necessary for normal blood coagulation because of its role in the synthesis of prothrombin (factor II) and several other clotting factors (see Section 1, p. 32). Evidence in both dogs and cats indicates very low dietary requirements for vitamin K, probably due to the ability of bacterial synthesis in the intestine to fully meet the animal's need for this nutrient. However, interference with vitamin K synthesis or absorption can cause a deficiency, with signs of hemorrhage and decreased levels of prothrombin in the blood.

Naturally occurring vitamin K deficiency has not been reported in dogs and has only been reported anecdotally in case studies of cats consuming diets containing high amounts of fish. In two separate situations, cats fed canned commercial cat foods containing either salmon or tuna developed clinical signs of vitamin K deficiency.[36] Signs included the development of gastric ulcers, increased coagulation times, and decreased serum concentrations of vitamin K–dependent clotting factors. Surprisingly, the vitamin K concentration in the diets was found to be 60 μg/kg diet, a level considered to be adequate for companion animals. Surviving animals responded positively to vitamin K supplementation and demonstrated normalized clotting times within 24 hours of vitamin K therapy. A subsequent series of studies by the same laboratory failed to induce vitamin K deficiency in cats fed various types of purified diets. The experimental diets contained low levels of vitamin K (4 to 30 μg/kg diet) and various factors with the potential to interfere with vitamin K synthesis or absorption. These results suggest that kittens fed purified diets have very low dietary vitamin K requirements and that there may be a factor present in some canned cat foods containing fish that interferes with vitamin K synthesis or absorption. Although this factor or underlying cause has not been identified, it is recommended that canned fish-based cat diets include supplemental vitamin K in the form of 1.0 milligrams (mg) menaquinone/kg food in a food containing 4000 kcal/kg.[4]

WATER-SOLUBLE VITAMINS

The water-soluble vitamins that are of importance to the dog and cat are all B-complex vitamins. Most of these vitamins are involved in the metabolism of food and the production of energy in the body (see Section 1, pp. 32-34). Because of the availability of well-formulated and well-balanced pet foods today, simple deficiencies of the B-complex vitamins are rare in companion animals. However, there are several situations in which B-vitamin nutrition may be of concern in the nutritional management of dogs or cats. Thiamin deficiency can occur when pets are fed certain types of raw fish containing an enzyme that destroys this vitamin, while biotin deficiency can be induced by feeding animals large amounts of raw egg whites (see Section 4, pp. 279-280 for complete discussions).[37-40] The requirement for vitamin B_6 (pyridoxine) is directly affected by the level of protein in the diet. As the protein level in

the diet increases, so does a dog's or cat's requirement for vitamin B_6.[41] Finally, genetics can also play a role in B-vitamin metabolism. An example is an inherited disorder in Giant Schnauzers that causes malabsorption of vitamin B_{12} (see Section 5, pp. 297-298).

MINERALS

As with most other nutrients, problems with mineral nutrition in dogs and cats are often a result of excesses or imbalances from interactions with other nutrients rather than a result of frank deficiencies in the diet. This section focuses on those minerals that are of most practical significance in the nutrition and feeding management of dogs and cats today.

Calcium and Phosphorus

Calcium and phosphorus are macrominerals necessary for the formation and maintenance of the skeleton. These nutrients are also involved in a wide range of metabolic reactions (see Section 1, pp. 37-40). When considering canine and feline requirements for all nutrients, availability in the diet must be taken into account. This is especially important for calcium and phosphorus because of the many factors that can affect the bioavailability of these minerals. The dietary requirement for available calcium is quite low. An early study reported that 0.37% available calcium or 0.5% to 0.65% total calcium was adequate for growing puppies.[42] Similarly, when cats are fed purified diets containing highly available nutrients, normal growth can be supported by as little as 150 to 200 mg of calcium/day.[43] However, up to twice this amount is needed when they were fed practical diets. The current AAFCO *Nutrient Profiles* for dogs and for cats recommend a minimum level of 1.0% calcium and 0.8% phosphorus for growth/reproduction, and 0.6% calcium and 0.5% phosphorus for adult maintenance.[5] The NRC recommends a minimum level of 0.8% calcium for all size puppies, noting that this level most likely exceeds the minimum needs of most dogs other than large and giant breeds.[4] Although there is evidence that adult cats can consume diets with a ratio as low as 0.6:1 with no adverse effects, dietary calcium/phosphorus ratios between 1.2:1 to 1.4:1 are considered optimal for animals by most nutritionists.[44]

When formulating rations, pet food manufacturers must account for differences in calcium and phosphorus availability in the various ingredients that are used. Absorption coefficients for calcium have been reported to vary between 0% and 90%, depending on the composition of the diet, the age of the animal, and the total calcium content of the diet.[45] Numerous studies have shown that, within limits, as the calcium content of a diet decreases, the dog's efficiency of absorption increases, and calcium availability gradually decreases as dogs mature.[46,47] In addition, calcium absorption coefficients decline with age as young growing animals reach maturity.[47] Another factor to consider in dogs is adult size. Recent data show that the minimum requirement for calcium may also vary with breed size in dogs; large-breed puppies have slightly higher requirements than small-breed ones. Studies with Great Dane puppies indicate that 0.55% total calcium was not adequate, while 0.82% supported normal growth.[48,49] Conversely, a study with growing Miniature Poodles found that small-breed puppies grew normally when fed as low as 0.36% and as high as 1.2% calcium.[50] Because large-breed puppies are also more sensitive to excessively high levels of calcium in the diet, dietary calcium levels for growing large- and giant-breed dogs must be carefully formulated to support healthy skeletal development (see Section 5, pp. 499-500 for a complete discussion).

In general, as the calcium content of a food decreases, the dog's efficiency of absorption increases. In addition, calcium absorption coefficients decline with age as young growing animals reach maturity. Finally, large-breed puppies have slightly higher calcium requirements than small-breed ones. Because large-breed puppies are also more sensitive to excessively high levels of calcium in the diet, dietary calcium levels for growing large- and giant-breed dogs must be carefully formulated to support healthy skeletal development.

A final consideration is the differing calcium and phosphorus availability among the ingredients that are commonly used in pet foods. In general, the calcium and phosphorus in plant products are less available than the minerals found in animal products. Cereal grains contain phytate, a phosphorus-containing compound that can bind other minerals, including calcium, and make them unavailable for absorption. Although phytate is very high in phosphorus, the availability of phytate phosphorus is only about 30%.[51] On the other hand, some of the animal-source proteins that are included in pet foods are high in phosphorus but relatively low in calcium; these products include fresh meat or poultry, meat or fish meals, and organ meats. As a result, pet foods must be carefully formulated to ensure that both adequate levels and a proper ratio of calcium to phosphorus are maintained.

Deficiencies of calcium and phosphorus are unusual today because of the production of well-formulated pet foods. Because phosphorus is present in so many foods, a dietary deficiency of this mineral is extremely rare. However, calcium imbalance in growing dogs or cats still occurs as a result of improper feeding practices. A calcium deficiency develops most commonly when puppies or kittens are fed unconventional diets that contain a high proportion of muscle or organ meats. This type of diet results in a syndrome called *nutritional secondary hyperparathyroidism*. The low calcium and extremely high phosphorus content of an all-meat diet leads to inadequate absorption of calcium and transient hypocalcemia. The lowered blood levels of calcium stimulate the release of parathyroid hormone (PTH). PTH causes increased production of calcitriol (active vitamin D) and thus increased bone resorption of calcium, resulting in a restoration of normal blood calcium levels. When calcium is deficient in the diet, chronically elevated levels of PTH maintain blood calcium levels within a normal range. However, these elevated PTH levels lead to bone demineralization and a loss of bone mass.[52] In dogs, the mandibles (jaw bones) show the earliest signs of bone demineralization; this leads to periodontal disease and loss of teeth. Over time, severe bone loss leads to compression of the spinal vertebrae and spontaneous fractures of the long bones. Affected dogs and cats exhibit joint pain and swelling, lameness, and a reluctance to move. Splaying of the toes, excessive sloping of the metatarsal and metacarpal bones, and lateral deviation of the carpus are also observed. Treatment involves correction of the diet through provision of a nutritionally complete and balanced ration. It is advisable to completely replace the deficient diet with a balanced commercially prepared pet food rather than attempt to balance the current diet through the addition of calcium supplements (see Section 4, p. 277).

A second problem that involves calcium homeostasis in the body is the occurrence of puerperal tetany or eclampsia in lactating bitches and queens. Eclampsia is a disease that is seen most frequently in small and toy breeds of dogs and, less frequently, in cats.[53] Its onset is immediately before or 2 to 3 weeks after parturition and is more common in dams of large litters. The disorder appears to be caused by the failure of the dam's calcium regulatory mechanisms to maintain serum-ionized calcium levels when there is a loss of calcium to the milk. One of the roles of ionized calcium in the body is to stabilize electrical charges across nerve and muscle cell membranes. In the absence of normal serum calcium levels, cell membranes become hyperexcitable, leading to convulsive seizures and tetany. Some dogs develop nonspecific signs such as excessive panting, changes in behavior, vomiting, or diarrhea.[54] Serum calcium levels may decrease to less than 7 mg/deciliter (dl). Normally, serum calcium is strictly maintained at a level of 9.5 to 10.5 mg/dl. Prompt medical care is necessary and consists of intravenous administration of calcium borogluconate.[55,56] Prognosis is very good if the disorder is treated at an early stage.

Although controlled studies have not been conducted with companion animals, research with dairy cattle has demonstrated that the consumption of a diet high in calcium during pregnancy actually increases the incidence of this disorder, and moderately low intakes of calcium can prevent its occurrence.[57] It is theorized that a relative hypercalcemia, caused by a high-calcium diet or calcium supplementation during pregnancy, exerts negative feedback on PTH synthesis and secretion by the parathyroid gland. This effect causes a decrease in both the body's capability to mobilize calcium stores from bone and its ability to increase calcium absorption in the intestine. When calcium is suddenly needed for lactation, the body's regulatory mechanisms are unable to adapt quickly enough to the sudden calcium loss. Calcium is diverted preferentially to milk production, and the animal's serum calcium decreases. Although a correlation between excess calcium during pregnancy and eclampsia has not been demonstrated in dogs or cats, it is prudent to avoid calcium supplements during pregnancy in these species. If a bitch or queen is being fed a high-quality commercial food that has been

formulated for feeding through gestation and lactation, calcium supplementation is not necessary and is probably contraindicated.

Just as too little calcium during growth can be detrimental to dogs and cats, so can excessive amounts. The most common cause of excess calcium in a pet's diet is supplementation of an already complete and balanced pet food with high-calcium foods or mineral supplements. Although adequate calcium is essential for normal bone growth and skeletal development, several health risks are associated with excessive dietary calcium. One of the most well-documented risk factors is the association between calcium intake and developmental skeletal disorders in large- and giant-breed dogs (see Section 5, pp. 497-499 for a complete discussion).

Magnesium

Magnesium is present in both soft tissues and bone. It is essential for normal muscle and nervous tissue functioning and plays a key role in a number of enzymatic reactions (see Section 1, p. 40). Although it has not been studied in dogs, magnesium absorption in growing kittens decreases with age. This reduction in efficiency is exacerbated when excessive dietary calcium is fed. Although uncommon, magnesium deficiency results in muscle weakness, ataxia, and, eventually, convulsive seizures. Naturally occurring magnesium deficiency has not been reported in dogs and cats. Conversely, excess magnesium is a risk factor in the development of certain types of feline lower urinary tract disease (see Section 5, pp. 362-365 for a complete discussion).

Copper

Copper is needed by the body for iron absorption and transport, hemoglobin formation, and normal functioning of the cytochrome oxidase enzyme system (see Section 1, p. 41). The normal metabolism of copper in the body involves the passage of excess copper through the liver and its excretion in bile. Disorders that affect bile excretion often result in an accumulation of copper in the liver, sometimes to toxic levels. In these cases, liver copper toxicosis is a secondary disorder that develops as an effect of the underlying liver disease. However, a primary hepatic copper-storage disease exists in certain breeds of dogs. In these cases, the underlying cause of the disease is an accumulation of copper in the liver that eventually results in degenerative liver disease (see Section 5, pp. 298-299).

Zinc

With the exception of iron, zinc is the most abundant micromineral present in the body's tissues. It is important for normal carbohydrate, lipid, protein, and nucleic acid metabolism, and it is necessary for the maintenance of epidermal integrity, taste acuity, and immunological functions.[58] Zinc is a cofactor for the enzyme delta-6-desaturase, and so is essential for the conversion of linoleic acid to arachidonic acid in the body. It is also a cofactor for ribonucleic acid (RNA) and deoxyribonucleic acid (DNA) polymerases, making it an important mineral for rapidly dividing cells, such as those found in the skin. These two functions have led researchers to study the synergistic use of zinc and supplemental fatty acid for the promotion of skin and coat health in dogs, and potentially for the treatment of certain types of inflammatory skin diseases (see Section 5, pp. 384-390).[59,60]

Zinc deficiency has been reported in a variety of animal species, including dogs and cats.[61-63] Clinical signs that are common to most species include growth retardation, abnormalities in hair and skin condition, gastrointestinal disturbances, and impaired reproductive performance. The disruption of normal cellular division and maturation processes is believed to be the underlying cause of many of these signs. Experimental studies of zinc deficiency in dogs and cats have found that skin and coat changes are usually the first clinical signs to develop in these species. Within 2 weeks of consuming a zinc-deficient ration, dogs will develop desquamating skin lesions on the foot pads, extremities, joints, and groin. Lesions first appear as small, erythematous areas that eventually enlarge and merge into dry, crusty, brown lesions. Microscopically, the lesions show parakeratosis, hyperkeratinization, and an inflammatory infiltration of neutrophils, lymphocytes, and macrophages.[64] Coat changes have also been reported to occur with zinc deficiency. Affected dogs develop a dry, harsh hair coat with fading coat color. When a diet containing adequate zinc is provided, these clinical signs rapidly resolve. Although not common, naturally occurring zinc deficiency has been reported in dogs fed poorly formulated, inexpensive, dry dog foods.[65] Young, rapidly growing dogs of the large and giant breeds seem to be most susceptible, but several cases have also been reported in adult animals (Figure 13-1) (see Section 3, pp. 168-169).[66] Another dietary cause of a relative zinc deficiency is feeding excessive calcium (see Section 5, pp. 497-499). An inherited disorder of zinc metabolism occurs in certain breeds of dogs and also causes clinical signs of zinc deficiency (see Section 5, pp. 299-300 for a complete discussion).

Sodium

The concern over the connection between sodium intake and essential hypertension in humans has resulted in interest in the sodium content of pet foods and its implications for companion animal health. An animal's requirement for sodium is primarily influenced by the unavoidable daily loss of this mineral from the body.[67] In adults, during maintenance, these losses are

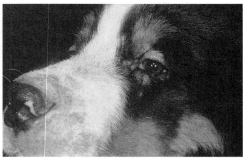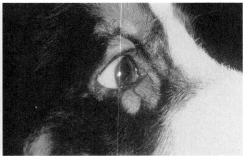

Figure 13-1   Zinc deficiency in a young, rapidly growing Bernese Mountain Dog due to increased requirements during growth. (Courtesy Candace Sousa, DVM, Animal Dermatology Clinic, Sacramento, California.)

usually quite low. The body's ability to conserve sodium results in a very low dietary sodium requirement in dogs and cats. Maintenance requirements of adults are estimated to range between 0.03% to 0.09% sodium (DM basis), with slight increases required during pregnancy and lactation. Most commercial pet foods contain well above these amounts of sodium.

In all animals, the immediate effect of increased salt intake is increased water consumption. Sodium balance in dogs is maintained primarily through changes in urinary excretion of the mineral.[68] An increase in intake above the body's requirement is accompanied by increases in urinary water and sodium excretion. The most important risk attributed to long-term salt excess is its effect on blood pressure. Although this association has been shown to be a causal factor in the development of essential hypertension in certain human subpopulations, there are no data supporting the existence of such a relationship in dogs and cats. Essential hypertension is infrequently seen in companion animals. Data from studies that examined the effect of salt intake on canine blood pressure indicate that this species is resistant to salt retention and hypertension.[69] Adult dogs that were fed high-sodium diets were able to resist very high levels of salt intake without weight gain or edema, and their renal systems adjusted quickly to changes in dietary sodium.[70] When hypertension does occur in dogs and cats, it is usually a secondary disorder occurring as a result of renal disease. Although additional controlled research needs to be conducted, the dog appears to be resistant to the development of salt-induced hypertension. In addition, companion animals readily adapt to the sodium levels in pet foods by altering urinary excretion of sodium.[71] These levels are probably of no harm when fed to animals that are healthy and have free access to fresh water.

References

1. Goodman DS, Huang HS, Kanai M, and others: The enzymatic conversion of all-trans beta-carotene into retinal, *J Biol Chem* 242:3543–3554, 1967.

2. Thompson SY, Braude R, Coates ME, and others: Further studies on the conversion of beta-carotene to vitamin A, *Br J Nutr* 4:398–420, 1960.

3. Gershoff SN, Andrus SB, Hegsted DM, and others: Vitamin A deficiency in cats, *Lab Invest* 6:227–239, 1957.

4. National Research Council: *Nutrient requirements of dogs and cats*, Washington, DC, 2006, National Academy Press.

5. Association of American Feed Control Officials (AAFCO): Official publication, 2008, AAFCO.

6. Hayes KC: On the pathophysiology of vitamin A deficiency, *Nutr Rev* 29:3–6, 1971.

7. Crimm PD, Short DM: Vitamin A deficiency in the dog, *Am J Physiol* 118:477–482, 1937.

8. Cline JL, Czarnecki-Maulden GL, Losonsky JM, and others: Effect of increasing dietary vitamin A on bone density in adult dogs, *J Anim Sci* 75:2980–2985, 1997.

9. Goldy GG, Burr JR, Longardner CN, and others: Effects of measured doses of vitamin A fed to healthy Beagle dogs for 26 weeks, *Vet Clin Nutr* 3:42–49, 1996.

10. How KL, Hazewinkel AW, Mol JA: Dietary vitamin D dependence of cat and dog due to inadequate cutaneous synthesis of vitamin D, *Gen Comp Endocrin* 96:12–18, 1994.

11. Morris JG: Ineffective vitamin D synthesis in cats is reversed by an inhibitory of 7-dehydrocholesterol-delta-7-reductase, *J Nutr* 129:903–908, 1999.

12. Hazewinkel HAW, Tryfonidou MA: Vitamin D3 metabolism in dogs, *Mol Cell Endocrinol* 197:23–33, 2002.

13. Tryfonidou MA, Holl MS, Vastenburg M, and others: Hormonal regulation of calcium homeostasis in two breeds of dogs during growth at different rates, *J Anim Sci* 81:1568–1580, 2003.

14. Campbell JR, Douglas TA: The effect of low calcium intake and vitamin D supplements on bone structure in young growing dogs, *Br J Nutr* 19:339–347, 1965.

15. Brickman AS, Chilumula RR, Coburn JW, and others: Biologic action of 1,25-dihydroxy-vitamin D3 in the rachitic dog, *Endocrinology* 92:728–734, 1973.

16. Morris JG, Earle KE: Vitamin D and calcium requirements of kittens, *Vet Clin Nutr* 3:93–96, 1996.

17. Hazewinkel HAW: Nutrition in relation to skeletal growth deformities, *J Small Anim Pract* 30:625–630, 1989.

18. Mellanby T: The part played by an "accessory factor" in the production of experimental rickets, *J Physiol* 52:1–14, 1918.

19. Morris JF: Vitamin D synthesis by kittens, *Vet Clin Nutr* 3:88–92, 1996.

20. Bahri LE: Poisoning in dogs by vitamin D3-containing rodenticides, *Compend Contin Educ Pract Vet* 12:1414–1417, 1990.

21. Murphy MJ: Rodenticides, *Vet Clin North Am Small Anim Pract* 32:469–484, 2002.

22. Peterson EN, Kirby R, Bovee KC: Cholecalciferol rodenticide intoxication in a cat, *J Am Vet Med Assoc* 199:904–906, 1991.

23. Mellanby RJ, Mee AP, Bery JL, Herrtage ME: Hypercalcaemia in two dogs caused by excessive dietary supplementation of vitamin D, *J Small Anim Pract* 46:334–338, 2005.

24. Sato R, Yamagishi H, Naito Y, and others: Feline vitamin D toxicosis caused by commercially available cat food, *J Jpn Vet Med Assoc* 46:577–581, 1993.

25. Sih TR, Morris JG, Hickman A: Chronic ingestion of high concentration of cholecalciferol in cats, *Am J Vet Res* 62:1500–1506, 2001.

26. Van-Vleet JF: Experimentally-induced vitamin E-selenium deficiency in the growing dog, *J Am Vet Med Assoc* 166:769–774, 1975.

27. Hayes KC, Nielsen SW, Rousseay JE: Vitamin E deficiency and fat stress in the dog, *J Nutr* 99:196–209, 1969.

28. Hayes KC, Rousseau JE, Hegsted DM: Plasma tocopherol concentration and vitamin E deficiency in dogs, *J Am Vet Med Assoc* 157:64–71, 1970.

29. Riis RE, Sheffy BE, Loew E, and others: Vitamin E deficiency retinopathy in dogs, *Am J Vet Res* 42:74–86, 1981.

30. Scott DW, Walton DK: Clinical evaluation of oral vitamin E for the treatment of primary canine acanthosis nigricans, *J Am Anim Hosp Assoc* 21:345–350, 1985.

31. Figueiredo C: Vitamin E serum contents, erythrocyte and lymphocyte count, PCV, and hemoglobin determinations in normal dogs, dogs with scabies, and dogs with demodicosis. In *Proceedings of the annual American Academy of Veterinary Dermatologists and the American College of Veterinary Dermatology*, 1985, p 8.

32. Hinchliff KW, Reinhart GA, Reynolds AJ, and others: Exercise and oxidant stress. In Reinhart GA, Carey DP, editors: *Recent advances in canine and feline nutrition, Iams nutrition symposium proceedings*, vol 2, Wilmington, Ohio, 1998, Orange Frazer Press.

33. Cordy DR: Experimental production of steatitis (yellow fat disease) in kittens fed a commercial canned cat food and prevention of the condition by vitamin E, *Cornell Vet* 44:310–318, 1954.

34. Gaskell CJ, Leedale AH, Douglas SW: Pansteatitis in the cat: a report of five cases, *J Small Anim Pract* 16:117–121, 1975.

35. Nize MM, Vilela CL, Ferreira LM: Feline pansteatitis revisited: hazards of unbalanced home-made diets, *J Feline Med Surg* 5:271–277, 2003.

36. Strieker MJ, Morris JG, Feldman BF, and others: Vitamin K deficiency in cats fed commercial fish-based diets, *J Small Anim Pract* 37:322–326, 1996.

37. Smith DC, Proutt LM: Development of thiamine deficiency in the cat on a diet of raw fish, *Proc Soc Exp Biol Med* 56:1–5, 1944.

38. Houston D, Hulland TJ: Thiamine deficiency in a team of sled dogs, *Can Vet J* 29:383–385, 1988.

39. Pastoor FJH, Herck H, van Klooster A, and others: Biotin deficiency in cats as induced by feeding a purified diet containing egg white, *J Nutr* 121:S73–S74, 1991.

40. Shen CS, Overfield L, Murthy PNA, and others: Effect of feeding raw egg white on pyruvate and propionyl CoA carboxylase activities on tissues of the dog, *Fed Proc* 36:1169, 1977.

41. Bai SC, Sampwon DA, Morris JG, and others: The level of dietary protein affects the vitamin B-6 requirement of cats, *J Nutr* 121:1054–1061, 1991.

42. Jenkins KJ, Phillips PH: The mineral requirements of the dog. II. The relation of calcium, phosphorus and fat levels to minimal calcium and phosphorus requirements, *J Nutr* 70:241–246, 1960.

43. Scott PP: Minerals and vitamins in feline nutrition. In Graham-Jones O, editor: *Canine and feline nutrition requirements*, London, 1965, Pergamon Press.

44. Kealy RD, Lawler DF, Ballam JM: Dietary calcium:phosphorus ratio for adult cats, *Vet Clin Nutr* 3:28, 1996.

45. Hedhammer A: Nutrition as it relates to skeletal disease. In *Proceedings of the Kal Kan symposium*, Columbus, Ohio, 1980.

46. Schoenmakers I, Hazewinkel H, van den Brom W: Excessive Ca and P intake during early maturation in dogs alters Ca and P balance without long-term effects after dietary normalization, *J Nutr* 129:1968–1974, 1999.

47. Tryfonidou MA, van den Broek J, van den Brom WE, Hazewinkel HAW: Intestinal calcium absorption in growing dogs is influenced by calcium intake and age but not by growth rate, *J Nutr* 132:3363–3368, 2002.

48. Hazewinkel HAW, van den Brom WE, van 'T Klooster AT, and others: Calcium metabolism in Great Dane dogs fed diets with various calcium and phosphorus levels, *J Nutr* 121:S99–S106, 1991.

49. Laflamme D: Effect of breed size on calcium requirements for puppies, *Compend Contin Educ Pract Vet* 23:66–69, 2000.

50. Nap RH, Hazewinkel H, van den Brom W: 45Ca kinetics in growing Miniature Poodles challenged by four different dietary levels of calcium, *J Nutr* 123:1826–1833, 1993.

51. Erdman J: Oilseed phytates: nutritional implications, *J Am Oil Chem Soc* 56:736–741, 1979.

52. Hintz HF, Schryver HF: Nutrition and bone development in dogs, *Comp Anim Pract* 1:44–47, 1987.

53. Smith FO: Postpartum diseases, *Vet Clin North Am Small Anim Pract* 16:521–524, 1986.

54. Brobat KJ, Casey KK: Eclampsia in dogs: 31 cases (1995-1998), *J Am Vet Med Assoc* 217:216–219, 2000.

55. Austad R, Bjerkas E: Eclampsia in the bitch, *J Small Anim Pract* 17:793–798, 1976.

56. Bjerkas E: Eclampsia in the cat, *J Small Anim Pract* 15:411–414, 1974.

57. Wiggers KD, Nelson DK, Jacobson NL: Prevention of parturient paresis by a low-calcium diet prepartum: a field study, *J Dairy Sci* 58:430–431, 1975.

58. Catalanotto FA: The trace metal zinc and taste, *Am J Clin Nutr* 31:1098–1103, 1978.

59. Kirby NA, Hester SL, Bauer JE: Dietary fats and the skin and coat of dogs, *J Am Vet Med Assoc* 230:1641–1644, 2007.

60. Marsh KA, Ruedisueli FL, Coe SL: Effects of zinc and linoleic acid supplementation on the skin and coat quality of dogs receiving a complete and balanced diet, *Vet Dermatol* 11:277–284, 2000.

61. Kane E, Morris JG, Rogers QR, and others: Zinc deficiency in the cat, *J Nutr* 111:488–495, 1981.

62. Wolf AM: Zinc-responsive dermatosis in a Rhodesian Ridgeback, *Vet Med* 82:908–912, 1987.

63. Van den Broek AHM, Thoday KL: Skin disease in dogs associated with zinc deficiency: a report of five cases, *J Small Anim Pract* 27:313–323, 1986.

64. Banta CA: The role of zinc in canine and feline nutrition. In Burger IH, Rivers JPW, editors: *Nutrition of the dog and cat*, New York, 1989, Cambridge University Press.

65. Sousa CA, Stannard AA, Ihrke PJ: Dermatosis associated with feeding generic dog food: 13 cases (1981-1982), *J Am Vet Med Assoc* 192:676–680, 1988.

66. Fadok VA: Zinc responsive dermatosis in a Great Dane: a case report, *J Am Anim Hosp Assoc* 18:409–414, 1982.

67. Mitchell AR: Salt intake, animal health and hypertension: should sleeping dogs lie? In Burger IH, Rivers JPW, editors: *Nutrition of the dog and cat*, New York, 1989, Cambridge University Press.

68. Smith RC, Haschem T, Hamlin RL, and others: Water and electrolyte intake and output and quantity of feces in the healthy dog, *Vet Med Small Anim Clin* 59:743–748, 1964.

69. Spangler WL, Gribble DH, Weiser MG: Canine hypertension: a review, *J Am Vet Med Assoc* 170:995–998, 1977.

70. Gupta B, Linden R, Mary D, Weatherill D: The influence of high and low sodium intake on blood volume in the dog, *J Exp Physiol* 66:117–128, 1981.

71. Kirk CA, Jewell DE, Lowry SR: Effects of sodium chloride on selected parameters in cats, *Vet Ther* 7:333–346, 2006.

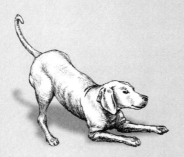

Section 3

Pet Foods

The previous two sections examined the basic principles of nutrition and the specific nutrient requirements of dogs and cats. The practical application of this information is the provision of optimal nutrition to companion animals throughout life. Section 3 provides information that enables pet owners and professionals to thoroughly evaluate and select appropriate foods for dogs or cats. The history and current regulation of commercial pet foods is examined, with special attention paid to current labeling requirements, measurements of nutritional adequacy, regulatory oversight, and pet food safety. A study of pet food labels and nutrient content in Chapters 15 and 16 includes overviews of the ingredients included in commercial pet foods and of methods used to measure nutrient content. Chapter 17, which examines the various types of available pet foods, facilitates easy categorization of foods for comparison purposes. Also, detailed information regarding the evaluation of pet foods allows owners and professionals to efficiently assess commercial products and select appropriate foods for individual animals.

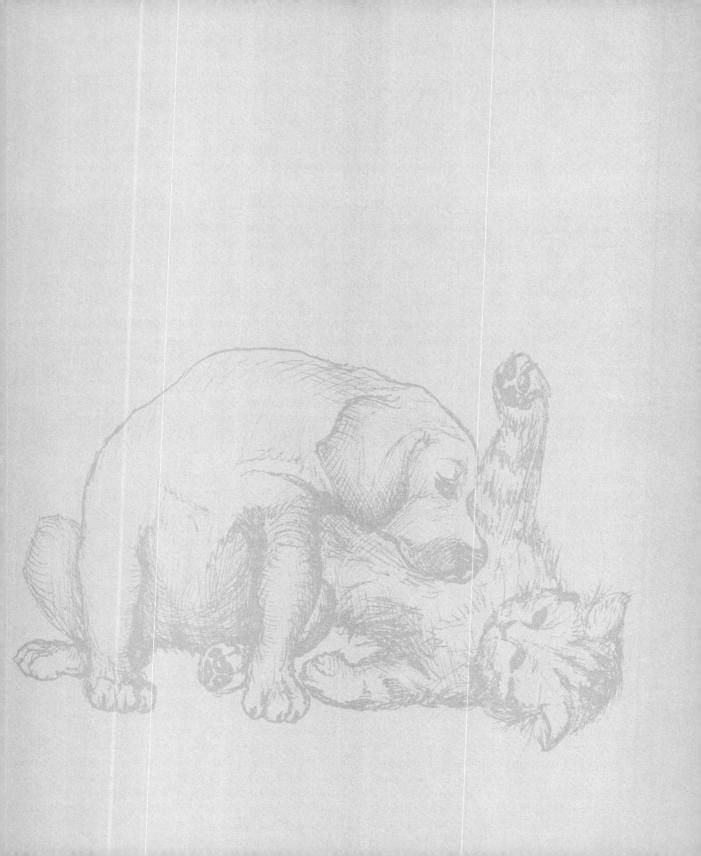

14

History and Regulation of Pet Foods

Pet owners generally have two options available when choosing the type of food to feed their companion animals. They may either prepare a homemade diet or purchase a commercially prepared dog or cat food. Today the majority of pet owners in the United States feed their companion animals commercially prepared foods.[1,2] The popularity of commercial products is evidenced by the growth of the pet food industry over the past 50 years. In 1958 total pet food sales in the United States were estimated to be $350 million. This amount increased to $1.43 billion in 1972, $5.1 billion in 1986, and almost $12 billion by 1996.[3] In recent years, as pet owners have become increasingly interested in the quality and safety of the foods that they feed their pets, pet supply growth has continued to reflect the importance that pets have in our lives. Between 2002 and 2007, the U.S. market for pet foods and supplies grew by more than 34% and saw the introduction of a wide variety of new types of foods that are formulated for different life stages, activity levels, and health conditions.[4]

HISTORY

Prior to the middle of the nineteenth century, foods for dogs and cats were not commercially prepared. Owners fed their pets table scraps or homemade formulas made from human foods and leftovers. The first commercial dog food to be marketed was in the form of a biscuit. It was produced and sold in 1860 by James Spratt, an American living in London.[5] Following success in England, Spratt began selling his product in the United States. In the early 1900s, several other groups observed Spratt's success and began to develop and sell pet foods. Milk-Bone, originally called "Maltoid" biscuits, was created by the F.H. Bennett Biscuit Company in 1908 as a convenient way to provide nutrition to dogs of varying sizes. Canned dog food was first introduced by the Chappel brothers of Rockford, Illinois in 1922. The Chappels named their product Ken-L-Ration and followed it with the introduction of a dry product several years later. Around the same time, Samuel

Gaines broke into the market with a new type of dog food called a "meal." The meal consisted of a number of dried, ground ingredients that were mixed together and sold in 100-pound (lb) bags. Pet owners enjoyed the convenience of this new product because they were able to buy fairly large quantities at one time and because the food required little preparation before feeding.

In the early 1900s, pet foods were marketed only through feed stores. The National Biscuit Company (Nabisco), which purchased Milk Bone in 1931, was the first group to attempt to sell its product in grocery stores. Selling pet food in human food markets initially met with much resistance. Because most pet foods were made from byproducts of human foods, customers and store owners considered it unsanitary to sell such products next to foods that were meant for human consumption. However, Nabisco persisted, and Milk Bones finally made it into the supermarket. The convenience and economy of purchasing pet foods at grocery stores rapidly overcame customer concerns. Improved distribution and availability resulted in increased sales and popularity of commercial pet foods. By the mid-1930s, many brands of dog food were sold in grocery stores. At this time, although some dry biscuits and meal products were available, canned pet foods were still the most popular type of pet food product sold in the United States.

Its popularity continued to grow and by 1941, canned dog food comprised 90% of the pet food market.[6] However, with the onset of World War II, government meat-rationing and the shortage of metal resulted in fewer resources being available for the processing of pet food. The pet food industry responded by producing and selling a larger proportion of dry foods. However, once the war was over, canned foods again became more popular with pet owners. It was not until the development of the extrusion process that dry pet foods increased in popularity. The extrusion process and expanded pet foods (foods produced through the extrusion process) were first developed by researchers at Purina laboratories in the 1950s. Extrusion involves first mixing all of the pet food ingredients together and then rapidly cooking the mixture and forcing it through an extruder (specialized pressure-cooker). This process causes a rapid expansion of the bite-sized food particles, resulting in increased digestibility and palatability of the food. After extrusion and drying, a coating of fat or other palatability enhancer is usually sprayed onto the outside of the food pieces. In 1957, Purina Dog Chow, an expanded product, was first introduced to grocery stores. Within 1 year, this new product had become the best-selling dog food in the United States. Today the majority of dry pet foods sold in the United States are extruded products, and dry pet foods make up the largest proportion of the U.S. market.[2,4]

Because little was known about the nutrient requirements of dogs and cats when pet foods were first manufactured, the same food was commonly marketed for both species. Manufacturers merely labeled the cans or bags differently. However, as more knowledge was acquired about the different nutrient needs of dogs and cats, and as cats became increasingly popular as pets, separate pet foods were formulated for each. Some of the first cat foods were comprised almost entirely of fish products and were sold in 1-lb cans. However, as pet food manufacturers learned more about the preferences of cats (and of their owners), they created more palatable products and sold the new "gourmet" products in smaller cans. Starting in the mid-1970s, in response to the growing interest in quality pet care, some companies created "premium" brands of foods that were marketed and sold exclusively through pet supply stores, feed stores, and veterinarians. These were the first products to target different stages of life in dogs and cats. During the same period, some manufacturers created breeder programs to encourage brand loyalty among purebred breeders. These breeders would then recommend the products to their puppy and kitten buyers.

During the new millennium, companies have continued to develop foods that are designed for specific stages of life, physiological states, and disease states.[6] Some of the most recent niche products include those produced from organic ingredients, various types of raw or grain-free diets, foods that target the health of specific body systems, and even foods that are patterned after popular human diet plans. These trends represent a response to the pet-owning public's desire to supply their companion animals with the best nutrition possible during all stages of life (see Chapter 17, pp. 167-173 for

a complete discussion). The public's increased interest in nutrition and health, coupled with the large number of commercial products available, has led many pet owners, hobbyists, and professionals to critically evaluate the type and the safety of the foods they select for their animals. An increasing number of pet owners are now interested in learning more about the regulation of the foods they buy and the formulation and nutrient content of these foods.

Pet foods designed for specific stages of life, physiological states, and disease states are available today. Some of the most recent niche products include those produced from organic ingredients, various types of raw or grain-free diets, foods that target the health of specific body systems, and even foods that are patterned after popular human diet plans. These trends represent a response to the pet-owning public's desire to supply their companion animals with the best nutrition possible during all stages of life.

GOVERNING AGENCIES

A number of agencies and organizations regulate the production, marketing, safety, and sales of commercial pet foods in the United States. Each agency has unique and sometimes overlapping responsibilities and varying degrees of authority. Although some regulations are mandatory, others are optional suggestions. The following discussion identifies the major agencies and their roles in pet food regulation and provides an overview of the current regulations that govern the production and sale of pet foods in the United States (Table 14-1).

Association of American Feed Control Officials

The Association of American Feed Control Officials (AAFCO) is the most instrumental agency in the regulation of commercial pet foods. AAFCO was first formed in 1909 and is an association of state and federal feed control officials that acts in an advisory capacity to provide models for state legislation. AAFCO produces its *Official Publication* (OP) each year, and this publication is the basis for pet food regulations in the

TABLE 14-1 GOVERNING AGENCIES OF COMMERCIAL PET FOODS

AGENCY	FUNCTION
Association of American Feed Control Officials (AAFCO)	Sets standards for substantiation claims and provides an advisory committee for state legislation; produces the AAFCO Official Publication annually; most important regulations are the *Model Pet Food Regulations* and *Model Feed Bill,* and the *Pet Food Nutritional Profiles*
National Research Council (NRC)	Collects and evaluates research and makes nutrient recommendations; prepared the publication *"2006 NRC Nutrient Requirements of Dogs and Cats"*
Food and Drug Administration (FDA)	Has authority over approval of new ingredients; enforces the Federal Food, Drug, and Cosmetic Act and oversees the Animal Feed Safety System to ensure the safety of pet foods; works with AAFCO during approval process for new ingredients and with state regulators regarding safety and contamination issues; regulates the inclusion of health claims on pet food labels
United States Department of Agriculture (USDA)	Regulates pet food labels and research facilities
Pet Food Institute (PFI)	Trade organization that represents pet food manufacturers; has no direct regulatory powers
State Feed Control Offices	Enforces the *Commercial Feed Law* within states
Environmental Protection Agency (EPA)	Regulates the use of pesticides in raw material and feeds; regulates processing plant discharges
Federal Trade Commission (FTC)	Regulates trade and advertising

United States and internationally. Most important for pet foods are AAFCO's *Model Pet Food Regulations* and *Model Feed Bill,* and the *Pet Food Nutritional Profiles* (see below). These regulations specify labeling procedures, ingredient definitions, and nomenclature for all animal feeds and pet foods. AAFCO is an association and not an official regulatory body but does operate within the guidelines of federal and state legislation including laws administered by the Food and Drug Administration (FDA) and the U.S. Department of Agriculture (USDA). Although a common misconception is that AAFCO is a trade association made up of industry representatives, members of AAFCO are required to be either state, federal, or foreign government employees. Members include representatives of each state's feed regulatory agencies, the FDA, and the USDA. All of AAFCO's policies must be voluntarily accepted by state feed control officials for actual implementation; many state governments have mandated AAFCO regulations into state law. Because pet food regulations can vary somewhat between states, AAFCO's policy statements and regulations serve to promote uniformity in feed regulations throughout the United States.

The Pet Food Committee of AAFCO acts as the liaison between AAFCO and the pet food industry, and has produced a manual entitled *AAFCO Pet Food and Specialty Pet Food Labeling Guide* to help explain the *Model Pet Food* and *Specialty Pet Food Regulations* and to facilitate compliance with regulations. AAFCO regulations help to ensure that nationally marketed pet foods are uniformly labeled and nutritionally adequate. Their services include providing interpretations of AAFCO's pet food regulations and suggestions to regulating agencies for uniform enforcement. A large proportion of AAFCO's regulations specify the type of information that manufacturers are allowed to include on their pet food labels (see Chapter 15 for a complete discussion of the pet food label). An important accomplishment of AAFCO during the 1990s was the development of practical *Nutrient Profiles* to be used as standards for the formulation of dog and cat foods. Committees consisting of canine and feline nutritionists from universities, government, and the pet food industry worked together to establish two sets of standard nutrient profiles: one for dogs and one for cats. The profiles are based on ingredients commonly included in commercial foods, and nutrient levels are expressed for processed foods at the time of feeding. Minimum nutrient levels to be included in the pet food are provided for two categories: (1) growth and reproduction and (2) adult maintenance. Maximum levels are suggested for nutrients that have been shown to have the potential for toxicity or for when overuse is a concern.

National Research Council

The National Research Council (NRC) is a private, nonprofit organization that collects and evaluates research that has been conducted by others. The NRC functions as the working arm of the National Academy of Sciences, National Academy of Engineering, and Institutes of Medicine, and it conducts services for the federal government, the scientific community, and the general public. The NRC includes a standing committee on animal nutrition that identifies problems and needs in animal nutrition, recommends appointments of scientists to subcommittees, and reviews reports. NRC subcommittees have been established for dog and cat nutrition. These groups develop reports that provide recommendations for the nutrient requirements of dogs and cats throughout various stages of life. Signs of nutrient deficiency and excess in these species are also included in these reports. Traditionally, two volumes were produced, the *Nutrient Requirements of Dogs* and the *Nutrient Requirements of Cats,* with the last editions published in 1985 and 1986, respectively.

In 2006, following almost 6 years of work, the current subcommittee produced a revised edition, a combined volume entitled *Nutrient Requirements of Dogs and Cats.* An important addition to the newest edition is the use of several different requirement classifications. A nutrient's *minimum requirement* represents the minimal concentration of a bioavailable nutrient that is needed as supported by published data. Conversely, *adequate intake* is presented as the amount of the nutrient that is presumed to support life when no minimum requirement has been established for the species or life stage. Therefore one of these two requirement recommendations (but not both) is provided for each species, nutrient, and life stage. The third measure, *recommended allowance,* represents the amount of a nutrient present in food that supports the relevant life stage. The recommended allowance includes a factor to account for

nutrient bioavailability and is calculated from either the nutrient's minimum requirement or adequate intake value. The final recommendation is *safe upper limit,* which represents the maximum concentration of a nutrient that has not been associated with adverse effects (when data are available). Nutrient requirements are expressed in terms of both the diet (amount per kilogram [kg] dry matter or per 1000 kilocalories [kcal]) and in terms of the animal's metabolic body weight.

Before the development and acceptance of the AAFCO's *Nutrient Profiles,* the NRC's reports on nutrient requirements for dogs and cats were the recognized authorities for pet food formulation and substantiation of nutritional adequacy claims on the labels of commercial pet foods. In 1991 the agency requested that their recommendations not be used to substantiate nutritional adequacy in dog and cat foods. AAFCO's *Nutrient Profiles* replaced the NRC recommendations as the standard to be used by pet food manufacturers, both for the formulation of pet foods and as label claims in the 1990s. The new NRC's *Nutrient Requirements for Dogs and Cats* is unlikely to replace the AAFCO profiles as a standard for pet food formulation and labeling. However, it can provide a detailed resource for future revisions of the profiles as well as valuable information for nutritionists, pet food companies, and pet owners.[7]

Food and Drug Administration

As a federal agency, the U.S. FDA in the Department of Health and Human Services has jurisdiction over all animal feeds, including pet foods, that are in interstate commerce. The FDA enforces the Federal Food, Drug, and Cosmetic Act (FFDCA) which requires that pet foods, like human foods, be pure and wholesome, be safe to eat, contain no harmful substances, and be truthfully labeled. Most recently, the FDA produced a draft framework of its Animal Feed Safety System (AFSS), a program designed to strengthen regulations that ensure the safety of animal feeds and pet foods. In August of 2007, the FDA signed a Memorandum of Understanding (MOU) with AAFCO that increases the FDA's involvement in the approval and definition process for new ingredients and provides for FDA authority over approved ingredients. The MOU specifically allows the FDA to take enforcement actions against foods that are found to contain prohibited ingredients. Shortly afterward, in September of 2007, the U.S Congress passed the Food and Drug Administration Amendments Act of 2007 (FDAAA). This legislation addresses both human and pet food safety issues and further strengthens the FDA's role (see Regulation of Pet Food Safety below).

Pet food manufacturers that ship their products across state lines (or that import products from out of the country) must follow FDA rules that specify proper identification of the product, a net quantity statement on the label, proper listing of ingredients, the manufacturer's name and address, and acceptable manufacturing procedures.[8] FDA regulations also specifically require that canned pet foods are processed in conformance with low-acid canned food regulations to ensure that these products are free of viable microorganisms. Feed control officials within each state are usually relied upon to inspect facilities and enforce these regulations, although the FDA is authorized to take direct action if necessary. Stipulations of the new law mandates cooperation and communication between the FDA and state regulators when dealing with pet food safety and contamination issues and also requires the FDA to rapidly investigate and communicate information to the public.[9]

Last, the FDA regulates the inclusion of health claims on pet food labels. One type of health claim, a drug claim, is defined as the assertion or implication that the consumption of a food may help in the treatment, prevention, or reduction of a particular disease or diseases. The Center for Veterinary Medicine (CVM), a department of the FDA, has primary regulatory authority over health claims on pet food labels. If a health claim is considered a drug claim, the CVM will not allow its use on the label. All new drugs are subjected to an FDA approval process before being marketed. New foods, on the other hand, are not required to undergo similar premarket testing and FDA authorization. Therefore the inclusion of any health claims on a pet food that indicates that the consumption of the product will treat or prevent a specific disease constitutes a drug claim, and such a product would be subject to the same series of tests required of all new drugs.

United States Department of Agriculture

The USDA is responsible for ensuring that pet foods are clearly labeled to prevent human consumers from mistaking these products for human foods. This role includes the inspection of the meat ingredients used in pet foods to ensure proper handling and guarantee that such ingredients are not included in the human food supply. A second important role that the USDA plays in the pet food industry is to inspect and regulate research facilities. All kennels and catteries that are operated by pet food companies, private groups, or universities must fulfill USDA requirements for physical structure, housing and care of animals, and sanitation. Once these facilities have passed initial certification, they are regularly inspected by USDA officials. Although many pet food companies maintain their own kennels, some contract their feeding trials out to private research kennels or universities. It is important that the facilities in which these tests are conducted maintain proper care of their animals and conform to sound sanitation practices.

Pet Food Institute

The Pet Food Institute (PFI) is a trade organization that represents manufacturers of commercially prepared dog and cat foods. The PFI works with the Pet Food Committee of the AAFCO to evaluate current regulations and make recommendations for changes. However, as a group, the PFI does not have any direct regulatory powers over the production of pet foods, pet food testing, or statements included on labels.

PET FOOD REGULATIONS

As stated previously, the FDA stipulates basic labeling requirements for animal feeds (including pet foods) that include a statement of identity (dog food or cat food), inclusion of an accurate and complete ingredient list, net weight declaration, and the name and address of the manufacturer or distributor. AAFCO regulations address the nutrient content of pet foods, ingredient nomenclature, and most types of label claims. The *Model Feed Bill* that AAFCO has developed and implemented is a template for state legislation; it specifies labeling procedures and ingredient nomenclature. Pet food regulations still vary somewhat from state to state, but adherence to AAFCO's regulations minimizes these differences. Each year AAFCO's OP includes a section containing the current regulations for pet foods. These regulations govern the definitions and terms, label formats, brand and product names, nutrient guarantee claims, accepted ingredients and food additives, statements of calorie content, and descriptive terms that are to be used with or included in commercial pet foods. In addition, AAFCO-sanctioned feeding protocols for proving nutritional adequacy and metabolizable energy (ME) are included.

Definitions, Terms, and Label Format

The definitions and terms section of the AAFCO's pet food regulations identify the Principal Display Panel (PDP) as the part of a container's label that is intended to be displayed to the customer for retail sales. This is followed by a section that defines the format to be used in the PDP and sets rules for ingredient and guaranteed analysis statements to be included on labels. Statements that are allowed on labels are described and strictly regulated; these are called *statements of nutritional adequacy* or *purpose of the product*. For example, the commonly used "complete and balanced nutrition for all stages of life" claim must be substantiated through one of several possible methods. The first method (option one) involves demonstrating through a series of feeding trials that the pet food satisfactorily supports health in a group of dogs or cats throughout gestation, lactation, and growth. The tests that the manufacturer uses must follow a set of feeding trial protocols that have been established and sanctioned by AAFCO. The second method (option two) requires that the food be formulated to contain ingredients in quantities that are sufficient to provide the estimated nutrient requirements for all stages of life for the dog or cat. This can be achieved either through calculation using standard ingredient tables or through laboratory analysis of nutrient levels. If the second option is used, the AAFCO's *Nutrient Profiles* for dog and cat foods are used as the standard against which to measure nutrient content. A third, less frequently used method is called the "family method of substantiation." A product that is shown to be nutritionally similar to a tested product, but has not been tested using feeding trials itself, may bear the same nutritional adequacy statement as the tested product (see Chapter 15, pp. 134-135 for a complete discussion of nutritional adequacy statements).

Limited label claims must be substantiated for the particular stage of life for which they are formulated.

Most commonly, limited claims signify feeding for adult maintenance only. In these cases, the food must either be shown to meet the AAFCO's *Nutrient Profiles* for adult maintenance or have passed AAFCO's feeding trials for maintenance. Foods that contain the statement "*intended for intermittent or supplemental use*" are not expected to meet requirements for either "complete and balanced" or for a limited claim. AAFCO also requires that all products labeled with the "complete and balanced" claim include specific feeding directions on the product label. If a secondary life stage is mentioned outside of the nutritional adequacy statement on the label, instructions for feeding pets in that life stage must also be included.

Statements and claims made on pet food labels, and even the name of the food itself, are regulated by the Association of American Feed Control Officials (AAFCO). For example, AAFCO requires that such claims as "complete and balanced nutrition for all stages of life" must be substantiated either through feeding trials or by formulating the food to meet the AAFCO's Nutrient Profiles for dog and cat foods.

Brand and Product Names

Brand name refers to the name by which a pet food manufacturer's products are identified and distinguished from the pet foods of other companies. AAFCO regulates both brand and product names. For example, if a pet food product name includes a flavor designation, the flavor must be shown to be detectable by a recognized testing method, and the source of the flavor must be designated in the ingredient list. Similarly, the use of the term "all" or "100%" must mean that only the designated ingredient, an amount of water necessary for processing, and trace amounts of preservatives and condiments are present in the product. The inclusion of one or more ingredient names in a descriptive product name is allowed if the ingredients constitute a minimum of 25% of the pet food, singularly or in combination. If in combination, none of the named ingredients can be less than 3% of the formula. For example, the use of the name "lamb and rice dinner" requires that 25% or greater of the formula is lamb meat and rice, with rice making up the lesser of the two ingredients while still providing at least 3% of the formula. When the phrase "with" is used to designate the inclusion of a specific ingredient, the identified ingredient must comprise at least 3% of the product's dry weight. The "3% rule" does not apply, however, to claims for specific nutrients such as vitamins, minerals, and fatty acids or to ingredients that are classified as condiments. Finally, any product claims of "new and improved" are only allowed to be stated on the PDP and can be used for a maximum period of 6 months after the introduction of the changes.

Nutrient Guarantees and Types of Ingredients

AAFCO identifies acceptable terms for designating the guaranteed analysis for prescribed nutrients on pet food labels. Comparisons that are made between nutrient levels in the pet food and the AAFCO's *Nutrient Profiles* must be listed in the same units as those used in the published profile. When such comparisons are made, it is also required that the product must meet the *Nutrient Profiles* to which the comparison is made. Foods that are formulated as vitamin or mineral supplements are regulated separately and must state nutrient levels in the units designated by AAFCO. Both the FDA and AAFCO require that all ingredients must be listed in the ingredient statement and shown in letters of the same font and size. The AAFCO also requires that no pet food, with the exception of those labeled as sauces, gravies, juices, or milk replacers, contain a moisture level greater than 78%. (For a complete discussion of the guaranteed analysis panel and ingredients included in pet foods, see Chapter 15, pp. 131-134 and Chapter 16, pp. 147-160.)

Drug and Food Additives

Artificial color may be added to pet foods only if it has been shown to be harmless to pets. Such additives are approved and listed by the FDA. Health claims, including the inclusion of drugs or the pharmacological use of nutrients, are regulated by the AAFCO through FDA state officials or through the FDA directly.

Statement of Caloric Content

Beginning in 1994, AAFCO accepted the inclusion of caloric content statement on pet food labels. Currently, this statement is optional for all products with the exception of dog and cat foods that are labeled with a claim of "less calories" or "lite." In these cases, a caloric content statement is mandatory. In 2005, the American College of Veterinary Nutrition submitted a proposal requesting that AAFCO mandate caloric content statements on most foods, with the intent of providing additional relevant information on pet food labels.[10] In 2008, AAFCO tentatively accepted this proposal, but had not yet determined specific regulations for inclusion on the label. As currently directed, a caloric content statement must be presented separately from the guaranteed analysis table, and energy must be expressed as ME in units of kcal per kg. The caloric content may also be expressed as kcal per lb, cup, or other commonly used household measuring unit. The calorie claim must be substantiated either by calculation using modified Atwater factors or through feeding trials specified by the AAFCO. Similar to nutritional adequacy substantiation, the method that is used must be stated on the label.

The caloric content of a pet food must be expressed as metabolizable energy (ME) in units of kilocalories (kcal) per kilogram (kg). Energy density may also be expressed as kcal per pound (lb), cup, or other commonly used household measuring unit.

REGULATION OF PET FOOD SAFETY

State feed agencies, the FDA, and the USDA provide guidelines, regulations, and oversight to ensure that pet foods are safe and wholesome. The FFDCA requires that pet foods are neither *adulterated* nor *misbranded*. Adulteration encompasses the presence of a chemical, physical, or microbiological contaminant in the product, or the use of an ingredient that is not sanctioned for use in pet foods. Pet food ingredients are included in the AAFCO *Feed Ingredient Definition* list that is published annually or are accepted as food additives. Per the MOA between AAFCO and the FDA, this list is maintained jointly by these two agencies. Any ingredient or additive that is not approved or that has not been accepted as safe via FDA regulatory discretion is considered to be prohibited, and its inclusion in a pet food constitutes adulteration. The term "misbranding" refers to the use of false or misleading claims or the failure to label a product in accordance with FDA and AAFCO regulations. In both types of infractions, manufacturers of adulterated or misbranded foods face seizure of their product, fines and injunctions, and possibly criminal prosecution. The degree of tolerance for the presence of pesticides in foods is established by the U.S. Environmental Protection Agency and these regulations are jointly enforced by the FDA and the USDA. The FDA maintains a monitoring program that tests pet foods and pet food ingredients for the presence of pesticides, mycotoxins, and heavy metals through its Feed Contaminants Program. In addition, most pet food companies have quality control programs that test both ingredients and finished products for nutrient level and for the presence of contaminants.

Several pet food recalls in recent years have led pet owners and professionals to question the effectiveness of quality and safety assurance programs that are currently in place. The most extensive recall to date occurred in 2007; it affected more than 150 brands of pet foods and numerous pet food companies.[11] In this case, economic adulteration of ingredients occurred at the supplier level. Melamine, a nitrogen-containing compound, had been added to wheat gluten and rice protein concentrate to artificially increase the analyzed protein content of these ingredients. Melamine is used in the manufacture of plastics and fertilizer and is not approved as a food ingredient in either human or animal foods in the United States. The laboratory measurement of nitrogen provides an estimate of protein concentration and is used by companies to confirm reported protein levels in ingredients. Therefore adding melamine would erroneously increase the apparent protein level of an ingredient. The adulteration was

not detected immediately because melamine had not been identified as a contamination risk and so was not routinely tested for. It was only when researchers discovered co-contamination with cyanuric acid in affected pet foods that the cause of illness was ascertained.[12,13] When present alone, neither melamine nor cyanuric acid is highly toxic. However, when present together and consumed orally, the two compounds form an insoluble complex in the kidneys, leading to crystallization in the renal distal tubules, tubular necrosis, and acute kidney failure.[14,15]

The 2007 recall led the governmental regulating agencies and the pet food industry to strengthen safety evaluation practices and to reexamine the risk profiles of all ingredients included in pet foods. The FDAAA, among other provisions, established an early warning system to alert the public about unsafe human and pet foods, and required state and federal authorities to work more closely together to improve food safety programs.[16] The new law specifically requires that companies report contamination of a product within 24 hours of discovery and provide records to the FDA to facilitate tracing the contamination to its origin. The legislation also includes provisions for increasing the timeliness of food recalls, alerts to the public, and notifications throughout the ingredient supply chain.[17] Last, although not related directly to pet food safety, the FDAAA requires the FDA to work with the AAFCO to create new FDA regulations pertaining to the nutritional information reported on the pet food label. Collectively, the strengthened regulations are intended to improve the FDA's and industry's ability to protect humans and companion animals from both foodborne illnesses and from foods adulterated with contaminants.

References

1. Zicker SC: Evaluating pet foods: how confident are you when you recommend a commercial pet food? *Top Companion Anim Med* 23:121–126, 2008.

2. Laflamme DP, Abood SK, Fascetti AJ, and others: Pet feeding practices of dog and cat owners in the United States and Australia, *J Am Vet Med Assoc* 232:687–694, 2008.

3. Harlow J: US pet food trends. In *Proceedings of the petfood forum*. Chicago, 1997, Watts Publishing.

4. Phillips T: US pet food sales go boom, *Pet Food Ind,* November 2007.

5. Lazar V: Dog food history, *Pet Food Ind* Sept/Oct:40-44, 1990.

6. Phillips T: Learn from the past, *Pet Food Ind,* October 2007.

7. Dzanis DA: Petfood insights: the new NRC is here, *Pet Food Ind*, August 2006.

8. Benz S: FDA's regulation of pet food, *FDA Vet,* XVI(Jan/Feb) 2000.

9. Dzanis DA: Recall update: regulatory changes, *Pet Food Ind*, February 2008.

10. Dzanis DA: Understanding regulations affecting pet foods, *Top Companion Anim Med* 23:117–120, 2008.

11. Rovner SL: Anatomy of a pet food catastrophe, *Chem Engineer News* 86:41–43, 2008.

12. Donovan L: Chemical combination in pet food proves lethal, *Vet Tech* 29:36–37, 2008.

13. Rosenthal M: Pet food recall: company plays integral role in cracking the case, *Vet Forum* 25:24–27, 2008.

14. Cianciolo RE, Bischoff K, Ebel JG, and others: Clinicopathologic, histologic and toxicologic findings in 70 cats inadvertently exposed to pet food contaminated with melamine and cyanuric acid, *J Am Vet Med Assoc* 233:729–737, 2008.

15. Puschner B, Poppenga RH, Lowenstine LJ, and others: Assessment of melamine and cyanuric acid toxicity in cats, *J Vet Diagn Invest* 19:616–624, 2007.

16. Nolen RS: Congress strengthens pet food safety regulations, *J Am Vet Med Assoc* 231:1320–1322, 2007.

17. Dzanis DA: Anatomy of a recall, *Top Companion Anim Med* 23:133–136, 2008.

Pet Food Labels

The pet food label is an important component of commercial pet foods because many consumers rely primarily on the label for information about the product's nutritional adequacy and palatability. Current regulations require that all labels of pet foods manufactured and sold in the United States contain the following items: product name; words "dog food" or "cat food"; net weight; name and address of the manufacturer; guaranteed analysis for crude protein, crude fat, crude fiber, and moisture; list of ingredients in descending order of predominance by weight; and a statement of nutritional adequacy or purpose of the product. Pet food manufacturers must also include a statement that indicates the method that was used to substantiate the nutritional adequacy claim, either through the Association of American Feed Control Officials's (AAFCO's) feeding trials or by formulating the food to meet the AAFCO's *Nutrient Profiles* (Box 15-1). An expiration date indicating the time span from the date of production to the date of expiration of the product is optional, as is a "best if used by" date. The "best if used by" date is the date at which the product is no longer considered fresh and should no longer be sold.

WHAT CONSUMERS CAN LEARN FROM THE PET FOOD LABEL

Guaranteed Analysis Panel

The guaranteed analysis panel on the pet food label is often one of the first places that consumers look for information about the product. This panel provides

---

BOX 15-1 TYPICAL COMMERCIAL PET FOOD LABEL

WUF-WUF DOG FOOD
Net weight 8 pounds (lb)

FEEDING INSTRUCTIONS	CUPS PER DAY
Toy breeds (5-10 lb)	0.5-1 cup
Small breeds (10-30 lb)	1-2 cups
Medium breeds (30-50 lb)	2-4 cups
Large breeds (50-80 lb)	4-5 cups
Giant breeds (80-120 lb)	5-7 cups

GUARANTEED ANALYSIS

Crude protein	Not less than 26%
Crude fat	Not less than 14%
Crude fiber	Not more than 4%
Moisture	Not more than 10%

Manufactured by Wuf-Wuf Inc., Bowserville, Ohio.
  Wuf-Wuf is formulated to meet the nutritional levels established by the Association of American Feed Control Officials' *Dog Food Nutrient Profiles* for all life stages.
  Ingredients: Chicken, chicken byproduct meal, ground corn, rice flour, fish meal, chicken fat (preserved with mixed tocopherols and citric acid), ground grain sorghum, dried beet pulp, chicken digest, dried egg product, brewer's dried yeast, flax, dicalcium phosphate, calcium carbonate, DL-methionine, potassium chloride, mineral supplement, vitamin supplement.

information regarding the amount of protein and fat contained in the pet food. Manufacturers are required to include minimum percentages for crude protein and crude fat and maximum percentages for moisture and crude fiber for both dog and cat foods. Optional guarantees that may be listed include, but are not limited to, magnesium (minimum percentage), taurine (minimum percentage), linoleic acid (minimum percentage), and ash (maximum percentage). It is important to recognize that these numbers represent only minimums and maximums and do not reflect the exact amounts of these nutrients in the product. For example, a pet food that has a label claim of "minimum crude fat: 11%" cannot have less than 11% fat, but may have more. Although one product with this claim may contain 13% fat, another carrying the same claim may have 11.5% fat. Assuming all other nutrients are comparable, the 1.5% difference in fat content can make a significant difference in a product's caloric density and palatability.

The terms *crude protein, crude fat,* and *crude fiber* all refer to specific analytical procedures used to estimate these nutrients in foodstuffs. On the average, protein contains 16% nitrogen. Crude protein is the estimate of total protein in a foodstuff that is obtained by multiplying its analyzed level of nitrogen by a constant. Slight inaccuracies in this estimate are caused by variations in nitrogen content between proteins and by the presence of nonprotein nitrogen compounds in the foodstuff. Crude fat is an estimate of the lipid content of a food that is obtained through extraction of the food with ether. In addition to lipids, this procedure also isolates certain organic acids, oils, pigments, alcohols, and fat-soluble vitamins. On the other hand, some complex lipids, such as phospholipids, may not be isolated with this method. Crude fiber represents the organic residue that remains after plant material has been treated with dilute acid and alkali solvents and after the mineral component has been extracted. Although crude fiber is used to report the fiber content of many commercial products, it usually underestimates the level of true dietary fiber in a product. It has been determined that the crude fiber method recovers only 50% to 80% of the cellulose, 10% to 50% of the lignin, and less than 20% of the hemicellulose in a given sample.[1] Consequently, crude fiber may be a measurement of most of the cellulose in a sample, but it underestimates all of the other dietary fiber components. Consumers can use the guaranteed

analysis panel to provide a rough estimate of protein, fat, and fiber content in a particular pet food. However, these numbers should only be considered as a starting point when comparing different products or brands, and they should not be assumed to represent the actual levels of these nutrients in the food.

When examining the guaranteed analysis panel of a pet food, consumers must always take into account the moisture (water) content of the product. The amount of water in a food significantly affects the values listed in the guaranteed analysis table, because most pet foods display nutrient levels on an "as-fed" (AF) basis, rather than a dry-matter basis (DMB). *As-fed* means that the percentages of nutrients were calculated directly, without accounting for the proportion of water in the product. Pet foods can vary greatly in the amount of water they contain. For example, dry cat and dog foods usually contain between 6% and 10% water, but canned foods contain up to 78% water.[2] In order to make valid comparisons of nutrients in foods with different amounts of moisture, it is necessary to first convert nutrients to a DMB. Similarly, the caloric content of a pet food also affects the interpretation of the guaranteed analysis panel. Caloric density must always be considered when comparing levels of protein, fat, carbohydrate, and other nutrients in different pet foods (see pp. 145-147).

When looking at the pet food label, many consumers read the guaranteed analysis panel. This includes minimum percentages of crude protein and crude fat and the maximum percentages of moisture and crude fiber. Consumers should be aware that these percentages do not represent actual amounts of protein and fat and that using these percentages to compare different products or brands may be misleading.

Ingredient List

The ingredient list is another important item that consumers examine when choosing a pet food. The terms used for ingredients in pet foods are limited to those assigned by AAFCO through AAFCO's Ingredients Definition process. This process includes oversight by the Food and Drug Administration (FDA), when applicable. The new FDA Amendments Act (FDAAA), passed in late 2007, requires increased involvement of the FDA in ingredient definition and standards (see Chapter 14, pp. 124-125). Cumulatively, these regulations mean that pet foods contain only those ingredients that are defined and accepted by these agencies. New ingredients can only be introduced following submission of data to AAFCO and the FDA and completion of the approval process. In addition to formally approved ingredient definitions, terms for ingredients that are considered to be "common and usual" are also allowed. Examples of these include ingredient designations that are also used in human foods, such as beef, wheat, oats, and water.

The pet food ingredient list must include all ingredients in the food, and the list is arranged in decreasing order by predominance by weight. The list may be quite simple, containing just one or two ingredients, such as in certain types of treats (i.e., freeze-dried liver or salmon). More commonly, pet foods contain multiple ingredients to provide a diet that is complete and balanced. In no case can any single ingredient be given undue emphasis in the list, nor can designations of the quality of ingredients be included. The ingredient list indicates where the principal components of a pet food come from—animal products or plant products. In general, if an ingredient from an animal source is listed first or second in a canned pet food or within the first three ingredients of a dry pet food, the food can be assumed to contain animal products as its principal protein source.

The list of ingredients may include just one or two ingredients, or 50 or more, depending on the product. Because ingredients are included to provide a needed nutrient and a dietary benefit, the belief that certain ingredients are included just to provide "filler" is usually false.

Most popular and generic brands of pet food are formulated as "variable-formula diets." This means that the ingredients used in the food will vary from batch to batch, depending on the availability and market prices of ingredients. In contrast, many premium foods are produced using fixed formulas. In this case, the company will not change the formulation in response to normal fluctuations in market prices. Checking the ingredient list of several bags of a particular pet food over a period of time can indicate whether the company is using fixed or variable formulation. Although the pet owner may pay slightly more for a fixed formulation diet, the consistency between batches of food is a distinct advantage to the dog or cat that is consuming the food.

Although the ingredient list can provide general information about the type of ingredients included in a food, it does not provide information about the quality of its components. Ingredients used in pet foods vary significantly in digestibility, amino acid content and availability, mineral availability, and the amount of indigestible material they contain. Unfortunately, there is usually no way of determining the quality of the ingredients by using the ingredient list. In fact, some premium foods with high-quality, highly available ingredients may have an ingredient list that is almost identical to that of a generic food that contains poor-quality ingredients with low digestibility and nutrient availability. Therefore the ingredient list alone should never be used to compare two pet foods because the differences in the qualities of ingredients are impossible to know from this information.

Like the guaranteed analysis, the list of ingredients can be deceptive, in some cases, because manufacturers are not required to list the ingredients on a DMB. This is usually not a problem in dry pet foods because most of the ingredients included in these diets have a relatively low moisture content. However, canned products may contain ingredients with vastly different amounts of moisture. As a result, an ingredient that actually contributes a low proportion of nutrients to the food may be listed first if it has a high water content, while an ingredient that contributes a large proportion of the nutrients to the food may be lower on the ingredient list if it has a low moisture content. A common example involves the use of texturized vegetable protein (TVP) in canned pet foods. TVP is composed of extruded soy flour that is dyed and shaped to resemble meat products. The actual meat ingredients in a product that contains TVP are usually listed high on the ingredient list because they have a very high moisture content. Conversely, TVP has very low moisture and so its total weight is much lower, and it is found much later in the ingredient list. This can be misleading because most of the protein in such a food comes from the TVP and not from the animal-source ingredients that are listed first.

A second way that the ingredient list can be confusing to consumers is the manner in which certain ingredients are presented. Manufacturers may separate different forms of similar ingredients so that they can be listed separately on the label and appear further down the list. For example, an ingredient list may include kibbled wheat, ground wheat, wheat flour, flaked wheat, wheat middlings, and wheat bran. These ingredients are called "split ingredients" and may in some cases represent two or more forms of the same product. Examples of split ingredients are ground wheat and wheat flour, which differ only in the fineness of the grind used during processing. Individually, these ingredients make up only a small fraction of the diet and therefore can be listed low on the ingredient list. As a whole, wheat actually constitutes a large proportion of this diet. Consumers should be aware that listing different forms of the same ingredient suggests a legal but purposeful misrepresentation of the product's ingredient content on the part of the manufacturer.

The ingredient list can tell consumers the principal components of the pet food and whether the components are from plant or animal sources. If an animal-source ingredient is listed first or second in a canned pet food or within the first three ingredients of a dry food, the food can usually be assumed to contain animal products as its principal protein source. However, the ingredient list does not provide information about the quality of the ingredients.

Nutritional Adequacy

Another item on the pet food label that can provide information to consumers is the claim of nutritional adequacy. With the exception of treats and snacks, the label of all pet foods that are in interstate commerce must contain a statement and validation of nutritional adequacy. Current AAFCO regulations allow four primary types of nutritional adequacy statements. The first and most common claim is "complete and balanced for all life stages." This statement signifies that the food has been formulated to provide complete and balanced nutrition for gestation, lactation, growth, and maintenance. A limited claim states that the food provides

complete and balanced nutrition for a particular stage of life, such as adult maintenance. A third claim is found on products that are intended for intermittent or supplemental feeding only. Last, products that are intended for therapeutic feeding, under the supervision of a veterinarian, bear the statement "use only as directed by your veterinarian" (Box 15-2).

When the "complete and balanced nutrition" claim is used for any or all life stages, manufacturers must indicate the method that was employed to substantiate this claim. AAFCO regulations require that the manufacturer either performs AAFCO-sanctioned feeding trials on the food (option one) or formulates the diet to meet AAFCO's *Nutrient Profiles* for dog and cat foods (option two).[3] The terminology for labels of pet foods that have passed the AAFCO feeding tests is as follows:

"Animal feeding tests using AAFCO procedures substantiate that (brand) provides complete and balanced nutrition for (life stages)."

Option 2 is commonly referred to as the "calculation method" because it allows manufacturers to substantiate the "complete and balanced" claim by calculating the nutrient content of the formulation of the diet using standard tables of ingredients or by analyzing the product through laboratory analyses. When option 2 is used, the label terminology will read as follows:

"(Brand) is formulated to meet the nutritional levels established by the AAFCO Dog (or Cat) Food Nutrient Profiles for (life stages)."

Though less frequently used, a company may also use an approach called the "family method of substantiation." A family consists of pet food products that contain similar ingredients, use the same processing method, are within the same moisture control and energy category, and are intended to have the same label claim. One product within a family will be required to pass complete AAFCO feeding trial protocols (option 1). This product is called the "lead product." If this product passes, it is assumed that the other products within the family will also pass because they are nutritionally similar to the lead product and contain similar ingredients. Once a particular nutritional claim

BOX 15-2 LABEL CLAIMS OF NUTRITIONAL ADEQUACY AND HOW TO INTERPRET THEM

Claim 1: "Wuf-Wuf is formulated to meet the nutrient levels established by the AAFCO's *Nutrient Profiles* for dog foods for all life stages."

Interpretation: This dog food has been formulated to meet the AAFCO's *Nutrient Profiles* for both growth and adult maintenance using either calculation or laboratory analysis of nutrient levels.

Claim 2: "Animal feeding tests using AAFCO procedures substantiate that Wuf-Wuf provides complete and balanced nutrition for all life stages."

Interpretation: This dog food has been subjected to AAFCO feeding studies, including those for gestation, lactation, and growth. This substantiation method shows that the food is complete for all life stages.

Claim 3: "Animal feeding tests using AAFCO procedures substantiate that Wuf-Wuf provides complete and balanced nutrition for adult maintenance."

Interpretation: This food has undergone AAFCO feeding protocol studies for maintenance only and has not been tested for gestation, lactation, or growth.

Claim 4: "Wuf-Wuf Veterinary Diet (Gastrointestinal Formula) is intended for intermittent or supplemental feeding only. Use as directed by your veterinarian."

Interpretation: This food is intended for special nutritional or dietary needs that require the involvement of a veterinarian for diagnosis, management, and follow-up.

AAFCO, Association of American Feed Control Officials.

---

is established for the lead product, pet foods within the same family are entitled to carry the same nutritional adequacy claim. When this type of substantiation method is used, the label statement will read as follows:

"(Brand) provides complete and balanced nutrition for (life stages) and is comparable in nutritional adequacy to a product which has been substantiated using AAFCO feeding tests."

Feeding Guidelines

AAFCO regulations require that dog and cat foods carrying the label claim of "complete and balanced" for any or all stages of life must include feeding directions on the product label. At a minimum, these instructions must state "Feed (weight unit) of product per (weight unit) of dog or cat."[4] The directions on a particular dog or cat food have been developed specifically for that particular formulation's energy and nutrient content and also consider the pet's life stage and activity level. However, because the guidelines reflect an average estimate, individual dogs and cats may require slightly more or less than the recommended feeding amount on the label.

Caloric Content Statement

In 1993 committee recommendations were made to AAFCO for the measurement of metabolizable energy (ME) and the inclusion of ME values on pet food labels. This new provision was accepted in 1994, making the inclusion of a caloric density statement on the label optional for pet food manufacturers. The inclusion of a caloric content statement, along with a breakdown of the percentage of calories that are contributed by fat, carbohydrate, and protein, provides information about the suitability of the food for different stages of a pet's life. For example, hard-working dogs may benefit from a diet with an increased proportion of ME calories supplied by fat and protein, while sedentary dogs benefit from foods containing moderately reduced fat. In addition, it is much more accurate to compare foods according to the percentage of calories that are contributed by carbohydrate, protein, and fat than to compare them by the percentage of these nutrients by weight (see Chapter 16, pp. 144-147 for a complete discussion).

The caloric content statement must be presented separately from the guaranteed analysis table, and energy must be expressed as ME in units of kilocalories (kcal) per kilogram (kg). The caloric content may also be expressed as kcal per pound (lb), cup, or other commonly used household measuring unit. Similar to the nutritional adequacy statement, the calorie claim must be substantiated either by calculation using modified Atwater factors or through a testing method specified by AAFCO. In 2005, the American College of Veterinary Nutrition submitted a proposal requesting that AAFCO mandate caloric content statements on most foods.[5] In 2008, AAFCO tentatively accepted this proposal, but has not yet determined specific regulations for the inclusion of this information on the label (Box 15-3).

ADDITIONAL LABEL CLAIMS

Together, AAFCO and FDA evaluate and regulate the addition of new descriptive terms on the pet food label. The challenge of this responsibility lies in providing consumers with as much factual information as possible and allowing only claims that can be reliably substantiated. For example, two terms that were evaluated and accepted in recent years for use on pet food labels are "natural" and "tartar control." AAFCO requires that the claim of "natural" can be used only when all of the food's ingredients and components of ingredients be derived solely from plant, animal, or mined sources (i.e., are not synthetic analogs), and do not contain synthetic additives or processing aids. If chemically synthesized vitamins or minerals are included, the product may be labeled "natural with added vitamins and minerals."[4] Acceptable "tartar control" claims include statements that a food or treat cleans teeth, freshens breath, or whitens teeth by virtue of its mechanical (abrasive) action during chewing. Likewise, label claims that imply pharmacological effects that prevent or control tartar are not permitted unless approved through established FDA protocols for new animal drugs or pharmaceuticals (see Chapter 34 for a complete discussion).

Statements that a food or treat can treat, prevent, or reduce risk of a specific disease are all considered to be drug claims by the FDA's Center for Veterinary Medicine (CVM) and are not permitted on pet foods. For example, a claim of "prevents itchy skin" or "hypoallergenic" is not allowed. Conversely, the claims of "promotes healthy skin" and "promotes glossy coat" are acceptable because they do not address a specific disease state.[2] When a specific nutrient or formulation claim is made, it is acceptable if the claim relates directly to the function that the nutrient has in the body but is not allowed if the claim relates to a function that is separate from nutritive value. For example, a claim of "contains taurine for heart health" in a cat food is acceptable, while a claim of "contains vitamin C to prevent infection" is not permitted.[6] A label claim controversy involved the formulation of cat foods intended to prevent a cat's risk of developing feline lower urinary tract disease (FLUTD). Any claim that a food, a food ingredient, or nutrient prevents or reduces the risk of FLUTD is disallowed because this constitutes a drug claim. However, the CVM has exercised regulatory discretion in the spirit of providing helpful information to pet owners by

---

BOX 15-3 INFORMATION PROVIDED BY THE PET FOOD LABEL

THE PET FOOD LABEL *DOES* PROVIDE INFORMATION ABOUT:	THE PET FOOD LABEL *DOES NOT* PROVIDE INFORMATION ABOUT:
Net weight of product	Exact levels of nutrients
Name and location of manufacturer or distributor	Digestibility and nutrient availability
Minimum crude protein and crude fat content	Quality of the ingredients
Maximum moisture and crude fiber content	
List of ingredients	
Nutritional adequacy statement	
Method of substantiation of adequacy claim	
Feeding instructions	
Caloric density (optional)	

allowing claims of "reduces urine pH to help maintain urinary tract health" and "reduced magnesium level for urinary tract health." However, in these cases, the CVM set limits for acidification and magnesium content, and companies are required to provide safety and efficacy data to the FDA for review. Additional regulations for these products include providing specific feeding instructions and having a nutritional adequacy statement for adult maintenance only (see Chapter 30, pp. 359-372 for a complete discussion of FLUTD).

AAFCO also closely regulates label descriptive terms for reduced calorie products. Acceptable terms include "light" (or "lite"), "less or reduced calories," "lean," "low-fat," and "less or reduced fat." Specific maximum energy contents are designated for all pet foods marketed using the term "light" (or "lite"). For example, a "light" dry dog food can contain no greater than 3100 kcal of ME/kg. Similarly, a dry dog food containing the designation of "less or reduced calories" must include the percentage of reduction from the product of comparison and a caloric content statement. The terms "lean" and "less fat" are regulated by designating the maximum percentages of fat within categories of dog and cat food. For example, a dry dog food that is labeled "lean" can contain no greater than 9% crude fat. As with the "reduced calories" term, the terms "less or reduced fat" must include the percentage of reduction from the product of comparison.

Another important category of foods that include label claims are veterinary medical foods (VMF). These foods are intended to be fed as a sole source of nutrition to pets that have specific medical conditions. They are typically sold by prescription only, through veterinarians. The label claim that identifies a VMF is "use only as directed by your veterinarian." VMF products are subject to all of the same labeling requirements and nutritional adequacy substantiation (for adult maintenance) as other dog and cat foods. Contrary to popular belief, because VMF products are foods, they cannot include drug claims. However, the CVM exercises regulatory discretion in allowing the use of informational brochures and other materials that are intended to educate veterinarians in the proper use of these foods when treating pets with various types of chronic disorders. The proper use of VMF products always includes continued veterinary supervision (see Section 5 for complete discussions).

PET FOOD ADVERTISING

Pet food manufacturers are in a unique situation when they consider the marketing techniques used to sell their products. Although it is the dog or the cat that is consuming the food and the animal's health that is directly affected by the product's quality, it is the pet owner who is making the decision to buy the product. Therefore manufacturers must not only consider what is nutritious for dogs and cats, they must also consider the pet owner's needs and perceptions. Although some pet owners are concerned primarily with providing the best nutrition for their companion animals, others are more interested in the cost of the food, its availability in stores, or the convenience of feeding it. In today's market, there are products that appeal to all of these needs and to the many different types of pet owners.

Most of today's marketing strategies are aimed toward convincing pet owners that a particular food offers some benefit to the pet above and beyond that of all other products.[7] Because most foods carry the "complete and balanced" label claim, offering complete nutrition is not perceived by many owners to be a unique selling point. Rather, acceptability and palatability, cost, feeding convenience, digestibility, and suitability of the food for the pet's lifestyle, age, or physiological state are all important considerations for today's owner. In recent years, as knowledge about canine and feline nutrition has advanced, pet food companies have started to produce foods that specifically meet the needs of companion animals during different stages of life, for different breeds and breed sizes, and for pets that live a variety of lifestyles. Examples of these foods include high-performance diets for working dogs, growth diets for large and small breeds, and reduced-calorie products for sedentary adults. The sale of these foods is accompanied by educational programs for pet owners about the nutrient needs of their companion animals during different stages of life.

Because there is no way to determine whether a food contains superior nutrition by examining it or by feeding it a few times, many pet owners rely on a product's palatability and acceptability as their chief selection criteria. Palatability is a subjective measure of how well an animal likes a particular food, and acceptability is an indication of whether the amount of food eaten is enough to meet the animal's caloric requirements (see Chapter 18, pp. 177-180 for a complete discussion of palatability). These are both important considerations because regardless of a food's nutritional value, it cannot nourish an animal if it is not eaten. Palatability and acceptability are also very powerful marketing tools. Most pet owners enjoy giving their companion animal a food that is eagerly accepted and eaten, and they will be inclined to buy a food that they know their pet relishes. However, many highly palatable foods are high in fat and as a result are energy dense. This increased palatability, coupled with a high energy density, can lead to overeating and obesity if the food is fed on a free-choice basis or if portion size is not carefully controlled. Owners should certainly pick a food that their pet enjoys, but they should be aware that extremely palatable foods can induce overeating.

In today's busy society, convenience and ease of preparation are also important to many pet owners. The convenience of feeding dry pet foods and the availability of these foods in supermarkets contributed greatly to their initial success. Dry foods keep well after opening, do not require refrigeration, and require little if any preparation before feeding. Packaging foods in portion-sized pouches or cans is another technique that attracts pet owners who desire convenience. Many canned cat foods and semimoist pet foods are marketed to provide one meal per package, therefore eliminating even the need to measure out a portion of food before feeding.

Although it is not the chief consideration for some pet owners, for others the cost of the food is very important. There are a number of commercial foods available today that are advertised as being more economical to feed while still providing superior nutrition. However, it is important for pet owners to know that to produce a low-cost product, ingredients that are of lower quality, and thus lower cost, must be used. Therefore a cheaper product is probably going to be a lower-quality food, even though the guaranteed analysis panel may not reflect this. In addition, when considering the price of a pet food, the actual cost of feeding the animal must be calculated, not just the cost per unit weight of the food. Most low-quality, cheap ingredients have significantly lower digestibilities than the ingredients used in premium foods. A greater quantity of a food with low digestibility must be fed to an animal to provide the same amount of nutrition as found in a food with higher digestibility and nutrient availability. As a result, owners may find that they have

to feed significantly larger portions of the cheaper food to their pet (see Chapter 18, pp. 177-180). Also, companies that produce inexpensive dog and cat foods may not dedicate the funds or possess the capability to conduct thorough testing of their products. In general, when pricing dog and cat foods, it is safe to assume that buyers usually "get what they pay for." Premium and super-premium products cost more primarily because they contain high-quality ingredients and because they have been subjected to more rigorous testing than inexpensive generic and name-brand products. Marketing techniques that promote low-priced foods as equivalent in value to more costly products may mislead the consumer into believing that the food offers the same benefits as a premium food but at a substantially lower cost.

Caveat emptor: Purchasing a low-cost pet food may seem economically practical, but low-cost pet foods usually contain low-quality, less-digestible ingredients. Therefore, more food must be fed to an animal to provide adequate nutrition than if the animal was being fed a high-quality, highly digestible food. Thus the per-meal cost of the inexpensive food may be higher.

Other commonly used marketing tools for pet foods include the development of products that resemble foods consumed by humans. This obviously appeals to the sense of taste of the pet owner, more so than that of the animal that will eat the food. These products are varied and creative. Some foods have the appearance of chunks of meat, and others look like stews, containing a variety of meat and vegetables. The actual content of these foods is usually not the ingredient that they are made to resemble. For example, TVP can be shaped and dyed to resemble chunks of meat. Flavor varieties are also a strong selling tool. Because owners enjoy variety in their diets, they believe that this is also important for their pets. Almost all of the pet foods and treats sold in grocery stores come in a variety of flavors. Although these differences may appeal to owners, it is unknown whether individual pets have strong preferences between certain flavors (see Chapter 18, pp. 177-180). Nonetheless, it is the owner who buys the food, and some will be induced to buy a food that looks like ground steak or pronounces itself to be "salmon-flavored."

Promoting the addition or deletion of a particular ingredient in a pet food is another tactic used to increase sales. Whether this information is grounded in fact is a moot point because there is always a segment of the pet-owning population that is willing to believe in the value or in the hazard of a given ingredient. For example, some owners believe that soy is a poor-quality ingredient, while others have targeted corn as an undesirable ingredient. Pet foods that are marketed as containing "no soy" or "no corn" capitalize on these beliefs, whether or not they are founded in fact. Similarly, the pet-owning public can be convinced that the presence of a particular ingredient may contribute to a superior product. The use of fish and fish meal in cat foods is an example. Cats are actually desert animals by ancestry and probably had very little access to fish in their original diets. However, the use of clever and cute advertisements has convinced pet owners that all cats inherently love the taste of fish. The presence of fish in certain cat foods is then promoted as a distinct benefit. Although it is true that cats enjoy the taste of fish, this ingredient is no more palatable to most cats than are several other high-protein ingredients included in cat foods.

References

1. Van Soest PJ: The uniformity and nutritive availability of cellulose, *Fed Proc* 32:1804–1808, 1973.

2. Bren L: Choosing pet food by the label, *FDA Consumer*, May/June 2001.

3. Michel KE: Expert summit on pet food, *Vet Forum* 25:12–18, 2008.

4. Association of American Feed Control Officials (AAFCO): Pet food regulations. In *AAFCO Official Publication*, Atlanta, 2008, AAFCO.

5. Dzanis DA: Understanding regulations affecting pet foods, *Top Companion Anim Med* 23:117–120, 2008.

6. Dzanis DA: Interpreting pet food labels; special use foods, *FDA Consumer*, Jan/Feb 1999.

7. Brown RG: Understanding advertising in pet nutrition, *Can Vet J* 35(4):246–250, 1994.

16

Nutrient Content of Pet Foods

The most important consideration in choosing a commercial pet food for a companion animal is its nutrient content. *Nutrient content* refers not only to the exact levels of nutrients in the food, but also to the digestibility and availability of all the essential nutrients. Nutrients can be supplied in commercial pet food through a large number of different ingredients. Commonly used pet food ingredients vary in form and quality, and it is this diversity that can make the selection of a suitable dog or cat food a challenging task. This chapter discusses the methods used to determine and express nutrient content in pet foods and examines many of the commonly used pet food ingredients and additives.

METHODS FOR DETERMINING NUTRIENT CONTENT

Laboratory Analysis

When pet food manufacturers formulate and produce pet foods, there are two ways they can determine the level of nutrients present in the food. The first and most accurate way is to conduct a laboratory analysis of the finished product. Proximate analysis is a commonly used panel of tests that provides information about a select group of nutrients. The laboratory procedures involved in proximate analysis provide the percentages of moisture, crude protein, crude fat, ash (minerals), and fiber that are contained in the food. Nitrogen-free extract (NFE), which represents a rough estimate of the soluble carbohydrate fraction of the food, can be calculated by subtraction. The guaranteed analysis panel of the pet food label is generated from the proximate analysis results. Association of American Feed Control Officials (AAFCO) regulations require that this panel reports only maximum or minimum levels of a select group of nutrients.[1]

Pet food companies that are producing high-quality products and are interested in the education of pet owners will provide consumers with additional information about the exact nutrient content of their foods. Because regulations do not currently allow the inclusion of these details on the pet food package itself, they are usually supplied to consumers in the form of informational brochures and through company websites. Such additional information may include the essential vitamin and mineral content and the energy density of the food.

> *Tip:* Additional information about the nutrient content and energy density of high-quality pet foods can be found in pamphlets obtained from the pet supply store or veterinarian where the food was purchased, or it can be obtained directly from the manufacturer via websites or telephone. Reputable manufacturers will readily supply information, and many have toll-free telephone numbers listed on the package.

Calculation

The second method that manufacturers may use to determine nutrient content is calculation of the average nutrient content of the food's ingredients using values reported in standard tables. The amount of essential nutrients contributed by each ingredient in the food are then summed. Standard tables contain average levels of essential nutrients in common feed ingredients. Although this method of nutrient determination is certainly less costly and time-consuming than laboratory analysis, there are several significant problems with using calculation alone to determine the nutrient content of pet foods.

First, there is a lack of complete and accurate data for the nutrient content of many ingredients included in commercial pet foods. As a result, manufacturers must rely upon tables that contain approximations of the types of ingredients they are using. These tables may contain information that is outdated or misleading. For example, as grain yields have increased in the United States, the average percentage of protein in corn and soybeans has decreased.[2] Standard tables do not always reflect these changes. A study conducted by the Office of the Texas State Chemist measured the protein content of corn, oats, and grain sorghum samples taken from different locations within the state.[3] The average crude protein content in 200 samples of yellow corn was 7.87%, with a range of 5.97% to 10.25%. Protein values were less than 8% in 62% of the samples, and 31.5% of the samples had protein contents below 7.5%. The National Research Council's (NRC's) 2006 standard value for corn used in the formulation of dog and cat foods is 9.1%.[4] If this value is used when formulating a pet food using the calculation method, the pet food might contain less corn protein than predicted. A similar trend of decreasing protein content was observed in oats and grain sorghum, which could lead to miscalculations with these grains. These discrepancies illustrate the need for pet food companies to directly analyze the nutrient content of their pet foods after formulation and not rely exclusively upon table values for the nutrient content of ingredients.

A second problem with the calculation method is that the quality of ingredients cannot be determined. Ingredient quality affects the level and availability of nutrients in finished pet foods. Standard tables represent averages and cannot reflect differences in ingredient quality among raw ingredients. The processing of a pet food further affects ingredient quality. Nutrient losses can occur during processing or storage, and studies have shown that the digestibility and nutrient availability of plant-based and animal-based ingredients may be significantly affected by processing methods.[5-7] For example, dogs digest soybean flour more efficiently than soybean grits when incorporated into a canned diet.[5] This difference is probably related to the smaller particle size of the flour. Subsequent work showed that dogs fed different forms of rice assimilate blended rice more efficiently than whole rice.[6] This difference was attributed to reduced food particle size and possibly to increased damage to starch granules in the blended product. In either case, it is apparent that the processing method used for plant ingredients significantly affects digestion and nutrient availability. Differences in the type of processing system and the cooking temperature for animal-based ingredients are also important. When the effects of cooking temperatures and processing systems on 46 sources of meat and bone meal or poultry byproduct meal were examined, it was found that higher processing temperatures caused decreases in the true digestibility values of

amino acids in the finished product.[7] Again, if table values alone are used to predict protein content, these effects cannot be predicted. Laboratory analysis of finished products, followed by feeding trials with animals, are the only methods for obtaining reliable information about nutrient availability after pet food processing.

Determination of Digestibility

Current AAFCO regulations do not require that companies determine the digestibility of their foods (see Chapter 18, p. 182). However, the digestibility of a pet food must always be considered. Digestibility provides a measure of a food's quality because it directly determines the proportion of nutrients in the food that are available for absorption into the body. Pet food companies evaluate the digestibility of their products through feeding studies (in vivo methodology). Digestibility estimates may also be obtained through the use of in vitro methods that have been developed or refined in recent years.[8-10] Feeding trials are the most accurate method and measure the disappearance of nutrients as they pass through the gastrointestinal tract and are absorbed into the body. The test diet is fed to a group of animals for a pretest period of 5 to 7 days to allow acclimation to the diet. Following this period, the amount of food consumed and the amount of fecal matter excreted are recorded for 3 to 5 days. The fecal matter that is collected represents the undigested residue of the food that was consumed. Laboratory analyses of both feed and fecal matter are conducted to provide the levels of nutrients in each, and amounts of digested nutrients are calculated by subtraction. These figures, expressed as percentages, are called *digestibility coefficients*. In this type of study, the figures that are derived are called "apparent" digestibility coefficients because the fecal matter also contains metabolic waste products that originated from the animal and not from the food (Table 16-1).

True digestibility can be determined by estimating the normal metabolic loss of the nutrient and deducting that value from the amount of the nutrient measured in the fecal matter. True digestibility trials are most commonly conducted for protein. The animals are fed a protein-free or very–low-protein diet for a short period, and a baseline level of protein excretion is measured. This figure can then be used to account for the endogenous metabolic loss of protein in the feces when

TABLE 16-1 PET FOOD DIGESTIBILITY COEFFICIENTS AND THEIR EFFECTS ON FECAL CHARACTERISTICS IN DOGS

	Diet		
	A	B	C
Protein digestibility (%)	70.25	80.99	85.86
Fat digestibility (%)	82.70	90.42	90.72
Fiber digestibility (%)	17.44	48.53	61.48
Fecal score*	3.95	4.47	4.48
Fecal volume	162.38	89.18	46.48

Data provided by Iams Technical Center, Lewisburg, Ohio, 1993.
*Based on a 1 to 5 rating: 1 = loose and watery; 5 = firm. Scores of 4 to 5 are considered normal.

BOX 16-1 EFFECT OF DIFFERENT DIGESTIBILITIES ON THE AMOUNT OF PROTEIN AVAILABLE TO THE DOG

DIET A

28% protein

70.25% of the protein is digestible

Therefore 70.25% of 28% protein = 0.7025 × 28 = **19.67%** digestible protein

DIET B

28% protein

85.9% of the protein is digestible

Therefore 85.9% of 28% protein = 0.859 × 28 = **24.05%** digestible protein

the digestibility trial is conducted. It can be argued that apparent digestibility is actually a better indication of a diet's ability to supply nutrients than is true digestibility. The endogenous losses that occur in the fecal matter represent cellular and enzymatic losses that are the result of the cost of digesting and absorbing food. Therefore apparent digestibility represents the actual net gain to the animal from the digestion of the food.

Information about the nutrient content of a food means little if the product's digestibility is not known. For example, laboratory analyses of two different dry dog foods reveal that they each contain 28% protein. If the protein digestibility of diet A is 70.25%, this means that the food actually provides less than 20% digestible protein. On the other hand, if the digestibility of diet B is 85.8%, it provides about 24% digestible protein (Box 16-1; also see Table 16-1). The amount of protein available to the animal is higher in diet B than in diet A, even though laboratory analyses indicate that they have similar total protein contents. Digestibility also affects fecal volume and form and defecation frequency (see Table 16-1). As a diet's digestibility increases, fecal volume decreases significantly. In addition, a highly digestible pet food produces firm and well-formed feces (see Chapter 18, p. 182 for a complete discussion of factors that affect nutrient digestibility in pet foods). Although manufacturers are not required to conduct digestibility trials on their feeds, reputable companies that produce quality products conduct these trials to ensure that their foods contain levels of nutrients that will meet animals' daily requirements for absorption into the body.

Determination of Metabolizable Energy

The metabolizable energy (ME) of a pet food is another important consideration when selecting a diet (see Chapter 1, pp. 4-6). ME indicates the amount of energy in a pet food that is available to the animal for use. Although digestible energy (DE) measures the amount of energy that is absorbed across the intestinal wall, ME accounts for digestibility and for losses of energy in the urine and through expired gases (flatus). Although expired gases account for a significant proportion of energy in most farm animals, it is an insignificant energy loss in dogs and cats. Therefore the analysis of the ME of foods for dogs and cats includes only urinary losses of energy.

ME is the preferred unit for analyzing the energy content of pet foods because unlike gross energy (GE), which is a measure of the total energy in the diet, ME provides an accurate representation of the amount of energy that is actually available to the animal. ME is determined most accurately through feeding trials with the target species. Studies in recent years have also provided in vitro methods for ME estimation and factorial equations for the calculation of ME using standard energy values for protein, carbohydrate and fat, and in some cases, dietary fiber.[11,12] Finally, a rough estimate of the ME of a pet food can be calculated using the values that are provided in the guaranteed analysis panel on the label (see Chapter 1, pp. 7-8).

The AAFCO allows (and may soon require) the inclusion of caloric claims on pet food labels (see Chapter 15, pp. 135-136). If an ME statement is included, it must be separate and distinct from the guaranteed analysis panel and must be identified as "calorie content." A pet food's ME must be expressed as kilocalories (kcal) per kilogram (kg) of product. Additional units such as kcal per measuring cup or pound (lb) may also be listed on the label. Like the "complete and balanced" statement on the pet food label, the ME statement must be accompanied by a substantiation claim. AAFCO regulations allow manufacturers to determine ME content using one of three possible methods:

1. Calculation using modified Atwater factors and values for crude protein, crude fat, and NFE obtained from proximate analysis. (Samples must be taken from at least four production batches of the product.)
2. Calculation from digestible nutrients or DE. (Data are obtained from digestibility trials without urine collection.)
3. Direct determination from digestibility trials (including urine collection).

EXPRESSION OF NUTRIENT CONTENT

The guaranteed analysis panel of a pet food usually reports nutrient levels on an "as-fed" (AF) basis. This means that the nutrient content in the diet is measured directly, without accounting for the amount of water in the product. This type of measurement is considered AF because it represents the level of nutrients in the food as they are consumed by the animal. For example, if 10 ounces (oz) of a semimoist cat food contains 2.5 oz of protein, it contains 25% ([2.5 ÷ 10] × 100) protein on an AF basis. Similarly, if 10 oz of a dry cat food also contains 2.5 oz of protein, it too has a protein content of 25% on an AF basis. Comparing these two foods on an AF basis would indicate that they contribute similar levels of protein to the cat. However, because of the large range in moisture content between different types of pet foods, the diluting effect of water makes comparisons between pet foods on an AF basis difficult to interpret.

Animals eat and are fed to meet their caloric needs. Therefore a food with high water content has its nutrients essentially "diluted" when compared with a food containing less water. Regardless of the amount of moisture in the diet, an animal still needs to eat a certain amount of dry matter (DM) to meet its daily caloric requirement. Conversion of nutrient data to a dry-matter basis (DMB) allows more accurate comparisons to be made between different types of pet foods. For example, the semimoist cat food discussed previously contains 25% water and 75% DM; the dry food contains 10% water and 90% DM. The percentage of protein on a DMB can be calculated by dividing the percentage of the nutrient on an AF basis by the proportion of DM in the diet. The protein content of the semimoist food on a DMB is approximately 33%, but the protein content of the dry diet is 28% (Box 16-2). Therefore, although their label guarantees indicate similar protein contents, the semimoist food actually contains a higher level of protein than does the dry food on a DMB.

One of the most accurate ways to compare foods is by calculating the levels of nutrients as a proportion of ME. This is called *nutrient density* and is the most accurate way to express a food's nutrient content because it allows an accurate comparison of nutrient content between all types of pet foods. Although the DM method eliminates

BOX 16-2 **CONVERTING NUTRIENTS FROM AN AS-FED (AF) TO A DRY-MATTER BASIS (DMB)**

FORMULA:

Percentage of nutrient on an AF basis ÷ proportion of DM in the diet

EXAMPLE:

Semimoist food contains: 25% protein

75% DM

Dry food contains: 25% protein

90% DM

For semimoist food: $(25 \div 75) \times 100 = $ **33%** protein on a DMB

For dry food: $(25 \div 90) \times 100 = $ **28%** protein on a DMB

differences in nutrient expression due to differences in water content, it does not account for differences in energy content. Nutrient density accounts for differences in both water content and caloric content, and it expresses nutrient levels in pet foods based upon the energy that is available for the animal to use (the ME). Because all animals eat or are fed to meet their energy needs, the amount of food consumed and thus the amount of nutrients taken in depends directly on the caloric content of the food. Nutrient density expresses the energy-containing nutrients such as protein, fat, and carbohydrate as a percentage of ME or as grams (g) per 1000 kcal of ME. The nutritional standard for nutrients that do not contain energy (vitamins and minerals) is units per 1000 kcal of ME.

For example, diets A and B contain the same amount of protein (26%) on a DMB. However, the two foods have different energy densities. Diet A contains 4000 kcal/kg and diet B contains 3500 kcal/kg. Because diet B is lower in calories, a greater quantity (volume of food) needs to be consumed to meet a particular animal's caloric needs. A dog that requires 2000 kcal/day would consume 500 g of diet A or approximately 570 g of diet B. If the two diets contain the same percentage of protein on a weight basis, the dog would consume more total protein when he was fed diet B than when he was fed diet A (Table 16-2). If the protein level is sufficiently high, excess protein will be consumed when the dog is fed diet B. Excess protein is invariably used directly for energy or converted to fat for the storage of energy. On the other hand, if the diets contain marginal levels of protein, the dog may be deficient in protein when consuming diet A, which had a higher caloric density. This example illustrates the need to increase nutrient density as the caloric density of a diet increases. Although protein is a commonly used example, this concept applies to all of the essential nutrients. Because an animal will be fed less of a calorically dense food, the percentage of nutrients by weight in these foods must be higher so that the animal can still meet its needs for all essential nutrients while eating a lower quantity of food. The nutrient level in pet foods must be carefully balanced so that when caloric requirements are satisfied, the requirements for all other nutrients are met at the same time.

The simplest way to solve the confusion of differences in caloric densities is to express nutrients as a percentage of ME or as units per 1000 kcal of ME, rather than as a percentage of weight. This is certainly the most accurate way to present nutrient content data and compare different foods. Nutrient densities of foods with different moisture contents can be compared because water does not contribute any calories to the distribution. In addition, foods with differing caloric contents are equalized using this method, allowing for accurate representation of nutrient levels. Although using DM calculations eliminates distortions that are the result of differences in moisture content, such comparisons do not take into consideration the calories of the foods or the amounts that must be consumed by the animal to meet energy needs. Comparisons using nutrient densities calculated on a caloric basis can be used with foods of different DM and energy content and with different weights or volumes.

Comparisons of caloric distribution are also important. The three nutrient groups that contribute energy to the diet are protein, carbohydrate, and fat. The relative contribution that each of these groups makes to a diet's energy content is an important consideration in choosing a suitable pet food for a particular animal. For example, a hard-working dog requires sufficient protein to supply needs for muscle development and maintenance and increased calories to supply the necessary energy for work. Diets for working dogs should contain slightly increased protein and a fairly high proportion of

TABLE 16-2 PROTEIN INTAKE RELATIVE TO DIETARY METABOLIZABLE ENERGY

	ENERGY REQUIREMENT (KCAL)		ENERGY DENSITY (KCAL/G)		FOOD INTAKE (G)		PROTEIN IN DIET (%)				PROTEIN CONSUMED (G)
Diet A	2000	÷	4.0	=	500	×	26	÷	100	=	130.0
Diet B	2000	÷	3.5	=	571	×	26	÷	100	=	148.5

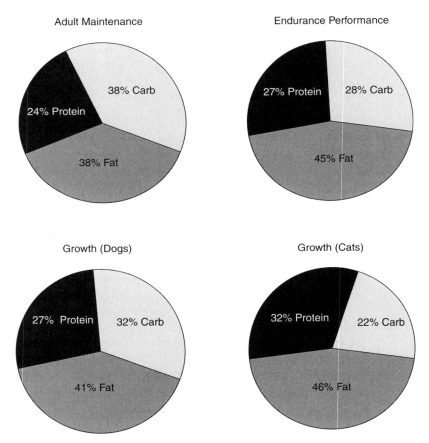

Figure 16-1 Recommended caloric distribution of pet foods.

fat. Recommended caloric distribution ranges for performance, expressed as a percentage of ME calories, are 25% to 30% protein, 40% to 45% fat, and 25% to 30% carbohydrate. In contrast, a diet formulated for normally active adult dogs during maintenance should have a lower proportion of fat and an increased proportion of digestible carbohydrates. A suggested distribution range for adult maintenance is 20% to 25% protein, 35% to 40% fat, and 35% to 45% carbohydrate, expressed as a

percentage of ME. A maintenance diet with this caloric distribution has an energy balance that is shifted from fat to digestible carbohydrate. This profile better meets the reduced energy needs of a less-active dog and makes weight gain less likely. The profile of ME distribution for growing dogs is 25% to 30% protein, 40% to 45% fat, and 30% to 35% carbohydrate, and a profile for growing cats is 30% to 35% protein, 45% to 50% fat, and 20% to 25% carbohydrate (Figure 16-1).

Pet food companies that provide nutritional information about their products to consumers through brochures and websites often include caloric distribution and nutrient density information. If the information is not available, pet owners can calculate a rough estimate of the food's ME and caloric distribution of protein, fat, and carbohydrate from the food's proximate analysis. If the proximate analysis is not known, the guaranteed analysis panel on the label can be used, although it is much less accurate. Calculations that can be used to estimate total ME per kg are provided in Section 1, pp. 4-6. The example used is a dry dog food that contains the following guaranteed analysis:

▸ Crude protein: not less than 26%
▸ Crude fat: not less than 15%
▸ Crude fiber: not more than 5%
▸ Moisture: not more than 10%

Mineral content is estimated to be about 7%, and carbohydrate content is determined by subtraction: 100% − 26% − 15% − 5% − 10% − 7% = 37%. Modified Atwater factors can be used to calculate the number of calories contributed by each nutrient in 100 g of food (see Chapter 1, Table 1-3, p. 8). The total calories in 100 g of food equals 348. The total calories of ME per kg of this food is 3480, or 1582 kcal/lb of food. The percentage of ME calories contributed by protein is approximately 26%. The proportions of calories contributed by fat and carbohydrate are 37% (Box 16-3). This pet food has a distribution that would be appropriate for an adult dog during maintenance.

If a pet food's caloric distribution is calculated from the guaranteed analysis panel, it is important to recognize that the calculated numbers represent only a rough estimate and not the actual caloric distribution of the food. Companies that produce quality products and are aware of the importance of nutrient density will make available the ME and caloric distribution information for companion animal professionals and consumers.

PET FOOD INGREDIENTS

The ingredient list on a pet food label contains all of the food sources included in the formulation of the diet. Pet food regulations require the actual

---

BOX 16-3 EXPRESSION OF NUTRIENTS AS A PERCENTAGE OF METABOLIZABLE ENERGY (ME)

TOTAL CALORIES IN 100 G OF FOOD:

Protein = 3.5 kcal/g × 26 g = 91 kcal

Fat = 8.5 kcal/g × 15 g = 127.5 kcal

Carbohydrate = 3.5 kcal/g × 37g = 129.5 kcal

Total kilocalories = 91 + 127.5 + 129.5 = 348 kcal/100 g of food

PERCENTAGE OF ME CONTRIBUTED BY EACH NUTRIENT (CALORIC DISTRIBUTION):

Protein = (91 kcal/348 kcal) × 100 = **26%**

Fat = (127.5 kcal/348 kcal) × 100 = **37%**

Carbohydrate = (129.5 kcal/348 kcal) × 100 = **37%**

---

ingredients in each food to conform to the label, and the ingredient list cannot contain any reference to the quality of the ingredients that were used. Every ingredient that is part of a commercial pet food is included for a specific purpose. A few of the major ingredients may contain only one major nutrient or nutrient group, and others may contribute several essential nutrients to the diet. For example, corn is an excellent source of starch and is a principal source of digestible carbohydrate in many dry pet foods. Although corn contains a small percentage of protein, the amount of protein that is contributed to the total diet is very low. Therefore corn is considered to be primarily a source of digestible carbohydrate when included in pet foods, rather than an important source of protein. Conversely, chicken contains high levels of protein and fat and is considered to be a source of both of these nutrients. A good rule for determining whether or not an ingredient in a pet food is a protein source is to compare the level of protein in the ingredient with the level of the ingredient in the food. Anything that has a protein content that is greater than its percentage in the diet is considered to be a source of protein for that ration. For example, if a pet food contains 20% chicken byproduct meal that has a protein content of 65%, chicken byproduct meal constitutes a protein source for that food.

BOX 16-4 COMMON PET FOOD INGREDIENTS

PRIMARY NUTRIENT CONTRIBUTION

Protein	Carbohydrate	Fat	Dietary Fiber
Beef	Alfalfa meal	Animal fat	Apple pomace
Brewer's dried yeast	Barley	Chicken fat	Barley
Chicken meal	Brewer's rice	Corn oil	Beet pulp
Chicken liver meal	Brown rice	Fish oil	Cellulose
Chicken byproduct meal	Carrots	Flax seed (full fat)	Citrus pulp
Chicken	Dried kelp	Poultry fat	Oat bran
Chicken byproducts	Dried whey	Safflower oil	Peanut hulls
Corn gluten meal	Flax seed	Soybean oil	Pearled barley
Dried egg product	Flax seed meal	Sunflower oil	Peas
Duck	Grain sorghum	Vegetable oil	Rice bran
Fish	Ground corn		Soybean hulls
Fish meal	Ground rice		Soybean mill run
Flax seed meal	Ground wheat		Tomato pomace
Lamb	Molasses		
Lamb meal	Oat meal		
Meat byproducts	Pearled barley		
Meat meal	Peas		
Meat and bone meal	Potatoes		
Poultry byproduct meal	Rice flour		
Rabbit	Wheat (ground)		
Salmon	Wheat flour		
Soy flour or grits			
Soybean meal			
Turkey			

To determine if an ingredient on the label is a protein source for the food, compare the level of protein in the ingredient with the level of the ingredient in the food. If the ingredient's protein content is greater than its percentage in the food, it is considered to be a source of protein for that ration.

When the ingredient list of a pet food is examined, the nutrient or nutrients contributed by each ingredient should be a primary concern. Both the amount and quality of the ingredient in the product determine how efficiently the ingredient can provide nutrition to animals consuming the complete diet. It is also important to consider that a pet food is made up of a number of ingredients, not just the first three or four provided at the start of the list. Nutrients that are contributed by all ingredients must be considered when evaluating a pet food. The following discussion reviews common pet food ingredients and the major nutrients that they contribute to pet foods (Box 16-4).

Protein Sources

The protein in dog and cat foods can be supplied by animal sources, plant sources (grains), or a combination of the two. In general, high-quality animal source proteins provide superior amino acid balances for companion animals when compared with the amino acid balances supplied by grain proteins. However, animal protein sources can range from excellent quality to poor quality.[13] In contrast, grain protein sources are comparatively consistent in their quality and ability to supply amino acids. The protein in grains is not as balanced or available as the protein in high-quality animal sources, but it is superior in these characteristics compared with poor-quality animal protein sources.

ANIMAL-SOURCE PROTEINS Animal protein sources that are commonly included in pet foods include beef, chicken, chicken meal, lamb, lamb meal, dried egg, fish, fish meal, meat and bone meal, meat byproducts, and meat meal. In recent years, novel protein sources such as rabbit, salmon, duck, turkey, and venison have also been included in some dog and cat foods (see Chapter 31, pp. 399-400). The term *meat*, as defined by AAFCO, can represent any species of slaughtered mammal. Most commonly, this includes the striated muscle of pork, beef, or sheep. The term *poultry* includes the flesh and skin of domestic poultry, most typically chicken, turkey, or duck. When a specific species is used, such as chicken, this must be identified as such. When the term *byproduct* is included in the ingredient name, this means that secondary products are included with the ingredient in addition to the principal product. Byproducts of meat and poultry products are the parts of these animals that are not typically used as human foods in the United States.[14] This includes organ meats, blood, fat tissue, stomach and intestines, but may *not* include hair, horns, teeth, hoofs, feathers, or fecal matter.[1] For example, when an ingredient is listed as "poultry," this means that it includes the clean combination of flesh and skin with or without bone derived from part or whole carcasses of poultry, exclusive of feathers, heads, feet, and entrails. On the other hand, "poultry byproduct" refers to the clean parts of carcasses of slaughtered poultry (flesh and skin), which may also contain bone, heads, feet, and intestines. If it includes heads and feet, poultry byproduct meal may be lower in nutritional value than fresh poultry; however, the inclusion of nutrient-rich internal organs may offset this. Another common term that is often part of an ingredient's name is *meal*. This term simply refers to any ingredient that has been ground or otherwise reduced in particle size. For example, "chicken meal" is the dry, ground, whole chicken, exclusive of heads, feet, viscera, or feathers, and "chicken byproduct meal" is the same processing method, but may include byproducts.

Depending on the supplier and the type of refining process that the pet food manufacturer uses, animal protein sources can vary greatly in quality and digestibility. Several factors influence this. Meat protein sources can contain varying amounts of bone. If meat and bone meal is included as an ingredient, the amount of bone contained in the product affects its quality as a protein source as well as the mineral balance of the entire diet. The matrix of bone is composed of the protein collagen. Collagen is very poorly digested by dogs and cats, yet it will be analyzed as protein in the pet food. All muscle meats are very low in calcium content and have calcium:phosphorus ratios between 1:15 and 1:26. When bone is included with a meat ingredient, the calcium level of the product is increased, and the calcium:phosphorus ratio may be normalized. However, inexpensive meat and bone meals often contain excess levels of minerals. In this case, the problem becomes one of supplying too much calcium, phosphorus, and magnesium, rather than an insufficient amount of these nutrients. An excessively high calcium level in a pet food that contains meat and bone meal, poultry meal, or fish meal is an indication that the meal included in the product may be of poor quality and contains excessively high amounts of bone.

Two other important factors are the form of the protein source and the degree of processing or cooking that was involved during the food's production. For example, the label of a dry dog food might include chicken, chicken meal, or chicken byproduct meal as its first ingredient. Although the animal source is the same for these three ingredients, their protein content and quality can differ significantly. There is a great deal of confusion among pet owners and professionals regarding the difference between "chicken" (or, sometimes "fresh chicken") and "chicken meal," when observed on the pet food label. Chicken is the "*clean combination of flesh and skin with or without accompanying bone, derived from the parts of whole carcasses of poultry or a combination thereof, exclusive of feathers, heads, feet, and entrails.*"[1] Following slaughter and processing, the resulting chicken is divided into blocks and frozen or chilled. Cooling is necessary because of the very high water content in whole chicken; chicken used in pet foods contains between 65% and 70% water.[15] Whole chicken is also typically very high in fat. Because of its high moisture content, the inclusion of whole chicken in a pet food may place the ingredient first on the ingredient list. However, chicken in this form contributes a very small proportion of the food's protein and may actually be a more substantial source of fat in the food. These facts are not necessarily shortcomings. There is evidence that poultry fat is a strong palatability enhancer for dogs and cats, and the protein that is contributed by fresh chicken is usually of high quality.[16,17] However, consumers must also be aware that when chicken is included as an ingredient, it may in fact be a minor contributor to the protein of the food and may be more important as a fat source.

In contrast, chicken *meals* are produced through the rendering of whole chicken (as defined by AAFCO, above). This cooking process is used to remove a high proportion of the animal fat.[14] The resultant mixture is dried and ground to a meal that has a consistency similar to that of corn meal. When protein meals are included in pet foods and are found high on the ingredient list, they comprise a principal protein source for the ration because of their low moisture and reduced fat content. Because rendering involves cooking, meals are heat-treated twice (once during rendering and again during extrusion), which may increase heat-related damage to protein and reduce digestibility when compared with the ingredient's fresh equivalent. However, studies of the effects of rendering and extrusion on animal-source proteins have found these reductions to be small, especially when the quality of the fresh product is high. Additionally, increased demand for high-quality pet food ingredients by pet food manufacturers has led to the production and increased availability of pet-food–grade animal source proteins that are higher in both protein and digestibility than are typical feed-grade sources.[18]

Finally, a *byproduct meal* refers to the meal produced from rendering and drying of an animal byproduct protein source. When chicken (or more commonly, poultry) byproduct meal is produced, the fresh chicken can include the byproducts identified previously. While the cooking process is the same as that used for just fresh chicken, the inclusion of feet and heads reduces protein quality and digestibility of the end product. When a byproduct meal is listed high on an ingredient list, it represents a primary protein source in the food as a result of its dry form. These same relationships and definitions apply to meat, meat meal, and meat byproduct meal and other animal source proteins such as lamb or fish.

Several factors influence the quality of animal source protein ingredients in dog and cat foods. These include the form and moisture content of the ingredient, the inclusion of less-digestible components such as collagen, and the processing methods used to prepare the ingredient. In addition, some protein sources also contribute a significant amount of fat to the food.

Last, animal source proteins are included in the diets of dogs and cats as a primary component of a homemade diet or as some form of treat or supplemental food. The category of *alternative pet foods* is one of the fastest growing sectors of the pet food market today. These products include raw food diets, organic foods, and rations that are promoted as "all natural" or holistic.[19] These are available as both commercial preparations and as homemade recipes. Even though the majority of pet owners still feed a commercial food as their pet's primary diet, table scraps, human foods, and raw foods made up at least a small proportion of the diets of many dogs and cats.[20] The most commonly fed animal-source protein ingredients that owners report feeding are beef and poultry. These ingredients may be purchased frozen from a commercial supplier, from a rendering plant, or from the owner's grocery store.[21,22] Other animal-source proteins that are fed to dogs and cats are commercial treats such as freeze-dried liver or salmon. These foods are highly palatable to most pets and can be used as potent primary reinforcers in training. However, they are not nutritionally balanced and so should not provide more than 5% of a pet's nutritional intake (see Chapter 17, pp. 173-174 for a complete discussion of alternative pet foods).

GRAIN-SOURCE PROTEINS   Grain sources of protein used in pet foods include corn gluten meal, various forms of soy (meal, flour, and grits), alfalfa meal, flax seed meal, and wheat germ. Pet foods that contain grain products as the major source of protein usually include a combination of soy products and corn gluten meal. Corn gluten meal is the dried residue that remains after most of the starch, fiber, and germ-containing portions of the corn grain have been removed. As a protein source, corn gluten meal is relatively consistent in quality, containing approximately 60% protein.[23]

This protein source is not as digestible as high-quality animal protein ingredients, but its protein is comparable to or more available than some meals and byproduct meals.[24,25] On a DMB, corn gluten meal contains a high proportion of protein, but its protein is deficient in the essential amino acids lysine, arginine, and tryptophan.

Soybean products have been included in pet foods for a number of years. Texturized vegetable protein (TVP), which contains approximately 50% crude protein, is the form that is often found in canned and semimoist foods. TVP is produced by the extrusion of defatted soy flour and has the advantage of retaining a meatlike texture and appearance through the high temperatures of the canning process.[26] Similar to tofu, a common human soy food, TVP has a bland flavor and aroma and absorbs the flavors of the ingredients with which it is cooked. A recent study of dogs' ability to digest TVP in canned foods reported that small intestinal digestion of TVP protein was just slightly lower than the digestibility of beef protein (73.4% vs. 77.0%).[27] As the proportion of TVP was increased, protein digestibility decreased slightly to about 70%. The decrease in digestibility was accompanied by increased fecal volume and the production of softer stools. Several forms of soy may be included in dry, extruded pet foods, but the most common forms are defatted soybean meal and soy flour. A study comparing the ability of adult dogs to digest soy products to poultry meal that were included in an extruded, dry food found that small intestinal and total tract protein digestibility of the soy products did not differ from each other but were all significantly more digestible than poultry meal.[28] Conversely, another study found that soybean meal protein had slightly lower small intestine and total tract digestibility coefficients when compared with low-ash poultry meal. The difference between these two studies reflects the different qualities of poultry meal that were tested (low-ash poultry meal had a higher digestibility coefficient), as soybean meal digestibility coefficients remained consistent. Because soy protein is limiting in the sulfur amino acid methionine but is rich in lysine, it is valuable as a complementary protein to corn gluten meal in commercial pet foods.

Although soy protein is well digested by dogs, soy carbohydrate is poorly digested in the canine small intestine. Soy flour and TVP contain approximately 30% carbohydrate, which is comprised principally of soluble oligosaccharides and polysaccharides.[29] These indigestible fibers travel to the large intestine, where they are fermented by colon bacteria, resulting in the production of short-chain fatty acids (SCFAs) and gas. SCFAs provide an important energy source for colonocytes and contribute to the health of the large intestine when produced at optimum levels. In addition, soybean oligosaccharides are assumed to be responsible for reduced postprandial insulin levels observed in dogs fed TVP diets, an effect that may be of benefit in the management of diabetes (see Chapter 29, pp. 348-352).[30] The osmotic action of the SCFAs and possibly increased electrolyte concentrations in the colon lead to increased fecal water content. This effect is not noticeable when moderate levels of soy are fed, but can be pronounced in diets containing 50% or more soy protein. This can cause loose stools and flatulence in some dogs.[27] Interestingly, investigations of the ability of dogs to digest and ferment soy carbohydrate found that when dogs were fed diets containing either conventional soybean (as whole beans or meal) or a low-oligosaccharide variety, they digested low-oligosaccharide soy as extensively as the conventional soybeans.[31,32] Although soy fibers cannot be digested by the enzymes of the small intestine, they are nearly 100% fermentable in the large intestine. This information is significant when considering the type and proportion of soy in a pet food because fecal consistency, defecation frequency, and colon health may be affected.

Soy also contains phytate and several metabolic inhibitors that affect an animal's ability to digest and absorb other nutrients. Soy trypsin inhibitors function to reduce the digestibility of protein in the diet. However, trypsin inhibitors, like many other antinutritional factors, are heat labile and are largely destroyed by heating during the processing of pet foods. Hemagglutinins in soy are lectins that are capable of binding carbohydrate and agglutinating red blood cells. However, these have not been shown to be toxic, and like trypsin inhibitors, they are heat labile. In contrast, phytate is not significantly affected by heat and is capable of interfering with the absorption of certain minerals even after processing. Therefore pet food manufacturers must account for the effects of phytate when balancing the mineral component of soy-containing foods.

Although soy is classified as a plant source of protein for pet foods, some forms of soy ingredients also contribute significant amounts of carbohydrate and fiber to the food. These components can have both benefits and potential drawbacks, depending upon their level in the food.

Carbohydrate Sources

Ingredients that contribute digestible carbohydrates to commercial pet foods include various forms of corn, rice, sorghum, wheat, and oats. Barley, carrots, flax seed, molasses, peas, and potatoes may also be included, but usually in lesser amounts. With the exception of molasses, all of these ingredients contribute varying amounts of complex carbohydrates in the form of starch. The source and the form of the grain significantly affects the amount of starch that it contributes to a food.[33] For example, whole wheat is comprised of approximately 50% starch, while wheat flour contains approximately 70%.[34] The difference is caused by the removal of the fiber-containing bran and protein-rich germ to produce flour from the complete grain. The form of the carbohydrate ingredient is also important. Grinding to produce a meal breaks open the grain's hard outer coating (the bran), making the starch more available and digestible. Cooking of plant starch greatly enhances its digestibility. Therefore heat treatment of these ingredients during processing ensures maximal use by companion animals. In dry pet foods, a certain proportion of the diet must be made up of starch to allow for proper expansion of the kibbles. During expansion, temperatures within the extruder come close to 150° C. This temperature increases the size of the starch granules and improves both digestibility and palatability.

COMMON GRAIN SOURCES The primary cereal grains that are included in pet foods are corn, wheat, and rice. Ground corn and corn grits are the two most common forms of corn that supply digestible starch to pet foods. Ground corn is also called *corn meal* on the pet food label; it is produced when the entire grain is chopped and then finely ground. Corn grits is ground corn without the outer coating of the corn kernel (the bran) or the protein-containing germ.

As a result, corn grits contains a higher proportion of digestible starch while corn meal is slightly higher in fiber and protein. The extruded corn starch in both ingredients provides an available and digestible source of energy to dogs and cats.[35]

Wheat and rice grains are usually processed and ground to produce flours for inclusion in pet foods. Cereal flours contain primarily the starch and protein from their respective grain, so are lower in fiber, fat, and ash than ground grains.[36] Wheat flour is often included as an ingredient in biscuits because its high gluten (protein) content contributes an appealing texture and palatability to baked products.[34] Wheat contains slightly more protein than other cereal grains; the principle wheat protein is gluten. Gluten is actually a mix of two proteins, glutenin and gliadin, and is often maligned as the cause of food hypersensitivity in dogs and cats. However, dietary hypersensitivity can develop to many different dietary proteins or protein-containing complexes, of which wheat gluten is just one possibility. Studies of dogs affected with dietary hypersensitivity have reported that the proteins found in beef, soy, and dairy products are the most common food allergens in dogs and cats.[37] The widespread perception of wheat as a potent food allergen is possibly related to a disorder called *gluten-induced enteropathy*.[38] Analogous to celiac disease in humans, this malabsorption disorder appears to have a strong genetic basis and is seen primarily in purebred Irish Setters.

Rice is one of the most highly digestible starches fed to dogs and cats. Its digestion leads to relatively rapid postprandial increases in blood glucose levels, when compared with other starch ingredients.[36,39] Interestingly, while wheat as a pet food ingredient has acquired an erroneous reputation as an "allergy-causing" ingredient, rice enjoys a reputation as the supposed "hypoallergenic" pet food ingredient. This perception developed because rice was used as a novel carbohydrate source in some of the first foods that were developed as elimination diets for pets with dietary hypersensitivity. As an ingredient, rice possesses no inherent "hypoallergenic" characteristics. Rather, it was initially selected because it provided a source of carbohydrate to which most pets had not been previously exposed. Regardless of this misconception, the rice starch that is supplied by finely ground rice flour provides a highly digestible source of energy for dogs and cats.

OTHER STARCH SOURCES   Oats, barley, sorghum (milo), and potatoes are other carbohydrate ingredients that are found in commercial pet foods today. Barley and sorghum are both grains that are ground and sometimes precooked prior to being added to a dry pet food. One of the benefits of these two starch sources is that they are more slowly digested than rice and corn and contribute to reduced or delayed postprandial glucose and insulin responses.[40] These attributes may make these grains suitable for starch mixes that are used in foods designed to aid in glycemic control (see Chapter 29, pp. 348-350 for a complete discussion). Peas and lentils have been studied as alternative starch sources of inclusion in pet foods, but tend to have lower digestibilities than conventional starches, even following extrusion.[40,41] This difference is attributed to the higher fiber content of these ingredients as well as to differences between grains and legumes in the predominant type of starch that they contain. However, these sources also modulate plasma fluctuations in blood glucose when compared with rice and corn and may have some benefit as ingredients for diabetic or older pets. Various forms of potatoes have been included in canned and dry pet foods in recent years.[42] Canned stews and dinners may contain potato cubes or pieces, which are visually appealing to pet owners and provide an excellent source of digestible starch. Potato starch is also used in canned products as a texture enhancer. Various forms of dried potatoes are found in dry pet foods, including potato flour, buds, starch, and isolated potato protein. Potato protein may also have use in elimination or alternative diets for pets with dietary hypersensitivity.[43]

> *The form and degree of heat treatment significantly affect how digestible and palatable a starch source is for dogs and cats, In addition, different starch sources vary in the type of starch that they provide, the level of indigestible fiber, and the rate at which they influence postprandial changes in blood glucose and insulin concentrations.*

FIBER SOURCES   Although it is not a digestible nutrient, dietary fiber is typically classified with carbohydrate ingredients. Dietary fiber is not digested by intestinal enzymes, but it is required in the diet to promote normal gastrointestinal tract functioning and health (see Section 1, pp. 14-16 and Section 5, pp. 465-470). Common sources of indigestible fiber in commercial pet foods include beet pulp; apple and tomato pomace; peanut hulls; citrus pulp; the bran of oats, rice, and wheat; peas; and cellulose.

Bran is a milling byproduct consisting of the outer coarse coat (pericarp) of cereal grains that was removed during the production of flour. The bran of several grains is used in pet foods and contains varying levels of fermentable and nonfermentable fiber, fat, and protein. The use of rice bran as a pet food ingredient has increased in recent years because it has been shown to be a palatable source of fermentable fiber, essential fatty acids (EFAs), and several naturally occurring antioxidants.[44] Rice bran contains an unusually high fat content for a cereal grain, with more than one third of the fat contributed by polyunsaturated fatty acids (PUFAs). However, when the bran is separated from the rice during the milling process, the cellular damage associated with breaking the seed coat results in the release of plant lipases. These enzymes immediately begin to hydrolyze the oil in the bran, which can lead to oxidative rancidity and loss of palatability. Therefore additional processing is necessary to denature the plant lipase and prevent destruction of the bran's fat. This is accomplished by rapidly cooking the bran immediately after its production. The resultant product is called *stabilized rice bran* and can be used as a fiber source for pet foods.[45]

Pulp is the solid residue that remains after juices are extracted from fruits or vegetables; pomace specifically refers to the pulp of fruit. The beet pulp that is included in pet foods is derived from sugar beets (not red beets) and is considered to be a high-quality fiber source. It contains 60% to 80% total dietary fiber, of which approximately 80% is insoluble.[46] Studies of the use of beet pulp as a fiber source for dogs and cats have found that including beet pulp in the food does not negatively affect palatability (as do some other fiber sources) and positively contributes to bowel regularity and stool quality.[47,48] When included at optimal levels in a food, the moderately fermentable fiber of beet pulp helps to provide adequate bulk for gastrointestinal tract functioning while also promoting gastrointestinal cell health through the production of SCFAs (see Section 1, pp. 14-16, and Section 5, pp. 465-467).

Fat Sources

The fat in a pet food contributes calories and EFAs and enhances palatability. Commonly used sources of fat in commercial pet foods include various types of animal fats and vegetable oils. The general term "animal fat" refers to fat that comes from the tissues of mammals and/or poultry. Animal fat must contain a minimum of 90% total fatty acids, not more than 2.5% unsaponifiable matter, and not more than 1% insoluble impurities.[1] The unsaponifiable portion of a fat contains lipid compounds other than triglycerides and fatty acids, such as sterols, pigments, and fatty alcohols. If the product is completely made up of a single type of fat, such as poultry or beef fat, a descriptive term denoting the species of the animal source can be used. Chicken fat and poultry fat are the two most common types of animal fat included in dog and cat foods. In recent years, fish oil has also been included in many pet foods because it is a rich source of n-3 fatty acids, specifically the long-chain PUFAs eicosapentaenoic acid (EPA) and docosahexaenoic acid (DHA). Similarly, the terms *vegetable fat* or *vegetable oil* refer to the product obtained from the extraction of the oil from seeds. If a specific plant is the exclusive source of the oil, this may be indicated on the label. Most commonly, corn, safflower, and soybean oils are used in commercial pet foods. Sunflower oil is also occasionally used, as it provides a concentrated source of linoleic acid.[49] Flax is an important plant source of fat because ground whole flaxseed is an excellent source of the omega-3 fatty acid alpha-linolenic acid.

In addition to specific fat sources, ingredients such as chicken, poultry, and various meat products also contribute a significant amount of fat to pet foods. Fish meal is an excellent protein source and also supplies fish oil, which contains long-chain omega-3 fatty acids. Finally, if an antioxidant has been added to the fat source as a preservative, this must be indicated following the listing of the product on the ingredient list (see pp. 155-158).

Vitamin and Mineral Sources

Almost all of the major ingredients discussed earlier also contribute vitamins and minerals to the diet. When a balanced ration is formulated, vitamin and mineral levels are made adequate through the addition of purified or semipurified forms of these nutrients. Because only small amounts of vitamins and minerals are required by animals and because other ingredients also supply these nutrients, purified forms of vitamins and minerals are present in small amounts in pet foods and are listed low on the ingredient list of the label.

Minerals vary greatly in their bioavailability, and many factors can affect the mineral availability within a diet. It is important not only to have adequate amounts of each mineral relative to the animal's requirement, but also to consider the relationship between minerals and the overall balance of the ration. Excess levels of any mineral may adversely affect the ability of the body to absorb other minerals in the diet. For example, excess levels of calcium, copper, and possibly vitamin D can all inhibit the absorption of zinc in dogs.[50] Manufacturers must always consider these relationships when balancing the mineral component of their pet foods. In recent years, there has been some interest in the use of chelated trace minerals in pet foods. These ingredients are also referred to as *organic minerals.* They are produced synthetically and consist of an organic ligand, such as an amino acid, peptide, or polysaccharide that is covalently linked to the trace mineral. It is theorized that chelated minerals are more bioavailable than naturally occurring minerals, either because digestion yields a more readily utilized ionic form or because the mineral and ligand are absorbed together as an intact molecule.[51] There is evidence that chelated minerals may confer some benefit to animals that are marginally deficient in the respective mineral (and so already have high absorption efficiency) and in diets that contain levels at or near requirements. However, because the body's efficiency of mineral absorption is dependent upon its mineral status, benefits of the inclusion of chelated minerals in pet foods are questionable. Per AAFCO guidelines, pet foods are formulated to include a buffer above minimum needs for essential nutrients and are also typically fed to replete animals. Therefore the small increment in increased bioavailability that may be conferred through organic chelating may not be of benefit to the majority of animals. However, some pet food companies do include chelated minerals in their foods, as an added "buffer" and because of pet owner perceptions of a benefit.

One of the biggest concerns about vitamins in commercial pet foods is their loss during processing and storage. Adequate quantities of vitamins that account for losses during processing and storage must be added to pet foods to ensure that sufficient levels are present at the time of feeding. The high heat and pressure used in the canning process result in losses of the B vitamins thiamin and folic acid. Compensatory levels of these vitamins must be added to maintain adequate postprocessing levels. In dry, extruded pet foods, there are considerable losses of vitamin A, riboflavin, folic acid, niacin, and biotin. However, if vitamin A is added as part of the fat coating that is sprayed onto the food after extrusion, there is little to no loss of the vitamin during storage. In semimoist foods, slight losses of vitamin A and riboflavin have been observed.[52] Studies have provided recommendations for levels of vitamins to add to preprocessed pet food to ensure that levels after processing and storage are still sufficient to meet an animal's nutrient needs. In addition, manufacturers who ensure thorough testing of their products conduct nutrient analyses of their finished products; this testing may not be done by manufacturers who use the calculation method for nutritional adequacy substantiation.

Ingredients that contribute vitamins and minerals to pet foods must be balanced in terms of their overall quantities, their bioavailability, and their relationships to each other. Commonly included sources of minerals in commercial pet foods include potassium chloride, calcium carbonate, dicalcium phosphate, monosodium phosphate, manganese sulfate or manganese oxide, copper sulfate, zinc oxide, sodium selenite, potassium iodide, ferrous sulfate, and cobalt carbonate. Examples of sources of vitamins include choline chloride, D-activated animal sterol (a source of vitamin D), alpha-tocopherol, thiamin or thiamin mononitrate, niacin, calcium pantothenate, pyridoxine hydrochloride, riboflavin, folic acid, biotin, menadione dimethylpyrimidinol (a source of vitamin K), vitamin A acetate, and vitamin B_{12}.

Additives and Preservatives

Additives are ingredients that are included in pet foods to enhance or preserve the product's color, flavor, texture, stability, or nutrient content. Preservatives are additives that are included with the express purpose of protecting nutrients in the food from oxidative or microbial damage. All preservatives are classified as additives, but not all additives have a function in food preservation.

One of the chief concerns in the production of commercial pet foods is safety. A product must be proven to be both nutritious and safe for consumption by companion animals throughout its designated shelf-life. The manufacturer must ensure that the food remains free of contamination with harmful bacteria and toxins and is protected from degradation and the loss of nutrients during storage. The method of preservation that is used for a pet food depends to some degree on the type of food. The low moisture content of dry pet foods inhibits the growth of most organisms. The heat sterilization and anaerobic environment of canned foods kills all microbes. Semimoist pet foods often have a low pH and contain humectants that bind water within the product, making it unavailable for use by invading bacteria or fungi. Frozen pet foods, although less common, are protected by storage at extremely low temperatures. Many commercial foods also contain added ingredients that aid in the preservation process. For example, potassium sorbate prevents the formation of mold and yeasts; glycerol and certain sugars act as humectants.

A primary nutrient in pet foods that requires protection during storage is dietary fat. The inclusion of high levels of fat in some dry pet foods has resulted in the need for methods of protecting these fats from oxidative destruction during storage. Foods that are formulated for dogs and cats contain vegetable oils, animal fats, and the fat-soluble vitamins A, D, E, and K. These nutrients all have the potential to undergo oxidative destruction during storage. This oxidative degradation, called *lipid peroxidation,* occurs as a three-stage process.[53] Initiation occurs when a free radical, usually oxygen, attacks a PUFA and results in the formation of a fatty acid radical. Exposure of the fat to heat, ultraviolet radiation, or certain metal ions such as iron and copper accelerate this process. The fatty acid radical continues to react with oxygen, resulting in the formation of peroxides. Peroxides react with other fatty acids to form more fatty acid radicals and hydroperoxides (Figure 16-2). This second phase is called *propagation* because the reaction is autocatalyzed and increases geometrically in rate. The reaction is only terminated when all of the available fatty acids and vitamins have been oxidized. The subsequent decomposition of the hydroperoxides produces offensive odors, tastes, and changes in the texture of the food. In addition, oxidation of lipids in pet foods results in a loss of caloric content and the formation of toxic

No Antioxidant

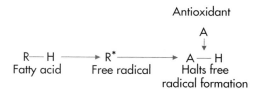

Antioxidant Added

Figure 16-2   Antioxidant action.

forms of peroxides that can be harmful to the health of companion animals.[54] For example, a study with growing Coonhounds found that dogs that consumed diets containing oxidized lipids had reduced serum vitamin E levels and compromised antioxidant status during growth.[55] Very high levels of oxidized lipids also caused decreased growth rates and negatively affected some measures of immune function.

Pet food manufacturers include antioxidants in commercial pet foods to prevent the autooxidation process. The Food and Drug Administration (FDA) defines antioxidants as substances that aid in the preservation of foods by retarding deterioration, rancidity, or discoloration as the result of oxidative processes.[56] Various types of antioxidants have been accepted for use in human and animal foods since 1947.[57] These compounds do not reverse the effects of oxidation once it has started; rather, they retard the oxidative process and prevent destruction of the fat in the food. Therefore, to be effective, antioxidants must be included in the diet when it is initially mixed and processed. The inclusion of antioxidant compounds in commercial pet foods prevents rancidity; maintains the food's flavor, odor, and texture; and prevents the accumulation of the toxic end products of lipid degradation.

Antioxidant ingredients can be categorized into two basic types—natural-derived products and synthetic products. Natural-derived antioxidants are commonly found in certain grains, vegetable oils, and some herbs and spices. While these compounds exist in nature, the term "natural" can be misleading to consumers because all of these compounds are processed in some way to make them available for use in commercial foods.[58] The mixed-tocopherols are probably the most widely distributed natural-derived antioxidant. These are composed of four homologues: alpha-tocopherol (vitamin E), beta-tocopherol, gamma-tocopherol, and delta-tocopherol. Physiologically, alpha-tocopherol (vitamin E) has the strongest biological function as an antioxidant in the body but has much lower activity as a food antioxidant. In contrast, gamma-tocopherol and delta-tocopherol both have low biological activity, but they are more effective than alpha-tocopherol as feed antioxidants. Generally, delta-tocopherol is more stable during processing and has greater carry-through than gamma-tocopherol. The mixed tocopherols that are used in foods are obtained primarily from the distillation of soybean oil residue and have the highest efficacy of the natural-derived antioxidants in protection of fats in pet foods. The tocopherols also have excellent consumer acceptance compared with some of the synthetic antioxidant preservatives. However, tocopherols are an expensive ingredient, have less antioxidant activity compared with synthetic antioxidants, and are rapidly decomposed as they protect fat from oxidation. As a result, the shelf-life of pet foods stabilized with tocopherols alone may be shorter than that of foods preserved with a mixture of several different antioxidants.[59]

Other natural-derived ingredients with antioxidant activity that may be included in pet foods include ascorbic acid (vitamin C), rosemary extract, marigold extract, and citric acid. Ascorbic acid functions naturally as an antioxidant by scavenging oxygen. However, it is a water-soluble compound and is not easily solubilized with the lipid fraction of foods, which affects its function as an antioxidant for the fat in commercial pet foods. Vitamin C has been shown to work synergistically with other antioxidants, such as vitamin E and butylated hydroxytoluene (BHT), and it is often included in pet foods for this reason. Ascorbyl palmitate is a compound that is similar in structure to ascorbic acid. Although ascorbyl palmitate is not normally found in nature, its hydrolysis yields ascorbic acid and the free fatty acid (FFA) palmitic acid, both of which are natural compounds. The antioxidant function of ascorbyl palmitate is the result of the ascorbic acid portion of the molecule.

Rosemary extract is a spice that is obtained from the dried leaves of an evergreen shrub, *Rosmarinus officinalis*. Although it is added to pet foods as a flavor enhancer, it also has effectiveness as a natural-derived preservative in high-fat diets and has been shown to enhance antioxidant efficiency when included in combination with tocopherols, ascorbic acid and citric acid.[59] As with the tocopherols, rosemary extract generally has high consumer appeal. Similarly, marigold extract is a source of lutein, a naturally occurring antioxidant that may also have positive effects on immune function. Citric acid is found in citrus fruits, such as oranges and lemons, and is often included in combination with other natural-derived antioxidants in pet foods. Lecithin, monoglycerides, and diglycerides are natural-derived compounds that are added to pet foods to act as emulsifying agents. In this capacity, they function to prevent separation of fat from other components of the diet, allowing greater contact between antioxidants and the lipid components in the food.

The natural-derived antioxidant formulations that are available for use in pet foods have improved greatly in recent years. However, they still have limited value when used as the only type of antioxidant in a commercially produced pet food because the concentration that must be included to provide an adequate level of protection is very high. Commercial pet foods undergo rigorous processing procedures that can include exposure to high heat, steam, and pressure. In addition, they must be protected from damaging oxidative reactions during varying lengths of storage. An effective antioxidant system must have high stability and retain its antioxidant functions after being subjected to the high heat, pressure, and moisture of food processing (i.e., have good carry-through). Most natural-derived antioxidants have lower carry-through than synthetic products, so high concentrations must be included in the food to compensate for losses during processing. When natural-derived antioxidants are used in pet foods, the products of choice are the mixed tocopherols, usually in combination with ascorbic acid and rosemary extract. In other cases, these ingredients are used to supplement the action of synthetic antioxidants that are also included in the food. Because these natural-derived compounds tend to be significantly more expensive than synthetic antioxidants, it can be difficult to attain the necessary level of natural-derived antioxidants without it becoming cost-prohibitive.

Effective synthetic antioxidants for pet foods include butylated hydroxyanisole (BHA), BHT, tertiary butylhydroquinone (TBHQ), and ethoxyquin. BHA and BHT are approved for use in both human foods and animal feeds and have a synergistic antioxidant effect when used together. BHA and BHT have good carry-through and a high efficacy in the protection of animal fats, but they are slightly less effective when used with vegetable oils.[57] TBHQ is an effective antioxidant for most fats and is approved for use in human and animal foods in the United States. However, this compound has not been approved in Canada or Japan, or by the European Economic Community, so it is not used in pet foods that have an international market. Ethoxyquin is approved for use in animal feeds and in human foods. Like BHT and BHA, ethoxyquin has good carry-through, and it has an especially high efficacy in the protection of fats. Ethoxyquin is more efficient as an antioxidant than BHA or BHT, which allows lower levels of the compound to be included in the feed. It is especially effective in the protection of oils that contain high levels of PUFAs and demonstrates synergistic protection when used in combination with BHA.[59,60]

Starting in the late 1980s, consumer concern was raised regarding the safety of synthetic antioxidants, specifically ethoxyquin, in pet foods. One of the arguments made against ethoxyquin was its use as an antioxidant in the rubber industry. The biochemical mechanism through which ethoxyquin prevents oxidation of rubber is exactly the same mechanism by which it works to protect the fat in pet foods. Similarly, BHA and BHT were both originally used to protect petroleum products from the oxidative changes that led to "gumming."[57] The fact that a compound acts as an antioxidant in other situations does not preclude it from being an effective antioxidant in foods. Like most compounds, ethoxyquin, BHA, and BHT have multiple uses.[61]

Ethoxyquin has been included in feeds for animals since 1959, and its safety in foods has been studied in rabbits, rats, poultry, and dogs. The original studies on which the FDA based approval for the inclusion of ethoxyquin in animal feeds included a 1-year chronic toxicity study in dogs. Data from this and other studies were used to determine a safe tolerance level of 150 parts per million (ppm) (150 milligrams [mg]/kg) of food.[62] Subsequently, the manufacturer of ethoxyquin conducted a 5-year, multigenerational study in dogs. The data from this study failed to show any adverse side effects of ethoxyquin when it was fed at a level of 300 mg/kg of the diet.[63] During the 1990s, an independent research facility conducted a study for the manufacturer of ethoxyquin on the effects of ethoxyquin upon the long-term health of dogs.[64] Two generations of male and female dogs were fed diets containing either 0, 180, or 360 ppm of ethoxyquin for a period of 42 months. During this time, the dogs mated and produced viable litters of puppies. There were no effects of the antioxidant upon the health or fertility of the adult dogs, or upon the health, growth, or mortality of their resultant puppies. However, liver pigmentation changes and increased liver enzymes were seen in some female dogs following lactation. These results led to a request by the FDA Center for Veterinary Medicine (CVM) to pet food manufacturers to voluntarily reduce the maximum level of ethoxyquin in their foods from 150 mg/kg to 75 mg/kg. The pet food industry has honored this request. However, there are no studies to date that support the contention that ethoxyquin is responsible for the variety of health problems that were originally reported by pet owners to the FDA.

It is important for pet owners to recognize that almost all products that humans and animals consume become toxic when consumed at high enough levels. The inclusion of antioxidants in commercial pet foods is necessary for the protection of dietary fat from detrimental oxidative changes. The proper use of all types of antioxidants prevents the occurrence of rancidity and the production of toxic compounds in pet foods. In most cases, synthetic antioxidants are included in foods because of their efficacy, good carry-through, and cost. In contrast, poor carry-through, instability, and high levels needed for effective protection make natural-derived antioxidants more challenging to use as the only type of antioxidant in a pet food (Table 16-3).

Pet foods also contain some additives that are included expressly to contribute to characteristics of color, texture, or palatability. For example, coloring agents are often added to enhance consumer appeal. Some examples include carotenoid pigments, iron oxide, tartrazine, sunset yellow, and allura red. Other coloring agents, such as nitrites, bisulfites, and ascorbate, are included to prevent discoloration of the pet

TABLE 16-3 COMMON ANTIOXIDANTS USED IN PET FOODS

	COST	AVAILABILITY	CARRY-THROUGH	EFFECTIVENESS
Natural-Derived				
Mixed tocopherols	High	Low	Poor	Low
Ascorbic acid	High	Low	Poor	Low
Ascorbyl palmitate	High	Low	Poor	Low
Synthetic				
BHA	Low	Moderate	Good	High
BHT	Low	Moderate	Good	High
TBHQ	Low	Poor	Good	High
Ethoxyquin	Low	Good	Excellent	High

BHA, Butylated hydroxyanisole; *BHT,* butylated hydroxytoluene; *TBHQ,* tertiary butylhydroquinone.

food. As with human foods, an artificial color can be used in a pet food only if it has been accepted as safe by the FDA. Flavor ingredients are included in some pet foods to support label claims regarding flavor. AAFCO regulations require that the designated flavor be detectable by a recognized testing method.[1] A related group of additives are those included to enhance palatability. These compounds are usually sprayed onto the outside of dry pet foods to make the food more appetizing to pets. A commonly used palatability enhancer is digest. The term *digest* refers to solutions that are produced through the enzymatic degradation of various types of meat or meat byproducts. This process is conducted under controlled conditions and is stopped when the protein in the mixture is partially digested. The resulting slurry of liquid is highly palatable to dogs and cats and is usually sprayed onto dry foods as an outer coating. In some cases, the digest is dried and added to the food as a powder following the application of a layer of fat. Digest can also be used as a means of designating the food's flavor. Other examples of palatability enhancers in commercial pet foods include garlic, onion, and various spices.

Finally, emulsifiers and thickening agents are important additives for the effect they have upon the pet food's texture. In canned pet foods, gums, glycerides, and modified starches are included for the production of a thick sauce or gravy. Examples of these ingredients are carrageenan, guar gum, gum arabic, and carboxymethylcellulose. These agents can also be sprayed onto the outside of a dry food so that when water is added to the food before feeding, they create a gravy or thick sauce.

Functional Ingredients

Functional ingredients are dietary components that are included in a food with the intent of providing a specific type of health benefit. These ingredients have become very popular in human diets, in part because of the passing of the Dietary Supplemental Health and Education Act (DSHEA) in 1994. This act limited the FDA's regulatory oversight of functional ingredients used in human foods, leading to an increase in these products in the human foods market. In recent years this interest has been expanded to companion animal diets.[65] Although the CVM argues that DSHEA does not apply to pet foods, it has tended to allow the inclusion of functional

ingredients that are comprised of AAFCO-approved ingredients or nutrients, and for which specific veterinary health claims are not made. Currently, all components in pet foods must be classified either as a feed ingredient (AAFCO-approved or -recognized) or as a drug. Therefore, if the CVM determines that a pet food's label claim for a functional ingredient constitutes a drug claim as opposed to a general health claim, they can intervene and require that the ingredient be classified as a drug and undergo requisite testing and approval.[66] For example, while the claim of "supports joint health" may be acceptable for foods that include chondroprotective agents such as chondroitin sulfate and glucosamine, a claim that states "reduces joint inflammation" or "decreases lameness" is not permissible.

Similar to human foods, a wide variety of micro- and macronutrients, nutrient combinations, and novel ingredients are included as functional ingredients in pet foods. Controlled studies providing empirical data for health benefits are available for some, but not all, of these compounds. In addition, because some nutrient combinations are proprietary, study results may not be published or are generally unavailable in the public arena. Pet food companies and nutritionists in academia continue to study functional uses for nutrient combinations and novel ingredients as they are identified. Currently, the primary categories of pet health effects that are targeted include joint health, skin and coat condition, gastrointestinal functioning, immune health, lower urinary tract health, and obesity.

Two functional ingredients that have been widely accepted as chondroprotective agents for joint health in human and pet foods are glucosamine and chondroitin sulfate. Others include green-lipped mussel powder (a source of glycosaminoglycans, omega-3 fatty acids, and other nutrients) and a type of collagen called *UC-II* (see Chapter 37, pp. 503-504 for a complete discussion). Feeding pets to promote a healthy skin and coat condition has been a focus of nutritionists and pet owners for many years. Owners may be particularly focused on coat condition because coat shine and skin health are perceived as a barometer of a pet's overall nutritional health. Functional ingredients that have been studied for their value in promoting skin health include modified levels of omega-3 and omega-6 fatty acids, conjugated linoleic acid, and formulas that combine various oils and B-vitamins (see Chapter 31, pp. 386-394 for a complete discussion). Gastrointestinal function can be supported through the inclusion of certain types of fiber combinations and select prebiotics such as fructooligosaccharide and mannanoligosaccharide.[67] Fiber combinations are also included in cat foods for the control of hairballs. Another approach to gastrointestinal health is the use of probiotics, which are preparations of specific bacterial species that function to favorably modify the microbial balance of the large intestine.[68] The effects of probiotics are influenced by numerous factors and their mode of action appears to be multifaceted. Published studies in human subjects, and increasingly in dogs and cats, show that probiotics have value as functional ingredients to promote gastrointestinal health and may also benefit skin health and immune function (see Chapter 35, pp. 470-472 for a complete discussion). Functional ingredients that support lower urinary tract health in cats include

agents that may control inflammation of the urinary tract and reduce the risk of urolith development (see Chapter 30). Finally, the high prevalence of overweight conditions in companion dogs and cats has led to the investigation of numerous functional ingredients that may help to prevent excessive weight gain and help to control glycemic response (see Chapters 28 and 29).

Functional ingredients are included in pet foods with the intent of providing specific health benefits. Similar to human foods, a wide variety of micro- and macronutrients, nutrient combinations, and novel ingredients are included as functional ingredients. The primary categories of pet health effects that are targeted include joint health, skin and coat condition, gastrointestinal functioning, immune health, lower urinary tract health, and obesity.

References

1. Association of American Feed Control Officials (AAFCO): Pet food regulations. In *AAFCO Official Publication*, Atlanta, 2008, AAFCO.

2. Weigel J: Changing values: reference vs. actual. In *Proceedings of the petfood forum*, Chicago, 1996, Watts Publishing.

3. Whitlock L: Ingredient changes: understanding the impact on your products. In *Proceedings of the petfood forum*, Chicago, 1995, Watts Publishing.

4. National Research Council: *Nutrient requirements of dogs and cats*, Washington, DC, 2006, National Academy Press.

5. Wiernusz CJ, Shields RG, Van Vlierbergen DJ, and others: Canine nutrient digestibility and stool quality evaluation of canned diets containing various soy protein supplements, *Vet Clin Nutr* 2:49–56, 1995.

6. Bisset SA, Guilford WG, Lawoko CR, and others: Effect of food particle size on carbohydrate assimilation assessed by breath hydrogen testing in dogs, *Vet Clin Nutr* 4:82–88, 1997.

7. Wang X: *Effect of processing methods and raw material sources on protein quality of animal protein meals, PhD thesis*, Urbana, Ill, 1996, University of Illinois.

8. Lankhorst C, Tran QD, Havenaar R, and others: The effect of extrusion on the nutritional value of canine diets as assessed by in vitro indicators, *Anim Feed Sci Tech* 138:285–297, 2007.

9. Smeets M, Minekus M, Havenaar R, and others: Description of a dynamic in vitro model of the dog gastro-intestinal tract and evaluation of various transit times for protein and calcium, *Altern Lab Anim* 27:L935–L949, 1999.

10. Gajda M, Flickinger EA, Grieshop CM, and others: Corn hybrid affects in vitro and in vivo measures of nutrient digestibility in dogs, *J Anim Sci* 83:160–171, 2005.

11. Laflamme DP: Determining metabolizable energy content in commercial pet foods, *J Anim Physiol Anim Nutr* 85:222–230, 2001.

12. Hervera M, Baucells MD, Torre C, and others: Prediction of digestible energy value of extruded dog food: comparison of methods, *J Anim Physiol Anim Nutr* 92:253–259, 2008.

13. Fahey G, Hussein SH: The nutritional value of alternative raw materials used in pet foods. In *Proceedings of the petfood forum*, Chicago, 1997, Watts Publishing.

14. Thompson A: Ingredients: where pet food starts, *Top Companion Anim Med* 23:127–132, 2008.

15. Aldrich G: Chicken first: marketing ploy or quality enhancement? *Pet Food Ind,* May 2007.

16. Cramer KR, Greenwood MW, Moritz JS, and others: Protein quality of various raw and rendered by-product meals commonly incorporated into companion animal diets, *J Anim Sci* 85:3285–3293, 2007.

17. Murray SM, Patil AR, Fahey GC Jr, and others: Raw and rendered animal by-products as ingredients in dog diets, *J Anim Sci* 75:2497–2505, 1997.

18. Dozier WA, Dale NM, Dove CR: Nutrient composition of feed-grade and pet-food-grade poultry by-product meal, *J Appl Poult Res* 12:526–530, 2003.

19. Phillips T: Alternative pet food sales booming in the US and Canada, *Pet Food Ind,* September 2008.

20. Laflamme DP, Abood SK, Fascetti AJ, and others: Pet feeding practices of dog and cat owners in the United States and Australia, *J Am Vet Med Assoc* 232:687–694, 2008.

21. Michel KE: Unconventional diets for dogs and cats, *Vet Clin North Am Small Anim Pract* 36:1269–1281, 2006.

22. Finley R, Ribble C, Aramini J, and others: The risk of salmonellae shedding by dogs fed *Salmonella*-contaminated commercial raw food diets, *Can Vet J* 48:69–75, 2007.

23. Aldrich G: Corn gluten meal, *Pet Food Ind,* April 2005.

24. Case L, Czarnecki GL: Protein requirements of growing pups fed practical dry-type diets containing mixed-protein sources, *Am J Vet Res* 51:808–812, 1990.

25. Yamka RM, Kitts SE, True AD, Harmon DL: Evaluation of maize gluten meal as a protein source in canine foods, *Anim Feed Sci Tech* 116:239–248, 2004.

26. Aldrich G: Textured vegetable protein: all about appearance, *Pet Food Ind*, September 2008.

27. Hill RC, Burrows CF, Ellison GW, Bauer JE: The effect of texturized vegetable protein from soy on nutrient digestibility compared to beef in cannulated dogs, *J Anim Sci* 79:2162–2171, 2001.

28. Clapper GM, Grieshop CM, Merchen NR, and others: Ileal and total tract nutrient digestibilities and fecal characteristics of dogs as affected by soybean protein inclusion in dry, extruded diets, *J Anim Sci* 79:1523–1532, 2001.

29. Aspinall GO, Begbie R, McKay JE: Polysaccharide components of soybeans, *Cereal Sci Today* 12:224–261, 1967.

30. Hill RC, Burrows CF, Bauer JE, and others: Texturized vegetable protein containing indigestible soy carbohydrate affects blood insulin concentrations in dogs fed high fat diets, *J Nutr* 136:2024S–2027S, 2006.

31. Zuo Y, Fahey GC Jr, Merchen NR, and others: Digestion response to low oligosaccharide soybean meal by ileal cannulated dogs, *J Anim Sci* 74:2441–2449, 1996.

32. Yamka RM, Kitts SE, Harmon DL: Evaluation of low-oligosaccharide and low-oligosaccharide low-phytate whole soya beans in canine foods, *Anim Feed Sci Tech* 120:79–91, 2005.

33. Heaton KW, Marcus SN, Emmett PM: Particle size of wheat, maize, and oat test meals: effects on plasma glucose and insulin responses and on the rate of starch digestion in vitro, *Am J Clin Nutr* 47:675–682, 1988.

34. Aldrich G: Wheat, *Pet Food Ind,* February 2005.

35. Twomey LH, Pethick DW, Borw JB, and others: The use of sorghum and corn as alternatives to rice in dog foods, *J Nutr* 132:1704S–1705S, 2002.

36. Murray SM, Fahey GC, Merchen NR, and others: Evaluation of selected high-starch flours as ingredients in canine diets, *J Anim Sci* 77:2180–2186, 1999.

37. Jeffers JG: Responses of dogs with food allergies to a single-ingredient dietary provocation, *J Am Vet Med Assoc* 209:608–611, 1996.

38. Garden OA, Pidduck H, Lakhani KH, and others: Inheritance of gluten-sensitive enteropathy in Irish Setters, *Am J Vet Res* 61:462–468, 2000.

39. Bouchard GF, Sunvold GD: Improving canine glycemic response to a meal with dietary starch, *Proc NAVC,* 1999, pp 16–19.

40. Carciofi AC, Takakura FS, do-Oliveria LD, and others: Effects of six carbohydrate sources on dog diet digestibility and postprandial glucose and insulin response, *J Anim Physiol Anim Nutr* 92:326–336, 2008.

41. Bednar GE, Patil AR, Murray SM, and others: Starch and fiber fractions in selected food and feed ingredients affect their small intestinal digestibility and fermentability in vitro in a canine model, *J Nutr* 131:276–286, 2001.

42. Aldrich G: Potatoes: common or novel carb? *Pet Food Ind,* October 2005.

43. Foster AP, Knowles TG, Moore AH, and others: Serum IgE and IgG responses to food antigens in normal and atopic dogs, and dogs with gastrointestinal disease, *Vet Immunol Immunopathol* 92:113–124, 2003.

44. Spears JK, Grieshop CM, Fahey GC: Evaluation of stabilized rice bran as an ingredient in dry extruded dog diets, *J Anim Sci* 82:1122–1135, 2004.

45. Aldrich G: Rice bran: filler or functional fiber? *Pet Food Ind,* February 2008.

46. Fahey GC Jr, Merchen NR, Corbin JE, and others: Dietary fiber for dogs. I. Effects of graded levels of dietary beet pulp on nutrient intake, digestibility, metabolizable energy and digesta mean retention time, *J Anim Sci* 68:4221–4228, 1990.

47. Sunvold GD, Fahey GC Jr, Merchen NR, and others: Dietary fiber for dogs. IV. In vitro fermentation of selected fiber sources by dog fecal inoculum and in vivo digestion and metabolism of fiber-supplemented diets, *J Anim Sci* 73:1099–1109, 1995.

48. Sunvold GD, Fahey GC Jr, Merchen NR, and others: Dietary fiber for cats: in vitro fermentation of selected fiber sources by cat fecal inoculum and in vivo utilization of diets containing selected fiber sources and their blends, *J Anim Sci* 73:2329–2339, 1995.

49. Aldrich G: Sunflower oil: flower power in a jug, *Pet Food Ind,* March 2007.

50. Kunkle GA: Zinc-responsive dermatoses in dogs. In Kirk RW, editor: *Current veterinary therapy VII*, Philadelphia, 1980, Saunders.

51. Aldrich G: Are chelated minerals worth it? *Pet Food Ind,* May 2008.

52. Adams CR: Stability of vitamins in processed dog food, *Pet Food Ind,* Jan/Feb:20–21, 1981.

53. Zicker SC, Wedekind KJ, Jewell DE: Antioxidants in veterinary nutrition, *Vet Clin North Am Small Anim Pract* 36:1183–1198, 2006.

54. Shermer WD: Effective use of antioxidants: optimizing ingredient quality. In *Proceedings of the petfood forum*, Chicago, 1995, Watts Publishing.

55. Turek JJ, Watkins BA, Schoenlein IA, and others: Oxidized lipid depresses canine growth, immune function, and bone formation, *J Nutr Biochem* 14:24–31, 2003.

56. Hilton JW: Antioxidants: function, types and necessity of inclusion in pet foods, *Can Vet J* 30:682–684, 1989.

57. Dziezak D: Preservatives: antioxidants—the ultimate answer to oxidation, *Food Tech* 9:94–102, 1986.

58. Coelho M, Parr J: The benefits of antioxidants. In *Proceedings of the petfood forum*, Chicago, 1996, Watts Publishing.

59. Reynhout GS, Berdahl DR: Natural antioxidant systems—experiences in the human food industry. In *Proceedings of the petfood forum*, Chicago, 1997, Watts Publishing.

60. Gross KL, Bollinger R, Thawnghmuch P, Collings GF: Effect of three different preservative systems on the stability of extruded dog food subjected to ambient and high temperature storage, *J Nutr* 124:2638S–2642S, 1994.

61. Coelho M: Ethoxyquin: science vs marketing, *Pet Food Ind,* Sept/Oct 1995.

62. Dzanis DA: Safety of ethoxyquin in dog foods, *J Nutr* 121:S163–S164, 1991.

63. Monsanto Chemical Company: A five-year chronic toxicity study in dogs with santoquin: report to FDA, 1964.

64. Monsanto Chemical Company: *Ethoxyquin Backgrounder*, December 1996.

65. Winter J: Pet foods get functional, *Functional Ingred Mag,* July 2006.

66. Phillips T: Functional fixes, *Pet Food Ind,* August 2008.

67. MacFarlane S, MacFarlane GT, Cummings JH: Review article: prebiotics in the gastrointestinal tract, *Aliment Pharmacol Ther* 24:701–714, 2006.

68. Trejo AV, Hayek MG, Kelley RL: Managing microbes for wellness. In *Proc NAVC Conf,* June 2008.

17

Types of Pet Foods

The majority of pet owners in the United States feed their companion animals commercially prepared pet foods. These products are available in several forms that vary according to the processing methods used, the ingredients included, and the methods of preservation. Foods can also be categorized according to their nutrient content, the purpose for which they are formulated, and the quality of ingredients they contain. One of the broadest classifications of commercial pet foods divides products according to processing method, methods of preservation, and moisture content; these categories are the dry, wet, and semimoist foods. In recent years, a variety of foods have been developed to meet specific needs of some pet owners. These include natural and organic foods, raw food diets, and vegetarian products. This chapter examines the various types of commercial pet foods, the advantages and disadvantages of each, and the use of homemade diets.

DRY PET FOODS

Dry pet foods contain between 6% and 10% moisture and 90% or more dry matter (DM). This category of pet foods includes baked kibbles, biscuits, meals, and expanded (extruded) products. Baked kibbles and biscuits are prepared in a similar manner, although the shape of the end product differs. In each case, all of the ingredients are mixed into a homogeneous dough, which is then baked. When biscuits are made, the dough is formed or cut into the desired shapes and the individual biscuits are baked much like cookies or crackers. When baked kibble is produced, the dough is spread onto large sheets and baked. After cooling, the large sheets are broken into bite-size pieces and packaged. Many dog and cat treats are baked biscuits, and a limited number of companies still produce complete and balanced baked kibble. Dry meals, the major type of dry pet food sold before 1960, are prepared by mixing together a number of dried, flaked, or granular ingredients. This type of product has almost completely disappeared from the commercial market.

The development of the extrusion process during the 1960s resulted in the almost complete replacement of meals and baked kibble with expanded pet foods. Today, expanded products represent the most common type of dry pet food produced and sold in the United States. The extrusion procedure involves mixing all of the ingredients together to form dough, which is then cooked under conditions of high pressure and temperature (80° to 200° C).[1] The machine that is used to cook and shape expanded foods is called an *extruder*. The dough moves very quickly through the extruder and is further mixed as it proceeds. The high cooking temperature, movement of the dough, and rising pressure causes cooking to occur very rapidly (within 10 to 270 seconds). When the cooked dough reaches the end of the extruder, it exits through a die (small opening). The die forces the soft product into the desired shape, and a rotating knife cuts the forms into the desired kibble size. Extrusion causes rapid cooking of the starches within the dough, resulting in increased digestibility and palatability. After cooling, a coating of fat or other palatability enhancer is usually sprayed on the expanded kibbles (a process called "enrobing"). Hot-air drying reduces the total moisture content of the product to 10% or less.

A certain level of starch must be included in expanded products to allow proper processing of the product. Similarly, baked biscuits often contain wheat as an ingredient because the starch and gluten of wheat contribute to the appealing texture and flavor of biscuits. The cooking process of both extruded and baked dry foods improves the digestibility of the complex carbohydrates in the product and enhances the food's palatability. Heat treatment and storage can result in minor losses of some vitamins, so compensatory amounts of these nutrients are included by manufacturers when the diet is formulated. The heat used in the extrusion process also sterilizes the product, and the low amount of moisture that is present in dry foods aids in the prevention of growth of bacteria or fungus.

Ingredients commonly used in dry pet foods include a variety of cereal grains, meat, poultry or fish products, some milk products, vegetable fats/oils, and vitamin and mineral supplements (see Chapter 16 for a complete discussion). The caloric density of dry pet foods typically ranges between 3000 and 4500 kilocalories (kcal) of metabolizable energy (ME)/kilogram (kg), or between 1300 and 2000 kcal/pound (lb) on a dry-matter basis (DMB). Dry cat foods are often slightly higher in energy density than dog foods. The energy density of dry pet foods is somewhat limited by the processing and packaging methods used. However, most dry pet foods can easily meet the energy needs of the majority of companion animals. Products that are formulated for adult maintenance will only be bulk limited if fed to hard-working dogs or puppies that have very high energy requirements. In these cases, foods have been developed to meet the specific energy requirements of working dogs and growing puppies. Depending on the purpose of the food, the DM content of dry dog foods ranges between 8% and 22% fat and 18% and 32% protein (Table 17-1). Cat foods of all types contain slightly higher levels of protein than dog foods.

Dry dog foods are very convenient for owners and continue to be the most common type of pet food bought by pet owners in the United States.[2] In general, these products are more economical to feed than wet or semimoist foods, and they store well because of their low moisture content. Large quantities of dry food can be purchased at one time, and dry products have a reasonably long shelf-life when stored under proper conditions. Many pet owners prefer feeding dry foods because they can leave a bowl of food available to their pet for a period of time without worrying about spoilage. In some cases, dogs and cats can be fed free-choice with a dry food and not overconsume. However, the high fat content and palatability of some of the foods marketed today coupled with the sedentary lifestyle of many pets preclude free-choice feeding for many dogs and cats. Dry pet food may also offer some dental hygiene advantages. The chewing and grinding that accompanies eating dry biscuits or pet food may aid in the prevention of plaque and calculus accumulation on teeth (see Chapter 34, pp. 442-445 for a complete discussion).[3]

TABLE 17-1   NUTRIENT CONTENT OF DRY, SEMIMOIST, AND WET DOG FOODS

	AF BASIS	DM BASIS
Dry		
Moisture (%)	6-10	0
Fat (%)	7-20	8-22
Protein (%)	16-30	18-32
Carbohydrate (%)	41-70	46-74
ME (kcal/kg)	2800-4050	3000-4500
Semimoist		
Moisture (%)	15-30	0
Fat (%)	7-10	8-14
Protein (%)	17-20	20-28
Carbohydrate (%)	40-60	58-72
ME (kcal/kg)	2550-2800	3000-4000
Wet		
Moisture (%)	75	0
Fat (%)	5-8	20-32
Protein (%)	7-13	28-50
Carbohydrate (%)	4-13	18-57
ME (kcal/kg)	875-1250	3500-5000

AF, As-fed; *DM*, dry matter; *ME*, metabolizable energy.

Dry dog foods are the most popular type of pet food purchased by consumers in the United States. Dry foods are economical and easy to store and feed, and they may be beneficial to dental hygiene. High-quality dry foods have high nutrient densities and digestibilities, meaning that less food can be fed, more nutrients will be absorbed and used, and stool volume will decrease.

A potential disadvantage of dry pet foods, when compared with semimoist or wet foods, is that dry foods may be less palatable to some dogs and cats. This disadvantage is especially true of foods that are low in fat or that contain poorly digestible or low-quality ingredients. However, dry pet foods that contain high-quality ingredients and moderate to high levels of fat do not demonstrate reduced acceptance in dogs and cats and are highly palatable to most companion animals. Because ingredients that are primarily low in moisture are used to formulate dry pet foods, harsh or improper processing of the ingredients can cause a reduction in nutrient availability and the loss of nutrients. As a result, poor-quality dry foods may have very low digestibilities and nutrient availabilities. Companies that manufacture high-quality, premium and super-premium foods only use properly treated ingredients and manufacturing methods to ensure that the digestibilities of their products remain high after processing.

WET PET FOODS

There are two primary types of wet pet foods—those that provide complete and balanced nutrition and those that provide a dietary supplement or treat in the form of a canned/pouched meat or meat byproduct. Complete and balanced wet foods may contain blends of ingredients such as muscle meats, poultry or fish meats or byproducts, cereal grains, texturized vegetable protein (TVP), and vitamins and minerals. Some of these products contain only one or two types of muscle meat or animal byproducts, with enough supplemental vitamins and minerals to make the product nutritionally complete. The second type of wet food, often referred to as "meat products," consists of the same types of meat listed earlier but without supplemental vitamins and minerals. These foods are not formulated to be nutritionally complete and are intended to be used only as a supplement to an already complete and balanced diet. For example, some pet owners add a small amount of wet food to their pet's complete and balanced dry food every day. The high fat content of the wet supplement enhances the texture and palatability of the pet's diet. Although many complete and balanced dry foods are also highly palatable and provide a balanced diet, some pet owners believe that a dry diet alone becomes boring or bland to their pet. Adding a spoonful or two of a product that looks like meat or stew makes many owners feel they are making the meal more enjoyable for their pet.

From a processing standpoint, there are three general types of wet foods—loaf, chunks or chunks in gravy, and a chunk-in-loaf combination. Wet pet foods are prepared by first blending the meat and fat ingredients with measured amounts of water. Measured amounts of dry ingredients are then added and the entire mixture is heated. Canning occurs on a conveyor line. Most pet foods are typically sold in either 3-, 5.5-, or 13.2-ounce (oz) cans. After filling, the cans are then sealed with a double seam, washed, and labeled with a manufacturer

code and date. Pressure sterilization of canned products is called *retorting*. Temperatures and times for retorting vary with the product and can size, but typically cans are held at around 250° C for 60 minutes. The high heat and pressure involved in processing canned foods kills harmful bacteria and causes some nutrient losses. Manufacturers of high-quality products conduct the research necessary to determine the extent of these losses and then adjust their formulations to compensate for them. After exiting the retort, the cans are cooled under controlled conditions to ensure the sterility of the product and the integrity of the sealed cans. To designate the product, paper labels are then applied during the final step of production. Wet foods are also sold in pouches and trays. These containers are more delicate and so retorting procedures are adjusted to prevent damage to package structures and seals. Generally, the cooking pressure is lower and more tightly controlled to ensure that rupture or shrinkage of the packaging does not occur.

In general, wet foods are more palatable and digestible than many dry pet foods, and they contain a higher DM proportion of protein and fat (see Table 17-1).[4] When measured on a DMB, the caloric content of wet pet foods generally ranges between 3500 and 5000 kcal/kg or about 1600 and 2300 kcal/lb. The fat content of wet pet foods ranges between 20% and 32%, and protein levels are usually between 28% and 50%. Most wet products contain a relatively small proportion of digestible carbohydrate when compared with that in other types of pet foods (see Table 17-1). Wet foods are also more expensive than dry pet foods. Although expense is often not a concern for owners of cats or small dogs, it can become significant when feeding large dogs or multiple pets. Nutrient and price comparisons between wet and dry pet foods should always be made on either a DMB or a caloric-density basis because wet foods contain a very large proportion of water (see Chapter 15, p. 132). In the United States the moisture content of pet foods can be as high as 78%, or equal to the natural moisture content of the ingredients used, whichever is greater.[5] On average, wet pet foods contain about 75% water; this amount can be compared with dry pet foods, which contain approximately 6% to 10% moisture.

Some advantages of wet pet foods include their long shelf-life and high acceptability. The sterilization and sealing of the cans and pouches allows these products to be kept for long periods before opening, without the need for special storage considerations. Because of their nutrient content and texture, wet foods tend to be highly palatable to dogs and cats. However, this can be a disadvantage for some companion animals. Dogs and cats that have moderate to low energy requirements may be predisposed to the development of obesity when fed exclusively wet pet foods. If fed free-choice, the high palatability of these products can override an animal's inherent tendency to eat to meet its caloric requirements, resulting in the overconsumption of energy. Conversely, dogs and cats that have increased energy needs or reduced interest in food because of illness may benefit from the high palatability and energy density of wet food. Feeding a wet diet is also an approach to ensuring adequate water intake in cats that are at high risk of developing lower urinary tract disease (see Chapter 30, pp. 365-366).

Gourmet-type wet cat foods are especially popular with cat owners. These products may or may not be nutritionally complete, and they contain primarily animal tissues such as fish, shrimp, tuna, or liver. These foods are often sold in small, one- or two-serving cans and appeal to owners' desires to give their cat "something special." There may some degree of risk in the exclusive feeding of these products to some cats. More so than dogs, which have an evolutionary history of scavenging and consuming a wide variety of food types, cats appear to be more susceptible to the development of neophobia, the rejection of foods that have not been previously encountered. This is more likely to develop if a cat is fed a diet of a certain type or that contains a single type of ingredient starting early in life and continuing for a long period of time.[6,7] Some cats eventually accept only this one food item and will refuse to eat any other type or flavor of food. This can be a problem if the food is not complete and balanced, or if the cat experiences a health condition that warrants a change in diet. Therefore, if wet foods are used with cats, it is advisable to feed complete and balanced rations that contain more than one principal ingredient and to occasionally offer different flavors of food. The gourmet products can be used as supplemental feeding, but they should not make up the entire diet.

Tip: There are two primary types of wet pet foods— those that provide complete and balanced nutrition and those that do not. Complete and balanced wet foods contain vitamins and minerals in addition to muscle meats, poultry, meat, or fish byproducts, cereal grains, and/or texturized vegetable protein. Foods that are not complete and balanced do not contain all the necessary vitamins and minerals and should be considered as a dietary supplement only.

SEMIMOIST PET FOODS

Semimoist pet foods contain 15% to 30% water and include fresh or frozen animal tissues, cereal grains, fats, and simple sugars as their principal ingredients. These products are softer in texture than dry pet foods, which contributes to their acceptability and palatability for some animals. Several methods of preservation are used to prevent contamination and spoilage of semimoist foods and permit an extended shelf-life. The inclusion of humectants such as salt, simple sugars, glycerol, or corn syrup reduces the water activity of the food, which prevents the growth of contaminating organisms.[8] Further protection is provided by preservatives such as potassium sorbate, which prevents the growth of yeasts and molds. Small amounts of organic acids may also be included to decrease the pH of products and inhibit bacterial growth.

The high simple sugar content of many semimoist dog foods and treats contributes to the palatability and digestibility of these products. Although dogs have been shown to enjoy the taste of simple sugars, cats are less likely to select sweet foods.[9-11] Semimoist pet foods that contain a high proportion of simple carbohydrates have digestibility coefficients that are similar to those of wet foods. However, because of their lower fat content, the caloric density of semimoist foods is usually less. The ME content of semimoist foods typically ranges between 3000 and 4000 kcal/kg on a DMB, or about 1400 to 1800 kcal/lb. Semimoist foods contain between 20% and 28% protein and between 8% and 14% fat on a DMB. The proportion of carbohydrate in semimoist foods is similar to that of dry foods (see Table 17-1). However, an important difference is that the carbohydrate in semimoist pet foods is largely in the form of simple carbohydrates, with a relatively small proportion present as starch.

Semimoist pet foods appeal to some pet owners because they generally are less odorous than wet foods, and many come in convenient single-serving packages. These foods are also available in a large variety of shapes and textures that often resemble different types of meat products, such as ground beef, meat patties, or chunks of beef. Although these different forms do not necessarily reflect nutrient content or palatability for the pet, they do appeal to the tastes of many pet owners. Semimoist foods do not require refrigeration before opening and have a relatively long shelf-life. The cost of these foods when compared on a DMB is usually between the cost of dry and wet products. However, products sold as single-serving packages are often comparable in price to wet pet foods. Because they are lower in energy density than wet foods, semimoist diets can be fed free-choice to some pets. However, these products dry out and lose appeal when left in a pet's bowl for an extended period of time.

SNACKS AND TREATS

Snacks and treats have become increasingly popular with pet owners in recent years. A survey conducted in 1965 showed that Nabisco's Milk Bones dominated the treat market, and the choice of snacks at that time was extremely limited. However, today almost every major pet food company markets one or more types of dog and cat snacks. This increase can be theorized to reflect some of the changing roles that dogs and cats have had in our society within the last few decades. Pet owners purchase treats not because of their nutritional value but as a way of showing love and affection to their pets. Feeding and caring for a pet is a nurturing process, and giving pets "special" snacks generates the positive feelings that accompany nurturing and the expression of affection. Pet owners also use treats as training aids to reinforce desired behaviors, at times of arrival or departure, as a means of providing a sense of variety in the pet's diet, and as an aid to proper dental health.[12]

Because emotional benefits are a primary motivator for buying treats, palatability to the pet is of chief importance. Owners are less concerned with the nutritional value of a snack than they are with its appearance and acceptability. In the early years, all dog treats were in the form of baked biscuits. Over time, different shapes, sizes, and flavors of biscuits were developed and marketed. Because treats are often purchased on impulse or because of novelty, owners are more likely to try a new flavor or type of treat than they are to completely switch dog or cat food. To capitalize on this, manufacturers have continued to develop new types of dog and cat snacks. Today, treats can be categorized into four basic types—semimoist, biscuits, jerky, and rawhide products. Cat treats are usually in the form of either semimoist or biscuit products, while rawhides and jerky products are highly palatable to many dogs. Many treats are made to resemble foods that humans normally eat, such as hamburgers, sausage, bacon, cheese, and even ice cream. Examples of several popular treat concepts include snacks that are made with all-natural ingredients, biscuits that promote dental health, and chews made from livestock body parts such as ears, hooves, and even noses.

Although treats and snacks do not have to be nutritionally complete, a significant proportion of these products are formulated to be complete and balanced, and some biscuits and semimoist treats carry the same nutritional label claims as dog and cat foods. In general, treats and snacks are highly attractive to pets and cost significantly more than other types of pet foods when compared on a weight basis. Part of this cost is a reflection of the larger amounts of marketing effort and money directed toward making the product attractive to pet owners.[13]

PET FOOD CLASSIFICATIONS

In addition to classifying pet foods according to the type of processing method that is used, they can also be classified with respect to overall quality, the types of ingredients that are included (or excluded), availability, and cost. A recent survey of the consumer habits of pet owners reported that the continuing devotion and commitment to companion animals is reflected in increased interest in "premium" and "super-premium" products, those that are on the higher end of the pet care spectrum.[14] A wide variety of new pet food products have also been introduced in recent years. Some of these target the needs of consumers in niche markets and are formulated to contain or eschew a specific type or quality of ingredient (organic foods, "natural" foods, and vegetarian food), while others employ a particular method of preparation or processing (raw diets and homemade diets). Pet owners select these foods for a variety of reasons. These may include beliefs about the wholesomeness and safety of foods; a desire to follow a prescribed "food philosophy" that reflects a religious, ethical or personal belief system; or beliefs about the therapeutic value of certain types of ingredients.[15] For example, according to a recent report, the market segment of raw, frozen, organic, and natural pet foods, while still relatively small, is growing at a rapid rate.[16] The primary motivator (or "driver") for this growth is a belief among pet owners that these foods are more healthful and of higher quality than more conventional products.

Today, pet owners enjoy a wide variety of pet foods to choose from. The premium and super-premium foods provide consumers with a guarantee of quality ingredients and high nutrient availability. Other foods are marketed to cater to pet owners' needs to provide a food that is all-natural, organic, vegetarian, or comprised of raw ingredients.

Premium and Super-Premium Brands

The term *premium pet food* refers to products developed to provide optimal nutrition for dogs and cats during different stages of life. These foods target companion animal owners, hobbyists, and professionals who are very involved with their companion animal's health and nutrition. In general, quality ingredients that are highly digestible and have good to excellent nutrient availability are used in these products. Manufacturers of most premium pet foods formulate and market products for different stages of life and lifestyles and for different breed sizes (dogs). For example, dog foods have been developed for hard-working dogs (performance diets), adult dogs during maintenance, growing dogs of different sizes, and for females during lactation and gestation. Super-premium foods are those that include high-quality ingredients along with various types of functional ingredients or nutrients that provide specific health benefits. Examples include foods that contain joint protective agents for large-breed dogs and foods

that are formulated to support immune health and proper body condition in senior pets. The companies that produce premium and super-premium foods also provide educational materials about their products and about companion animal nutrition and feeding to pet owners and professionals. Although some of these products can be found in grocery stores, many are only available through pet supply stores, feed stores, or veterinarians.

Most of the premium and super-premium brands of pet food are produced using fixed formulations. This means that the manufacturer does not change the ingredients composition from batch to batch based on ingredient availability or market price. In addition, manufacturers of these products conduct research and feeding studies to ensure the wholesomeness of their foods and to validate the use of new ingredients and formulations. These studies confirm to the pet owner that the food has been adequately tested and is based upon sound nutritional principles. Premium and super-premium pet foods are usually more costly on a weight basis than basic nutrition brands because of the high-quality ingredients that are used and the level of testing and research that is conducted on these products. However, because these foods are usually very digestible and nutrient dense, smaller amounts can be fed, and the cost per serving is often comparable to many basic nutrition brands of pet food.

Basic Nutrition and Economy Brands

Basic nutrition brands include foods that are marketed nationally or regionally and sold in grocery store chains and through mass-merchant stores. The companies that produce these foods devote a substantial amount of energy and finances to advertising, which results in high name recognition of their products among consumers. The principal marketing strategies used to sell these products relate either to the diet's palatability and appeal to the pet owner (basic nutrition brands), or to its price (economy brands). Many of these brands are produced using variable formulations. This means that the ingredients included in a particular brand may vary from batch to batch, depending on ingredient availability and cost to the manufacturer. For example, poultry meal may be the primary protein source in

Happy Pal dog food the first time a pet owner purchases a bag. However, because of changes in market prices, the second bag may include lower amounts of poultry meal and higher amounts of other protein sources such as poultry byproduct meal or a cereal grain. When variable formulation is used, the guaranteed analysis panel will not change, but the source and the quality of the ingredients may be altered without notice. This alteration can result in variable product quality and digestibility and may cause gastrointestinal upset in some pets when a new bag of food is fed. In general, basic nutrition brands of pet food that are marketed for palatability have high brand-recognition among pet owners and have an appearance that appeals to owners' perceptions of wholesome food for their dog or cat. These foods tend to have lower digestibilities than the premium and super-premium brands of foods, but they typically contain higher-quality ingredients and have higher digestibilities than do the economy brands. Ingredients, palatability, and digestibility may vary significantly among brands, as well as among different products produced by the same manufacturer.

Economy brands are those foods that are formulated on a least-cost basis and are priced substantially lower than other comparable brands. They include generic brands (no label) and some private-label brands of food (see below). Generic products represent the least expensive and typically the poorest quality of pet foods commercially available to pet owners. Many of these are produced and marketed locally or regionally. Because the manufacturers of economy brands are chiefly concerned with producing a low-cost product, inexpensive, poor-quality ingredients are often used, and few, if any, feeding studies are conducted. Some of the generic products are not formulated to be nutritionally complete and will not carry a label claim. Feeding studies with dogs have shown that generic products have significantly lower digestibilities and nutrient availabilities than premium and popular brands of food.[18] Another study reported the development of zinc-responsive dermatosis in dogs that were fed generic pet foods.[19] Poor-quality ingredients and a low fat content can result in low palatability, leading to reduced acceptance of these foods by some dogs. Altogether, problems with ingredient quality, nutrient balance and availability, and the uncertainty of adequate testing and quality control generally make economy and generic brands a poor choice for pet owners when selecting a commercial pet food.

Premium and super-premium pet foods contain high-quality ingredients, are backed by nutritional research, and target specific life stages and health benefits. Basic nutrition brands focus on owner appeal and palatability to the pet, while economy brands are marketed for owners who are most concerned with the cost of a product. Finally, because generic pet foods are produced on a least-cost basis, contain lower-quality ingredients, and may not be formulated to be complete and balanced, they are not a good choice for most pets.

Private-Label Brands

Private-label pet foods are products that carry the house name of the grocery store chain or mass-merchant retailer in which they are sold. Some of these products are produced on a least-cost basis while others are produced to reflect the pet care philosophy of the sponsoring store or outlet. Because some of these products are produced by the same companies that make generic foods, they can be similar in quality to generic pet foods. In addition, private-label foods often claim to be comparable to premium foods, although they sell for a much lower price. As in any industry, "clone" products are marketed that may imitate the name, packaging, bag colors, and/or ingredient lists of premium foods.

Organic and Natural Brand Labels

Although organic foods still account for just over 5% of total pet food sales, these foods experienced an increase in retail sales of almost 50% between 2003 and 2007.[16] This increase suggests a rapidly expanding level of interest, similar to that which is occurring in the human foods marketplace. Pet owners' interest in and concern about the source of pet food ingredients is a primary reason for this increase. In 2002 the U.S. Department of Agriculture (USDA) established the National Organic Program, which provides a set of standards for organic human foods. These regulations require that animal-source ingredients come only from animals that received no antibiotics or growth hormone, and plant-source foods cannot be treated with pesticides, synthetic fertilizers, or ionizing radiation. Bioengineered products are also prohibited. The USDA inspects and certifies producers and human food processors, but has not extended their organic certification program to pet foods. Although the Association of American Feed Control Officials (AAFCO) does not have written labeling regulations for organic pet foods, it does recognize the term *organic* and requires compliance with USDA standards for pet food ingredients that are labeled as organic.[5]

Related to organic products are the "natural" foods, which are formulated to include no artificial additives (particularly preservatives), coloring agents, or flavors. In addition, these foods are usually promoted as being free of unintentional contaminants such as pesticides and heavy metals. Natural foods are preserved using combinations of natural-occurring antioxidants, such as the mixed tocopherols, ascorbic acid, and rosemary extract (see Chapter 16, pp. 156-157). Because the natural-occurring antioxidants are generally not as effective as synthetic preservatives, the shelf-life of most natural foods is shorter that the shelf-life of foods that include synthetic preservatives. Therefore, it is important that both retailers and consumers monitor the "best used by" dates of these products to avoid selling or purchasing an unsafe product. Finally, although organic and natural pet foods are often discussed together, the label of "natural" is not synonymous with "organic." While an organic pet food is by definition "natural," foods that are marketed as "all natural" are not necessarily organic, because all of the USDA standards for organic certification may not have been followed.

Raw Food Diets

Raw food diets have become popular in recent years with a small proportion of pet owners and enthusiasts. Although the majority of people continue to feed commercially available foods as their pet's primary diet, a recent survey of owners in the United States and Australia found that approximately 25% of dogs were fed raw meat or bones on a regular basis to supplement their normal diet.[20] The number of pet owners who fed raw diets as their pet's primary diet was much smaller, comprising less than 3% of owners. A primary motivation for feeding a raw diet relates to beliefs about the dog's

evolutionary history as a carnivore. Proponents of raw diets assert that because the dog's wild ancestors hunted and consumed prey species, present day dogs are best fed foods that are not heat-treated or processed. These claims may also reflect prevailing perceptions about the hunting behavior and eating patterns of wild wolves and the relationship between the dog and its wild ancestors.[21] Proponents of raw food diets for dogs also make numerous claims for the health benefits of raw meat diets. These include, but are not limited to, improved immune function, enhanced vitality and overall health, increased energy, decreased body odor, and improvements in skin and coat condition. However, with the exception of testimonial anecdotes, there are no objective data to support or refute any of these claims. Although raw diets can be formulated to be complete and balanced, there is no evidence that they promote superior health or cure disease in dogs or cats.

Raw diets come in several forms. Commercially available products include complete rations that are sold frozen or less commonly, as slightly cooked (pasteurized) or dehydrated refrigerated foods. Other companies provide a grain or supplement mix, which the owner then adds to raw meat that is purchased locally. Another approach is to prepare homemade raw food diet using recipes obtained through popular books or through the Internet. Regardless of the source or type of raw food diet that is fed, there are two primary categories of concerns that are raised about these diets. The first is nutritional adequacy and the second focuses on food safety. In one report, food samples from five raw food diets for dogs were analyzed for nutrient content.[22] Three of the products were homemade and two were commercially prepared. All three of the homemade diets had numerous nutrient deficiencies and excesses when compared with the AAFCO nutrient profile for dogs. The two commercial products also had several nutrient imbalances. When compared with AAFCO nutrient profiles for adult dogs, one commercial food was deficient in calcium and phosphorus, and had a calcium:phosphorus ratio that was dangerously low (0.15). This food also contained excessively high levels of zinc. Both commercial raw foods contained excessive levels of vitamin D. Although additional studies that examine a wider range of commercial and homemade raw diets are necessary, these results suggest that the risk of nutrient imbalance is a valid concern when feeding a raw food diet. It is also likely that home-prepared raw diets vary most dramatically in nutrient content because of variation in the types of ingredients that are used, the potential for using substitutions, and the untested adequacy of some recipes.[23]

Food safety concerns with raw food diets include the danger of gastrointestinal obstruction or perforation that is associated with feeding any type of bone. However, the most prevalent concern is the risk of meat contamination with foodborne pathogens and transmission of these pathogens to both pets and to people.[24] Proponents of raw food diets counter these concerns by claiming that bacterial pathogens do not cause illness in dogs because of a unique adaptation of the canine intestinal tract that protects dogs from infection.[25] However, there is no evidence to support this claim, and there are documented cases of fecal shedding of *Salmonella* spp. and of salmonellosis in dogs and cats that were fed raw meat.[24,26,27] Moreover, such a claim does not address risks associated with fecal microbe shedding in pets fed raw meat or the risk of transmission of raw food pathogens to humans.

Several studies have examined the prevalence of microbial contamination in raw food diets. In a small pilot study, 8 out of 10 samples of chicken-based, home-prepared raw diets for dogs were contaminated with *Salmonella* species.[28] The raw food diets were significantly more likely to be contaminated than were the commercial dry dog foods in the control group. A second study evaluated 25 commercially available raw pet diets and found coliform bacteria in all 25 foods.[29] In all cases, coliform level, which is used as an index of sanitation, exceeded the maximum allowable concentration for raw meat of 10,000 colony-forming units (CFU)/gram (g). Although chicken is most commonly cited as the primary meat fed in home prepared raw diets, the commercial foods in this study contained a wide variety of meats, including chicken, beef, lamb, rabbit, ostrich, venison, and salmon. Another study of commercially prepared raw foods collected 240 samples from 20 different commercially prepared raw meat diets for dogs.[30] Samples were collected on four occasions, every 2 months, and were tested for the presence of enteric pathogens. More than 50% of the raw diet samples were contaminated with non–type-specific *Escherichia coli*. At least one positive culture was found in products from all vendors and manufacturers

whose products were tested. *Salmonella enterica* was also found, but in a lower incidence rate than that reported in other studies (7.1% of the raw meat samples).

Collectively, these studies indicate that homemade and commercially prepared raw meat diets for pets present a risk to both pets and their owners of exposure to potentially pathogenic bacterial species. Contamination with enteric bacteria has been found in a wide variety of animal-source meats, with chicken representing a frequent source of *Salmonella* species. Although human-grade meats are often used with homemade raw diets, this is not necessarily the case with commercially prepared raw pet foods. This is an important consideration because of the difference in regulatory oversight between human-grade and non–human-grade meats. There are currently no regulations that monitor bacterial contamination of raw meat pet foods in either the United States or Canada.[31] In the United States, the USDA's Food Safety Inspection Service is responsible for ensuring that the domestic meat supply of meats consumed by humans is not contaminated. However, their oversight does not extend to bacterial contamination in meats that are non–human grade and which can be included in raw pet foods. Because of this regulatory omission, the Food and Drug Administration (FDA) has produced a set of guidelines for manufacturers to promote safe manufacturing practices of raw pet foods.[32] The FDA guidelines recommend including only animal meats from USDA-inspected sources and which have passed USDA inspections for meats intended for human consumption. However, compliance with these guidelines is voluntary and the FDA has no official authority to either track or enforce conformity. Therefore, when consumers purchase a raw pet food that has been produced from meats that were not intended for human consumption, there is no assurance that these meat sources were inspected for bacterial contamination.

The presumed risks of microbial transmission to humans from raw pet foods can come either from handling the diet during preparation and feeding or from exposure to feces of an animal that is shedding foodborne microbes. Fecal shedding of *Salmonella* spp. has been associated with feeding as little as a single contaminated raw food meal.[33] In addition, dogs that are fed raw meat are significantly more likely to shed *Salmonella* spp. than are dogs that are fed commercial dry dog foods.[34] Salmonellosis is a significant health risk to humans, with more than one million people infected annually in the United States.[35] The overwhelming majority of these infections are associated with foodborne contamination. Although the proportion of infections that occur as a result of owners handling raw meats intended for pets is unknown, this is a potential mode of transmission. Other potential pathogens that could be transmitted from raw pet food diets to humans include *E. coli, Campylobacter* spp., *Toxoplasma* spp., and *Clostridium* spp.[24] The transmission of enteropathogenic bacteria to humans is of greatest concern for high-risk populations such as the elderly, infants, and immunocompromised individuals. For example, because of the increased risk of fecal shedding of foodborne pathogens in dogs fed raw diets, animal-assisted therapy programs in Canada are cautioned to exclude these dogs from programs that visit immunocompromised populations.[34]

If an owner decides to feed a raw diet, it is advisable to select a product that carries a guarantee of the inclusion of human-grade meats and compliance with AAFCO nutrient profiles. Another approach that may reduce risk of nutrient imbalances and foodborne illness is a compromise in which the pet is fed a high-quality conventional pet food that is supplemented with fresh, but cooked, vegetables, grains, and meats. Cooking meat lightly to sear the surface will significantly reduce bacterial contamination because most foodborne pathogens reside on the surface of raw meat products. (If a ground meat is fed, this is not the case, and the entire meat should be lightly cooked.) Finally, if owners insist upon feeding raw meat, they must practice meticulous hygiene and thoroughly disinfect all surfaces, utensils, and feeding bowls after use. Although these are the same recommendations that are promulgated for the preparation of meats meant for human consumption, those foods, unlike raw pet diets, are eventually cooked thoroughly, reducing risk. Therefore, additional precautions are needed when raw meat is handled, prepared, and fed to pets. Because many of the pathogens found in raw meat will grow in meat left at room temperature, unconsumed raw foods should be promptly discarded and should never be left in a bowl. For the same reason, raw diets should never be fed on an ad libitum basis. Finally, the proper handling and disposing of feces from pets that are fed raw meat

is crucial because of increased risk of the pet shedding foodborne microorganisms.

If an owner chooses to feed a raw diet to his or her pet, risks can be reduced by selecting a product that complies with Association of American Feed Control Officials' Nutrient Profiles and that is guaranteed to contain only human-grade ingredients. Another way to reduce risk is to supplement a complete and balanced dry pet food with small amounts of fresh, but cooked, vegetables, grains, and meats. Cooking meats slightly can reduce risk of bacterial contamination because most foodborne pathogens reside on the surface of raw meat products.

Vegetarian Diets

A wide range of dietary practices are included under the umbrella term of *vegetarianism*. For example, ovo-vegetarians consume plants and eggs, lactovegetarians consume plants and dairy products, and ovolactovegetarians consume plants, eggs, and dairy products. One of the most restrictive forms is veganism, in which only foods of plant origin are consumed and no animal products are included in the diet. Pet owners may decide to feed a vegetarian or vegan diet to their pets for a variety of reasons. In many cases, an owner's decision to feed his or her pet a vegetarian diet follows directly from personal religious beliefs, ethical concerns, or health considerations that dictate the owner's diet choices. Although there are limited studies available, one report found that 32 of 34 owners who were feeding their cat a vegetarian diet were vegetarian themselves, and the majority (82%) cited ethical reasons for choosing this dietary regiment for their cats.[36] Owners who were feeding a vegetarian diet to their cat were more likely to believe that a vegetarian diet had health benefits for cats and that conventional commercial pet foods were not healthful or wholesome.

Commercial vegetarian diets are available for both dogs and cats. For dogs, creating a vegetarian and even a vegan food that is complete and balanced is not particularly difficult given the more omnivorous nature of the canid species. A number of plant-based dry and wet foods that carry the complete and balanced label claim are available for dogs and have been shown to be nutritionally adequate.[15] However, as an obligate carnivore, the cat has several nutrient requirements that impose a requirement for animal-source ingredients in the diet (see Section 2, pp. 57-58). Specific nutrients that are of concern in a vegetarian diet formulated for cats are taurine, preformed vitamin A, and arachidonic acid. These nutrients are found principally in animal tissues and are deficient in plant-source ingredients. When a vegetarian or vegan diet is formulated for cats, it is necessary to include synthetic forms of some or all of these nutrients. One type of commercial product that is marketed for cats is a supplemental mix that purportedly supplies all of the nutrients that are deficient in a vegetarian diet.[36] This mix is than added to a homemade vegetarian diet. Recipes for the homemade portion of the diet are supplied by the manufacturer of the supplement. There are also several vegan wet cat foods that are marketed as providing complete and balanced nutrition to cats. Although this is theoretically possible, studies that have analyzed vegetarian cat foods and compared their nutrient content with AAFCO nutrient profiles for cats have reported numerous nutrient deficiencies in both the homemade/supplemental mix and the complete ration varieties.[37,38] The most common nutrient inadequacies found were low taurine content, insufficient protein, and low preformed vitamin A.

A primary concern for cats that are fed vegetarian diets is long-term health in response to a diet that may be marginal or even deficient in these essential nutrients. Because of the many factors that can affect a cat's taurine status and the documented and serious health risks associated with deficiency, this nutrient has received the most attention. When whole blood and plasma taurine levels were assessed in cats that were being fed vegan diets, 3 of 17 cats had whole blood taurine levels that were lower than the reference range.[36] However, the blood levels were not considered to be within the critical concentration for taurine deficiency, and none of these cats showed clinical signs of deficiency. Serum cobalamin levels were also measured in this study. Cobalamin (vitamin B_{12}) is only found in animal tissues or fermented products and so must be added as a supplement to vegetarian cat foods. Although one of the diets in the study contained marginally low cobalamin levels, none of the cats showed compromised cobalamin status. However, the body has the ability to conserve cobalamin for long periods of time, so status might not be compromised until after cats had received a deficient diet for months or years. Finally, while vitamin A deficiency is also of concern in cats fed vegetarian foods and has been shown to be deficient in at least one vegan product, there is currently no reliable blood assay that reflects vitamin A status in animals. Therefore, vitamin A status could not be assessed in the cats that were fed vegetarian diets.

The results of these studies demonstrate the difficulties inherent in creating a vegetarian diet for cats that supplies all of the cats' needed essential nutrients. Because clinical signs of taurine, cobalamin, and vitamin A deficiencies can develop over periods of months and years, a response to a diet that contains marginally low concentrations of these nutrients may take years to manifest. Therefore owners who wish to feed a vegetarian food to their cats should take great care in pet food selection and carefully monitor their cat's health status through frequent veterinary examinations. Periodic measurement of target nutrients such as whole blood taurine levels and serum cobalamin should be conducted. Although dietary taurine is not a concern for the majority of healthy dogs, the fact that a vegetarian diet may contain marginal levels of taurine dictates that dogs fed vegetarian diets should also be monitored periodically for taurine status (see Chapter 12, pp. 99-100).

Creating a complete and balanced vegetarian food for dogs is not difficult, given the more omnivorous nature of the canid species. A number of plant-based dry and wet foods that carry the complete and balanced label claim are available for dogs today. However, this is not true for the cat, an obligate carnivore. Specific nutrients that are of concern in a vegetarian diet formulated for cats are taurine, preformed vitamin A, and arachidonic acid. These nutrients are found principally in animal tissues and are deficient in plant-source ingredients.

Homemade Diets

Although the majority of pet owners in the United States enjoy the convenience, economy, and reliability of commercially produced pet foods, some owners prefer to prepare homemade diets for their pets. A recent survey of pet feeding practices of pet owners in the United States and Australia reported that 93% of dogs and 98% of cats were fed commercial pet foods for at least half of their daily intake.[20] Of the owners who fed a homemade diet to their dog or cat, less than 30% used a recipe that was specifically designed for dogs or cats. Of these recipes, half had been obtained from the owner's veterinarians and the other 50% were either found on the Internet or obtained from unidentified sources. These results suggest that while the number of owners who rely completely upon homemade pet foods is relatively small, the use of inadequate recipes is relatively common among them.

Owners may choose to prepare a homemade diet for their pet for a variety of reasons. In recent years, increased concerns about the use of additives and artificial preservatives in commercial pet foods has led to a desire by some owners to avoid commercially prepared foods. There is also a perception in some owners of reduced nutrient quality that results from food processing techniques. Most recently, distrust in the safety of commercial pet foods has increased in response to pet food recalls.[36] These beliefs have led to an increasing number of owners seeking to supplement or completely replace their commercial pet food with a homemade diet.[23]

A principal problem with feeding a homemade diet is that many of the recipes that are available have not been adequately tested for nutritional adequacy or even for nutrient content. Interestingly, most of the recipes that are available contain too much, rather than not enough, protein. This anomaly is attributed to the common belief that, as carnivores, dogs and cats should be fed diets that are comprised almost completely of meat products. As a result, these recipes often contain an inverse Ca:P ratio. Reported imbalances with homemade cat diets are inadequate levels or inappropriate sources of fat.[23] Homemade recipes are also often not balanced for essential vitamins and minerals.[39] Although many owners attempt to correct for these imbalances by feeding a vitamin-mineral supplement, the majority of pet supplements that are sold for this purpose are not balanced themselves.[23] Balanced recipes for homemade diets for dogs and cats can be obtained from veterinary nutritionists and from several online services provided through the American College of Veterinary Nutrition. However, because of the cost of these services, many owners may continue to use recipes that are available

free-of-charge via various Internet sources. Even when an adequate recipe is acquired, owners may begin to use ingredient substitution over time as a result of availability, cost, or owner's beliefs about an ingredient's wholesomeness. Such substitutions may or may not imbalance the end product.

When a properly formulated and tested recipe is used, there can be benefits of homemade diets for some owners and their pets. For some owners, preparing a homemade food for their pet provides an additional outlet for caretaking and management of their pet's health. Although preparing a homemade diet tends to be time consuming and costly, engaging in this activity and believing that they are doing a good thing for their pet is highly rewarding for many pet owners. A homemade diet may also be the best choice for some types of medical conditions. For example, a homemade ration produced from a single protein and single carbohydrate source can be used for the initial diagnosis of food allergies or intolerances. The flexibility of such a diet allows for single item substitutions as various ingredients are tested for the pet's allergic response. A properly formulated therapeutic diet can also be easily modified to alter nutrient levels to closely meet an individual pet's needs. However, it is imperative to keep in mind that these benefits all rely upon the identification of a suitable and pretested recipe as well as long-term compliance with preparation and feeding instructions.

If an owner wishes to prepare a homemade food, the first step is to obtain a recipe that has been proven to be nutritionally adequate and complete. Once an adequate recipe is found, the ingredients that are purchased should conform as closely as possible to the recipe and should be consistent between batches of food. Most recipes allow the owner to prepare a relatively large volume at one time and freeze small portions for extended use. Ingredients should never be substituted or eliminated from the recipe because of the danger of imbalancing the ration. Pet owners should also be aware of the dangers of feeding single-food items in lieu of a prepared diet. Foods that owners enjoy are not necessarily the most nutritious foods to feed to their pets. Similarly, projecting current human nutritional guidelines such as a reduction in fat and sodium are usually not appropriate for healthy dogs and cats.

Veterinary (Therapeutic) Diets

In the past several decades, a host of human health claims have become associated with the consumption of certain types of foods, ingredients, and nutrients. Examples include the relationship between fiber consumption and dietary fat intake and heart and gastrointestinal health. As a direct result of this trend in human foods, companion animal nutritionists and pet food manufacturers have begun to investigate the use of diet and dietary ingredients for the nutritional management of disease conditions in dogs and cats. This has resulted in a rapid increase in the number of therapeutic, or veterinary, diets that are available to veterinarians and pet owners. These foods can be distinguished from pet foods formulated for healthy animals by their mode of sale and the manner in which they are labeled. Specifically, veterinary diets are sold only through veterinary clinics and are labeled for use only under the direction of a veterinarian.[40,41]

Companion animal professionals should critically evaluate any therapeutic diets that they are considering, paying specific attention to the type and quantity of research that supports the clinical benefits. Well-controlled, randomized clinical studies in which the diet was fed to pets with naturally occurring diseases are the most desirable. Results from clinical trials can also be supported by studies performed in a laboratory or kennel setting that uses an appropriate model for the disease in question. In all cases, the diet or dietary component should be demonstrated to provide a realistic level of benefit and an acceptable level of risk to justify its use. Examples of veterinary diets that are currently available to small-animal veterinarians include diets for animals recovering from trauma or severe illness, foods designed to manage kidney or gastrointestinal disease, and products for the diagnosis and management of adverse reactions to food (food allergies). As more knowledge is acquired concerning the benefits of diet and certain nutrients in the management of companion animal disease, more veterinary diets are expected to become available (see Section 5 for complete discussions).

References

1. Lankhorst C, Tran QD, Havenaar R, and others: The effect of extrusion on the nutritional value of canine diets as assessed by in vitro indicators, *Anim Feed Sci Tech* 138:285–297, 2007.

2. Harlow J: US pet food trends. In *Proceedings of the petfood forum*, Chicago, 1997, Watts Publishing.

3. Samuelson AC, Cutter GR: Dog biscuits: an aid in canine tartar control, *J Nutr* 121:S162, 1991.

4. Kallfelz FA: Evaluation and use of pet foods: general considerations in using pet foods for adult maintenance, *Vet Clin North Am Small Anim Pract* 19:387–403, 1989.

5. Association of American Feed Control Officials (AAFCO): Pet food regulations. In *AAFCO Official Publication*, Atlanta, 2008, AAFCO.

6. Bradshaw JWS, Healey LM, Thorne CJ, and others: Differences in food preferences between individuals and populations of domestic cats, *Felis sylvestris catus, Appl Anim Behav Sci* 68:257–268, 2000.

7. Stasiak M: The effect of early specific feeding on food conditioning in cats, *Dev Psychobiol* 39:207–215, 2001.

8. Carter B, Fontana A Jr: Water activity: the key to pet food quality and safety, white paper, *Pet Food Ind*, 2008.

9. Ferrell F: Preference for sugars and nonnutritive sweeteners in young Beagles, *Neurosci Biobehav Rev* 8:199–203, 1984.

10. Li X, Li W, Wang H, and others: Cats lack a sweet taste receptor, *J Nutr* 136:1932S–1934S, 2006.

11. Bradshaw JWS: The evolutionary basis for the feeding behavior of domestic dogs (*Canis familiaris*) and cats (*Felis catus*), *J Nutr* 136:1927S–1931S, 2006.

12. Morgan T: Treat trends, *Pet Food Ind,* pp 32–37, September/October 1997.

13. Lazarus C: Resealable treats, *Pet Food Ind,* pp 8–12, November/December 1996.

14. Phillips T: US pet food sales go boom, *Pet Food Ind,* November 2007.

15. Michel KE: Unconventional diets for dogs and cats, *Vet Clin North Am Small Anim Pract* 36:1269–1281, 2006.

16. Alternative pet food sales booming in the US and Canada, *Pet Food Ind,* September 2008.

17. Kallfelz FA: Evaluation and use of pet foods: general considerations in using pet foods for adult maintenance, *Vet Clin North Am Small Anim Pract* 19:387–403, 1989.

18. Huber TL, Wilson RC, McGarity SA: Variations in digestibility of dry dog foods with identical label guaranteed analysis, *J Am Anim Hosp Assoc* 22:571–575, 1986.

19. Sousa CA, Stannard AA, Ihrke PJ, and others: Dermatosis associated with feeding generic dog food: 13 cases (1981–1982), *J Am Vet Med Assoc* 192:676–680, 1988.

20. Laflamme DP, Abood SK, Fascetti AJ, and others: Pet feeding practices of dog and cat owners in the United States and Australia, *J Am Vet Med Assoc* 232:687–694, 2008.

21. Case LP: Perspectives on domestication: the history of our relationship with man's best friend, *J Anim Sci* 86:3245–3251, 2008.

22. Freeman LM, Michel KE: Evaluation of raw food diets for dogs, *J Am Vet Med Assoc* 218:705–709, 2001.

23. Remillard RL: Homemade diets: attributes, pitfalls, and a call for action, *Top Companion Anim Nutr* 23:137–142, 2008.

24. LeJeune JT, Hancock DD: Public health concerns associated with feeding raw meat diets to dogs, *J Am Vet Med Assoc* 219:1222–1225, 2001.

25. Billinghurst I: *Feeding the adult dog: give your dog a bone*, Alexandria, Australia, 1993, Bridge Printery, pp 265–280.

26. Stiver SL, Frazier KS, Mauel MJ: Septicemic salmonellosis in two cats fed a raw-meat diet, *J Am Anim Hosp Assoc* 39:538–542, 2003.

27. Stone GG, Chengappa MM, Oberst RD: Application of polymerase chain reaction for the correlation of *Salmonella* serovars recovered from Greyhound feces with their diet, *J Vet Diagn Invest* 5:378–385, 1993.

28. Joffe DJ, Schlesinger DP: Preliminary assessment of the risk of *Salmonella* infection in dogs fed raw chicken diets, *Can Vet J* 43:441–442, 2002.

29. Weese JS, Rousseau J, Arroyo L: Bacteriological evaluation of commercial canine and feline raw diets, *Can Vet J* 46:513–516, 2005.

30. Strohmeyer RA, Morley PS, Hyatt DR, and others: Evaluation of bacterial and protozoal contamination of commercially available raw meat diets for dogs, *J Am Vet Med Assoc* 228:537–542, 2006.

31. Finley R, Reid-Smith R, Weese JS: Human health implications of *Salmonella*-contaminated natural pet treats and raw pet food, *Clin Infect Dis* 42:686–691, 2006.

32. Food and Drug Administration (FDA) Center for Veterinary Medicine: Manufacture and labeling of raw meat foods for companion and captive non-companion carnivores and omnivores, *Guidance for industry #122*, Washington DC, 2005, FDA.

33. Finley R, Ribble C, Aramini J, and others: The risk of salmonellae shedding by dogs fed *Salmonella*-contaminated commercial raw food diets, *Can Vet J* 48:69–75, 2007.

34. Lefebvre SL, Reid-Smith R, Boerlin R, Weese JS: Evaluation of the risks of shedding salmonellae and other potential pathogens by therapy dogs fed raw diets in Ontario and Alberta, *Zoonoses Public Health* 55:470–480, 2008.

35. Voetsch AC, Van Vlider TJ, Angulao FJ: FoodNet estimate of the burden of illness caused by nontyphoidal *Salmonella* infections in the United States, *Clin Infect Dis* 38:S127–S134, 2004.

36. Wakefield LA, Shofer FS, Michel KE: Evaluation of cats fed vegetarian diets and attitudes of their caregivers, *J Am Vet Med Assoc* 229:70–73, 2006.

37. Gray CM, Sellon RK, Freeman LM: Nutritional adequacy of two vegan diets for cats, *J Am Vet Med Assoc* 225:1670–1675, 2004.

38. Kienzle E, Engelhard R: A field study on the nutrition of vegetarian dogs and cats in Europe, *Compend Contin Educ Pract Vet* 23:81, 2001.

39. Streiff EL, Zwischenberger B, Butterwick RF, and others: A comparison of the nutritional adequacy of home-prepared and commercial diets for dogs, *J Nutr* 132:1698S–1700S, 2002.

40. Dzanis DA: When pet foods are drugs, *FDA Vet* 8:4–5, 1993.

41. Kronfeld DS: Health claims for pet foods: particulars, *J Am Vet Med Assoc* 205:174–177, 1994.

18

Evaluation of Pet Foods

The large variety of pet foods produced and sold in the United States can make the selection of a proper diet a complex and confusing process. The information presented earlier in this section illustrates the need for pet owners and professionals to critically evaluate a product before feeding it to their pets. Because many pet foods are intended to provide the primary source of nutrition for a pet, it is extremely important that owners select a product capable of providing optimal nutrition and promoting long-term health. This chapter provides tools that companion animal owners and professionals can use to evaluate pet foods. These criteria aid in distinguishing between products that are inadequate, acceptable, or optimal in their ability to provide proper nutrition to a companion animal (Box 18-1).

COMPLETE AND BALANCED

The phrase "complete and balanced" is used by the pet food industry to signify that a pet food contains all of the essential nutrients at levels that meet the target animal's requirements. Because animals eat or are fed to meet their energy requirements, nutrient levels in a food must be balanced so that when an animal meets its caloric needs, its requirements for all other nutrients are fulfilled at the same time. The regulations of the Association of American Feed Control Officials (AAFCO) allow pet food manufacturers to include the complete and balanced claim

on their label if they have substantiated this claim using one of two possible methods. Option one requires that the pet food be successfully evaluated through a series of AAFCO-sanctioned animal feeding trials, and option two requires that the food is formulated to meet the minimum and/or maximum levels of nutrients established by the AAFCO's *Nutrient Profiles* for dog and cat foods (see pp. 134-135). Companies that use option 2 may also conduct feeding tests on their products, but may not be using AAFCO protocols for those studies.

The first criterion that a pet owner should use when evaluating a food is a check for the complete and balanced claim. The most important criterion is that the life stage(s) designated in the claim corresponds to the pet's stage of life and activity level. Examples of common claims are "Supplies complete and balanced nutrition for all stages of a cat's life" or "This food provides complete and balanced nutrition for growing puppies." Pet food manufacturers are required to include the method of substantiation that was used for the complete and balanced claim on the pet food label. If a statement that AAFCO feeding trials were conducted is included, this means that the food was adequately tested using AAFCO feeding trials with dogs and cats. If the statement claims that the food meets the AAFCO's *Nutrient Profiles,* this signifies that the food was formulated to meet the nutrient profile for the intended stage of life (adult maintenance or growth/reproduction).

When selecting a pet food, owners should first check for a "complete and balanced" label claim. The food should also be appropriate for their pet's breed size, age, and activity level.

PALATABILITY

The palatability and acceptability of a pet food is a crucial consideration because a food must be acceptable to the pet in order for it to provide optimum nutrition.

> **BOX 18-1 FACTORS TO CONSIDER IN THE EVALUATION OF PET FOODS**
>
> Complete and balanced nutrition
> Palatability
> Digestibility
> Metabolizable energy content
> Feeding cost
> Reputation of manufacturer
> Dental health contribution
> Taurine content (cats)
> Urinary health properties (cats)

A pet's daily intake of essential nutrients is a function of the quantity of food eaten and the concentration of available nutrients in the food. Because of this relationship, the amount of food that is eaten is as important as the food's nutrient and energy content. An unpalatable food will be rejected by a dog or cat regardless of the level or balance of nutrients that it contains. Similarly, a diet can be palatable but still not contain adequate levels of some nutrients. Contrary to popular belief, dogs and cats are not capable of detecting specific nutrient deficiencies or imbalances in their diets and will continue to consume an imbalanced diet until the physiological effects of the deficiency or excess cause illness or a reduction in food intake. Following this, learned aversions to imbalanced diets can develop. For example, an arginine-deficient diet rapidly leads to emesis, hyperammonemia and severe illness in cats. When cats were fed a single arginine-free meal, they demonstrated single-trial aversive responses to the deficient food when presented with the food on a subsequent occasion.[1]

Animal-Related Factors

Palatability is defined as the subjective pleasure that an individual experiences in association with eating a particular food.[2] Therefore palatability should not be considered to be an intrinsic property of the food, but rather a property of an animal's perception of the food and the tendency to select one particular food over another. Historically, palatability in dogs and cats has been measured using food acceptability and preference tests. A food acceptance test (also called a "one-pan test") examines initial response to a new food and may also record the time that it takes an animal to taste and consume the new food. Because no choice is involved in this initial screening, this test only provides information about whether or not the dog or cat finds the new food to be appealing and is willing to eat it. Factors that can affect initial acceptability include the animal's degree of hunger and an individual's response to novelty. Food preference tests (also called "two-pan tests") are based upon the assumption that a greater intake of one food over another is an indication of higher palatability.[3] Using this approach, animals are offered the simultaneous choice of two foods for a predetermined number of days and intake is recorded. One food will be ranked higher in palatability than a second food if a greater volume of the first food is

eaten. However, limitations of this approach include the confounding effects of satiety when foods of differing caloric density are fed and the inability to discern short- or long-term effects of novelty (see below).

In recent years, the assessment of food preferences and palatability in dogs and cats has become significantly more sophisticated as methods have been developed to measure animals' responses to the smell, taste, and texture of foods.[4] Because of the highly developed olfactory acuity of dogs and cats, it is not a surprise that the odor of a food significantly influences food preferences in both species.[5,6] When presented with more than one food choice, cats first smell the foods and will preferentially consume the food with the most attractive odor, usually without tasting the less attractive food(s).[7] Olfaction is intrinsically linked to taste, which appears to be second in importance to dogs and cats during food selection.[8] For example, when cats cannot discriminate among foods using olfaction, they will then use taste to make a choice.[7] The sense of touch is involved in food selection when dogs and cats react to a food's shape and texture. Together with the size of kibble pieces, these sensations make up the "mouth feel" of a food. For example, increasing the size of kibble pieces generally decreases rate of eating in dogs, because they spend more time chewing and masticating the food pieces than they do when fed foods with small kibble sizes. Cats are especially sensitive to the size and shape of kibble pieces because of their tendency to eat slowly and because they chew foods less thoroughly when compared with dogs. For example, cats tend to reject kibble pieces with sharp edges, presumably because these pieces have an uncomfortable "mouth feel."[9] Other animal-related factors that may influence a pet's acceptance of a particular food include past experiences, age, and breed. The feeding environment and an owner's behavior can also affect a pet's response to a new food. Most reputable pet food manufacturers recognize this and conduct controlled palatability tests both with kenneled animals and within a wide variety of home environments.

An individual dog's or cat's perception of a new food is affected by the food's smell, taste and "mouth feel." Because their olfactory sense is very sensitive, the odor of a food is a very important component of palatability for dogs and cats.

Two conflicting effects that can significantly influence an individual dog or cat's food selection are the primacy effect and novelty effect.[10] The primacy effect occurs when an animal is fed a specific type or flavor of food for a long period of time (most commonly beginning at weaning) and the individual shows an enhanced preference for that food to the exclusion of novel foods. For example, an early series of studies found that limiting the flavor experiences of puppies and kittens at an early age led to fixed food preferences in which all novel foods are rejected later in life.[11] When the same experimenters fed foods of varying flavors and textures early in life, the dogs and cats showed increased acceptance of novel foods as adults. This form of neophobia is most commonly reported as a problem when a cat has been fed one type or flavor of food for many years and a change in nutrient needs or health status suddenly requires a change in food. Although neophobia can also occur in dogs, it is less common, possibly because the dog's scavenging nature and more omnivorous diet make dogs more resistant to the development of fixed food preferences. Although it has been speculated that there are breed-specific differences in dogs in the tendency to accept or reject novel foods, there is currently little evidence to support or refute this.[6]

Paradoxically, the novelty effect can also occur with animals that are fed a single food item for a long period. In these cases, instead of rejecting novel foods, the individual shows an enhanced (though sometimes transient) preference for a new food or treat when it is offered.[12,13] In another early study, puppies that had been fed a single type of canned food starting at weaning and continuing until they were 16 weeks of age showed a strong preference for novel foods when they were offered.[14] Dog trainers regularly capitalize on this tendency by using treats that differ from a dog's daily food or by varying the type of treats that are used as food reinforcers during consecutive training sessions. It is possible that the attraction to a new food (novelty) in some animals is actually a reflection of a mild aversion to or boredom with a food that has been fed for a long period of time. This has been called the "monotony effect" and has been used to explain attraction to novel foods in cats more often than dogs.[15,16] It is theorized that cats may have an evolutionary bias toward selecting more than a single food choice or prey species to avoid nutrient deficiencies from developing.

Although the primacy and the novelty effects have both been observed in dogs and cats, the incompatibility of these two responses and factors that determine which behavior an individual animal will show are not completely understood. Recently, a series of studies with cats led investigators to speculate that these opposing responses may be explained by cats possessing certain innate flavor preferences. When a varied diet is fed to kittens, being exposed to multiple food flavors would tend to "mask" inborn flavor or food preferences; conversely, feeding a limited diet early in life would be more likely to allow expression of inborn flavor preferences.[17] Cats in this study appeared to possess an innate preference for the flavor of tuna when compared with beef. This preference was only expressed when kittens that were raised on a beef-flavored food were presented with tuna as the novel flavor. Conversely, other investigators argue against the existence of a select set of innate flavor preferences in cats and suggest that observed differences in preference are a result of early learning from the mother and possibly litter-specific predispositions.[15] More studies are needed to explore innate and learned flavor preferences and to further elucidate the importance of primacy and novelty in food selection in both dogs and cats.

Food Properties Affecting Palatability

There are several properties of food components that can directly affect palatability and food selection in dogs and cats.[18] The quality of ingredients, and the way that they are cooked, processed, and stored, significantly affects acceptability and palatability. For example, the extrusion of grain starches imparts a desirable texture and flavor to dry pet food kibbles. However, if mold growth has occurred or if the product has not been properly extruded, grains will be perceived as highly unacceptable. Poorly extruded starches cause food particles to have high bulk densities, which negatively affect the texture and chewiness of the product. Poorly processed or poorly stored foods may also contain high levels of oxidized oils and fats. High concentrations of aldehydes produced by fat oxidation are unpalatable to animals. Food palatability for both dogs and cats is positively correlated with protein level. Animal-source proteins are generally considered to be more palatable than plant-source proteins, although the extrusion process significantly increases the palatability of plant-based protein sources such as soybean.[19,20] However, just as with starch, the overprocessing of protein or the inclusion of poor-quality protein sources in a food can lead to compounds that are perceived as unpalatable.

Low-quality pet foods may have decreased palatability as a result of the inclusion of poor-quality ingredients or harsh processing methods. Although not the only factors involved, proper processing, handling, and storage of pet foods containing high-quality ingredients contribute to a food's acceptability and palatability. Once an acceptable degree of palatability has been met, however, the owner must evaluate other diet characteristics that are important for the delivery of optimal nutrition. Because most commercial pet foods available today are highly palatable to dogs and cats, problems of overconsumption and weight gain are more common than are problems of diet rejection. Therefore, although palatability is important, it should not be used as the sole criterion when evaluating a food.

DIGESTIBILITY

The digestibility of a pet food is an important criterion because it directly measures the proportion of nutrients in the food that are available for absorption. True and apparent digestibility can only be measured through controlled feeding trials (see pp. 142-143). The results of these trials provide digestibility coefficients for a food's dry matter (DM), crude protein, crude fat, and nitrogen-free extract (NFE), which is a measure of the carbohydrate fraction in a food. A series of early studies of commercial brands of dog foods reported average digestibility coefficients for crude protein, crude fat, and NFE of 81%, 85%, and 79%, respectively.[21] Premium and super-premium pet foods usually have slightly higher digestibility coefficients than these values, while basic nutrition products have similar or lower digestibilities. Digestibilities as high as 89%, 95%, and 88% for crude protein, crude fat, and carbohydrate, respectively, can occur in dry premium and super-premium pet foods. As the quality of ingredients included in the food increases, so will the food's DM and nutrient digestibility.

Food Properties

A pet food that is low in digestibility contains a high proportion of ingredients that cannot be digested by the enzymes of the gastrointestinal tract. These components pass through to the large intestine, where they are partially or largely fermented by colonic bacteria. Rapid or excessive bacterial fermentation leads to the production of gas (flatulence), loose stools, and occasionally diarrhea. In addition to these side effects, a greater quantity of a poorly digested food must be fed to the animal because the pet is absorbing a smaller proportion of nutrients from the food. As the quantity of food that is consumed increases, rate of passage through the gastrointestinal tract also increases. A more rapid passage of food through the intestines further contributes to poor digestibility, high stool volume, and gas production. A food's digestibility is decreased by the presence of high levels of nonfermentable fiber, ash, phytate, and poor-quality protein. Improper processing or excessive heat treatment can also adversely affect digestibility. In contrast, pet food digestibility is increased by the inclusion of high-quality ingredients and increased levels of fat, as well as the use of proper processing techniques.

In general, dogs and cats digest foods of animal origin better than those of plant origin. This difference is primarily the result of the presence of lignin, cellulose, and other nonfermentable fibers in plant ingredients. However, it is important for owners and professionals to recognize that low-quality animal products containing high amounts of skin, hair, feathers, and connective tissue are also not well digested by dogs and cats. Although a pet food that contains high-quality animal products has a higher digestibility than a plant-based food, pet foods that contain poor-quality animal ingredients may have lower digestibilities than plant-based products with similar nutrient profiles.[22]

Digestibility represents the proportion of nutrients in a food that is available for absorption by an animal's body. Factors that can negatively affect a food's digestibility include the inclusion of poor quality ingredients and high levels of fiber, ash, and phytate. Improper processing and excessive heat treatment also adversely affect digestibility. In contrast, pet food digestibility is increased by the inclusion of high-quality ingredients and the use of proper processing techniques.

Animal-Related Factors

There is some evidence that apparent digestibilities of the major organic nutrients in commercial pet foods are higher for dogs than for cats.[23,24] Both the dog and the cat belong to the order Carnivora and are classified as simple-stomached carnivores. The cat is a strict carnivore, but the dog is more omnivorous in nature. One way in which this difference is reflected is in the abilities of the two species to digest certain types of dietary components. A study comparing the digestive capabilities of dogs and cats found that when fed the same dog or cat food, dogs had higher apparent digestibility coefficients and obtained more digestible nutrients per unit of food eaten than cats for almost all nutrients and types of foods.[24] It was suggested that some of these differences could be explained by a greater ability of the dog to digest (ferment) certain types of fiber in the large intestine. Data from studies of the fermentative capacities of canine and feline colonic microflora support this. While both dogs and cats are capable of fermenting certain fiber types, the cat is less tolerant of wide ranges of fiber fermentability than the dog.[25-27]

Within species, animal-related factors that may affect digestibility include body size, breed, age, and physiological state. Size effects may occur in dogs because of the wide range in body size and body types that occur in the domestic dog. The relative weight of a dog's gastrointestinal tract decreases with increasing body size, which may influence the digestion efficiency.[28,29] While the empty intestinal tract comprises 6% to 7% of the body weight of small dogs, it decreases to 3% to 4% in large- and giant-breed dogs. One group of researchers examined the apparent digestibilities of canned and dry commercial foods in 10 breeds of dogs that ranged in body size between 9 and 115 lb.[30] The large-breed dogs tended to have looser stools and higher fecal moisture when compared with small- and medium-size dogs, but there were no significant differences in organic matter digestibility coefficients among dogs of different sizes or breeds. In addition, the giant breed of dog that was tested in this study, the Irish Wolfhound, had lower fecal moisture than other breeds, suggesting that body weight alone was not responsible for the observed differences in fecal scores.

Another study measured apparent digestibility in four breeds of dogs fed a dry extruded diet starting shortly after weaning and continuing until the dogs were 15 months of age.[31] These investigators also found that large- and giant-breed dogs (Giant Schnauzers and Great Danes) had consistently looser stools that contained higher fecal moisture, and that the reduced fecal quality was not related to lower diet digestibility. In fact, in this study, the large- and giant-breed dogs had significantly higher digestibility coefficients than the smaller breeds, regardless of age. These differences did not appear to be due to a difference in the volume of food that was consumed because food intake did not differ significantly among breeds when expressed as a function of metabolic body size. Because the large dogs also showed higher total fiber digestibility, it was speculated that the higher fecal water in large dogs may have been caused by greater colonic fermentation of carbohydrate and protein fractions of the diet. Higher microbial mass and increased organic acid production in the colon can contribute to increased fecal water.[32] Another possible explanation for the higher fecal water is reduced absorption of electrolytes in the large intestine of large breed dogs. A strong relationship between poor stool quality (i.e., high water content) and reduced sodium and chloride absorption in the colon has been reported in dogs, and Great Danes have been shown to have lower apparent absorption of sodium and potassium when compared with Beagles.[33,34]

It is important to recognize that the use of purebred dogs to represent different body sizes in all of the aforementioned studies may confound the potential effects of size and breed, making it difficult to separate differences that are primarily due to size from those that may have a genetic component. The breeds used to represent the large and giant breeds were Giant Schnauzers, Great Danes, and Irish Wolfhounds. Other studies have examined digestibility efficiencies among different breeds of dogs of the small- and medium-size categories and have found no differences in digestibility efficiencies within size categories and among breeds.[35,36] However, with the exception of the three breeds identified previously, no studies to date have been conducted that compare digestive capacity among the many large and giant breeds of dogs. Given the results suggesting differences in these dogs, especially those pertaining to electrolyte absorption, such research would be helpful in fully elucidating the underlying causes of differences in fecal quality that have been reported.

Although a limited number of studies have been conducted, it appears that a dog's and cat's digestibility efficiency increases gradually from weaning until adolescence, and then remains stable in healthy animals throughout adulthood.[37] The lower digestibility values observed in puppies and kittens may be caused by the increased food consumption, relative to body size, that is needed to meet increased energy and nutrient needs of growth, or could reflect a true difference in digestive efficiency (for a complete discussion, see Chapter 22, p. 231).[31,38,39] The fact that there are age-related changes in digestive enzyme activities suggests that newly weaned and young puppies and kittens may have lower capacities to digest certain nutrients. For example pancreatic amylase activity is lower in puppies than in young adult dogs and increases gradually with age.[40] There is also indirect evidence that young kittens may have reduced pancreatic lipase activity.[41] These differences may impact the young puppy's and kitten's ability to digest dietary starch and fat, respectively. Conversely, similar to many other species, intestinal lactase activity is high in young dogs and decreases with maturity, signifying an adaptation to milk consumption early in life. Finally, nutrient digestibility does not generally change in healthy older dogs, but may decrease in older cats (see Chapter 25, p. 265 for a complete discussion).[42]

Differences among Commercial Pet Foods

Regardless of differences in the digestive capabilities of dogs and cats and among animals of different breeds and ages, it is important to be aware that commercial pet foods can differ significantly in digestibility and nutrient availability. The labels of two products may have the same ingredient lists and guaranteed analysis panels, but when the products are fed, they may have different digestibilities. This variability will directly affect the ability of each diet to provide adequate levels of nutrients to an animal. A greater quantity of a poorly digested diet must be fed to an animal in order to meet its nutrient requirements. This fact is illustrated by a study with growing dogs that compared two commercial dry dog foods (R1 and R2) using feeding trials that followed the AAFCO feeding test protocols.[43] Chemical analysis of the two diets showed that they contained identical levels of nutrients. However, when fed to a

group of dogs, the effect of each diet on growth and development was significantly different. Dogs that were fed the R2 diet grew significantly less and ate less food than did the R1-fed dogs. The R2-fed dogs became anorexic, had significantly lower body weights and body lengths, and showed poor coat quality and graying of the hair coat. These dogs also had depressed hemoglobin and hematocrit values and lower serum cholesterol, alkaline phosphatase, calcium, and phosphorus levels. The authors of the study concluded that the R2 diet had a lower palatability and that its nutrients were less available than those in the R1 diet. Subsequent digestibility trials found that the R2 diet was 18% lower in apparent digestibility than diet R1. In another study, digestibility trials of four commercial dog foods with identical guaranteed analysis panels showed that the national brand of food had a significantly higher digestibility than did the three price brands that were examined.[44] It is important to note that in both of these studies the analytical values obtained through chemical analysis provided no information that would indicate differences in the digestibility of the foods.

Currently, AAFCO regulations do not allow pet food manufacturers to include quantitative or comparative digestibility claims on their labels.[45] This information can only be obtained by actually feeding the food. Many manufacturers of premium and super-premium brands of foods include information about ingredient and product digestibility with the educational materials they give to the retailers, pet supply stores, and veterinarians, as well as on their websites. However, most basic nutrition brands of pet food do not provide information regarding digestibility. If digestibility information is not readily available, this information may be obtained by writing or calling the company directly. As a general rule of thumb, pet owners should choose foods that have a DM digestibility of 80% or greater and should reject any foods that have digestibilities lower than 75%.

Finally, buying a package of pet food and actually feeding it to a pet can also provide valuable information about a food's digestibility. A product that is highly digestible and contains available nutrients will produce low stool volumes and well-formed, firm feces. In addition, the fecal matter will not contain mucus, blood, or any recognizable components of the pet food. Defecation frequency should be relatively low, and bowel movements should be regular and consistent. Normal growth rates and body weight should be easily maintained by the food without the need to feed excessive quantities, and long-term feeding should result in healthy skin and hair coat. Although these observations do not provide quantitative information about digestibility, they are a reasonably accurate measure of a diet's ability to supply absorbable nutrients to a companion animal.

When fed to companion animals, pet foods that are highly digestible and contain available nutrients will produce well-formed, firm feces and low stool volume and defecation frequencies. Long-term feeding should support optimal growth and body condition along with healthy skin and hair coat condition.

METABOLIZABLE ENERGY CONTENT

The ME of a pet food represents the amount of energy that is available for an animal for use (see pp. 143-144). The energy density of pet foods is typically expressed as kilocalories (kcal) of ME per unit weight (kilogram [kg] or pound [lb]). ME can be determined either through feeding trials or through calculation using standard energy values for protein, carbohydrate, and fat (see Section 1, pp. 4-6).

Energy density should be considered when evaluating a pet food because it will directly affect the quantity of food that must be fed to meet the pet's energy requirement. For example, two dry dog foods that are advertised as performance diets for working dogs have ME values of 4500 kcal/kg (diet A) and 3600 kcal/kg (diet B). If a sled dog that is training in mild weather conditions requires 4500 kcal/day, it will need to consume 1 kg of diet A or 1.25 kg of diet B (Table 18-1).

The consumption of 25% more of diet B is necessary to meet this dog's daily caloric requirement. Hard-working dogs and lactating bitches and queens all have high energy requirements. These requirements are often best met by feeding a food that is relatively high in energy and nutrient density. On the other hand, a diet with a lower energy density facilitates weight maintenance in adult pets that lead sedentary lifestyles. However, if the ME content of a pet food is too low, the quantity of food that the pet needs to eat in order to meet its requirement may exceed the physical capacity of the gastrointestinal tract. The consumption of an excessive quantity of food leads to increased rate of passage through the gastrointestinal tract and decreased digestibility. In general, pet owners should select a pet food that contains between 3000 and 5000 kcal/kg on a dry-matter basis (DMB), depending on the needs of the animal.

Before 1994, AAFCO regulations prohibited the inclusion of statements of caloric density on pet food labels. But in 1994 the AAFCO passed a regulation allowing voluntary label claims of ME content. In 2008, AAFCO accepted a proposal to make calorie statements mandatory (see pp. 135-136). The caloric density regulation requires companies that include ME claims to substantiate the ME content through either a calculation method using modified Atwater factors or through data collected from a series of digestibility trials with animals. As in the case of complete and balanced claims, the method that the company uses to substantiate the ME claim must be stated (see pp. 134-135). In addition to knowing the caloric density of the pet food, it is also helpful for pet owners to know the relative energy contributions that are provided by the carbohydrate, protein, and fat fractions of the food. The dietary proportion of fat should be higher for hard-working animals and lower for sedentary adult or elderly animals. Similarly, the proportion of calories supplied by digestible carbohydrate should be increased in diets that are intended for adult maintenance or for elderly animals.

TABLE 18-1 DETERMINATION OF COST PER SERVING

	METABOLIZABLE ENERGY REQUIREMENT		KCAL/KG		QUANTITY/DAY	PRICE/LB	PRICE/KG	COST/DAY
Diet A	4500	÷	4500	=	1 kg (2.2 lb)	$1.28	$2.82	$2.82
Diet B	4500	÷	3600	=	1.25 kg (2.75 lb)	$1.06	$2.33	$2.92

FEEDING COST

As the quality of the ingredients included in a pet food increases, so does the cost to the manufacturer. Therefore, as a product's quality increases, so does its price per unit weight. When making price comparisons between foods, it is important to consider the cost of actually feeding the food as opposed to the cost per unit weight. The cost per serving of a premium or super-premium product is often equal to or just slightly higher than that of an inferior product because a smaller quantity of the high-quality pet food is fed. Using the previous example, the price of diet A is $45 for a 40-lb bag and the price of diet B is $37 for a 40-lb bag. Although a bag of diet A is actually more expensive than that of diet B, the cost of feeding diet B to a hard-working dog is higher because of its lower energy density (see Table 18-1). When evaluating a food for the first time, owners can record the purchase date and the price of the food. When the package is empty, dividing the cost of the product by the number of days that the bag lasted provides the cost per day to feed that particular food. A second product with the same net weight can then be compared in the same manner.

Although some economy or private-label (store brand) foods may appeal to pet owners because of their low cost, owners are cautioned that the cost is usually a reflection of the inexpensive, low-quality ingredients used and the lack of thorough feed-trial testing.

REPUTATION OF THE MANUFACTURER

The reputation of the pet food manufacturer should always be considered when selecting a pet food. Companies that have a national reputation for producing consistent, high-quality products and devoting resources to consumer education about proper nutrition for companion animals should be selected. The inclusion of a toll-free phone number on the product's package and a customer service website indicate a company that welcomes inquiries about their products. In addition, the manufacturer's response to questions should be timely, thorough, and direct. A pet food manufacturer should be expected to readily supply information about the pet food's ingredients, types of testing, digestibility information, ME content, and nutrient content. Pet food manufacturers that produce quality products are concerned with their reputations and with serving the needs and concerns of the pet owners who buy their pet foods. This concern will be evidenced by the company's accessibility to consumers and their response to questions about their products.

OTHER FACTORS

Several other factors may be considered when evaluating commercial pet foods. A cat food's taurine content should be noted. The availability of taurine in a diet is influenced by a number of factors, including other nutrients and the type of processing that is used. Therefore the adequacy of the taurine level of a diet can only be assessed through actual feeding trials. Pet food manufacturers should be able to show that their product will maintain normal blood taurine levels in cats when it is fed on a long-term basis. Whole-blood taurine should be maintained in adult cats at a level of 250 nanomole per milliliter (ml) or greater.[46] Generally, extruded dry foods that contain at least 1000 milligram (mg)/kg (0.10%) and canned cat foods that contain at least 2000 mg/kg (0.20%) on a DMB are adequate.

Cat foods also should be evaluated with regard to their ability to support urinary tract health. A urinary pH of 7 or higher is an important risk factor for the development of struvite-induced feline urolithiasis (see Chapter 30, pp. 362-365 for a complete discussion). Feeding a diet that maintains a urinary pH between 6 and 6.8 when fed ad libitum may inhibit the development of the struvite crystals that may cause this disorder. However, a diet that produces an overly acidified urine (less than 6) can put the cat at risk of metabolic acidosis and skeletal decalcification. Pet owners who have concerns about their cats' urinary tract health can select a diet that has been formulated to promote an appropriate acidic urine pH. Although magnesium was once implicated as an important risk factor for struvite urolithiasis, it is now known that magnesium levels in the diet only become significant when urinary pH is maintained at too high a level.[47] However, it is still wise to avoid products that have magnesium contents greater than 0.1% of the diet's DM. Currently, pet food manufacturers in the United States are not allowed to include information about urinary pH on the cat food label. This information can be obtained through educational literature produced by the company or by contacting the manufacturer directly.

Another factor that may be assessed is a pet food's ability to contribute to dental health. Some dry pet foods and hard biscuits may contribute to dental health because the type of formulation that they use enhances chewing abrasion and reduces plaque and calculus formation (see Chapter 34, pp. 442-446 for a complete discussion). In addition, there are numerous oral chewing devices available that are designed to improve dogs' dental health or maintain healthy gingivae. Most research indicates that diet alone is unable to maintain clinically healthy gingivae or prevent periodontal disease in the absence of regular tooth-brushing and other types of oral cleansing.[48,49]

Although dry pet foods and the feeding of hard biscuits as treats may contribute to dental health and reduce calculus formation, feeding dry pet food should not be considered an alternative to regular dental care and teeth cleaning.

The overall best judge of a commercial pet food is the animal itself. Once a pet food has been evaluated and selected, pet owners should feed the product for a minimum of 2 months before evaluating its total effect on their pet's health. A food that provides optimal nutrition supports normal development and body condition, healthy skin, a shiny coat, normal fecal volume and consistency, and overall vitality in the pet. Signs of a poor diet include weight loss or poor growth, poor coat quality, the development of skin problems, and a lack of vigor. Whenever any of these signs are observed, a thorough examination by a veterinarian should be conducted. Although changing the diet may be warranted, other medical causes of these problems should always be investigated.

References

1. Morris JG, Rogers QR: Arginine: an essential amino acid for the cat, *J Nutr* 108:1944–1953, 1978.

2. Araujo JA, Studzinski CM, Larson BT, Milgram NW: Comparison of the cognitive palatability assessment protocol and the two-pan test for use in assessing palatability of two similar foods in dogs, *Am J Vet Res* 65:1490–1496, 2004.

3. Thorne CJ: Behaviour and palatability testing. In *Proceedings of the petfood forum*, Chicago, 1997, Watts Publishing.

4. Thombre AG: Oral delivery of medications to companion animals: palatability considerations, *Adv Drug Delivery Rev* 56:1399–1413, 2004.

5. Mugford RA: External influences on the feeding of carnivores. In Kare MR, Maller O, editors: *The chemical senses and nutrition*, New York, 1977, Academic Press.

6. Bradshaw JW: Sensory and experiential factors in the design of foods for domestic dogs and cats, *Proc Nutr Soc* 50:99–106, 1991.

7. Hullar I, Fekete S, Andrasofszky E, and others: Factors influencing the food preference of cats, *J Anim Physiol Anim Nutr* 85:205–211, 2001.

8. Houpt KA, Hintz HF, Shepherd P: The role of olfaction in canine food preferences, *Chem Senses* 3:281–290, 1978.

9. Trivedi N, Benning J: Total palatability: the triangle of success: ingredients, processing and palatants, *Pet Food Ind*, pp 12–14, May/June 1999.

10. Stasiak M: The development of food preferences in cats: the new direction, *Nutr Neurosci* 5:221–228, 2002.

11. Kuo ZY: *The dynamics of behaviour development: an epigenetic view*, New York, 1967, Random House.

12. Griffin RW, Scott GC, Cante CJ: Food preferences of dogs housed in testing-kennels and in consumers' homes: some comparisons, *Neurosci Biobehav Rev* 8:253–259, 1984.

13. Mugford RA: Comparative and developmental studies of feeding in dogs and cats, *Br Vet J* 133:98, 1977.

14. Ferrel F: Effects of restricted dietary flavour experience before weaning on post weaning food preferences in puppies, *Neurosci Biobehav Rev* 8:191–198, 1984.

15. Bradshaw JWS: The evolutionary basis for the feeding behavior of domestic dogs (*Canis familiaris*) and cats (*Felis catus*), *J Nutr* 136:1927S–1931S, 2006.

16. Thorne CJ: Feeding behavior of the cat: recent advances, *J Small Anim Pract* 23:555–562, 1982.

17. Stasiak M: The effect of early specific feeding on food conditioning in cats, *Dev Psychobiol* 39:207–215, 2001.

18. Kestrel-Rickert D: What constitutes palatability? In *Proceedings of the petfood forum*, Chicago, 1995, Watts Publishing.

19. Zaghini G, Biagi G: Nutritional peculiarities and diet palatability in the cat, *Vet Res Comm* 29:39–44, 2005.

20. Hullar I, Fekete S, Szocs Z: Effect of extrusion on the quality of soybean-based cat food, *J Anim Physiol Anim Nutr* 80:201–206, 1998.

21. Kendall PT, Holme DW, Smith PM: Methods of prediction of the digestible energy content of dog foods from gross energy value, proximate analysis and digestible nutrient content, *J Sci Food Agric* 3:823–828, 1982.

22. Case L, Czarnecki GL: Protein requirements of growing pups fed practical dry-type diets containing mixed-protein sources, *Am J Vet Res* 51:808–812, 1990.

23. Kendall PT: Comparable evaluation of apparent digestibility in dogs and cats, *Proc Nutr Soc* 40:45a, 1981.

24. Kendall PT, Holme DW, Smith PM: Comparative evaluation of net digestive and absorptive efficiency in dogs and cats fed a variety of contrasting diet types, *J Small Anim Pract* 23:577–587, 1982.

25. Sunvold GD, Fahey GC Jr, Merchen NR, and others: Dietary fiber for cats: in vitro fermentation of selected fiber sources by cat fecal inoculum and in vivo utilization of diets containing selected fiber sources and their blends, *J Anim Sci* 73:2329–2339, 1995.

26. Sunvold GD, Titgemeyer EC, Bourquin LD, and others: Fermentability of selected fibrous substrates by cat faecal microflora, *J Nutr* 124:2721S–2722S, 1994.

27. Sunvold GD, Fahey GC Jr, Merchen NR, and others: Dietary fiber for dogs. IV. In vitro fermentation of selected fiber sources by dog fecal inoculum and in vivo digestion and metabolism of fiber-supplemented diets, *J Anim Sci* 73:1099–1109, 1995.

28. Kirkwood JK: The influence of size on the biology of the dog, *J Small Anim Pract* 26:97–110, 1985.

29. Meyer H, Kienzle E, Zentek J: Body size and relative weights of gastrointestinal tract and liver in dogs, *J Vet Nutr* 2:31–35, 1993.

30. Meyer H, Zentek J, Habernoll H, Maskell I: Digestibility and compatibility of mixed diets and faecal consistency in different breeds of dog, *J Vet Med* 46:155–165, 1999.

31. Weber M, Martin L, Biourge V, and others: Influence of age and body size on the digestibility of a dry expanded diet in dogs, *J Anim Physiol Anim Nutr* 87:21–31, 2003.

32. Zentek J: Influence of diet composition on microbial activity in the gastro-intestinal tract of dogs. III. In vitro studies on the metabolic activities of the small-intestinal microflora, *J Anim Physiol Anim Nutr* 74:62–73, 1995.

33. Rolfe VE, Adams CA, Butterwick RF, Batt RM: Relationships between fecal consistency and colonic microstructure and absorptive function in dogs with and without nonspecific dietary sensitivity, *Am J Vet Res* 63:617–622, 2002.

34. Zentek J, Meyer H: The normal handling of diets—are all dogs created equal? *J Small Anim Pract* 36:354–359, 1995.

35. James WT, MacCay CM: A study of food intake, activity, and digestive efficiency in different type dogs, *Am J Vet Res* 11:412–413, 1950.

36. Kendall PT, Blaza SE, Smith PM: Influence of level of intake and dog size on apparent digestibility of dog foods, *Br Vet J* 139:361–362, 1983.

37. Fahey GC, Barry KA, Swanson KS: Age-related changes in nutrient utilization by companion animals, *Ann Rev Nutr* 28:425–445, 2008.

38. Shields RG: Digestibility and metabolizable energy measurement in dogs and cats. In *Proceedings of the petfood forum*, Morris, Ill, 1993, Watts Publishing, pp 21–35.

39. Harper EJ, Turner CL: Age-related changes in apparent digestibility in growing kittens, *Reprod Nutr Dev* 40:249–260, 2000.

40. Kienzle E: Enzymeaktivitaet in pancreas, darmwand und chymus des hundes in abhangigkeit von alter und futterart, *J Anim Physiol Anim Nutr* 60:276–288, 1988.

41. National Research Council: *Nutrient requirements of dogs and cats*, Washington, DC, 2006, National Academy Press.

42. Burkholder WJ: Age-related changes to nutritional requirements and digestive function in adult dogs and cats, *J Am Vet Med Assoc* 215:625–629, 1999.

43. Sheffy BE: The 1985 revision of the National Research Council nutrient requirements of dogs and its impact on the pet food industry. In Burger IH, Rivers IPW, editors: *Nutrition of the dog and cat*, New York, 1989, Cambridge University Press.

44. Huber TL, Wilson RC, McGarity SA: Variations in digestibility of dry dog foods with identical label guaranteed analysis, *J Am Anim Hosp Assoc* 22:571–575, 1986.

45. Association of American Feed Control Officials (AAFCO): Pet food regulations. In *AAFCO Official Publication*, Atlanta, 2008, AAFCO.

46. Douglass GM, Fern EB, Brown RC: Feline plasma and whole blood taurine levels as influenced by commercial dry and canned diets, *J Nutr* 121:S179–S180, 1991.

47. Tarttelin MF: Feline struvite urolithiasis: factors affecting urine pH may be more important than magnesium levels in food, *Vet Rec* 121:227–230, 1987.

48. Gorrel C, Rawlings JM: The role of tooth brushing and diet in the maintenance of periodontal health in dogs, *J Vet Dent* 13:139–143, 1996.

49. Rawlings JM, Gorrel C, Markwell PJ: Effect of two dietary regimens on gingivitis in the dog, *J Small Anim Pract* 38:147–151, 1997.

Feeding Management Throughout the Life Cycle

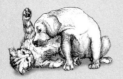

The previous sections have examined basic nutritional principles, the nutrient requirements of dogs and cats, and the different types of diets that can be fed to companion animals. Although knowledge of nutrient requirements and pet foods is essential, an understanding of feeding methods, feeding behavior, and dietary management is also necessary for the provision of optimal nutrition and care. The following section provides practical guidelines for feeding healthy dogs and cats throughout all stages of life. Proper dietary management and care that begins at birth and continues throughout life supports optimal health and vitality in companion animals and ultimately contributes to a quality life and a rewarding human/companion animal relationship.

This section examines feeding management for each stage of life and for different levels of physical activity. Guidelines are provided that help pet owners to properly select the best food for their particular dog or cat during each stage of life. These recommendations provide a starting point for feeding dogs and cats. However, it is important to remember that every dog and cat is an individual. For example, two adult animals of the same breed, age, and relative size in the same household may have significantly different energy and nutrient needs. Pet owners should use general guidelines coupled with regular assessments of their pet's weight, health status, and vigor to evaluate the best way to feed their particular dog or cat.

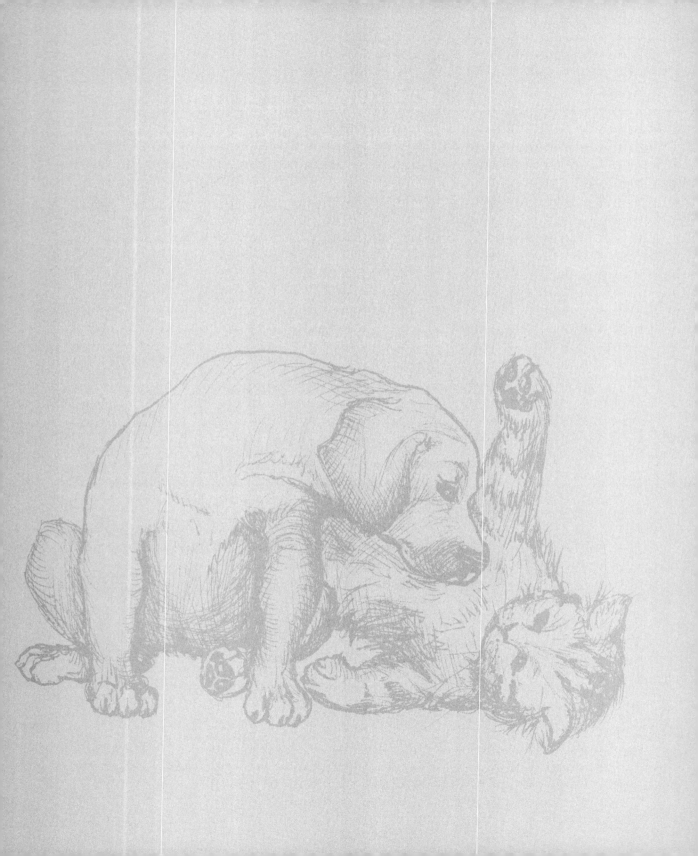

19

Feeding Regimens for Dogs and Cats

NORMAL FEEDING BEHAVIOR

An examination of the way that the wild ancestors of the dog and cat hunted and consumed food provides insight into the normal eating behaviors exhibited by domesticated pets. Both dogs and cats are classified in the order Carnivora, but only cats are true carnivores; dogs are more omnivorous in nature. This difference is manifested by unique anatomical and metabolic characteristics, as well as in the differing ways the two species prefer to obtain and ingest food.

An obvious difference between the domestic dog and cat and their progenitor species is that wild canids and felids were required to expend considerable amounts of energy locating and capturing prey and did not have a reliable source of nutrition. In contrast, our domestic pets are provided with a consistent source of palatable and nutritious foods and they do not generally expend energy to obtain their meals. Despite this difference, domestic dogs and cats still exhibit some of their ancestral hunting and feeding behavior patterns and these behaviors certainly affect mealtime behaviors and interactions with owners.[1]

Dogs

The wolf, the dog's wild relative, obtains much of its food supply by hunting in a pack. Cooperative hunting behaviors allow the wolf to prey on large prey species that would otherwise be unavailable to a wolf hunting alone. As a result, most wolf subspecies tend to be intermittent eaters, gorging themselves immediately after a kill and then not eating again for an extended period of time. Competition between members of the pack at the site of a kill leads to the rapid consumption of food and the social facilitation of eating behaviors. Many wolves and other wild canids also exhibit food hoarding behaviors; small prey or the remainder of a large kill are buried when food is plentiful and later dug up and eaten when food is not readily available.

Like their ancestors, domestic dogs tend to eat rapidly. Although it has been suggested that rapid eating

may be more common in some breeds than in others, there is little empirical evidence for this and a wide range of feeding behaviors are observed among individual dogs, even within breeds.[2] The tendency to eat rapidly can be a problem for some dogs because it may predispose them to choke or swallow large amounts of air. If social facilitation is the cause of rapid eating, feeding the dog separately from other animals, thus removing the competitive aspect of mealtime, often normalizes the rate of eating. In other cases, changing the diet to a food that is less palatable or to one that is difficult to consume rapidly solves the problem. For example, some dogs readily gorge themselves on canned or semimoist foods but return to eating at a normal rate when fed a dry food. The size of kibble pieces can also affect rate of eating, with larger piece size tending to slow rate of eating. Finally, if a dog attempts to eat dry food too quickly, adding water to the dog's food immediately before feeding decreases the rate of eating and minimizes the chance of swallowing large amounts of air. Other approaches include adding a large ball to the bowl or purchasing a feeding bowl that includes a center hub that functions to slow eating rate.

Eating too rapidly can be a problem for some dogs because it may predispose them to choke or swallow large amounts of air. In multiple dog homes, feeding dogs individually to remove the competitive aspect of mealtime helps to normalize the rate of eating. In other cases, adding water to a dry food before feeding, using a specially designed feeding bowl, changing to a food that is less palatable, or feeding a food with larger kibble pieces can decrease rate of eating.

Social facilitation is observed in domestic dogs that are fed together as a group. The most common manifestation of social facilitation occurs when the presence of another animal at mealtime stimulates another dog to consume more food or to eat more rapidly. For example, it is not unusual for a pet owner to comment that his dog was a poor eater until a second dog was introduced into the family. Studies have shown that puppies and dogs usually consume more food when fed as a group, compared with when they are fed alone.[3] If food is available at all times, the effects of social facilitation eventually become minimal. On the other hand, if dogs are fed their meals as a group and have not been trained to eat only from their own bowl (and not to steal from others), competitive interactions and resource guarding behaviors may occur. Training dogs in multiple dog homes to eat only from their own bowls prevents this problem (Box 19-1).

Another form of social facilitation in dogs relates to food preferences and selection. Although there are limited published data available, there is evidence that dogs are capable of learning preferences for novel flavors from other familiar dogs.[4] Dogs also react to human pointing gestures during food selection and some will even select a smaller quantity of food over a larger quantity if their owner directs more attention toward the smaller pile of food.[5] Given the large number of homes today that include more than one dog, the influence that the behavior of other dogs and of the owner may have upon an individual dog's food choice is an important consideration.

Vestiges of the wolf's food hoarding behaviors are often observed in domestic dogs. For example, some dogs frequently bury bones in their yard or hide coveted food items such as biscuits or chew bones in furniture or under beds. However, unlike their wild ancestors, many domestic dogs forget about outdoor hidden caches and rarely return to dig them up. Related activities that are common in dogs are scavenging and coprophagy (stool eating).[6] Many dogs readily consume garbage, carrion, insects, and feces that they encounter in the yard or while out walking.[7,8] Plant eating, in particular grass eating, is also frequently reported by owners. Contrary to popular beliefs, there is no evidence that grass/plant eating in dogs is a sign either of illness or nutrient deficiency.[9,10] Rather, grass eating appears to be a normal canid behavior as it is widespread among wolves and has not been shown to be associated with gastrointestinal upset or the onset of vomiting.[9,11] It has been suggested that plant eating in canid and felid species may play a role similar to that described in chimpanzees, who consume entire leaves from various plants, which then function to purge intestinal parasites as they travel through the gastrointestinal tract.[10,12] It is possible that plant eating evolved in dogs and cats to serve the same function. Although scavenging garbage and coprophagy are considered to be normal behaviors in dogs, these behaviors can present a health and sanitation risk and generally should be prevented. Keeping the yard picked up, using supervision, and teaching dogs a reliable "leave it" command are the best approaches to controlling scavenging and stool-eating behaviors.

The dog's ancestry suggests that an intermittent feeding schedule consisting of large meals interrupted by periods of fasting is the most natural way to feed dogs. However, when dogs are given free access to food, they will consume many small meals frequently throughout the day. This pattern is similar to that seen in cats, with the exception that dogs tend to eat only during the daytime.[3] The domestic dog is quite capable of adapting to a number of different feeding regimens. These regimens include portion-controlled feeding, time-controlled feeding, or free-choice (ad libitum) feeding. These regimens, and the advantages and disadvantages of each, are discussed later in this chapter.

Cats

It is common to think of the domestic cat as a descendant of the wild felid species that prey on large, grazing animals. However, the primary ancestor of the cat is the small, African wild cat, *Felis libyca*. This cat's primary prey are small rodents that are similar in size to field mice.[13] Therefore the immediate ancestor of the cat

---

BOX 19-1   PRACTICAL FEEDING TIPS: METHODS TO DECREASE THE RATE OF EATING

Feed a less palatable food.

Feed a food with larger kibble pieces to encourage chewing.

Add water to the dry food just before serving.

Use a feeding bowl that is designed to slow rate of eating.

Train adult animals to eat only from their own bowl.

Feed puppies from several pans and in different areas.

is not an intermittent feeder like the larger wild cats; rather, it is an animal that feeds frequently throughout the day by catching and consuming a large number of small rodents. Like the majority of wild felids, the African wild cat is a solitary animal, living and hunting alone for much of its life and interacting with others of its species only during mating season. This solitary nature has resulted in an animal that tends to eat slowly and is generally uninhibited by the presence of other animals.

Most domestic cats living in homes consume their food slowly and do not respond to other cats by either increasing the rate of eating or consuming a higher volume of food. In multiple cat homes, cats often eat peaceably from the same bowls either together or at different times of the day. When problems do occur, they are often very subtle, with one or more cats intimidating a less assertive cat and not allowing access to the food bowl or supplanting the cat if he or she was already eating.[14] To prevent this type of feeding problem, several feeding stations located in different areas of the home should always be provided in multiple-cat homes.

If fed free-choice, most cats will nibble at their food throughout the day, as opposed to consuming a large amount of food at one time. Several studies of eating behavior in domestic cats have shown that if food is available free-choice, cats eat frequently and randomly throughout a 24-hour period.[2,15] It is not unusual for a cat to eat between 9 and 16 meals per day, with each meal having a caloric content of only about 23 kilocalories (kcal). (Interestingly, the caloric value of a small field mouse is approximately 30 kcal.) It has been suggested that the eating behaviors observed in domestic cats are similar to those of feral domestic cats eating rodents or other small animals.[16] However, just like the dog, the cat is capable of adapting to several types of feeding schedules.[17]

Domestic cats tend to eat slowly and do not respond to other cats by either increasing the rate of eating or consuming a higher volume of food. In multiple cat homes, cats often eat peaceably from the same bowls either together or at different times of the day. If fed free-choice, cats nibble at the food throughout the day, as opposed to consuming a large amount of food at one time.

WHAT TO FEED

Pet owners have a choice of feeding a commercially prepared food or a homemade diet. Most pet owners prefer the convenience, cost-effectiveness, and reliability of feeding commercial products. The decision of what type of commercial product to feed can be made with an understanding of the advantages and disadvantages of each type of food (see Section 3, pp. 163-167). If a homemade diet is fed, care must be taken to ensure that a complete and balanced ration is prepared, that all ingredients and the final diet are stored safely to avoid spoilage, and that there is consistency of ingredients and nutrient content between batches of food. Surveys have shown that more than 90% of pet owners in the United States continue to feed commercially prepared pet foods as the primary component of their pet's diet.[18] Therefore most of the discussion in this section concerns feeding commercial diets to pets; reference is made to homemade diets in special situations.

One of the most important considerations when choosing a dog or cat food is the pet's stage of life and lifestyle. Nutrient and energy needs differ according to an animal's age, activity level, reproductive status, and health. As knowledge about these needs has increased, specific diets have been developed to efficiently meet the needs of pets during different ages and physiological states.

Several important factors must be considered when selecting a food for dogs and cats in all physiological states. Nutrient content and bioavailability are of primary importance:

▸ The food should provide all of the essential nutrients in adequate amounts and in the proper balance to meet the needs of the pet's lifestyle and stage of life.
▸ The food must supply sufficient energy to maintain ideal body weight or support optimal tissue growth. Caloric needs must be met when the food is fed in an amount that is well within the limits set by the animal's appetite and by the storage and digestive capacity of its gastrointestinal tract.
▸ The food must be appetizing to the dog or cat and should be acceptable when fed as the primary diet over an extended period of time. The form and texture of the food must be appealing and should be easily chewed and ingested.

▶ Feeding the pet food for extended periods of time should support proper gastrointestinal tract functioning and consistently result in the production of regular, firm, and well-formed stools.

▶ The long-term effects of feeding the food must be assessed. The food should support those measurements of vitality and health that are somewhat subjective, such as good coat quality, healthy skin condition, proper body physique and muscle tone, and high energy level (Box 19-2).

WHEN AND HOW TO FEED: FEEDING REGIMENS

There are three primary types of feeding regimens that may be used when feeding dogs and cats. These regimens are called *free-choice* (also called *ad libitum* or *self-feeding*), *time-controlled feeding*, and *portion-controlled feeding*. One method of feeding may be preferred over another, depending on the owner's daily schedule, the number of animals being fed, and the acceptability of the method by the pet or pets.

Free-Choice Feeding

Free-choice feeding involves having a surplus amount of food available at all times. The pet is able to consume as much food as is desired at any time of the day. This type of feeding relies on the animal's ability to self-regulate food intake so that energy and nutrient needs are met. Dry pet food is most suitable for this type of feeding because it will not spoil as quickly as canned food or

---

BOX 19-2 FACTORS TO CONSIDER WHEN SELECTING A PET FOOD

Nutrient content and bioavailability

Palatability and acceptance

Effect on gastrointestinal tract functioning

Caloric density

Diet digestibility

Long-term feeding effects on body condition, skin and coat health and vitality

---

dry out as easily as semimoist products. However, even if dry food is used, the food bowl or dispenser should be cleaned and refilled with fresh food daily. Compared with other feeding methods, free-choice feeding requires the least amount of work and knowledge on the part of the owner. The food and water supply is replenished only one time daily, and it is not necessary to determine the pet's exact daily requirements.

If dogs are fed free-choice in a kennel setting, the kennel noise that usually occurs in response to mealtime will be decreased or eliminated; this fact is considered a distinct advantage by many kennel owners. In addition, the constant presence of food in the kennel can help to relieve boredom that may be associated with confinement and to minimize undesirable behaviors such as coprophagy (stool eating) and excessive barking. Another feeding approach that can help to reduce kennel-related behavior problems is to use food delivery toys. These consist of hard rubber or plastic balls, disks, or other odd shapes that are designed with compartments that hold kibble or soft foods. Depending on the type of toy that is used, the dog must either push the toy around or manipulate the toy with his paws and teeth to obtain the food. These interactive toys can be used to provide part or even most of a dog's daily food and have been used as a form of environmental enrichment in shelters and kennels. Although limited studies of this type of enrichment have been conducted, results suggest that the inclusion of food delivery toys to kenneled dogs who are housed individually relieves boredom, improves activity, and reduces barking.[19,20] Free-choice feeding can also be used in homes or kennels where a group of dogs are housed together and have access to several food dispensers. Feeding in this way ensures that all of the dogs will be able to consume adequate food, because there is always surplus food available. It is important that food dispensers are spaced far enough apart to allow all dogs to eat and to reduce the risk of resource-guarding behaviors.

When dogs are fed free-choice, they tend to consume frequent, small meals throughout the day. This pattern may have an energy balance advantage because a greater meal-induced energy loss occurs when many small meals are consumed, as compared with when one or two large meals are eaten per day.[21] However, this loss is usually more than compensated for by the tendency of dogs that are fed free-choice to increase their total daily food intake. This effect of a free-choice regimen can be an advantage for dogs or cats that are "poor keepers" and do not eat enough to meet their energy needs when fed one or two meals per day. Animals with very high energy needs may also benefit from consuming frequent meals on a free-choice regimen. Feeding numerous small meals per day is often prescribed for pets with dysfunctions in the ability to digest, absorb, or utilize nutrients, and for dogs that have a history of gastric dilatation. However, because free-choice feeding allows the animal rather than the owner to decide when it is time to eat, animals that require frequent feeding as a treatment for medical conditions are better fed on a portion-controlled, rather than a free-choice, basis.

Although free-choice feeding is convenient for the owner, problems such as anorexia or overconsumption may go undetected with this method. If an animal is sick, or one or more dogs are prevented from eating in a group, a change in food intake may not be noticed until the dog has lost substantial weight. If the decreased intake is the result of a medical problem, valuable time may be lost before the problem is diagnosed. The opposite situation, overconsumption and the development of obesity, is fairly common in dogs and cats that are fed free-choice. Although almost all animals are capable of eating to meet their caloric needs, the regulatory mechanisms that control food intake can be overridden if an animal is leading a relatively sedentary lifestyle and is fed a highly palatable and energy-dense food. In this situation, a dog or cat often consumes more energy than is required to meet its daily needs. In growing animals this can result in an accelerated growth rate and increased deposition of body fat; in adult animals it leads to obesity.

Most dogs and cats overconsume when they are first introduced to a free-choice feeding regimen. However, over time many can adjust their intake to meet caloric needs. It is advisable to begin free-choice feeding by setting out a dish of food immediately after the dog or cat has consumed a meal. This extra food helps to prevent engorgement by the pet the first time that a surplus amount of food is available. The ability to adapt to free-choice feeding depends on the physiological state, energy level, temperament, and lifestyle of a pet. Although some adult dogs and cats maintain optimal weight and condition on this type of regimen, others habitually overeat and should not be fed free-choice.

Time-Controlled Meal Feeding

Meal feeding involves controlling either the amount of time that the pet has access to food or the portion size that is fed. Similar to a free-choice regimen, time-controlled feeding relies somewhat on the pet's ability to regulate its daily energy intake. At mealtime, a surplus of food is provided and the pet is allowed to eat for a predetermined period of time. Most adult dogs and cats that are not physiologically stressed are able to consume enough food to meet their daily needs within 15 to 20 minutes. Although one meal per day can be sufficient for feeding adult pets during maintenance, providing two meals per day is healthier and more satisfying. There is some evidence that feeding a large volume of food at one time is a risk factor for with gastric dilatation in large breeds of dogs, so dividing food into two smaller portions per day may be prudent.[22] Moreover, feeding two times per day reduces hunger between meals and minimizes food-associated behavior problems, such as begging and stealing food.

As in the case of free-choice feeding, there are some dogs and cats that do not adapt well to time-controlled feeding. Pets that are very fastidious may not consume enough food within the allotted period. In contrast, other pets use the opportunity to eat voraciously throughout the allotted period. A time-controlled feeding program may actually exacerbate gluttonous behavior because a pet may quickly learn that he must "beat the clock" whenever a meal is offered.

Portion-Controlled Meal Feeding

Portion-controlled feeding is the feeding method of choice in most situations. This procedure allows the owner the greatest amount of control over their pet's diet. One or several meals are provided per day, and meals are premeasured to meet the pet's daily caloric and nutrient needs. As in the case of time-controlled feeding, many adult pets can be maintained on one meal per day, but providing two or more daily meals is preferable. Portion-controlled feeding enables the owner to carefully monitor the pet's food consumption and immediately observe any changes in food intake or eating behavior. The pet's growth and weight can be strictly controlled with this method by adjusting either the amount of food or the type of food that is fed. As a result, conditions of underweight, overweight, or inappropriate growth rate can be corrected at an early stage. Meal feeding is also often preferred by owners because it represents a time of pleasurable interaction with their pets, characterized by daily and familiar feeding routines of communication, petting, and handling.

A disadvantage to portion-controlled feeding is that it demands the greatest time commitment and knowledge on the part of the owner. Guidelines for feeding are provided on the bags or containers of most pet foods; these can be used as a starting point when determining the amount to feed. Additional advice can be obtained from veterinarians, breeders, and pet food companies. The time commitment of portion-controlled feeding is usually not an issue with most pet owners unless very large numbers of animals are involved. Most owners coordinate their pets' meals with their own and find that mealtime becomes an enjoyable routine for both their pets and themselves.

Both dogs and cats are capable of adapting to several types of feeding schedules. The type of feeding regimen used depends on several factors: the owner's schedule, the number of animals being fed, and the pet's acceptance of the feeding method. Meal feeding is often preferred by owners and their pets, because it allows owners to carefully monitor their pet's intake and represents a time of pleasurable interaction each day.

DETERMINING HOW MUCH TO FEED

In all animals, food intake is governed principally by energy requirement. When companion animals are fed free-choice, the underlying control over the amount of food consumed is primarily the animal's need for energy. Although highly palatable or energy-dense foods can override the natural tendency to eat to meet energy needs, energy is still the dietary component that most strongly governs the amount of food consumed. When companion animals are fed on a portion-controlled

basis, owners select a quantity of food based primarily on their pet's weight and appearance, thereby feeding to meet energy needs. If the pet gains too much weight (energy surplus), the owner decreases the amount that is fed. Conversely, if weight is lost, an increased amount of food is provided.

Commercial pet foods are formulated to contain the proper amount of essential nutrients when a quantity is fed that meets the pet's energy requirement. Balancing energy density with nutrient content ensures that when an animal's caloric needs are met, its needs for all other essential nutrients are met by the same quantity of food. Therefore the best way to determine how much to feed a particular animal is to first estimate the animal's energy needs and then calculate the amount of a particular pet food that must be fed to meet that need.

A number of factors affect an individual dog's or cat's energy requirement. These factors include age, reproductive status, body condition, level of activity, breed, temperament, environmental conditions, and health. When determining a pet's energy requirement, these factors are accounted for by adding or subtracting calories from the quantity of food that is determined to support the maintenance energy requirement of the adult pet (see Chapter 9, p. 67). The *maintenance requirement* refers to the amount of energy (kcal/day) necessary to support a normally active adult animal that is not reproducing and is living in a temperate climate. For example, energy needs during the latter stage of gestation in dogs and cats increase from 1.25 to 1.5 times the female's maintenance requirement. If an active 15-kilogram (kg) (33-pound [lb]) bitch is estimated to require 991 calories per day for maintenance, she would require approximately 1239 to 1486 kcal/day at the end of gestation. Using the lower estimate, if a food containing 4500 kcal/kg is fed, this would correspond to approximately 2¾ cups of food per day during gestation, an increase of approximately ½ cup of food (Table 19-1). The information presented later in this section provides estimates for accounting for these factors when estimating the energy requirements of a given animal.

Another way to determine the amount to feed a dog or cat is to use the guidelines included on the commercial pet food label. All pet foods that carry a "complete and balanced" claim are required to include feeding instructions on the product label.[23] These guidelines

TABLE 19-1 DETERMINATION OF QUANTITY TO FEED DURING MAINTENANCE AND GESTATION (15-KG DOG)

	ENERGY REQUIREMENT (KCAL OF METABOLIZABLE ENERGY)		ENERGY DENSITY*		QUANTITY (KG)				LB		OZ				CUPS PER DAY
Maintenance	991	÷	4500	=	0.220	×	2.2	=	0.48	=	7.8	÷	3.5†	=	2.21
Gestation	1239	÷	4500	=	0.275	×	2.2	=	0.60	=	9.7	÷	3.5	=	2.76

*Energy density (kcal/kg) can be obtained from product literature or by contacting the pet food manufacturer.
†An 8-oz measuring cup contains approximately 3.5 oz of dry food.

usually provide estimates of the quantity to feed for several different ranges in body size. Such instructions provide only a rough estimate that can be used as a starting point when first feeding a particular brand of food. Adjustments in these estimates should be made based on the owner's knowledge of the individual animal and on the animal's response to feeding.

Determining how much to feed a dog or cat is based on age, reproductive status, body condition, level of activity, breed, temperament, and environmental conditions. Commercial pet food labels provide general guidelines, but every pet must be evaluated and fed as an individual.

References

1. Bradshaw JWS: The evolutionary basis for the feeding behavior of domestic dogs *(Canis familiaris)* and cats *(Felis catus), J Nutr* 136:1927S–1931S, 2006.

2. Mugford RA: External influences on the feeding of carnivores. In Kare MR, Maller O, editors: *The chemical senses and nutrition,* New York, 1977, Academic Press.

3. Houpt KA: Ingestive behavior: the control of feeding in cats and dogs. In Voith VL, Borchelt PL, editors: *Readings in companion animal behavior,* Trenton, NJ, 1996, Veterinary Learning Systems.

4. Lupfer-Johnosn G, Ross J: Dogs acquire food preferences from interacting with recently fed conspecifics, *Behav Proc* 74:104–106, 2007.

5. Prato-Previde E, Marshall-Pescini S, Valsecchi P: Is your choice my choice? The owners' effect on pet dogs' *(Canis lupus familiaris)* performance in a food choice task, *Anim Cogn* 11:167–174, 2008.

6. Wells DL: Comparison of two treatments for preventing dogs eating their own faeces, *Vet Rec* 153:51–53, 2003.

7. Svartberg K, Forkman B: Personality traits in the domestic dog *(Canis familiaris), Appl Anim Behav Sci* 79:133–155, 2002.

8. Gazzano A, Mariti C, Sighieri C, and others: Survey of undesirable behaviors displayed by potential guide dogs with puppy walkers, *J Vet Behav* 3:104–114, 2008.

9. Sueda KLC, Hare BL, Cliff KD: Characterization of plant eating in dogs, *Appl Anim Behav Sci* 111:120–132, 2008.

10. Hart BL: Why do dogs and cats eat grass? *Vet Med* (Dec 2008):648-649, 2008.

11. Anderson Z: Food habits of wolves *(Canis lupus)* in Latvia, *Acta Theriologica* 49:357–367, 1998.

12. Huffman MA, Canton J: Self-induced increase of gut motility and the control of parasitic infections in wild chimpanzees, *Int J Primatol* 22:329–346, 2001.

13. Serpell JA: The domestication and history of the cat. In Turner DC, Bateson P, editors: *The domestic cat: the biology of its behaviour*, Cambridge, UK, 1988, Cambridge University Press, pp 151–158.

14. Knowles RJ, Curtis TM, Crowell-Davis SL: Correlation of dominance as determined by agonistic interactions with feeding order in cats, *Am J Vet Res* 65:1548–1556, 2004.

15. Kanarek RB: Availability and caloric density of diet as determinants of meal patterns in cats, *Physiol Behav* 15:611–618, 1975.

16. Hart BL, Hart LA: *Canine and feline behavioral therapy*, Philadelphia, 1985, Lea & Febiger.

17. Bradshaw JW, Cook SE: Patterns of pet cat behaviour at feeding occasions, *Appl Anim Behav Sci* 47:61–74, 1996.

18. Laflamme DP, Abood SK, Fascetti AJ, and others: Pet feeding practices of dog and cat owners in the United States and Australia, *J Am Vet Med Assoc* 232:687–694, 2008.

19. Schipper LL, Vinke CM, Schilder MBH, Spruijt BM: The effect of feeding enrichment toys on the behaviour of kenneled dogs (*Canis familiaris*), *Appl Anim Behav Sci* 114:182–195, 2008.

20. Gainew SA, Rooney NJ, Bradshaw JWS: The effect of feeding enrichment upon reported working ability and behavior of kenneled working dogs, *J Forensic Sci* 53:1400–1404, 2008.

21. Leblanc J, Diamond P: The effect of meal frequency on postprandial thermogenesis in the dog (abstract), *Fed Proc* 44:1678, 1985.

22. Raghavan M, Glickman N, McCabe G, and others: Diet-related risk factors for gastric dilatation-volvulus in dogs of high-risk breeds, *J Am Anim Hosp Assoc* 40:192–203, 2004.

23. Association of American Feed Control Officials (AAFCO): Pet food regulations. In *AAFCO official publication*, Atlanta, 2008, AAFCO.

20

Pregnancy and Lactation

It has been observed that successful gestation and lactation in companion animals is the result of a combination of factors. These factors include selection of healthy breeding animals, use of correct breeding management techniques, maintenance of a healthy environment, and the consistent and long-term provision of a proper diet.[1-3] Ideally, the correct feeding and management of reproducing animals begins during growth and development of the dam and sire and continues throughout mating, gestation, and lactation (Boxes 20-1 and 20-2).

PREBREEDING FEEDING AND CARE

The selection of breeding animals should include screening for any faults or anomalies that are believed to be genetically transmissible.[4,5] All animals should also undergo a thorough assessment of temperament, structure, and health before being admitted into a breeding program. Conformation shows and various types of performance tests can be used by breeders to evaluate their animals and compare them to established breed standards. Once an adult dog or cat has been selected for breeding, a complete physical examination should be administered. This should include a fecal check for internal parasites, serological tests for brucellosis and herpesvirus in dogs, and the administration of any required vaccinations.

Before breeding, both the sire and the dam should be in excellent physical condition, well-exercised, and not overweight or underweight. It is especially important that the dam be at optimum weight and in prime condition. If the dam is underweight, she may be unable to consume enough food during gestation to provide for her own nutritional needs as well as the needs of her developing fetuses. Lack of proper nutrition in the dam can result in decreased birth weight and increased neonatal mortality. Conversely, an overweight condition in the dam can lead to the development of very large fetuses and dystocia.

At least 2 weeks prior to breeding the queen or bitch should be transitioned (if needed) to a high-quality, highly digestible food that is adequate for gestation and lactation. Changing to this diet early in the dam's reproductive cycle allows her to be fully adjusted to the new food when breeding takes place and prevents the need to abruptly change diets during either gestation or lactation. Pet foods that have increased nutrient density are needed because of the increased nutrient and energy requirements of reproduction. Feeding a nutrient-dense food allows these needs to be met without excess food consumption, thus avoiding the likelihood of gastrointestinal upset or weight loss. The bitch or queen should be fed this food throughout pregnancy and lactation. For dogs, the food should contain animal-based protein as the primary protein source at a level of 28% to 30% (as fed).[6] Protein level for a reproducing queen should be slightly higher (~32%).[3] Energy density of the food should be relatively high; generally at least 20% fat (as fed) is recommended.

Both omega-6 and omega-3 fatty acids should be supplied in the diet, ideally balanced in a ratio between 5:1 and 10:1. This is important because a female's essential fatty acid (EFA) status is negatively influenced by the physiological stress of pregnancy and lactation.[7] This risk is greatest in females who have had multiple litters.[8] This occurs because an increased supply of EFAs are needed during gestation and lactation to supply fetal tissues with fatty acids via the placenta and after birth through the milk. Of particular importance to reproducing females and their developing fetuses is the n-3 fatty acid docosahexaenoic acid (DHA). DHA is essential for normal neurological and retinal development in puppies and kittens (see Chapter 21, p. 211).[9] Because adult animals have a limited ability to synthesize DHA from alpha-linolenic acid, the best way to supply developing fetuses and neonates with DHA (and other essential long-chain polyunsaturated fatty acids) is through enrichment of the mother's diet during pregnancy and lactation.[10,11]

BOX 20-1   PRACTICAL FEEDING TIPS: GESTATION

Feed a food that is highly digestible and energy- and nutrient-dense.

Do not increase feed intake until the fifth or sixth week of gestation (dogs).

Provide several small meals per day during late gestation.

Increase feed intake to approximately 1.25 to 1.5 times maintenance by the end of gestation.

Dams should gain no more than 15% to 25% of body weight by the end of gestation.

Dams should weigh 5% to 10% above normal body weight after whelping.

BOX 20-2   PRACTICAL FEEDING TIPS: LACTATION

Feed a diet that is highly digestible and energy- and nutrient-dense.

Provide adequate calories to prevent excess weight loss.

Provide clean, fresh water on a free-choice basis.

Feed two to three times maintenance during peak lactation.

Provide free-choice feeding or several small meals per day during peak lactation.

Slowly reduce dam's intake after fourth week of lactation.

A final consideration is the level of antioxidants in the food. During gestation, females experience increased oxidative stress as a result of the increased oxygen consumption and altered metabolism that is associated with pregnancy.[12,13] Although limited studies have been conducted with companion animals, one study reported reduced antioxidant status in female dogs during gestation.[14] These changes, when considered in combination with recommendations to increase dietary EFAs during pregnancy, suggest that antioxidant nutrients such as vitamin E, vitamin A, and magnesium should also be increased in foods that are selected for pregnant bitches.

A high-quality, highly digestible food with slightly increased protein and a relatively high energy density should be selected for reproducing bitches and queens. Optimal levels of omega-6 to omega-3 fatty acids are needed, and should be balanced in a ratio ranging between 5:1 and 10:1 and should contain adequate levels of docosahexaenoic acid and other essential fatty acids. The food should also contain sufficient concentrations of antioxidants to offset the oxidative stress that is associated with pregnancy.

FEEDING MANAGEMENT DURING GESTATION AND PARTURITION

Bitches

In pregnant bitches, less than 30% of fetal growth in size occurs during the first 5 weeks of pregnancy.[15] Although the fetuses are developing rapidly, they are very small until the last third of the 9-week gestation (Figure 20-1). As a result, there is only a slight increase in the dam's weight and total nutritional needs during the first 5 weeks of gestation (Figure 20-2).[16] After the fifth week, fetal weight and size increase rapidly for the remaining 3 to 4 weeks of gestation. In the dog, more than 75% of weight, and at least half of fetal length, is attained between the fortieth and fifty-fifth day of gestation.[17] Although optimal nutrition is important throughout reproduction, it is especially crucial during the last few weeks of gestation to ensure optimal fetal growth and development.

If a bitch is at ideal weight at the time of breeding, no increase in food intake is necessary until the fifth week of gestation. Contrary to popular belief, a bitch should not receive a greater amount of food immediately after she has been bred. An increase of food at this time is unnecessary and could lead to excessive weight gain during pregnancy. It is not unusual for bitches to undergo a transient period of appetite loss at approximately 3 weeks of gestation. However, this change lasts for only a few days and is usually not a health concern. After the fifth or sixth week of pregnancy, the bitch's food intake should be increased gradually so that at the time of whelping her daily intake is approximately 25%

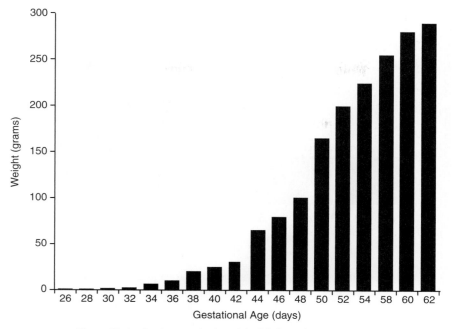

Figure 20-1   Fetal puppy body weight (g) throughout gestation.

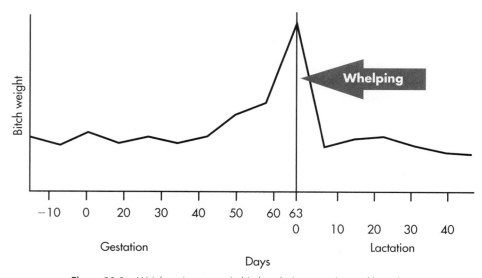

Figure 20-2   Weight gain pattern in bitches during gestation and lactation.

to 50% higher than her normal maintenance needs, depending on the size of the litter and the size of the bitch (Figure 20-3). Her body weight should increase by approximately 15% to 25% by the time of whelping. Using the previous example, a bitch whose optimum

weight is 15 kilograms (kg) (33 pounds [lb]) should weigh between 17 and 19 kg (37 and 41 lb) at the end of her pregnancy.

As the developing puppies increase in size, there is a reduction in the abdominal space available for expansion

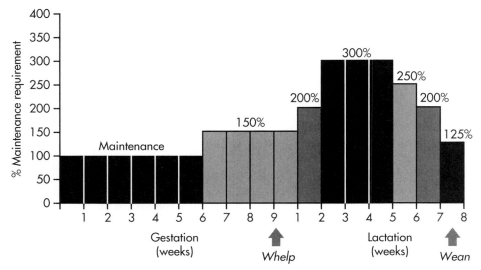

Figure 20-3   Nutritional needs of the bitch during gestation and lactation.

of the bitch's digestive tract after a meal. Therefore it is helpful to provide several small meals per day during the last few weeks of gestation so that abdominal space does not limit the bitch's ability to consume an adequate quantity of food. It is important to provide enough food during this period because dams that are underweight during middle and late gestation may have difficulty maintaining body condition for the high demands of milk production that occur during lactation. Likewise, it is also important not to overfeed pregnant bitches. Excessive intake and weight gain will be reflected in heavier fetuses and may result in complications at the time of whelping.

> *During the later stages of gestation, it is advisable to feed females several small meals per day to ensure that she is able to consume an adequate quantity of food. It is important to provide enough food during this period because dams that are underweight during middle and late gestation may have difficulty maintaining body condition for the high demands of milk production that occur during lactation.*

Mammary gland development and milk production occur 1 to 5 days before parturition, and many bitches refuse all food approximately 12 hours before whelping.

A slight drop in body temperature, occurring 12 to 18 hours before the start of labor, is a fairly reliable indicator of impending parturition.

Once the bitch has whelped the litter and expelled all of the fetal placentas, and when her puppies are resting normally, she should be provided with fresh water and food. Most bitches will begin eating within 24 hours of whelping. If necessary, the dam's appetite can be stimulated by moistening her food with warm water. Adding water to the food also ensures that adequate fluid is consumed, which is an important consideration. If the bitch has been adequately prepared for lactation, she should have a postwhelping weight that is 5% to 10% above her prebreeding maintenance weight (Table 20-1).

Queens

The weight gain pattern that occurs in pregnant queens is slightly different from that observed in bitches (Figure 20-4).[18] Although most of the bitch's weight increase occurs during the last third of gestation, pregnant queens exhibit a linear increase in weight beginning around the second week of gestation. A second difference between bitches and queens involves the type of weight that is gained during pregnancy. In dogs, almost all of the preparturition gain is lost at whelping. In contrast, weight loss immediately following parturition in

TABLE 20-1 RECOMMENDED FEEDING GUIDELINES FOR REPRODUCING BITCHES

PERIOD	ENERGY INTAKE RELATIVE TO MAINTENANCE	FEEDINGS PER DAY	COMMENTS
Maintenance	100%	2	Maintenance intake = kcals needed to maintain optimal body condition
Prebreeding	100%	2	Bitches should be fed to maintain optimal condition (i.e., no weight gain)
Gestation (Weeks 1-4)	100%	2-3	Gradually increase to 3 portions per day by the fourth or fifth week
Gestation (Week 5)	Gradual increase to 125%-150%	2-3	Gradually increase to 3 portions per day by the fourth or fifth week
Gestation (Week 6 to whelping)	125% -150%	3-4	By end of gestation, female's BW increase should be ~15%-25% above optimal BW
Lactation (Week 1)	150%-200%	4-6	Postwhelping BW should be ~10-15 above optimal BW
Lactation (Weeks 2-5)	200%-300%	4-6	If 4 or more feedings per day are not possible, female should be fed free-choice
Lactation (Week 6 to weaning)	Gradual reduction to 150%	4-6	Puppies are consuming primarily solid food by the end of week 6
Postweaning (Weeks 1-2)	125%-150%	2-3	Feed to regain any weight that was lost during lactation
Postweaning (Week 3 and after)	100%	2	Feed to attain and maintain optimal body weight and condition

Adapted from Coffman M, Kelley RL: Managing the brood bitch. In *Raising beagle puppies: Iams open brace beagle championship,* Camden-Hamilton, Ohio, June 15-16, 2001, Iams, p 16.
BW, Body weight.

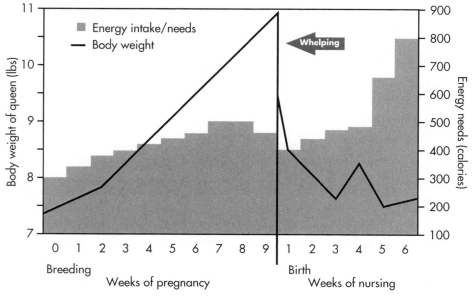

Figure 20-4   Weight gain pattern in queens during gestation and lactation.

the cat accounts for only 40% of the weight that was gained during pregnancy. The remaining 60% of the queen's weight gain is body fat and is gradually lost during lactation. Thus it appears that the queen is able to prepare for the excessive demands of lactation by accumulating surplus body energy stores during gestation.

Similar to dogs, female cats should be fed a diet, that is intended for reproduction throughout gestation and lactation. Litter size is positively influenced by the provision of adequate fat in the queen's diet, and fat in the diet should provide optimal levels of EFAs, particularly arachidonic acid.[19] Taurine is also an important nutrient to consider because both conception rate and kitten birth weight are reduced in queens when dietary taurine is limiting.[3,20] The amount of food that the queen receives should be gradually increased beginning the second week of gestation and continuing until parturition (see Figure 20-4). At the end of gestation, the queen should be receiving approximately 25% to 50% more food than her normal maintenance needs. Because most cats adapt well to free-choice feeding, this is often the best way to provide the pregnant queen with adequate nutrition during pregnancy. The queen's weight gain should be monitored closely to prevent excessive weight gain during this time. Queens typically gain between 12% and 38% of their prepregnancy body weight by the end of gestation.[21]

FEEDING MANAGEMENT DURING LACTATION

For both bitches and queens, the most important nutritional considerations during lactation are calories and water. Ample energy intake allows for sufficient milk production and prevents drastic weight loss in the dam. For example, Beagle puppies require approximately 5.5 ounces of milk per day. For an average litter size, this translates to the production of more than a quart of milk per day in a Beagle bitch.[22] Large-breed dogs produce substantially more than this volume. In addition, because milk is 78% water, a female's water requirement increases drastically during lactation. Ample water intake is essential for the production of a sufficient volume of milk. The high water turnover rate of newborn puppies and kittens adds further to the mother's daily water requirements.[23]

The degree of stress that lactation imposes on the bitch or queen depends on the dam's nutritional status and weight at parturition, her litter size, and her stage of lactation. Females with large litters and those that have minimal body energy stores at parturition are at greatest risk for excessive weight loss and malnourishment during lactation. Because a lactating bitch or queen will sacrifice her own body condition to continue to produce an adequate quantity of nutrient-rich milk, feeding females to prevent loss of condition and nutrient depletion is of utmost concern.

Depending on the size of the litter, a bitch or queen will consume two to three times her maintenance energy requirement during lactation (see Figures 20-3 and 20-4). A general guideline is to feed 1.5 to 2 times the mother's maintenance needs during the first week of lactation, 2 times maintenance during the second week, and 2.5 to 3 times maintenance during the third to fourth week of lactation.[24] Peak lactation occurs at 3 to 4 weeks postpartum and is followed by the introduction of solid or semisolid food to the litter. After the fourth week, the amount of milk consumed by the puppies and kittens will decrease as their solid food intake gradually increases. Many pet foods formulated for adult maintenance do not provide sufficient nutrient density for a bitch or queen during lactation. For example, early studies with lactating bitches found that when a diet containing approximately 4200 kilocalories (kcal)/kg (1900 kcal/lb) was fed, little or no weight loss occurred during the entire period of lactation. However, bitches with four or more puppies that were fed a diet with a lower energy density (3100 kcal/kg) lost weight during lactation.[25]

A highly digestible, nutrient-dense diet should be fed to all lactating queens and bitches, regardless of litter size. Premium pet foods that are formulated for growth, performance, or high activity are recommended because these foods are formulated to provide optimal levels of energy and nutrients to pets that are experiencing conditions of physiological stress. Even when a premium-quality food is fed, the quantity of food that the dam requires during peak lactation may exceed the capacity of her gastrointestinal tract. Therefore the daily ration should be divided into several meals or should be fed free-choice. After 3 weeks, it is advisable to feed the bitch and queen separately from the litter to prevent the puppies and kittens from consuming the dam's food.

Fresh, cool water should always be readily accessible to the lactating queen and bitch.

By 3 to 4 weeks of age, puppies and kittens begin to be interested in solid food. At the same time, the dam's interest in nursing starts to decline. As this occurs, the dam's daily food intake should be slowly reduced. By the time that the puppies and kittens are of weaning age (7 to 8 weeks), the dam's food consumption should be less than 50% above her normal maintenance needs (see Table 20-1).

The most important nutritional considerations for reproducing females during lactation are calories and water. Providing enough calories and free access to plenty of fresh water will support optimal milk production and prevent drastic weight loss in the mother during the physiological stressful period of lactation.

FEEDING THE DAM DURING WEANING

Bitches and queens naturally begin the gradual process of weaning when their puppies and kittens are about 5 to 6 weeks of age. Most breeders impose complete weaning by 7 to 9 weeks of age so that the puppies and kittens can be transferred to their new homes. Puppies and kittens that begin eating solid food at 3 to 4 weeks of age are usually consuming the major portion of their diet in the form of solid food by the time they are 6 to 7 weeks old (see Chapter 21, pp. 212-213).

If the dam continues to produce milk immediately before weaning, several days of limited feeding aids in decreasing milk production. If milk production is allowed to continue at a high level during weaning, there is an increased chance for the dam to develop mastitis. All food should be withheld from the dam on the day of weaning, provided she is in good physical condition. The dam's daily ration should then be gradually reintroduced at 25%, 50%, 75%, and, finally, 100% of her maintenance level on successive postweaning days (see Table 20-1).

In general, bitches and queens lose some weight during lactation, but the amount should not exceed 10% of their normal body weight. Proper feeding and management during gestation and lactation ensure that weight loss is minimized, even when large litters are raised. The condition of the bitch or queen at the time of breeding influences her ability to withstand the stresses of gestation and lactation and significantly affects her body condition at the end of the reproductive cycle. An animal that is in poor condition when bred loses greater amounts of weight than is desirable and will require an extended period of repletion after weaning. The repletion period allows the dam's body to regain stores of nutrients lost during gestation and lactation. Continuing to feed the nutrient and energy dense food that was used for gestation and lactation for at least 3 weeks after weaning will support optimal nutrient repletion in the bitch and queen.[26]

SUPPLEMENTATION DURING GESTATION AND LACTATION

It is not unusual for dog and cat breeders to add nutrient supplements to the diets of their females during gestation and lactation. Regardless of the belief that this can be helpful, it is important to understand that an animal will only show a positive health response to supplementation when the food that is being fed fails to supply optimal nutrition. Therefore, it is safer (and often more economical) to instead select a food that is designed to support optimal health of a female and her fetuses throughout breeding, gestation, and lactation, as opposed to feeding a suboptimal food and attempting to correct nutrient deficiencies through supplementation.

The most common essential nutrient that is supplemented during pregnancy, especially in dogs, is calcium. Breeders may supply calcium either through mineral supplements or by adding calcium-containing foods, such as cottage cheese or other dairy products, to their dog's food. The added mineral is believed to ensure healthy fetal development during pregnancy and aid in milk production during lactation. However, lactating bitches naturally regulate the deposition and mobilization of their body's calcium reserves in response to the need for milk production. Calcium homeostasis is tightly controlled by several hormones, most importantly parathyroid hormone (PTH) and calcitonin. PTH is secreted in response to decreased serum calcium concentrations during periods of high need (i.e., milk production).

It functions to increase skeletal resorption of calcium by promoting osteoclastic activity and also increase the efficiency of calcium absorption in the small intestine.

Dietary supplementation with calcium maintains serum calcium levels and causes down-regulation of PTH synthesis and secretion. Ultimately this reduces the pregnant female's ability to meet the high demands for calcium mobilization that occur with the onset of lactation. If this effect is severe, especially in small or toy breeds, the mother is at risk of developing eclampsia (also called *puerperal tetany*). Eclampsia most commonly occurs at parturition or 2 to 3 weeks later and is caused by a failure of the female's calcium-regulating mechanisms to maintain serum calcium levels when calcium is being lost via milk during lactation. Hypocalcemia develops and the dog develops ataxia, muscular tetany,

and convulsive seizures. Dogs respond well to intravenous treatment with calcium borogluconate, but the disorder can be life-threatening if not detected and treated promptly. Although calcium needs are high during both gestation and lactation, the bitch and queen normally obtain the additional nutrient requirements through consumption of higher amounts of the normal diet. Therefore calcium supplementation is unnecessary and, given the risk for developing eclampsia, contraindicated.

During pregnancy, supplementation with calcium or any other mineral is not necessary or recommended if a well-balanced, high-quality commercial food is fed.

References

1. Kelley R: Nutritional management of the bitch: pre-breeding to whelping. In *Proc Symp Canine Repro for Breeders*, Westminster Kennel Club Dog Show, New York, February 2001, pp 14-17.

2. Lawler DF, Bebiak DM: Nutrition and management of reproduction in the cat, *Vet Clin North Am Small Anim Pract* 16:495–519, 1986.

3. Kelley RI: The effect of nutrition on feline reproduction. In *Proceedings of the society for theriogenology*, 2003, pp 354–361.

4. Battaglia CL: Selecting sires. In *Proc Tufts Anim Expo Symp*, Boston, 2001, pp 20–23.

5. Giger U: Diagnosis and management of hereditary disease in the dog. In *Proceedings of the society for theriogenology*, 1996, pp 152–154.

6. Kelley RL: Factors influencing canine reproduction and nutritional management of the pregnant bitch. In *Proc Tufts Anim Expo Symp*, Boston, 2001, pp 9–14.

7. Holman RT, Johnson SB, Osburn PL: Deficiency of essential fatty acids and membrane fluidity during pregnancy and lactation, *Proc Natl Acad Sci U S A* 88:4835–4839, 1991.

8. Kelley RL, Lepine AJ, Ruffing J, and others: Impact of maternal dietary DHA and reproductive activity on DHA status in the canine. In *Proc 6th Cong Internat Soc Study Fatty Acids Lipids*, 2004, p 149.

9. Lauritzen L, Hansen HS, Jorgensen MH, Michaelson KE: The essentiality of long-chain n-3 fatty acids in relation to development and function of the brain and retina, *Prog Lipid Res* 40:1–94, 2001.

10. Bauer JE, Heinemann KM, Bigley KE, and others: Maternal diet alpha-linolenic acid during gestation and lactation does not increase canine milk docosahexaenoic acid, *J Nutr* 134:2035S–2038S, 2004.

11. Heinemann M, Waldron MK, Bigley KE: Long-chain (n-3) polyunsaturated fatty acids are more efficient than alpha-linolenic acid in improving electroretinogram responses of puppies exposed during gestation, lactation, and weaning, *J Nutr* 135:1960–1966, 2005.

12. Poston L, Raijmakers TM: Trophoblast oxidative stress, antioxidants and pregnancy outcome—a review, *Placenta* 25:S72–S78, 2004.

13. Liurba E, Garatacos E, Martin-Gallan P, and others: A comprehensive study of oxidative stress and antioxidant status in pre-eclampsia and normal pregnancy, *Free Radical Biol Med* 37:557–570, 2004.

14. Vannucchi CI, Jordao AA, Vannucchi H: Antioxidant compounds and oxidative stress in female dogs during pregnancy, *Res Vet Sci* 83:188–193, 2007.

15. Bebiak DM, Lawler DF, Reutzel LF: Nutrition and management of the dog, *Vet Clin North Am Small Anim Pract* 17:505–533, 1987.

16. Lepine A: Feeding management of the reproductive cycle. In *Proc North Am Vet Conf,* 1997, pp 27–29.

17. Moser D: Feeding to optimize canine reproductive efficiency, *Probl Vet Med* 4:545–550, 1992.

18. Loveridge GG: Bodyweight changes and energy intake of cats during gestation and lactation, *Anim Tech* 37:7–15, 1986.

19. MacDonald ML, Anderson BC, Rogers QR, and others: Essential fatty acid requirements of cats: pathology of essential fatty acid deficiency, *Am J Vet Res* 45:1310–1317, 1984.

20. Jayawickrama L, Jacobsen K, Lepine AJ, and others: Factors affecting milk intake of kittens, *FASEB J* 12:A836, 1998.

21. Kustritz MVR: Clinical management of pregnancy in cats, *Theriogenology* 66:145–150, 2006.

22. Oftedal O: Lactation in the dog: milk composition and intake by puppies, *J Nutr* 114:803–812, 1984.

23. Lepine AJ: Nutritional considerations affecting canine reproduction. In *Proc NAVC,* 1997, pp 23–27.

24. Coffman M: Care and feeding of the lactating bitch. In *Proc Symp Canine Repro for Breeders,* Westminster Kennel Club Dog Show, New York, February 2001, pp 21–24.

25. Ontko JA, Phillips PH: Reproduction and lactation studies with bitches fed semi-purified diets, *J Nutr* 65:211–218, 1958.

26. Kelley R: Managing the brood bitch. In *Vital health care and management of competitive dogs, Proc Iams breeders' symposium series,* 2003, pp 22–28.

21

Nutritional Care of Neonatal Puppies and Kittens

The neonatal period in puppies and kittens is considered to be the first 2 weeks after birth. The offspring of dogs and cats are *altricial*, which means that puppies and kittens are born in a relatively immature state and are completely dependent upon their mother's care. Because of this immature state, preweaning mortality estimates for puppies and kittens are estimated to be as high as 40%, and the vast majority of deaths occur during the neonatal period.[1] As more information has become available about the needs of newborns, it is apparent that proper nutritional support during this time is essential for maintaining health and preventing neonatal illness and mortality.

The first 36 hours of a puppy's or kitten's life are a critical time because the process of birth and the sudden environmental changes that newborns experience are physiologically stressful. Therefore every effort should be made during this time to minimize stress and variations in the environment. A quiet, warm whelping/queening area should be provided, and human visitors outside of the immediate family should be prevented from disturbing the litter during the first few days.

COMPOSITION OF NATURAL MILK

Like all mammals, female dogs and cats produce a special type of milk called *colostrum* during the first few days following parturition. Colostrum provides both specialized nutrition and passive immunity to newborn puppies and kittens. Passive immunity is provided in the form of immunoglobulins (antibodies) and other bioactive factors that are absorbed across the intestinal mucosa of newborns. Most of these factors are large, intact proteins. Once absorbed into the body, passively acquired antibodies offer protection from a number of infectious diseases. Because the immune system of puppies and kittens is not fully developed until they are about 16 weeks of age, the transfer of this protective immunity from the mother to newborns via colostrum

is important for their survival. In addition to antibodies, examples of bioactive factors found in colostrum include lysozyme, a bacteriolytic enzyme that prevents the growth of certain types of bacteria, and bile salt–activated lipase, which aides in the digestion of fat.[2,3]

In some species, such as humans, rats, rabbits, and guinea pigs, a significant proportion of passive immunity is acquired prior to birth (in utero). In contrast, puppies and kittens, like pigs, horses, and ruminant species, obtain the greatest proportion of maternally derived antibodies through the colostrum. These differences are due to the types of placentas found in different species, reflecting the number of placental layers that antibodies must transverse to reach developing fetuses. The dog and cat have an endotheliochorial placenta consisting of four layers. This type of placenta allows only about 10% to 20% of passive immunity to be transferred in utero. Therefore, for puppies and kittens, the major proportion of passive immunity is acquired after birth via the colostrum. This emphasizes the importance of immediate nursing and the provision of colostral antibodies and bioactive factors to puppies and kittens immediately after birth.

In older neonates and adult animals, normal digestive processes would result in the complete digestion of the immunological compounds found in colostrum, making them unavailable to the body as immune mediators. However, the intestinal mucosa of newborn dogs and cats is capable of absorbing intact immunoglobulins provided by colostrum. The time during which the newborn's gastrointestinal tract is permeable to the intact immunoglobulins in colostrum is very short. The term *closure* refers to the change in the gastrointestinal tract's absorptive capacity that precludes further absorption of large, intact proteins. The mechanisms behind closure are not fully understood, but they appear to be hormonally mediated, possibly related to increased circulating insulin that appears after the initiation of suckling.[4] This limits the ability of the neonatal intestine to absorb intact proteins to about the first 48 hours of life.[5] Therefore it is vitally important that newborn puppies and kittens receive adequate colostrum as soon as possible during the first day after birth.

Within the first 24 hours after birth, colostrum provides intact immunoglobulins and other bioactive factors which function to protect puppies and kittens from infectious diseases. The nutrient content of colostrum differs significantly from mature milk, and its protective components are absorbed for just a short period of time following birth.

In addition to the immunological benefits of colostrum, the volume of fluid ingested immediately after birth contributes significantly to postnatal circulating volume.[1] A lack of adequate fluid intake shortly after birth can contribute to circulatory failure in newborns. Water turnover is very high in neonates, necessitating high fluid intake to maintain normal blood volume throughout the neonatal period.[5] For this reason, the consistent ingestion of adequate fluids by neonates and the production of sufficient milk volume by the mother are as important as the milk's nutrient content.

Like the milk of many mammalian species, dog and cat mammary secretions change during lactation to effectively meet the needs of their developing young. Several forms of colostrum are produced during the first 24 to 72 hours after birth, after which the composition slowly transforms to mature milk. The protein content in cat colostrum that is produced on the first day of lactation is very high (greater than 8%); however, protein rapidly declines to about half this value by the third day of lactation.[6,7] Protein concentration then slowly increases throughout lactation to again reach a concentration of about 8%. Lipid concentration in cat milk follows a similar pattern. On the first day of lactation, the total lipid concentration is relatively high, but rapidly decreases until the third day of lactation. Values then gradually increase until the forty-second day of lactation, after which they decline slightly.[6,8] In addition to the stage of lactation, the queen's diet can also affect the fat content of queen's milk. For example, queens fed a food that contained 22% crude fat (dry-matter [DM] basis) produced milk containing up to 17% fat.[9] Lastly, lactose concentrations in cat milk stay relatively constant or increase slightly throughout lactation (Table 21-1).

TABLE 21-1 AVERAGE NUTRIENT COMPOSITION OF DOG AND CAT MILK

	DOG MILK	CAT MILK
Protein (%)	8-10	7-8
Lactose (%)	3-4	3-4
Fat (%)	11-13	5-7
Calcium (mg/L)	1400-2200	700-1800
Magnesium (mg/L)	90-100	65-70
Iron (mg/L)	2-7	8-9
Zinc (mg/L)	4-6	6-7
Copper (mg/L)	1.0-1.4	1.0
Energy (kcal/L)	1500-1800	850-1600

Adapted from Adkins Y, Lepine AJ, Lonnerdal B: Changes in protein and nutrient composition of milk throughout lactation in dogs, *Am J Vet Res* 62:1266–1272, 2001; and Dobenecker B, Zottmann B, Kienzle E, Zentek J: Investigations on milk composition and milk yield in queens, *J Nutr* 128:2618S–2619S, 1998.

The nutrient pattern of dog's milk is somewhat different. The most recent study reported that while milk protein is very high on the first day of lactation (>10%), it decreases gradually for the following 3 weeks and then, after day 21, increases slightly until weaning.[10] This is in contrast to an earlier study that reported a pattern of change that was similar to that of cat's milk.[11] The lipid content of dog's milk is higher than that reported for cat's milk and does not show the dramatic decrease early in lactation that is reported for cat mammary secretions. Because of this higher fat content and possibly due to its slightly higher protein concentration, dog's milk is higher in energy than cat's milk. In both species the total energy content of the milk decreases gradually from colostrum to the milk that is produced during midlactation. Energy concentration then increases until weaning in both species. Lactose concentration in dog's milk is lowest in colostrum and increases gradually until midlactation (see Table 21-1).

The type of protein found in the milk is also an important consideration. In cats, colostrum protein has a casein-to-whey ratio of about 40:60.[6] This ratio shifts to a slight predominance of casein as the colostrum transitions to mature milk, with a final ratio of about 60:40. This shift from a predominance of whey early in lactation to a predominance of casein is also seen in humans and horses. It is significant because the amount of casein in the milk may affect protein digestion, mineral utilization, and the milk's amino acid composition.[12] In contrast, the casein-to-whey ratio in dog's milk is more similar to that of humans and cows in that casein predominates throughout lactation and remains relatively constant at a ratio of 70:30.[10]

Calcium concentrations in dog and cat milk are similar, increasing in both species over the course of lactation. The concentrations of protein and calcium in milk are highly correlated during lactation because casein has a high calcium-binding capacity.[10,11] The milk of both dogs and cats also has a relatively high iron concentration. These two species are similar to the rat and several marsupial species in their ability to concentrate iron in their milk at a level that is substantially higher than the concentration found circulating in the mother's plasma. The high iron content in milk may reflect a high requirement for this mineral early in life. Similar to other nutrients, iron concentration is strongly influenced by the stage of lactation, with values increasing slightly during the first 2 days of lactation and then gradually declining (see Table 21-1).[13]

The fatty acid profile of mother's milk has received considerable interest in recent years in response to recognition of the importance of long-chain polyunsaturated fatty acids (PUFAs) to fetal and neonatal development. As discussed in Chapter 20, maternal essential fatty acid (EFA) status is depleted during reproduction, and this effect is exacerbated by an increasing number of parities.[14] When maternal EFA status is supported by feeding a diet with an improved fatty acid profile, litter size is positively affected.[15] This effect is most pronounced in females who have had several litters. The same series of studies found that puppies of mothers who were fed a high EFA food that was balanced for both linoleic acid (n-6) and alpha-linolenic acid (n-3) PUFAs had a higher EFA status at birth than did puppies born to mothers fed a diet containing a less favorable EFA profile. This effect was most pronounced for the n-3 PUFA docosahexaenoic acid (DHA), which is necessary for normal retinal and neurological development in neonates.

Enrichment of milk with long-chain PUFAs is dependent upon the types of EFAs that are included in the maternal diet. A study of the effect of the maternal diet on fatty acid profiles in canine mammary secretions found that concentrations of the two 18-carbon parent fatty acids, n-6 and n-3, in milk increased in parallel with an increase in these fatty acids in the maternal diet.[16]

However, an important finding of this study was that the milk did not become enriched with the respective derived fatty acids, arachidonic acid (AA) from linoleic acid, and DHA, eicosapentaenoic acid (EPA), or docosapentaenoic acid (DPA) from alpha-linolenic acid. These findings are in agreement with those reported in humans and suggest that supplementation of maternal diets with linoleic acid and alpha-linolenic acid does not provide an effective approach for increasing the long-chain PUFAs in milk.[17] Recent studies have shown that while newborn puppies can convert milk alpha-linolenic acid to DHA early in life, they lose this ability after weaning.[18] Even prior to weaning, the efficiency of conversion is very low, so very large doses of alpha-linolenic acid are necessary to see a significant increase in tissue DHA levels.[19] Both AA and DHA are essential during perinatal life; DHA is especially crucial for normal neurological and retinal development.[20,21] Therefore it is prudent to provide a food to the mother that contains n-3 and n-6 long-chain PUFAs during gestation and lactation to ensure adequate enrichment of her milk with these EFAs. This is the best approach to ensuring a supply of AA and DHA to puppies and kittens during the perinatal period (see Chapter 22, pp. 228-229 for additional information about DHA and development).

NORMAL DEVELOPMENT OF PUPPIES AND KITTENS

The two primary activities of all newborns are eating and sleeping. During the first few weeks of life, puppies and kittens should nurse every few hours, at a minimum of four to six times per day. The frequent intake of small amounts of milk is necessary because of the small size of the neonate's stomach. Infrequent or weak nursing often signifies chilling, illness, or congenital problems and should be attended to immediately by a knowledgeable breeder or veterinarian. The eyes of puppies and kittens open between 10 and 16 days after birth and their ears begin to function between 15 and 17 days after birth. Normal body temperature for puppies is 94° Fahrenheit (F) to 97° F for the first 2 weeks of life. Normal kitten temperature during this time is about 95° F. By 4 to 5 weeks of age, body temperatures have reached the normal adult temperature in both species (approximately 101.5° F).

Because puppies and kittens have no shivering reflex for the first 6 days of life, an external heat source is necessary.[22] The dam is the best source of this warmth. After 6 days the puppies and kittens are able to shiver, but they are still very susceptible to chilling. Keeping the environment warm and free from drafts is of utmost importance during the first few weeks of life to prevent hypothermia. It is recommended that the environmental temperature be kept at 70° F during this period, assuming the dam is providing an adequate amount of warmth and protection to the newborns. Newborns should be weighed daily during the first 2 weeks and then every 3 to 4 days until weaning. A helpful guideline is for puppies to gain between 1 and 2 grams (g) per day for every pound (lb) of anticipated adult weight for the first 3 to 4 weeks of life. For example, if the anticipated adult weight of a dog is 25 lb, the puppy should be gaining between 25 and 50 g/day (0.9 to 1.8 ounces [oz]). Kittens usually weigh between 90 and 110 g at birth and should gain between 50 and 100 g (1.8 to 3.5 oz) per week until they are 5 to 6 months of age.

The gastrointestinal tracts of newborn puppies and kittens are uniquely suited to digest and absorb the milk produced by the mother dog and cat, respectively.[23] Immediately after birth, the ingestion of milk is a potent stimulator for enteric growth and for the development of the intestinal mucosal cells.[24,25] Fat and lactose are the primary sources of energy in milk; puppies and kittens have high intestinal lactase activity and are capable of digesting milk fat very early in life.[23] Similarly, both the type and amount of protein found in the milk are intricately matched to the developmental state of life. Gastric acid production is low in puppies and kittens until they are about 3 weeks of age. However, this does not appear to inhibit their ability to digest milk proteins. The renal capacity of neonates is also not fully developed and is sensitive to excessive or poor quality protein intake. Milk protein is of high quality and at a concentration that is closely matched to the metabolic capabilities of the developing young. Lastly, at birth, the gastrointestinal tract of puppies and kittens is sterile. Microbial colonization begins within the first day of life as the newborns ingest milk. This continues to evolve when solid food is introduced at 3 to 4 weeks of age and as the young attain adulthood.[26]

Volume of milk intake is affected by age, rate of growth, and for dogs, breed size. An early study of neonatal Beagle puppies reported that puppies consumed between 160 and 175 g (5 to 6 oz) of milk per day.[27] However, the technique used in the study may underestimate intakes by up to 30%, suggesting that daily intake was substantially higher than this.[28] Naturally, puppies of larger breeds are expected to consume a greater volume of milk, with smaller breeds and kittens consuming less volume. Similarly, the volume of milk that a female dog produces varies with her size. German Shepherds produce about 900 g (32 oz) of milk per day in early lactation, with increases of up to 1700 g (60 oz) per day during peak lactation.[29] In contrast, a much smaller breed, the Dachshund, produces between 100 and 180 g (3 to 6 oz) of milk per day in early lactation. Other influences upon the volume of milk produced are litter size, the age at which supplemental food is introduced, and age of weaning. In healthy puppies and kittens, the dam's milk supports normal growth until the young are 3 to 4 weeks old. Supplemental feeding with commercial milk replacer is usually not necessary, with the exception of unusually large litters. Even in those cases, dividing the litter into two groups and allowing each group to feed every 3 to 4 hours can often allow adequate intake for all of the puppies or kittens.[23]

After 4 weeks, milk alone no longer provides adequate calories or nutrients for normal development. At approximately the same time, puppies and kittens become increasingly interested in their environment and begin to spend more time awake and playing with each other. The time at which the dam's milk is no longer solely able to meet the nutrient needs of the offspring corresponds to the time at which the young are becoming interested in trying new foods and when they are developmentally capable of handling the introduction of semisolid food.

INTRODUCTION OF SOLID FOOD

Supplemental food should be introduced to puppies and kittens when they are 3 to 4 weeks of age. A commercial food made specifically for weaning puppies or kittens can be used, or a thick gruel can be made by mixing a small amount of warm water with the mother's food. Cow's milk should not be used to make the gruel because it is higher in lactose than bitch's and queen's milk and may cause diarrhea. Puppies and kittens should also not be fed a homemade "weaning formula." Although the foods that are used to make these formulas are usually of high nutrient value, many homemade formulas are not nutritionally balanced or complete. The use of this type of formula should be avoided unless its exact nutrient composition is known.

The semisolid food should be provided in a shallow dish, and puppies and kittens can be allowed access to fresh food several times per day. The bowl should be removed after 20 to 30 minutes. At first, little of the semisolid gruel will be consumed, and the litter's major food source will continue to be the dam's milk. However, by 5 weeks of age, puppies and kittens are readily consuming semisolid food. The deciduous teeth erupt between 21 and 35 days after birth. By 5 to 6 weeks of age, puppies and kittens are able to chew and consume dry food. Nutritional weaning is usually complete by 6 weeks of age, although some bitches and queens continue to allow their young to nurse for 8 weeks of age or longer (Box 21-1). Puppies will suckle occasionally and will continue to interact with the mother dog at 7 weeks of age even when offered free access to solid food.[30] It is believed that the psychological and emotional benefits of suckling may be as important as the nutritional benefits in puppies that are older than 5 weeks of age. For this reason, complete weaning (behavioral weaning) should not be instituted until puppies and kittens are at least 7 to 8 weeks of age.

Puppies and kittens can be introduced to semisolid food when they are 3 to 4 weeks of age. A commercial food made specifically for weaning puppies or kittens can be used, or a thick gruel can be made by mixing a small amount of warm water with the mother's food. Nutritional weaning is usually complete by 6 weeks of age, but complete weaning should not be instituted until puppies and kittens are at least 7 to 8 weeks of age.

NUTRITIONAL CARE OF ORPHANS

The bitch and queen normally supply warmth, stimulus for elimination and circulatory functions, passive immunity, nutrition, maternal attention, and security to their puppies and kittens. Technically, an orphan is any young animal that does not have access to the milk or care of its mother. Circumstances that may render young puppies and kittens orphans include the death of the dam, the production of an inadequate quantity or quality of milk, or rejection of the young by the dam. Whatever the underlying circumstance, once puppies or kittens are orphaned they depend on humans for the provision of maternal care, proper nutrition, and a suitable environment. Although it is difficult, if not impossible, to fully compensate for the absence of the mother, the use of proper diet, management techniques, and feeding techniques can result in the development of normal, healthy puppies and kittens.

Maintaining the Proper Environment

Orphaned animals must be kept in a warm, draft-free, and clean environment. Maintaining the appropriate temperature is of the utmost importance because chilling can decrease the survivability of newborns. When a bitch or queen is present, her body heat provides an excellent heat source and protection against drafts. In her absence, the ambient temperature must be increased. For the first week of life, the ambient temperature should be kept between 85° F and 90° F. This temperature can be decreased slightly to between 80° F and 85° F during the second to fourth weeks and to between 70° F and 75° F during the fifth week. After the litter reaches 5 to 6 weeks of age, a room temperature of approximately 70° F can be maintained (Table 21-2). Generally, newborn kittens and small puppies require

TABLE 21-2	PROPER ROOM TEMPERATURE FOR ORPHAN PUPPIES AND KITTENS	
AGE (WEEKS)		**TEMPERATURE (° F)**
0-1		85°-90°
2-4		80°-85°
5-6		70°-75°
More than 6		70°

TABLE 21-3	NUTRIENT COMPOSITION OF MILK FROM VARIOUS SPECIES (%)			
SPECIES	**FAT**	**PROTEIN**	**LACTOSE**	**DRY MATTER**
Dog	5.0	5.0	4.5	22.8
Cat	7.0	7.5	4.0	18.5
Cow	3.8	4.7	4.7	12.4
Goat	4.5	4.6	4.6	13.0

Adapted from Baines FM: Milk substitutes and the hand rearing of orphan puppies and kittens, *J Small Anim Pract* 22:555–578, 1981; Adkins Y, Zicker SC, Lepine A, and others: Changes in nutrient and protein composition of cat milk during lactation, *Am J Vet Res* 58:370–375, 1997; and Keen CL, Lonnerdal B, Clegg MS, and others: Developmental changes in composition of cats' milk: trace elements, minerals, protein, carbohydrate and fat, *J Nutr* 112:1763–1769, 1982.

slightly higher ambient temperatures than do large puppies. A heating pad or heat lamp may be used to provide heat, although a pad is often preferred because it allows for the maintenance of a normal day/night light cycle. Regardless of the type of heater used, the heat source should provide a temperature gradient within the whelping box so that the puppies and kittens can move to warmer or cooler areas as needed. Humidity must also be considered. If the environment is too dry, neonates are subject to dehydration. If dry heat is used to keep the whelping box warm, pans of water should be placed near the heaters to maintain room humidity. A relative humidity of approximately 50% is effective in preventing dehydration and maintaining moist nasal and respiratory passages in newborn puppies and kittens.[31] Drafts in the room can be controlled by providing a whelping box or incubator with high sides.

Orphaned puppies and kittens represent a challenge to breeders and foster homes. They depend completely on humans for maternal care, proper nutrition, and a suitable environment. Maintaining proper warmth, normally provided by body heat from the bitch or queen, is critical to ensure survival of the newborn puppies and kittens.

What to Feed

One of the greatest challenges involved in raising orphaned puppies and kittens is providing them with adequate nutrition. Because the best possible nutrition for young animals comes from their dam, foster mothering is the best solution for orphaned newborns. Unfortunately, a foster mother of the same species is usually not available. The alternative is to provide nutrition through a well-formulated milk replacer. A milk replacer will nourish the puppies and kittens for the first few weeks of life until their digestive and metabolic functions develop to the point at which semisolid food can be introduced. It is important that the chosen formula closely approximates the composition of the natural milk of the bitch or queen. Feeding a formula that is not similar in composition to the species' natural milk can result in diarrhea and digestive upsets and has the potential to compromise growth and development.

Several commercially produced canine and feline milk replacers are available. Most of these products are composed of cow's milk that has been modified to simulate the composition of bitch's and queen's milk (based on crude protein and crude fat levels). A comparison of the compositions of the milk of different species shows that bitch's and queen's milk have larger proportions of their calories from fat and protein and lower proportions from lactose than the milk of ruminant species such as the cow and goat. Although the percentages (by weight) of these nutrients only differ slightly, the more dilute composition of ruminant milk exaggerates the relative differences between these values. This is reflected by the lower DM content of goat's and cow's milk as compared to the milk of dogs and cats (Table 21-3).[32] For example, when converted to a calorie basis, the lactose content of cow's milk is nearly three times that found in bitch's milk.[33] For this reason, puppies that are fed straight cow's milk will develop severe diarrhea. Evaporated cow's milk is occasionally recommended for raising orphans because it has levels of protein, fat, calcium, and phosphorus that are similar to bitch's milk. However, the lactose content of evaporated milk is still much too high for young puppies and kittens. In addition, the casein-to-whey protein ratio in cow's milk is not ideal for puppies, and cow's milk contains an excessive proportion of casein for neonatal kittens.[34]

There are numerous recipes available for the formulation of homemade milk replacers. Most of these use a combination of cow's or goat's milk and eggs. Eggs are added to increase the protein content and dilute the lactose concentration of the ruminant milk. Regardless of the popularity of a homemade formula, breeders should be advised that most of these recipes were originally developed through trial-and-error, and their actual nutrient compositions are not known. A published analysis of several commonly used homemade formulas found that these recipes contain a wide range of nutrient compositions.[33] Although some formulas seem to be adequate for feeding puppies and kittens, many contain a nutrient composition that is drastically different from that of natural bitch's and queen's milk. A homemade formula should only be used if its nutrient composition is known and if the formula has been proven to be safe and effective for raising orphaned puppies or kittens. If a well-researched product that is formulated for puppies and kittens is available, this is preferable to a homemade formula.

Commercial milk replacers are the preferred source of nutrition for orphans. A product that has been tested for the specific purpose of raising neonatal puppies and kittens should be selected. In addition, unlike homemade formulas, the nutrient content and the biological integrity of commercial preparations is guaranteed. However, some commercial formulas can vary in their ability to provide orphans with adequate nutrition and calories. For example, a study that compared feeding queen's milk, a commercial milk replacer for cats, and an experimental milk replacer to kittens ranging from 2 to 6 weeks of age found that the commercial product caused chronic diarrhea and the development of lens opacities and cataracts.[35] Suboptimal levels of the essential amino acid arginine in the commercial formula appeared to be the cause of the cataracts, and an unusually high crude fiber content may have been the cause of the diarrhea. When the kittens were switched to a growth diet at 6 weeks of age, the lens opacities resolved almost completely, and diarrhea subsided during the sixth week of feeding. Additional studies of the nutrient composition of dog and cat milk have led to

the development of replacers that closely conform to the nutrient profiles of natural milk and that promote growth rates that are close to those of nursing neonates.[36,37]

Because the Association of American Feed Control Officials (AAFCO) does not currently provide detailed guidelines for testing milk replacers, it is essential that breeders obtain information from manufacturers about a replacer's nutrient composition, nutritional integrity, and feeding efficacy. Also, it is important to note that even a well-formulated commercial milk replacer cannot provide newborns with the antibodies that are normally found in colostrum. Therefore, if newborns are orphaned before they have received colostrum, extra care must be taken to maintain a clean environment and prevent the transmission of disease.

Because most homemade formulas have not been thoroughly tested for nutritional adequacy, commercial milk replacers are preferred for feeding orphaned puppies and kittens. A replacer that closely matches dog's or cat's milk in nutrient composition and performance should be chosen. Cow's milk or goat's milk should never be used as a puppy or kitten milk replacer.

How Much to Feed

Calorie and fluid intake must be adjusted so that the puppies and kittens are able to consume enough formula to meet their nutrient needs for growth and, at the same time, not underconsume or overconsume fluid volume. During the first few weeks, the food intake of the neonate is largely limited by stomach volume. Most newborn puppies can handle only 10 to 20 milliliters (ml) of milk per feeding. Kittens are able to handle approximately $\frac{1}{3}$ to $\frac{1}{2}$ of this amount.[33] Therefore the concentration of the formula is extremely important. The milk replacer for puppies should have a caloric value of between 1400 and 1800 kilocalories (kcal) of metabolizable energy (ME) per liter (L), a concentration that is similar to that of bitch's milk.[10] Queen's milk has a caloric density of approximately 850 to 1600 kcal ME/L.[6] If the energy concentration is lower than this, more feedings per day will be necessary to meet the neonate's needs. In this case, the intake of excess fluid would adversely affect water balance and may stress the immature kidneys.

Conversely, if the energy density of the formula is too high, digestive upsets and diarrhea may occur.

There are various estimates of the caloric needs of newborn puppies. A generally accepted guideline suggests that during the first 3 weeks of life, orphaned puppies need to receive between 130 and 150 kcal of ME per kilogram (kg) of body weight per day. After 4 weeks of age, caloric needs increase to 200 to 220 kcal/kg of body weight.[33] Less is known about the optimal energy intake of newborn kittens, but one guideline suggests feeding 20, 25, 30, and 35 ml/100 g of body weight during the third, fourth, fifth, and sixth week of life, respectively.[34] In all cases, these figures should be used only as guidelines because the individual requirements of puppies and kittens can vary greatly. Orphans should be weighed daily to ensure that they are receiving enough nourishment to support normal weight increases. General guidelines for determining the volume to feed are provided in Tables 21-4 and 21-5.

Once determined, the total volume of formula should be divided equally among the daily feedings.

If the concentration of the formula is correct, neonates that are bottle-fed should be able to self-regulate their formula intake. Feeding orphans four to six times per day is usually practical, with the feedings spaced at even time intervals. This schedule is often reasonable for human caretakers, and it also allows the neonates to obtain their needed hours of uninterrupted sleep.

Methods of Feeding

Two possible methods may be used to feed orphaned puppies: bottle-feeding with a small animal nursing bottle or delivering the formula directly into the stomach using a stomach tube. If puppies and kittens are bottle-fed, they should be held in a natural nursing position with the head tilted slightly upward. The bottle should be held in a manner that minimizes air intake by the puppy or kitten. To allow proper nursing and suckling behavior, a nipple that fills the puppy's or kitten's mouth should be selected.[38] When bottle-fed, orphans usually reject the bottle when their stomachs

TABLE 21-4 VOLUME OF MILK REPLACER TO FEED ORPHAN PUPPIES (GENERAL GUIDELINES)

Body weight (oz)	Body weight (g)	Volume/Day (oz)	Volume/Day (tbsp or cup)	Volume/Day (g)
5	140	1.5	3 tbsp	45
10	285	2.5	⅜ cup	75
20	570	5.0	⅝ cup	150
30	850	8.0	1 cup	235
50	1420	12.0	1½ cup	355
70	1990	17.0	2⅛ cup	505
100	2840	25.0	3⅛ cup	740

Data from P&G Pet Care, Lewisburg, Ohio.

TABLE 21-5 VOLUME OF MILK REPLACER TO FEED ORPHAN KITTENS (GENERAL GUIDELINES)

Body weight (oz)	Body weight (g)	Volume/Day (oz)	Volume/Day (tbsp or cup)	Volume/Day (g)
4	115	1.00	2.0	30
6	170	1.50	3.0	45
8	225	1.75	3.5	50
10	285	2.25	4.5	65
12	340	3.00	6.0	90
14	440	3.75	7.5	110

Data from P&G Pet Care, Lewisburg, Ohio.

are full. However, the correct volume of formula should still be estimated and measured for each feeding. This step aids in record keeping and minimizes the risk of overfeeding.

Some breeders prefer to use a feeding tube with orphans. This method of feeding is faster and, if conducted properly, reduces the risk of formula aspiration. However, caution is advised because repetitive placement of a feeding tube can cause irritation to the esophagus.[5] In addition, tube feeding does not allow neonates to engage in normal suckling behaviors. The necessary equipment is an infant feeding tube attached to a syringe. For puppies and kittens that weigh less than 300 g (10 oz), a number 5- or 8-French–sized tube can be used. For larger puppies, a number 10-French tube is appropriate. The depth of insertion can be estimated by measuring the distance from the puppy or kitten's nose to the last rib. This length is marked on the tube and should be readjusted every 2 to 3 days to account for growth. The syringe is filled with a measured volume of warm formula, and extra air in the syringe and tube is expelled. To insert the tube, the puppy or kitten is held upright, the mouth is opened slightly and the tube is gently inserted over the tongue to the back of the throat. This contact will induce a swallow reflex, and the tube should pass easily down into the stomach. If any resistance is felt, this indicates that the tube may be in the trachea, and should be removed and reinserted. When the tube is inserted properly into the stomach, the puppy or kitten will be breathing normally and not crying or showing distress. Formula should be administered slowly over a 2- to 3-minute period. Because the neonate cannot self-regulate intake when tube-fed, formula volume must always be carefully measured to avoid overfeeding or underfeeding.

Fresh formula should be made up daily and warmed to approximately 100° F before feeding. A slightly restricted quantity of formula should be fed for the first two to three feedings; this allows gradual adjustment to the milk replacer. If puppies and kittens are overfed during the first few days, diarrhea may result, leading to dehydration and increased susceptibility to infection. After each feeding, and several times daily, the anal/genital area of the newborns should be massaged gently with a damp cloth. This action simulates the dam's licking and stimulates urination and defecation.

Grooming, cleaning, and feeding of the orphans should be conducted on a regular basis, and the box should be cleaned several times per day.

Orphans should be weighed regularly. There may be a small decrease in body weight during the first 2 to 3 days because of the restricted feeding of the new formula. After this, if a well-formulated milk replacer is used, growth will closely approximate that of dam-raised puppies and kittens.[36,37]

Orphans show an increased demand and tolerance for food once their eyes open and they are on their feet. At this time, a small shallow bowl of formula should be provided before each bottle-feeding. The puppies and kittens should be encouraged to lap formula from the bowl. The bowl of formula should not be left out for more than 20 or 30 minutes at a time. Once the litter readily initiates lapping at each meal, they can begin to take entire feedings from the bowl. In general, puppies adjust to lapping at an earlier age and more rapidly than kittens.

When the orphans are 3 to 4 weeks old, a gruel can be made using milk replacer and dry dog or cat food or a puppy or kitten weaning formula. Once semisolid food is introduced, fresh water should be available at all times. The thickness of the gruel can be gradually increased with time. This gradual change allows the puppies and kittens to become accustomed to chewing and swallowing solid food and enables their gastrointestinal tracts to adapt to the new food. By 6 to 8 weeks of age, puppies and kittens should be consuming normal dry food (Box 21-2).

BOX 21-2   PRACTICAL FEEDING TIPS: ORPHAN PUPPIES AND KITTENS

Provide a warm, draft-free, clean environment.

Feed a milk replacer that closely approximates the nutrient composition of bitch's or queen's milk.

Estimate the correct amount of formula based on the orphan's age and weight.

Divide the formula into four to five equal feedings per day.

Bottle-feed or use a feeding tube.

Weigh orphans regularly: one time per day for the first week and one to two times per week thereafter.

Introduce semisolid food at 3 to 4 weeks.

Wean to dry pet food by 6 to 8 weeks.

References

1. Hoskins JD: Puppy and kitten losses. In Hoskins JD, editor: *Veterinary pediatrics: dogs and cats from birth to six months*, Philadelphia, 1995, Saunders.

2. Halliday JA, Bell K, Shaw DC: Feline and canine milk lysozymes, *Comp Biochem Physiol* 106B:859–865, 1993.

3. Iverson SJ, Kirk CL, Hamosh M: Milk lipid digestion in the neonatal dog: the combined actions of gastric and bile salt stimulated lipases, *Biochem Biophys Acta* 1083:109–119, 1991.

4. Donovan SM, Odle J: Growth factors in milk as mediators of infant development, *Ann Rev Nutr* 14:147–167, 1994.

5. Lepine AJ: Nutrition of the neonatal puppy. In *Proc Canine Reprod for Breeders*, Symposium at Westminster Kennel Club Dog Show, February 2001, pp 26–30.

6. Adkins Y, Zicker SC, Lepine A, and others: Changes in nutrient and protein composition of cat milk during lactation, *Am J Vet Res* 58:370–375, 1997.

7. Dobenecker B, Zottmann B, Kienzle E, Zentek J: Investigations on milk composition and milk yield in queens, *J Nutr* 128:2618S–2619S, 1998.

8. Keen CL, Lonnerdal B, Clegg MS, and others: Developmental changes in composition of cats' milk: trace elements, minerals, protein, carbohydrate and fat, *J Nutr* 112:1763–1769, 1982.

9. Jacobsen KL, DePeters EJ, Rogers QR, Taylor SJ: Influences of stage of lactation, teat position and sequential milk sampling on the composition of domestic cat milk *(Felis catus)*, *J Anim Physiol Anim Nutr* 88:46–58, 2004.

10. Adkins Y, Lepine AJ, Lonnerdal B: Changes in protein and nutrient composition of milk through out lactation in dogs, *Am J Vet Res* 62:1266–1272, 2001.

11. Lonnerdal B, Keen CL, Hurley LS, and others: Developmental changes in the composition of Beagle dog milk, *Am J Vet Res* 42:662–666, 1981.

12. Kunz C, Lonnerdal B: Re-evaluation of the whey protein/casein ratio of human milk, *Acta Pediatr* 81:107–112, 1992.

13. Lonnerdal B: Lactation and neonatal nutrition in the dog and cat. In *Proc North Am Vet Conf*, 1997, pp 13–16.

14. Kelley RL, Lepine AJ, Ruffing J, and others: Impact of maternal dietary DHA and reproductive activity on DHA status in the canine. In *Proc 6th Cong Internat Soc Study Fatty Acids Lipids*, 2004, p 149.

15. Lepine AJ, Kelley RL: Effect of fatty acids on canine reproductive health. In *WSAVA Proc*, 2004, pp 34–39.

16. Bauer JE, Heinemann KM, Bigley KE, and others: Maternal dipha-linolenic acid during gestation and lactation does not increase docosahexaenoic acid in canine milk, *J Nutr* 134:2035S–2038S, 2004.

17. Francois CA, Connor SL, Wander RC, Connor WE: Supplementing lactating women with flaxseed oil does not increase docosahexaenoic acid in their milk, *Am J Clin Nutr* 77:226–233, 2003.

18. Bauer JE, Heinemann KM, Lees GE, Waldron MK: Docosahexaenoic acid accumulates in plasma of canine puppies raised on alpha-linolenic acid-rich milk during suckling but not when fed alpha-linolenic acid-rich diets after weaning, *J Nutr* 136:2087–2089, 2006.

19. Heinemann KM, Bauer JE: Docosahexaenoic acid and neurologic development in animals, *J Am Vet Med Assoc* 228:700–705, 2006.

20. Heinemann KM, Waldron MK, Bigley KE, and others: Long-chain (n-3) polyunsaturated fatty acids are more efficient than alpha-linolenic acid in improving electroretinogram responses of puppies exposed during gestation, lactation, and weaning, *J Nutr* 135:1960–1966, 2005.

21. Bauer JE, Heinemann KM, Lees GE, Waldron MK: Retinal functions of young dogs are improved and maternal plasma phospholipids are altered with diets containing long-chain n-3 polyunsaturated fatty acids during gestation, lactation, and after weaning, *J Nutr* 136:1991S–1994S, 2006.

22. Pownall R, Crighton GW: Factors influencing body temperature in newborn dogs, *Br Vet J* 133:191–196, 1977.

23. Zentek J: Nutrition and physiology of the young dog and cat. In *WSAVA Proc*, 2004, pp 16–20.

24. Paulsen DB, Buddington KK, Buddington RK: Dimensions and histologic characteristics of the small intestine of dogs during postnatal development, *Am J Vet Res* 64:618–626, 2003.

25. Heird WC, Schwarz SM, Hansen IH: Colostrum-induced enteric mucosal growth in Beagle puppies, *Pediatr Res* 18:512–515, 1984.

26. Buddington RK: Postnatal changes in bacterial populations in the gastrointestinal tracts of dogs, *Am J Vet Res* 64:646–651, 2003.

27. Oftedal OT: Lactation in the dog: milk composition and intake by puppies, *J Nutr* 114:803–812, 1984.

28. Hendriks WH, Wamberg S: Milk intake of suckling kittens remains relatively constant from one to four weeks of age, *J Nutr* 130:77–82, 2000.

29. Russe I: Laktation der Hundin, *Zentralbl Veterinarmed* 8:252–282, 1961.

30. Malm K, Jensen P: Weaning in dogs: within—and between—litter variation in milk and solid food intake, *Appl Anim Behav Sci* 49:223–235, 1996.

31. Monson WJ: The care and management of orphaned puppies and kittens, *Vet Tech* 8:430–434, 1987.

32. Monson WJ: Orphan rearing of puppies and kittens, *Vet Clin North Am Small Anim Pract* 17:567–576, 1987.

33. Baines FB: Milk substitutes and the hand rearing of orphan puppies and kittens, *J Small Anim Pract* 22:555–578, 1981.

34. Lepine AJ: Nutrition of the neonatal canine and feline. In Reinhart GA, Carey DP, editors: *Recent advances in canine and feline nutrition, Iams nutrition symposium proceedings*, vol 2, Wilmington, Ohio, 1998, Orange Frazer Press.

35. Remillard RL, Pickett JP, Thatcher CD, and others: Comparison of kittens fed queen's milk with those fed milk replacers, *Am J Vet Res* 54:901–907, 1993.

36. Lepine AJ, Kelley RL, Bouchard G: Effect of feline milk replacers on growth and body composition of nursing kittens (abstract). In *Proc Am Coll Vet Intern Med Forum*, 1998, p 737.

37. Kelley RL, Lepine AJ, Bouchard G: Effect of milk composition on growth and body composition of puppies (abstract), *FASEB Proc* 12:A837, 1998.

38. Kelley RK, Coffman M: Hand-rearing orphan pups. In *Proc Iams Open Brace Beagle Champ*, 2001, pp 28–30.

22

Growth

Most puppies and kittens are fully weaned and ready to be placed in their new homes by 7 to 9 weeks of age. For puppies, this represents an ideal time to enter a new home because the primary socialization period occurs between 5 and 12 weeks of age. At 7 weeks of age the puppies have spent sufficient time with their litter to allow proper canine socialization. The remainder of this important developmental period can then be spent bonding to their new owners. The primary socialization period for kittens occurs between 2 and 7 weeks of age. Although this period is not as well defined in kittens as it is in puppies, this means that early handling while kittens are still with their litter mates is important. Like puppies, 7 to 9 weeks appears to be the best age for kittens to go to their new homes.

GROWTH PATTERNS

By the time they reach their adult weight, most dogs and cats have increased their birth weight by fortyfold to fiftyfold. Enormous variation exists in the mature size, body type (conformation), body weight, coat type, and temperament of different breeds and types of dogs. For example, a 5-pound (lb) Chihuahua and a 150-lb Newfoundland both achieve complete development and growth within relatively similar periods of time. The thirtyfold difference in mature size between these two dogs means that the Newfoundland's rate of growth and amount of tissue accretion far exceeds that of the Chihuahua. Such dramatic differences in body size and type are not observed in cats, which vary relatively little in mature size.

In both dogs and cats, the most rapid growth period occurs during the first 3 to 6 months of life. Patterns of growth differ among dog breeds of different sizes, with larger breeds experiencing a longer growth period than small breeds. While both large and small dogs show exponential growth rates during the first several months of life, this period of rapid growth is shorter in small breeds and ends earlier, at about 3 months of age.[1] Conversely, exponential growth continues for another month in large breeds and for another

2 months in giant breeds. Toy, small, and medium breeds of dogs attain adult body weight by approximately 9 to 10 months of age, while large and giant breeds attain adult weight when they are between 11 and 15 months old.[1,2] Although body weight stabilizes at these ages, development continues for several more months. Toy- and small-breed dogs and cats reach mature body size when they are between 9 and 12 months old, while the large and giant breeds of dogs are not typically considered to be mature until they are 18 to 24 months of age (Figures 22-1 and 22-2).[3,4] Although the mature size of many breeds has changed since they were initially constructed, the growth curves shown in Figure 22-2 illustrate the relative growth rate differences among dog breeds of different sizes.

> Large and giant dog breeds experience a longer growth and maturation period than the small and toy breeds. Although body weight stabilizes several months earlier, toy- and small-breed dogs and cats reach mature body size when they are between 9 and 12 months old. Body size and conformation of the large and giant breeds of dogs continue to develop until they are 18 to 24 months of age.

Dog breeds also differ in conformation. For example, breeds such as the Greyhound and Irish Wolfhound were developed to chase prey species while acting as hunting aids. The long legs, deep chest and relatively slender conformation of these breeds contributes to speed and agility. In contrast, other large breeds such as Mastiffs and Newfoundlands were selected for strength and endurance and have heavier body conformations that reflect their original working functions. Because different breeds of dogs have different rates of growth, mature weights, and body types, the food that is fed during growth should reflect these differences. In recent years, pet food companies have recognized these differences and have developed products that provide

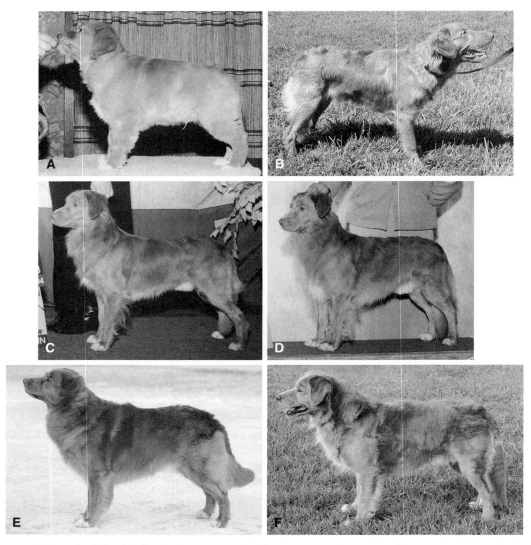

Figure 22-1   **A**, Nova Scotia Duck Tolling Retriever at 9 weeks of age. **B-E**, Same dog at 7 months, 2 years, 5 years, and 7 years. **F**, Same breed, different dog, at 11 years of age. (**A-E**, Am/Can CH skylark's Rowdy Riverdancer UD can CDX RA WC VC CGC, Jean and Jon Gravning, owners, and Laurie Geyer, breeder. **F**, Can/Int'l CH Skylark's Pistol Pete CD OA NAJ WC VC ROM, Laurie Geyer, breeder/owner.)

optimal nutrition for growing dogs of different mature sizes and weights, and in some cases different breeds. Although there is some evidence that growth patterns may differ among similarly sized breeds with differing body compositions, the most important nutritional distinction during growth is that observed between the large and giant breeds and small and toy breeds.

Large- and Giant-Breed Dogs

The genetic selection for breeds of dogs that have a large mature size has concurrently selected for the potential to grow very rapidly. Although the genetic potential for rapid growth is not in itself a health risk, feeding practices that allow maximal growth

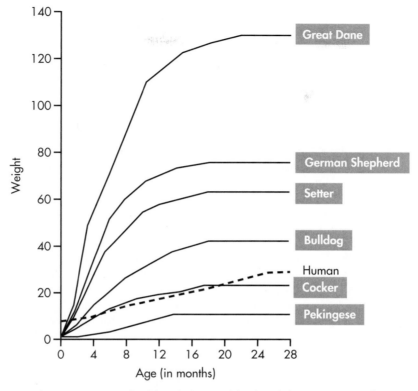

Figure 22-2   Rate of weight gain in several dog breeds from 0 to 28 months.

rate contribute to risk for developmental orthopedic diseases such as osteochondrosis, hypertrophic osteodystrophy and hip dysplasia.[5-7] The most important nutrient that affects growth rate is energy. Large-breed puppies that are overfed or fed energy-dense (high-fat) foods during periods of rapid growth are able to reach their maximum genetic growth potential. Growing at a rapid rate is incompatible with healthy skeletal development. For example, when Great Dane puppies were either allowed to eat ad libitum or were limit-fed to 60% to 70% of ad libitum intake, the dogs that were limit-fed grew more slowly and showed a dramatic reduction in skeletal abnormalities when compared with the ad libitum–fed dogs.[8] Conversely, controlling rate of growth supports healthy skeletal development. A longitudinal study with Labrador Retrievers found that dogs that were limit-fed to maintain a lean body condition grew at moderate rates and showed a reduced

incidence and severity of hip dysplasia when compared with dogs that were fed ad libitum.[9]

Although the underlying causes of developmental skeletal diseases are multifaceted and vary with the type of disorder, it is without question that excess energy intake and the resultant rapid growth rate in large dogs can contribute to aberrations in normal bone and cartilage development. During rapid growth, the bone that supports developing cartilage in joints becomes less dense and weaker than normal, causing the bone matrix to inadequately support the overlying joint cartilage.[10] The damaged cartilage surface, coupled with disturbances to the normal function and metabolism of cartilage-forming cells in the joint, lead to joint defects such as those seen in osteochondrosis. These changes are exacerbated by the mechanical stress of a heavier body weight on the developing skeleton. Similarly, increased weight bearing on developing hips and a growth disparity between soft tissue and skeletal tissue are considered to be factors in the development of canine hip dysplasia (for a complete discussion, see Chapter 37, pp. 491-494).

In addition to the food's energy density, another nutrient that is important for skeletal health in large and giant breeds is calcium. Active calcium absorption mechanisms are not fully mature in growing puppies until they are about 6 months of age.[11,12] Prior to this age, up to 70% of the calcium that is absorbed from the diet enters the body through passive absorption in the small intestine. Because passive absorption cannot be down-regulated, the amount of calcium that is absorbed is directly proportional to its concentration in the diet.[13] Active absorption is functional in growing puppies, but cannot effectively down-regulate in response to excess dietary calcium. As a result, puppies are unable to protect themselves from absorbing excess (and unneeded) calcium when it is present in the diet. As puppies mature, active absorption mechanisms become tightly regulated through the actions of vitamin D_3, parathyroid hormone, growth hormone, and calcitonin.[14] Together, these hormones tightly regulate the amount of calcium that is absorbed, protecting the older puppy from excessive calcium uptake. However, the time at which the body's calcium absorption mechanisms mature is too late to protect puppies from excessive dietary calcium uptake during the most rapid growth period between 3 and 5 months of age. As a result, puppies from weaning to 6 months are highly susceptible to excessive dietary calcium and its effects on the developing skeleton.

Several studies have shown that an excessive level of dietary calcium or supplementation with this mineral during the rapid growth period negatively affects skeletal development in large breeds of dogs (most frequently, Great Danes).[6,12,15] Great Dane puppies fed a food containing 3.3% calcium from weaning until 6 months of age showed an increased incidence of osteochondritic lesions when compared with puppies fed a food that contained 1.1% calcium.[16] Interestingly, although small and medium breeds of dogs have the same patterns of passive and active calcium absorption during growth, these breeds are not as susceptible to developmental skeletal disease when exposed to dietary calcium excess.[17,18] Neither do all large and giant breeds respond as dramatically to excess dietary calcium as do Great Danes. There is some evidence that such differences may be related to genetic differences among breeds in calcium uptake and metabolism

early in life.[19] Regardless of possible differences among breeds, including more calcium than the body needs, either through diet or supplementation, is unnecessary and poses significant risk for the development of several types of skeletal disease in large- and giant-breed dogs (for a complete discussion, see Chapter 37, pp. 497-500).

Two other nutrients that are of interest when feeding large-breed dogs during growth are protein and vitamin D. Although high protein intake was identified as a potential contributor to rapid growth rate in early studies, it was subsequently discovered that the apparent protein effect was actually caused by excess energy intake and was not related to the protein level in the food. When growing Great Dane puppies were fed foods that had identical caloric densities (3600 kilocalories (kcal) metabolizable energy/kilogram (ME/kg) but varied in protein content (31.6%, 23.1%, or 14.6%), dietary protein did not affect skeletal development.[20] However, the lowest protein diet (14.6%) was not sufficient to promote optimal growth and health. Although it is important that adequate level of protein is provided and that protein level is balanced with the food's energy density, protein by itself does not negatively affect growth rate or skeletal development in large-breed dogs.

Because of its role in calcium metabolism and homeostasis, the impact of dietary vitamin D on skeletal development in dogs has been examined in recent years.[21] As discussed in Chapter 13 (pp. 108-110), dogs and cats require a dietary source of vitamin D_3 (cholecalciferol) because they are unable to produce adequate amounts of the vitamin from its precursor, 7-dehydrocholesterol, found in skin. Dietary vitamin D_3 is converted to 24-dihydroxycholecalciferol in the liver. Blood concentrations of this metabolite closely parallel dietary intake. 24-dihydroxycholecalciferol is converted in the kidney into one of the two biologically active forms of vitamin D; 1,25-dihydroxycholecalciferol or 24,25-dihydroxycholecalciferol. The biologically active forms of vitamin D influence calcium homeostasis by regulating calcium absorption in the intestine and resorption in the kidney, and bone formation and resorption. The first compound, 1,25-dihydroxycholecalciferol, is recognized as the most biologically active form and exerts its effects on all three tissues (intestine, kidney, and bone). The less active form, 24,25-dihydroxycholecalciferol, works principally at the skeletal level to promote the formation of new bone. As a species, dogs are relatively tolerant of excess dietary vitamin D_3 and possess effective mechanisms to maintain normal calcium homeostasis even when fed excess levels of the vitamin during growth.[22,23] However, Great Dane puppies raised on foods containing nontoxic but excess concentrations of vitamin D_3 (10- and 100-fold greater than recommended levels) developed abnormal changes to growth plates and skeletal remodeling, even though they maintained normal calcium homeostasis.[24] The higher concentration caused the development of radius curvus syndrome in some dogs. These changes were not caused by calcium, but rather by a direct effect of vitamin D_3 on developing growth plates.

It was theorized that differences in vitamin D metabolism may exist between large- and small-breed dogs. Studies to test this found that concentrations of 24,25-dihydroxycholecalciferol in the plasma of growing large-breed dogs (Great Danes) were significantly lower than the levels observed in small-breed puppies (Miniature Poodles).[14] Concentrations in the Great Danes were found to be negatively correlated with the activity of growth hormone.[25] Great Dane puppies also had lower plasma levels of 25-dihydroxycholecalciferol and slightly lower 1,25-dihydroxycholecalciferol levels. Despite these differences, intestinal absorption of calcium did not differ between the two breeds of puppies; however, Great Dane puppies showed irregularities in growth plate development that were not seen in the Poodle puppies.[26] Differences in vitamin D_3 metabolism between large and small breeds may be another factor that influences an individual dog's susceptibility to developmental skeletal disease. Further studies are needed to examine effects of different levels of dietary vitamin D on the production of biologically active vitamin D metabolites during growth in large and small breeds, and the effects on the developing skeleton. Currently, commercial dog foods contain vitamin D_3 (cholecalciferol) to supply the needed source of this vitamin since dogs cannot produce cholecalciferol from 7-dehydrocholesterol in the skin. Additional research may support adjustments in these levels with enhanced understanding of its role in skeletal health in growing large-breed dogs.

Multiple factors, including genetics and husbandry practices, influence a dog's risk for developing skeletal disease. Breeders can help to reduce the incidence of developmental skeletal disease through careful screening and selection of breeding animals. In addition, feeding an appropriate diet and using proper feeding practices throughout the growth period reduces risk and supports healthy skeletal growth (see pp. 231-233). The time period that is of greatest importance is the period of rapid growth, between 3 and 5 months of age. An appropriate food for large- and giant-breed puppies has reduced fat and energy density, a balanced level of high-quality protein that is adjusted to energy density, and a level of calcium and phosphorus that is slightly less than that found in puppy foods intended for small breeds of puppies. A recommended nutrient profile for a growth diet formulated for large and giant breeds is one that contains 26% to 28% protein, 14% to 16% fat, 0.8% to 0.9% calcium, 0.6% to 0.8% phosphorus, and a caloric density between 360 and 400 kcal per cup.[27] Feeding practices are equally important. Puppies should be meal-fed two or three times daily, and portions should be premeasured. Limit-feeding should be closely adjusted to maintain a lean, not plump, body condition, throughout growth (see pp. 231-233). Although rate of growth will be lower than that of a dog who is fed a more energy-dense food, ultimate adult size will not be compromised and risk of skeletal disease will be reduced (Table 22-1).

Large and giant breeds of dogs have the potential to grow very rapidly during their first 6 months of life. However, allowing these dogs to achieve their genetic potentials for growth rate is not compatible with healthy skeletal development. An appropriate food for large- and giant-breed puppies has reduced fat and energy density, a balanced level of high-quality protein that is adjusted to energy density, and a level of calcium and phosphorus that is slightly less than that found in puppy foods intended for small breeds of puppies.

Small- and Toy-Breed Dogs

Dogs of the small and toy breeds have higher energy requirements per unit of body weight than do the large and giant breeds. This occurs because basal metabolic rate is related to total body surface area. Small and toy breeds have higher ratios of surface area to body weight than do large breeds and so have higher energy needs per unit of weight (lb or kg). In addition to their

TABLE 22-1 SUMMARY OF PROTEIN, ENERGY, AND CALCIUM EFFECTS ON SKELETAL DEVELOPMENT AND NUTRITIONAL RECOMMENDATIONS FOR LARGE AND GIANT BREEDS

| | EFFECT OF NUTRIENT LEVEL ON SKELETAL DEVELOPMENT | | | NUTRITIONAL |
NUTRIENT	Low	MEDIUM	HIGH	RECOMMENDATION
Protein	Decreased growth rate (if deficient)	Normal growth rate	Normal growth rate	26%-28%
Energy	Decreased growth rate (if deficient)	Normal growth rate	Increased growth rate and risk of skeletal disease	360-400 kcal/cup
Calcium	Decreased growth rate Decreased bone mineral content and strength	Increased bone mineral content and strength Proper conformation Reduced risk of HOD	Increased bone mineral content and strength Poor conformation Increased risk of HOD	0.8%-0.9% (Ca:P ratio = 1.2:1)

Adapted from Lepine AJ: Optimal nutrition for the growing retriever and upland dog. In *Nutrition and care of the sporting dog*, Dayton, Ohio, 2002, The Iams Company, pp 17–22.
HOD, Hypertrophic osteodystrophy.

relatively high energy needs, small breeds of puppies also have small stomachs that hold limited amounts of food. A dog food formulated for growing small and toy breeds should be higher in energy and nutrient density than a food formulated for large dogs, and it should contain ingredients that are highly digestible and available. The size and shape of the kibble pieces should be designed for small mouths to facilitate easy chewing and consumption.

Small- and toy-breed puppies should be fed foods that are higher in energy (and nutrient) density than foods designed for large-breed puppies. The food should also contain ingredients that are highly digestible and available, and kibble pieces should be small enough for small mouths.

NUTRIENT NEEDS DURING GROWTH

Energy

For all dogs and cats, regardless of size or breed, nutrient and energy needs during growth exceed those of any other stage of life except lactation. During the period of rapid growth the energy needs of growing puppies are approximately twice those of adult dogs of the same size. After 6 months of age, these needs begin to decline as growth rate decreases. After weaning, growing puppies require approximately twice the energy intake per unit of body weight as adult dogs of the same weight.[28] When puppies reach about 40% to 50% of their adult weight, this requirement declines to about 1.6 times maintenance levels. When 80% of adult weight is achieved, energy needs are approximately 1.2 times maintenance levels. As discussed previously, the age at which a puppy will attain these proportions of adult weight will vary with the adult size of the dog. Although all puppies grow most rapidly when they are between 3 and 5 months of age, large breeds of dogs reach maturity at a later age than do small breeds.[1] With the exception of the giant breeds, most puppies achieve 40% of their adult weight between 3 and 4 months of age and 80% of adult weight between 4 ½ and 8 months. Very large breeds of dogs do not attain adult size until they are 10 months of age or older.[29] General guidelines for determining energy needs for growing dogs are provided in Table 22-2.

Similarly, growing cats have energy needs that are significantly higher than are the maintenance needs of adult cats. The energy and nutrient requirements of growing kittens are highest per unit of body weight at about 5 weeks of age. Young, rapidly growing kittens require approximately 200 to 250 kcal of ME per kg of body weight. This requirement declines to 130 kcal/kg by 20 weeks of age and to 100 kcal/kg by 30 weeks of age. An example of energy needs for a growing kitten is provided in Table 22-3.

TABLE 22-2   CALCULATION OF ESTIMATED ENERGY REQUIREMENTS FOR GROWING DOGS

Age	Adjustment factor (× adult ME)	Example
Small and medium breeds		ME requirement = $130 \times W_{kg}^{0.75}$
Weaning to ~4 months	2	7-lb puppy: $[2 \times (130 \times 3^{0.75})]$ = **590 kcal/day**
4-6 months	1.6	16-lb puppy: $[1.6 \times (130 \times 7.3^{0.75})]$ = **923 kcal/day**
6-10 months	1.2	22-lb puppy: $[1.2 \times (130 \times 10^{0.75})]$ = **877 kcal/day**
~10-12 months	1 (Adult)	26-lb dog: $130 \times 11.8^{0.75}$ = **827 kcal/day**
Large and giant breeds		
Weaning to ~4 months	2	16-lb puppy: $[2 \times (130 \times 7.3^{0.75})]$ = **1151 kcal/day**
4-8 months	1.6	34-lb puppy: $[2 \times (130 \times 15.4^{0.75})]$ = **1617 kcal/day**
9 to ~12 months	1.4	52-lb puppy: $[(1.4 \times (130 \times 23.6^{0.75})]$ = **1948 kcal/day**
~12-18 months	1.2	58-lb dog: $[(1.2 \times (130 \times 26.4^{0.75})]$ = **1815 kcal/day**
18-24 months	1 (Adult)	64-lb dog: $130 \times 29^{0.75}$ = **1624 kcal/day**

ME, Metabolizable energy.

TABLE 22-3   CALCULATION OF ENERGY REQUIREMENTS FOR GROWING CATS

Age	kcal/kg body weight	Example
6-20 weeks	250	3-lb kitten: 250×1.4 = **350 kcal/day**
4-6½ months	130	5-lb kitten: 130×2.3 = **299 kcal/day**
7-8½ months	100	6-lb kitten: 100×2.7 = **270 kcal/day**
9-11 months	80	7-lb kitten: 80×3.2 = **256 kcal/day**
12 months	60	7.5-lb cat: 60×3.4 = **204 kcal/day**

Protein

The protein requirement of growing puppies and kittens is higher than the protein requirement of adult animals. In addition to normal maintenance needs, young animals also need more protein to build the new tissue that is associated with growth. Because young animals consume higher amounts of energy and thus higher quantities of food than adult animals, the total amount of protein that they consume is naturally higher. Pet foods fed to growing puppies and kittens should contain slightly higher protein levels than foods developed for maintenance only. More importantly, the protein included in the diet should be of high quality and highly digestible. This type of protein ensures that sufficient levels of all of the essential amino acids are being delivered to the body for use in growth and development. The actual percentage of protein in the diet is not as important as is the balance between protein and energy. The minimum proportion of energy that should be supplied by protein in foods for growing dogs is 22%

of the ME kcal, and the minimum for growing cats is 26%.[30] Optimal levels are between 25% and 29% of ME kcal for puppies and 30% and 36% for kittens. As discussed previously, the percentage of protein in foods formulated for growing large- and giant-breed dogs will be slightly lower (~26%) than the percentage of protein found in foods for small- and medium-breed puppies because of the lower energy content and the need to balance protein with energy.

To support the growth of new tissues, foods for growing puppies and kittens should have slightly higher protein content than foods formulated for adult maintenance. The protein in the food should be of high quality and levels must be adjusted to be balanced with the food's energy density.

Calcium and Phosphorus

Diets for growing dogs and cats should contain optimal, but not excessive, amounts of calcium and phosphorus. The Association of American Feed Control Officials's (AAFCO's) *Nutrient Profiles* recommends that dog and cat foods formulated for growth contain a minimum of 1% calcium and 0.8% phosphorus on a dry-matter basis (DMB).[30] These recommendations are based upon diets containing 3500 and 4000 kcal/kg. Some commercially available pet foods contain slightly more than the recommended levels of calcium and phosphorus. These levels are not considered excessive but might not be optimal for large- and giant-breed dogs during periods of rapid growth. Growth diets formulated for large breeds should contain lower percentages of calcium and phosphorus because of the lower energy densities of these diets and the need to carefully control calcium intake to support proper skeletal development. Dietary calcium and phosphorus supplements should never be added to a balanced, complete food that has been formulated for growing dogs or cats (see Section 5, pp. 497-500).

Contrary to popular belief, calcium and phosphorus supplements are not necessary for growing pets and can be harmful in large and giant breeds of dogs, contributing to the development of certain developmental skeletal disorders.

Docosahexaenoic Acid

Long-chain n-6 and n-3 polyunsaturated fatty acids (LCPUFAs) are essential early in life for normal neurological development (see Chapter 11, pp 84-85 and Chapter 21, p. 211). The two fatty acids of greatest significance are arachidonic acid (AA), derived from linoleic acid, and docosahexaenoic acid (DHA), derived from alpha-linolenic acid. Both of these fatty acids are essential during perinatal life; DHA is especially crucial for normal neurological and retinal development.[31,32] In human fetuses, AA and DHA rapidly accumulate in brain and retinal tissues during the latter half of gestation and together make up approximately 50% of the total fatty acids found in the brain's grey matter.[33] The analogous period of brain growth and maturation in puppies occurs between 1 and 60 days of age.[34] Both a prenatal and postnatal supply of DHA is considered to be essential for puppies and kittens.[35-37]

Recent studies have shown that newborn puppies can convert milk alpha-linolenic acid to DHA early in life, but this ability is lost or greatly reduced after weaning.[35] Even prior to weaning, the efficiency of conversion is very low, so very large doses of alpha-linolenic acid are necessary to see a significant increase in tissue DHA levels.[36] However, the dog, like other species, does seem capable of converting alpha-linolenic acid to an intermediate LCPUFA, docosapentaenoic acid (DPA). When adult dogs were fed a diet that was enriched with alpha-linolenic acid, DPA, but not DHA, accumulated in plasma phospholipids.[38] Because DHA is highly conserved in retinal tissue and is important for normal functioning of the retina, it is theorized that the retina and other neural tissues of dogs can convert circulating DPA to DHA and that plasma DPA acts as the reservoir for this fatty acid. Together, these studies show that DHA may be provided to growing dogs either as alpha-linolenic acid (the most inefficient route), as DPA (either from hepatic conversion of alpha-linolenic acid or directly via diet), or as preformed DHA in the diet.

Because conversion is inefficient and is affected by age, supplying DHA directly in the food of growing puppies and kittens is the most effective approach to ensure adequate intake. Tests of retinal function and sensitivity in 12-week-old puppies improved more dramatically when puppies were exposed to diets containing preformed DHA throughout fetal and postnatal life than when they were exposed to a food containing alpha-linolenic acid but not DHA.[31] The effects of DHA on neural development have also been examined in growing dogs by testing learning ability and memory. Both the ability to learn a new task and memory of learned tasks were significantly improved in puppies fed a food containing high DHA throughout gestation, lactation, and weaning when compared with puppies that had been exposed to a low-DHA food during the same period.[39] Puppies exhibited these responses when they were tested daily between 10 and 16 weeks of age, illustrating the postweaning effects of DHA. Although a limited number of studies have been conducted with growing dogs, these recent results, together with corroborating evidence in other species, suggest that the provision of DHA early in life is essential for optimal neurological development in growing dogs.[40,41] Although dogs (and presumably cats) are capable of some conversion of alpha-linolenic acid to its long-chain derivatives, this conversion is not highly efficient. Therefore, it is prudent to include at least small amounts of the preformed LCPUFAs, especially DHA, in foods that are formulated for growing dogs and cats.

Docosahexaenoic acid (DHA) is a conditionally essential fatty acid that has an important role in early neurological development. Although dogs (and presumably cats) are capable of some conversion of alpha-linolenic acid to its long-chain derivatives, this conversion is not highly efficient. Therefore at least small amounts of the preformed long-chain polyunsaturated fatty acids, especially DHA, should be included in foods that are formulated for growing dogs and cats.

Antioxidant Nutrients and Immune Function

Puppies and kittens are born with functional but immature immune systems.[42] For example, day-old puppies are capable of developing an immune response to vaccination, but the response is lower in magnitude than that of an adult dog and will not confer complete protection when maternal antibodies are present. Lymphocytes, specifically T-cell populations, are smaller in kittens and are less responsive to antigenic challenge than those of adults.[43,44] In young puppies and kittens, immune cell numbers and their distribution continues to develop for the first 4 months of life. Therefore the consumption of an adequate volume of colostrum shortly after birth is essential for protection against infectious disease during the first several months of life (see Chapter 21, pp. 209-210 for a complete discussion of colostrum).

Vaccination programs are typically initiated when puppies and kittens are between 6 and 8 weeks of age. Following the initial vaccination, repeated vaccines (boosters) are administered every 3 to 4 weeks until animals are 16 weeks of age. (Orphaned neonates that did not receive colostrum should receive their first vaccination much earlier, starting at 2 to 3 weeks.) The purpose of vaccinations is to deliberately stimulate humoral (antibody-producing) and cell-mediated immune responses to specific (attenuated) antigens without causing disease. Successful vaccination produces immune memory that will protect the animal from subsequent exposure to actual infectious agents.

The importance of nutrition for proper immune function has been studied in many species. Most dramatically, frank deficiencies of energy, protein, essential fatty acids, and certain vitamins and minerals are known to negatively affect an animal's immune competency.[45] In recent years, focus has shifted to specific nutrients that support the immune system and have the potential to enhance an animal's immune response. Antioxidant nutrients have been targeted because of their role in scavenging the free radicals (also called *reactive oxygen species*) that are produced during oxidative metabolism and immune system functioning. Examples of free radical compounds include superoxide, hydrogen peroxide, and hydroxyl radicals. Lymphocytes (B and T cells) are highly active cells and produce a high number of free radicals during normal cellular activity. In addition, the cell-mediated immune response uses a mechanism called the "respiratory burst" that generates free radicals, which are then converted to bactericidal agents to destroy invading antigens. Although free radicals are produced as part of the body's normal and necessary immune defenses, excess production is harmful to the host animal, causing oxidative damage to cells and tissues. Because the membranes of immune cells contain an unusually high proportion of PUFAs and because these cells produce more free radicals than other cells, immune cells are especially vulnerable to injury and loss through excess free radical production. The body has several endogenous mechanisms that scavenge free radicals and maintain an optimal oxidant to antioxidant ratio in tissues. These mechanisms work in conjunction with exogenous antioxidant nutrients that are supplied in the diet. For growing dogs and cats, including an optimal concentration of these nutrients in their diet may help the developing immune system to respond optimally to vaccination. The most widely used nutrients that have antioxidant activity in the body are vitamin E, beta-carotene (provitamin A), lutein (another carotenoid antioxidant), vitamin C, flavonoids, zinc, and selenium.

Of the group of tocopherols that make up vitamin E, alpha-tocopherol has the highest biological activity in the body (see Chapter 5, p. 31). It is needed to maintain cell membrane fluidity and protects cellular components from oxidative damage. Immune cells contain higher amounts of alpha-tocopherol than other cells, which is suggestive of the need for additional antioxidant protection by these cells. Both supplemental and intramuscular injections of vitamin E have been shown to improve measures of immune function and reduce damage to blood cells in several species, including dogs and cats.[46,47] There appears to be an effective dietary range for this vitamin, because studies with human subjects have shown that excessive supplementation with vitamin E can cause a reduced antibody titer response to vaccination.[48] Similarly, a study with cats found that while moderate supplementation with vitamin E enhanced the immune response, high levels did not have a significant impact.[46]

Beta-carotene and lutein are carotenoid plant pigments that have antioxidant properties and have been shown to modulate the immune response in humans and other animals.[49] Supplementation with beta-carotene (provitamin A) modulates nonspecific cellular defense mechanisms and increases the number and function of immune cells. Adult dogs that were supplemented with 20 mg of beta-carotene per day had increased antibody levels and an enhanced delayed-type hypersensitivity (DTH) response after 8 weeks of supplementation.[50] (A test of DTH is used as a measure of an animal's cell-mediated immunity.) A subsequent study corroborated the DTH results and also reported that supplementing adult dogs with beta-carotene increased T- and B-cell proliferation responses.[51] Although immune responses

to beta-carotene have not been reported in cats, adult cats readily absorb dietary beta-carotene and rapidly incorporate it into circulating immune cells.[52] These results suggest that the immune system of cats also may benefit from this nutrient. Another carotenoid pigment, lutein, has been shown to have membrane-protecting effects similar to alpha-tocopherol and beta-carotene, and has a synergistic effect when fed with other carotenoid pigments.[53,54] Feeding adult dogs supplemental lutein showed benefits similar to those observed with beta-carotene, specifically enhanced DTH and lymphocyte proliferation responses.[55]

Vaccination programs for puppies and kittens are timed to coincide with the period that colostrum-derived immune protection is decreasing and the young animal's active immune system is maturing. Serial vaccination programs are designed to ensure that the puppy and kitten's developing immune system has adequate exposure to vaccine antigens to allow production of antibodies and to generate the immune memory that is needed to protect the animal from subsequent exposure to infectious agents. Identifying nutrients that may support or enhance a healthy immune response during initial vaccination in puppies and kittens is an important area of study because young animals are especially vulnerable to infection as their immune systems are maturing and because vaccination presents an immune challenge to growing animals.

Although limited studies have been conducted with dogs and cats during the period of initial vaccination, there is evidence that dietary antioxidants support healthy immune responses. In one study, 40 puppies were fed either a control puppy food or the same food supplemented with vitamin E, lutein, and beta-carotene.[42] Puppies were fed the test foods starting at weaning (6 weeks) and continuing for 4 months, and were vaccinated according to a standard protocol (see p. 229). The group of puppies fed the antioxidant-supplemented food showed significantly greater lymphocyte proliferation responses when compared with unsupplemented puppies. The enhanced response became more pronounced the longer the puppies were fed the supplemented food. Following vaccination, the supplemented group also had higher antibody titers to distemper, parainfluenza, and parvovirus, and a higher immunoglobulin M response to an antigenic challenge than the nonsupplemented group. Another study examined the response of growing puppies to supplementation with vitamin E, vitamin C, beta-carotene, and selenium between 7 weeks and 13 weeks of age.[56] Following completion of their vaccination series, puppies fed the supplemented foods had higher antibody titers to distemper virus when compared with titers of puppies fed nonsupplemented foods. In addition supplementation with antioxidant nutrients increased the number of memory T cells and related lymphocyte proliferation response to vaccine antigens. These studies provide evidence that the immune function of growing puppies (and presumably kittens) may benefit from the provision of certain antioxidant nutrients during growth to support immune function during periods of immune challenge.

PET FOOD DIGESTIBILITY AND ENERGY DENSITY

Diet digestibility and energy density are important considerations when feeding growing pets because of the quantity of food necessary to meet the requirements for growth and development. Growing dogs and cats have higher requirements for energy and essential nutrients than adults, but they also have less digestive capacity, smaller mouths, and smaller and fewer teeth. This is especially true for small and toy breeds of dogs. These differences limit the amount of food that a young animal can consume and digest within a meal or a given amount of time. If a diet is low in digestibility or energy density, a larger quantity must be consumed. The effects of low digestibility are exacerbated by the fact that as increasing amounts of a food must be fed, diet digestibility decreases further. When a poor-quality food with a very low-energy density is fed to growing puppies and kittens, the limits of the pet's stomach may be reached before adequate nutrients have been consumed. The result is compromised growth and impaired muscle and skeletal development. Young animals benefit from eating a food that is properly balanced for both essential nutrients and energy so that it is not necessary for them to consume an excessive volume of food at each meal and so that intake will not be limited by the size of the animal's stomach. Although the energy density of foods that are formulated for large-breed dogs should have lower energy densities, this reduction is

not excessive enough to impact stomach fill, provided quality ingredients are included and nutrients are properly balanced to energy.

It is equally important that growing dogs and cats not be overfed. Overfeeding during growth leads to an accelerated growth rate and can predispose the animal to obesity later in life. As discussed previously, rapid growth rate is an important risk factor in the development of skeletal disease (see pp. 222-225). One of the most common causes of overnutrition in growing puppies and kittens is the addition of supplemental foods to a balanced diet that has been formulated for growth. Supplementation is unnecessary and may be detrimental; therefore it is not recommended.

FEEDING MANAGEMENT DURING GROWTH

Once a puppy or kitten has been placed in a new home, the owner may wish to feed a food that is different from the food that was fed to the litter. If the puppy or kitten's diet is going to be changed, the new food should be introduced very gradually. No dietary change should be made at all within the first few days that the puppy or kitten is in the new home. Moving to a new home and leaving the dam and litter mates is very stressful, and providing a brand new diet at the same time can exacerbate this stress. Most breeders send a small package of food along with the puppy or kitten. This food should be fed for the first few days that the animal is in the new home. After 2 or 3 days, the new food can be introduced by mixing it in quarter increments with the original diet. The proportion of the new food should be increased for 4 successive days until the puppy or kitten is consuming only the new diet.

Dogs

Proper feeding of young dogs supports normal muscle and skeletal development and a rate of growth that is typical for the dog's particular breed. All dogs grow and develop rapidly during the first year of life, but small and toy breeds reach maturity at a younger age than large breeds (see Figure 22-2). Still, the most rapid period of growth for all dogs occurs between 3 and

5 months of age. Overfeeding for maximal growth rate and early maturity should be avoided in all dogs, but is crucial in large- and giant-breed puppies. In addition to negative effects upon skeletal development (see pp. 222-225), overnutrition early in life results in an increased number of fat cells and higher total body fat during adulthood.[57,58] Conversely, the mild restriction of calories during growth and throughout life contributes to increased longevity.[59,60]

AVOID OVERWEIGHT BODY CONDITION

When obesity occurs in a young animal, there is often an increase in both the size and number of fat cells in the body. This condition, called *hyperplastic obesity,* is believed to be more resistant to treatment than is hypertrophic obesity, which involves only an increase in fat cell size.[61] The presence of additional numbers of fat cells results in a higher percentage of body fat, even if the animal is not yet overweight. Thus an animal with fat cell hyperplasia has a higher percentage of total body fat than an animal that weighs the same amount but has a normal number of fat cells.[62,63] Normal adipocyte hyperplasia occurs during specific critical periods of development in growing animals.[64,65] The exact age that these periods occur in dogs and cats is not known. However, data in other species indicate that adipose tissue growth normally occurs during either infancy or adolescence.[62,66,67] If these data are true for the dog and cat, it is probable that the level of nutrition provided to growing pets is of importance in determining the number of fat cells that the animal has at maturity.

It has been postulated that superfluous fat cell hyperplasia during the critical periods of adipose tissue growth may produce a long-term stimulus to gain excess weight in the form of excess adipocytes that require lipid filling.[68] The existence of excess numbers of adipocytes results in both an increased predisposition toward obesity in adulthood and an increased difficulty in maintaining weight loss when it occurs. This theory has been supported by several studies showing that early overnutrition results in increased numbers of fat calls and increased total body fat throughout adult life.[58,62] The use of proper feeding techniques that allow judicious control of a growing dog's weight are therefore important for long-term weight control (see Section 5, Chapter 28, for a complete discussion of overweight conditions in dogs).

FEED FOR MODERATE GROWTH RATE As discussed previously, the second reason that overfeeding for maximal growth rate and development is not desirable relates to its potential to affect skeletal development. A concern for skeletal development is important when feeding large and giant breeds of dogs, which generally exhibit a higher incidence of developmental bone disorders. The two most important nutritional factors that can negatively affect skeletal development are feeding an energy- and nutrient-dense food at a level that leads to maximal growth rate and feeding excess amounts of calcium (see pp. 494-500). Feeding growing dogs moderately restricted levels of a well-balanced diet to achieve a lean body condition and moderate rate of growth does not affect either final body size or development. Dogs that are fed restricted levels of food that support a slower growth rate still attain normal adult size, but they do so at a slightly later age. It is advisable to feed growing dogs enough to attain an average, rather than a maximal, growth rate for the dog's particular breed. This goal can best be achieved through portion-controlled feeding of a food that is formulated for the dog's size and body type, and the frequent assessment of growth rate, weight gain, and body condition.

FEEDING MANAGEMENT Growing dogs have a very steep growth curve, and their total daily energy needs do increase as they grow. The amount of food that is fed should be adjusted in response to a weekly or biweekly assessment of the dog's body condition and weight. A dog that is too thin has easily palpable ribs with little or no overlying fat layer. The tail base may be prominent, and the overhead profile will be an exaggerated hourglass. A dog that is overweight has a moderate to heavy layer of fat overlying the ribs. In very overweight puppies, the ribs may be difficult to even feel. There may be a thickening around the base of the dog's tail due to fat stored in that area. The dog's profile will show only a slight hourglass shape, and in very overweight dogs, there is no waist at all. Overweight dogs that are older than 6 months lose their abdominal tuck and may show abdominal distention. Growing dogs that are at their ideal weight have ribs that are easily palpable with just a thin layer of overlying fat. The bony prominences of the hips are easily felt but not prominent. The dog's profile from above has an hourglass shape with a well-defined waist. Owners should assess body condition regularly and adjust the amount of food that is fed to maintain the dog's ideal body condition throughout the growth period.

Portion-controlled feeding is the recommended feeding regimen for growing dogs. A puppy's daily portion of food should be divided into at least two but preferably three meals per day until the puppy is 4 to 6 months of age. After 6 months, two meals per day can be fed. Some large and giant breeds of dogs may benefit from three or more feedings per day as a precaution against the development of gastric dilatation-volvulus (see Section 5, pp. 459-461). Free-choice feeding is not recommended for growing dogs because this type of feeding regimen makes it difficult to monitor and control weight gain and growth rate and has been associated with a greater incidence of developmental bone disease. If a pet owner eventually wishes to switch a dog to a free-choice regimen, this should be done only after the dog has achieved mature size.

Portion-controlled feeding is the recommended feeding regimen for growing dogs. This feeding regimen allows control of the puppy's weight and rate of growth. Young puppies do best when fed three meals a day. This can be reduced to twice daily feeding after 4 to 6 months. The amount of food that is fed should be adjusted in response to a weekly or biweekly assessment of the dog's body condition and weight. Maintaining a lean and well-muscled body condition throughout growth supports a moderate rate of development and prevents overweight conditions.

Although this is becoming less common, some breeders continue to recommend feeding an adult maintenance food rather than a growth diet to large- and giant-breed puppies. It is erroneously believed that owners can more easily achieve a lower rate of growth in their puppy by feeding an adult food because maintenance diets typically have lower energy densities than growth diets. However, adult maintenance foods are not formulated for growth, and their nutrients are not balanced with the energy of the diet for the needs of growing dogs. Because a growing puppy requires up to twice the amount of energy per day as an adult of the same weight, the puppy may need to consume a larger volume of an adult food to meet its energy needs. This may result in the inadvertent consumption of excess amounts of other nutrients (such as calcium). If very large volumes of food are fed to meet the puppy's energy needs, this can also lead to digestive upsets, gastric discomfort, or diarrhea. It is therefore best to choose a highly digestible growth diet in which the nutrient and energy levels are specifically formulated for the growing dog's size and body type (or breed).

In addition to controlling food intake, owners should also provide regular periods of exercise for their growing dog. Exercise aids in the achievement of proper energy balance and supports normal muscle development. Young dogs should be exercised at a level that maintains a lean, well-muscled body condition throughout their growing period. Daily running, swimming, or retrieving for 20 to 40 minutes is adequate for most dogs. High-impact activities such as playing with other dogs, wrestling with owners, or prolonged periods of running should be strictly supervised and provided only in moderation. There is evidence that exercise that is overly vigorous or intense may predispose young dogs to skeletal abnormalities such as osteochondritis dissecans (OCD).[69] Care should always be taken to avoid excessive periods of exercise involving prolonged concussion to developing joints in growing dogs, especially dogs of the large or giant breeds (see Box 22-1).

Cats

Like dogs, growing cats should be fed to achieve normal growth and development. A high-quality, commercial cat food that has been formulated for growing kittens is recommended. Supplementation of this diet is not necessary and can be detrimental. Normal feline feeding behavior results in the frequent consumption of many small meals throughout the day (see Chapter 19, pp. 192-193). If adequate exercise is provided, most growing cats can self-regulate their energy intake when fed free-choice and will not overeat. In general, excessive caloric intake and accelerated growth rate are not common problems in growing cats. However, if inadequate exercise is provided or a highly palatable diet is fed, excessive weight gain can result. In these situations, portion-controlled feeding should be used (Box 22-1).

BOX 22-1   PRACTICAL FEEDING TIPS: GROWING DOGS AND CATS

Feed a highly digestible, nutrient-dense food formulated for growth.

Meal-feed using a portion-controlled regimen.

Feed three to four meals per day until 4 to 6 months of age; feed two or more meals per day after 6 months.

Feed to achieve an average rate of growth for a pet's breed and to support a lean body condition.

Avoid overfeeding to promote maximal growth rate.

Energy density and calcium should be carefully controlled in foods selected for large- and giant-breed puppies.

Provide regular daily exercise.

Do not add nutrient supplements to a pet's balanced diet.

References

1. Hawthorne AJ, Booles D, Nugent PA, and others: Body-weight changes during growth in puppies of different breeds, *J Nutr* 134:2027S–2030S, 2004.

2. Trangerud C, Grondalen J, Indrebo A, and others: A longitudinal study on growth and growth variables in dogs of four large breeds raised in domestic environments, *J Anim Sci* 85:7–83, 2007.

3. Douglass GM, Kane E, Holmes EJ: A profile of male and female cat growth, *Comp Anim Pract* 2:9–12, 1988.

4. Allard RL, Douglass GM, Kerr WW: The effects of breed and sex on dog growth, *Comp Anim Pract* 2:15–19, 1988.

5. Lauten SD: Nutritional risks to large-breed dogs: from weaning to the geriatric years, *Vet Clin North Am Small Anim Pract* 36:1345–1359, 2006.

6. Hedhammer A, Wu F, Krook L, and others: Overnutrition and skeletal disease: an experimental study in growing Great Dane dogs, *Cornell Vet* 64(Suppl 5):1–159, 1974.

7. Kealy RD, Olsson SE, Monti KL, and others: Effects of limited food consumption on the incidence of hip dysplasia in growing dogs, *J Am Vet Med Assoc* 201:857–863, 1992.

8. Dammrich K: Relationship between nutrition and bone growth in large and giant dogs, *J Nutr* 121:S114–S121, 1991.

9. Smith GK, Paster ER, Powers MY, and others: Lifelong diet restriction and radiographic evidence of osteoarthritis in the hip joint in dogs, *J Am Vet Med Assoc* 229:690–693, 2006.

10. Lepine AJ: Optimal nutrition for the growing retriever and upland dog. In *Nutrition and care of the sporting dog*, Dayton, Ohio, 2002, The Iams Company, pp 17–22.

11. Dobenecker B: Influence of calcium and phosphorus intake on the apparent digestibility of these minerals in growing dogs, *J Nutr* 132:1665S–1667S, 2002.

12. Hazewinkel HAW, Goedegebuure SA, Poulos PW, and others: Influences of chronic calcium excess on the skeletal development of growing Great Danes, *J Am Anim Hosp Assoc* 21:377–391, 1985.

13. Tryfonidou MA, van den Broek J, van den Brom WE: Intestinal calcium absorption in growing dogs is influenced by calcium intake and age but not by growth rate, *J Nutr* 132:363–368, 2002.

14. Tryfonidou MA, Holl MS, Oosterlaken-Dijksterhuis MA: Growth hormone modulates cholecalciferol metabolism with moderate effects on intestinal mineral absorption and specific effects on bone formation in growing dogs raised on balanced food, *Domest Anim Endocrinol* 25:155–174, 2003.

15. Goodman SA, Montgomery RD, Fitch RB, and others: Serial orthopedic examinations of rowing Great Dane puppies fed three diets varying in calcium and phosphorus. In Reinhart GA, Carey DP, editors: *Recent advances in canine and feline nutrition, Iams nutrition symposium proceedings*, vol 2, Wilmington, Ohio, 1998, Orange Frazer Press.

16. Goedegebuure SA, Hazewinkel HA: Morphological findings in young dogs chronically fed a diet containing excess calcium, *Vet Pathol* 23:594–605, 1986.

17. Nap RC, Hazewinkel HAW, van den Brom WE: Calcium kinetics in growing Miniature Poodles challenged by four different levels of calcium, *J Nutr* 123:1826–2833, 1993.

18. Stephens LC, Norrdin RW, Benjamin SA: Effects of calcium supplement and sunlight exposure on growing Beagle dogs, *Am J Vet Res* 46:2037–2042, 1988.

19. Dobenecker B: Apparent calcium absorption in growing dogs of two different sizes, *J Nutr* 134:2151S–2153S, 2004.

20. Nap RC, Hazewinkel HAW, Vorrhout G, and others: The influence of the dietary protein content on growth in giant breed dogs, *J Vet Comp Orthop Trauma* 6:1–8, 1993.

21. Hazewinkel HAE, Tryfonidou MA: Vitamin D_3 metabolism in dogs, *Mol Cell Endocrinol* 197:23–33, 2002.

22. Tryfonidou MA, Oosterlaken-Dijksterhuis MA, Mol JA, and others: 24-hydroxylase: potential key regulator in hypervitaminosis D_3 in growing dogs, *Am J Physiol Endocrine Metab* 284:E505–E513, 2003.

23. Tryfonidou MA, Stevenhagen JJ, van den Bernd GJ, and others: Moderate cholecalciferol supplementation depresses intestinal calcium absorption in growing dogs, *J Nutr* 132:2644–2650, 2002.

24. Tryfonidou MA, Holl MS, Stevenhagen JJ, and others: Dietary 135-fold cholecalciferol supplementation severely disturbs the endochondral ossification in growing dogs, *Domest Anim Endocrinol* 24:265–285, 2003.

25. Tryfonidou MA, Hazewinkel HAW: Different effects of physiologically and pharmacologically increased growth hormone levels on cholecalciferol metabolism at prepubertal age, *J Steroid Biochem Mol Biol* 89/90:49–54, 2004.

26. Tryfonidou MA, Holl MS, Vastenburg M, and others: Hormonal regulation of calcium homeostasis in two breeds of dogs during growth at different rates, *J Anim Sci* 81:1568–1580, 2003.

27. Lepine AJ: Nutritional management of the large breed puppy. In Reinhart GA, Carey DP, editors: *Recent advances in canine and feline nutrition, Iams nutrition symposium proceedings*, vol 2, Wilmington, Ohio, 1998, Orange Frazer Press.

28. National Research Council: *Nutrient requirements of dogs and cats*, Washington DC, 2006, National Academy Press.

29. Allard RL, Douglass GM, Kerr WW: The effects of breed and sex on dog growth, *Companion Anim Pract* 2:15–19, 1988.

30. Association of American Feed Control Officials (AAFCO): *Official publication*, Atlanta, 2008, AAFCO.

31. Heinemann KM, Waldron MK, Bigley KE, and others: Long-chain (n-3) polyunsaturated fatty acids are more efficient than alpha-linolenic acid in improving electroretinogram responses of puppies exposed during gestation, lactation, and weaning, *J Nutr* 135:1960–1966, 2005.

32. Bauer JE, Heinemann KM, Lees GE, Waldron MK: Retinal functions of young dogs are improved and maternal plasma phospholipids are altered with diets containing long-chain n-3 polyunsaturated fatty acids during gestation, lactation, and after weaning, *J Nutr* 136:1991S–1994S, 2006.

33. O'Brien JS, Fillerup DL, Mead JF: Quantification and fatty acid and fatty aldehyde composition of ethanolamine, choline, and serine glycerophosphatides in human cerebral grey and white matter, *J Lipid Res* 5:329–338, 1964.

34. Arant BS Jr, Gooch JM: Developmental changes in the mongrel canine brain during postnatal life, *Early Hum Dev* 7:179–194, 1982.

35. Bauer JE, Heinemann KM, Lees GE, Waldron MK: Docosahexaenoic acid accumulates in plasma of canine puppies raised on alpha-linolenic acid-rich milk during suckling but not when fed alpha-linolenic acid-rich diets after weaning, *J Nutr* 136:2087–2089, 2006.

36. Heinemann KM, Bauer JE: Docosahexaenoic acid and neurologic development in animals, *J Am Vet Med Assoc* 228:700–705, 2006.

37. Bauer JE: Metabolic basis for the essential nature of fatty acids and the unique dietary fatty acid requirements of cats, *J Am Vet Med Assoc* 229:1729–1732, 2006.

38. Bauer JE, Dunbar BL, Bigley KE: Dietary flaxseed in dogs results in differential transport and metabolism of n-3 polyunsaturated fatty acids, *J Nutr* 128:2641S–2644S, 1998.

39. Kelley R, Lepine AJ: Improving puppy trainability through nutrition. In *Proc NAVC*, 2005, pp 21–26.

40. Suzuki H, Park SJ, Tamura M, Ando S: Effect of the long-term feeding of dietary lipids on the learning ability, fatty acid composition of brain stem phospholipids and synaptic membrane fluidity in adult mice: a comparison of sardine oil diet with palm oil diet, *Mech Ageing Dev* 101:119–128, 1998.

41. Lim SY, Suzuki H: Dose-response effect of docosahexaenoic acid ethyl ester on maze behavior and brain fatty acid composition in adult mice. *Int J Vitam Nutr Res* 72:77–84, 2002.

42. Massimino SP, Daristotle L, Ceddia MA, Hayek MA: The influence of diet on the puppy's developing immune system. In *Proc WASVA*, 2004, pp 51–55.

43. Bortnick SJ, Orandle MS, Papadi GP, Johnson CM: Lymphocytes subsets in neonatal and juvenile cats: comparison of blood and lymphoid tissues, *Lab Anim Sci* 49:395–400, 1999.

44. Somberg RL, Robinson JP, Felsburg PJ: T lymphocyte development and function in dogs with X-linked severe combined immunodeficiency, *J Immunol* 153:4006–4015, 1994.

45. Gershwin ME, German BJ, Keen CL, editors: *Nutrition and immunology: principles and practice*, Totowa, NJ, 2000, Humana Press.

46. Hayek MG, Massimino SP, Burr JR, Kearns RJ: Dietary vitamin E improves immune function in cats. In Reinhart GA, Carey DP, editors: *Recent advances in canine and feline nutrition, Iams nutrition symposium proceedings*, vol 3, Wilmington, Ohio, 2000, Orange Frazer Press, pp 555–564.

47. Heaton P, Reed CF, Mann SJ: Role of dietary antioxidants to protect against DNA damage in adult dogs, *J Nutr* 132:1720S–1724S, 2002.

48. Meydani SN, Meydani M, Blumberg JB, and others: Vitamin E supplementation and in vivo immune response in healthy elderly subjects: a randomized controlled trial, *JAMA* 277:1380–1385, 1997.

49. Chew BS, Park JS: Carotenoid action on the immune response, *J Nutr* 134:257S–261S, 2004.

50. Chew BP, Park JS, Wong TS, and others: Importance of beta-carotene nutrition in the dog and cat: uptake and immunity. In Reinhart GA, Carey DP, editors: *Recent advances in canine and feline nutrition, Iams nutrition symposium proceedings*, vol 2, Wilmington, Ohio, 1998, Orange Frazer Press, pp 513–533.

51. Kearns RJ, Loos KM, Chew BP, and others: The effect of age and dietary beta-carotene on immunological parameters in the dog. In Reinhart GA, Carey DP, editors: *Recent advances in canine and feline nutrition, Iams nutrition symposium proceedings*, vol 3, Wilmington, Ohio, 2000, Orange Frazer Press, pp 389–401.

52. Chew BP, Park JS, Weng BC, and others: Dietary beta-carotene absorption by blood plasma and leukocytes in domestic cats, *J Nutr* 130:2322–2325, 2000.

53. Sujak A, Gabrielska J, Grudzinski W, and others: Lutein and zeaxanthin as protectors of lipid membranes against oxidative damage: the structural aspects, *Arch Biochem Biophys* 371:301–307, 1999.

54. Stahl W, Junghans A, de Proer B, and others: Carotenoid mixtures protect multilamellar liposomes against oxidative damage: synergistic effects of lycopene and lutein, *FEBS Lett* 427:305–308, 1998.

55. Kim HW, Chew BP, Wong TS, and others: Dietary lutein stimulates immune response in the canine, *Vet Immunol Immunopathol* 74:315–327, 2000.

56. Khoo C, Cunnick J, Friesen K, and others: The role of supplementary dietary antioxidants on immune response in puppies, *Vet Ther* 6:43–56, 2005.

57. Faust IM, Johnson PR, Hirsch J: Long-term effects of early nutritional experience on the development of obesity in the rat, *J Nutr* 110:2027–2034, 1980.

58. Johnson PR, Stern JS, Greenwood MRC, and others: Effect of early nutrition on adipose cellularity and pancreatic insulin release in the Zucker rat, *J Nutr* 103:738–743, 1973.

59. Ross MH: Length of life and caloric intake, *Am J Clin Nutr* 25:834–838, 1972.

60. Kealy RD, Lawler DF, Ballam JM, and others: Effects of diet restriction on life span and age-related changes in dogs, *J Am Vet Med Assoc* 220:1315–1320, 2002.

61. Bjorntorp P, Sjostrom L: Number and size of fat cells in relation to metabolism in human obesity, *Metabolism* 20:703–706, 1971.

62. Faust IM, Johnson PR, Hirsch J: Long-term effects of early nutritional experience on the development of obesity in the rat, *J Nutr* 110:2027–2034, 1980.

63. Faust IM, Johnson PR, Stern JS, and others: Diet-induced adipocyte number increase in adult rats: a new model of obesity, *Am J Physiol* 235:E279–E286, 1978.

64. Bertrand HA, Lynd FT, Masoro EJ, and others: Changes in adipose mass and cellularity through the adult life of rats fed ad libitum or a life-prolonging restricted diet, *J Gerontol* 35:827–835, 1980.

65. Hirsch J, Knittle JL: Cellularity of obese and non-obese adipose tissue, *Fed Proc* 29:1516–1521, 1970.

66. Etherton TD, Wangsness PJ, Hammers VM, and others: Effect of dietary restriction on carcass composition and adipocyte cellularity of swine with different propensities for obesity, *J Nutr* 112:2314–2323, 1982.

67. Lewis DS, Bertrand HA, Masoro EJ: Pre-weaning nutrition on fat development in baboons, *J Nutr* 113:2253–2259, 1983.

68. Vasselli JR, Cleary MP, van Itallie TB: Modern concepts of obesity, *Nutr Rev* 41:361–373, 1983.

69. Slater MR, Scarlett JM, Donoghue S, and others: Diet and exercise as potential risk factors for osteochondritis dissecans in dogs, *Am J Vet Res* 53:2119–2124, 1992.

23

Adult Maintenance

A dog or cat that has reached mature adult size and is not pregnant, lactating, or working strenuously is defined as being in a maintenance state. This category includes most of the dogs and cats kept as household pets. Primary nutritional concerns during this period of life are the provision of a nutritionally complete and balanced food that supplies adequate energy and all of the pet's daily nutrient needs. Feeding proper amounts of a high-quality, well-formulated food throughout a dog or cat's adult life contributes to optimal health and the maintenance of ideal body weight and condition.

The majority of dogs and cats kept as household pets are in the adult maintenance state. Proper nutrition and activity levels throughout adulthood are important factors in the healthy maintenance of pets.

Adult dogs should be fed food that is formulated for their life stage, activity level, and if appropriate, breed size. Although canned, semimoist, or dry food can be fed, dry foods are often preferred for this stage of life. In general, canned and semimoist foods have higher caloric densities on a dry-matter basis (DMB) than dry foods (see Chapter 17, p. 164). When canned or semimoist foods are fed to adult dogs, they may contribute to the development of overweight conditions if intake is not closely monitored. Dry dog foods are less calorically dense, and they can also help to maintain proper tooth and gum hygiene (see Chapter 34, p. 442 for a complete discussion). Dry foods are also easier and more economical to feed to large groups of dogs than are other types of foods.

The availability of highly palatable pet foods coupled with the sedentary lives of many dogs has resulted in a high incidence of obesity in the adult dog population. It is estimated that 20% to 40% of American dogs and cats are either overweight or obese.[1,2] Similar incidence rates are reported in other industrialized countries.[3] The two most effective ways to prevent obesity in adult dogs are to provide daily exercise and to closely regulate food intake. Exercise can be in the form of daily walks or runs or several sessions of vigorous games such as fetch or hide and seek. Swimming is also an excellent form of exercise. Most dogs enjoy swimming if introduced to water at an early age and in a gradual manner. There are also many types of organized dog activities and dog sports available to interested owners. Popular examples include agility, rally, flyball, freestyle, obedience competitions, and tracking. These sports are enjoyable activities for both owners and their dogs and provide mental stimulation along with the benefits of physical activity.

Monitoring an adult dog's daily food intake is best accomplished through portion-controlled feeding (see Chapter 19, pp. 195-196). Some dogs are able to self-regulate their food intake when fed free-choice. However, many dogs tend to overconsume and gain weight. Providing two or more premeasured meals at regular times each day is a simple way to carefully regulate a dog's food intake. The feeding guidelines printed on pet food labels provide an estimate of the amount needed to feed an average adult dog that is living indoors and provided with a moderate amount of exercise. Alternatively, an estimate of the amount to feed can be calculated using the dog's ideal body weight (see Chapter 9, pp. 66-68, and Table 9-2, p. 67). Although each of these approximations can be used as a starting point, every dog should be fed as an individual. Adjustments are made in accordance with the dog's activity level, temperament, body condition, and weight status. Body condition scoring systems provide a reliable method for owners and veterinarians to use when assessing body condition in dogs and cats.[4,5] Because body weight alone is not necessarily a reliable indicator of a dog's body condition, these visual tools have been developed as aids for determining optimal body condition and for the diagnosis of obesity in companion animals. Examples of body scoring systems for dogs and cats are provided in Figures 23-1 and 23-2, respectively. The use of body scoring is discussed in detail in Chapter 28, pp. 322-326.

Body Condition Scores

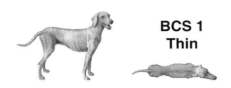

BCS 1 **Thin**		• Ribs, lumbar vertebrae, and pelvic bones visible at a distance and felt without pressure • No palpable fat over tail base, spine, or ribs • Diminished muscle mass • Extreme concave abdominal tuck when viewed from side • Severe hourglass shape when viewed from above

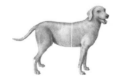

BCS 2
Underweight

- Ribs palpable with little pressure; may be visible
- Minimal palpable fat over ribs, spine, tail base
- Increased concave abdominal tuck when viewed from side
- Marked hourglass shape to waist when viewed from above

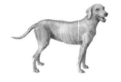

BCS 3
IDEAL

- Ribs and spine palpable with slight pressure but not visible; no excess fat covering
- Ribs can be seen with motion of dog
- Good muscle tone apparent
- Concave abdominal tuck when viewed from side
- Hourglass shape to waist when viewed from above

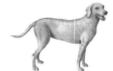

BCS 4
Overweight

- Ribs palpable with increased pressure; not visible and have excess fat covering
- Ribs not seen with motion of the dog
- General hefty appearance
- Abdominal concave tuck is reduced or absent when viewed from the side
- Loss of hourglass shape to waist with back slightly broadened when viewed from above

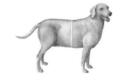

BCS 5
Obese

- Ribs and spine not palpable under a heavy fat covering
- Fat deposits visible over lumbar area, tail base, and spine
- Loss of hourglass shape to waist
- Complete loss of abdominal tuck with rounded abdomen
- Back is markedly broadened

Figure 23-1 Assessment of body conditions in the dog.

(Copyright © Procter & Gamble Co., Cincinnati, Ohio, 2009.)

Body Condition Scores

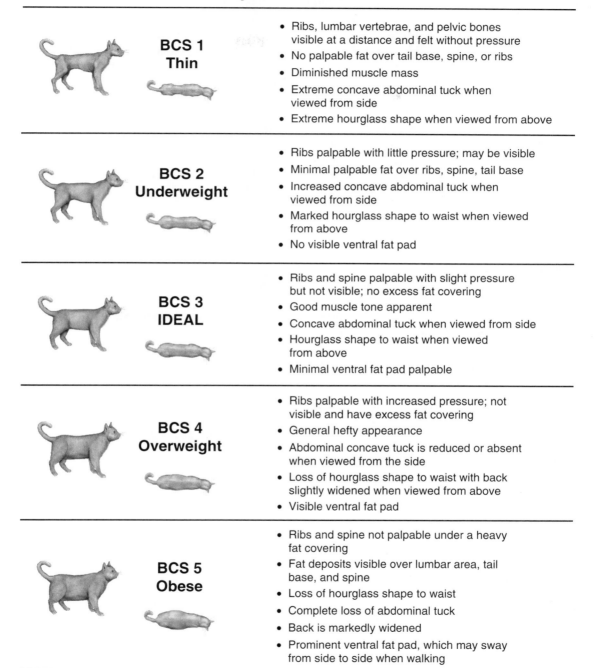

BCS 1
Thin

- Ribs, lumbar vertebrae, and pelvic bones visible at a distance and felt without pressure
- No palpable fat over tail base, spine, or ribs
- Diminished muscle mass
- Extreme concave abdominal tuck when viewed from side
- Extreme hourglass shape when viewed from above

BCS 2
Underweight

- Ribs palpable with little pressure; may be visible
- Minimal palpable fat over ribs, spine, tail base
- Increased concave abdominal tuck when viewed from side
- Marked hourglass shape to waist when viewed from above
- No visible ventral fat pad

BCS 3
IDEAL

- Ribs and spine palpable with slight pressure but not visible; no excess fat covering
- Good muscle tone apparent
- Concave abdominal tuck when viewed from side
- Hourglass shape to waist when viewed from above
- Minimal ventral fat pad palpable

BCS 4
Overweight

- Ribs palpable with increased pressure; not visible and have excess fat covering
- General hefty appearance
- Abdominal concave tuck is reduced or absent when viewed from the side
- Loss of hourglass shape to waist with back slightly widened when viewed from above
- Visible ventral fat pad

BCS 5
Obese

- Ribs and spine not palpable under a heavy fat covering
- Fat deposits visible over lumbar area, tail base, and spine
- Loss of hourglass shape to waist
- Complete loss of abdominal tuck
- Back is markedly widened
- Prominent ventral fat pad, which may sway from side to side when walking

Figure 23-2   Assessment of body conditions in the cat.

(Copyright © Procter & Gamble Co., Cincinnati, Ohio, 2009.)

Like dogs, adult cats should be fed a food that has been formulated for maintenance. Cats are generally nonvoracious feeders and prefer to eat many small meals frequently throughout the day (see Chapter 19, pp 192-193). Some cats adapt well to free-choice feeding and can maintain their normal body weight on this type of regimen, while others do best if fed several premeasured meals per day. Although any type of food can be fed to adult cats, dry cat foods are best suited for free-choice feeding because they keep fresh longer than other foods. In addition, cats are less likely to overconsume dry foods when fed free-choice. In general, cats that live entirely indoors have less opportunity or inclination to exercise than do cats that have access to the outdoors.

As a result, indoor cats are more prone to overweight conditions. A variety of interactive cat toys, designed to stimulate chase and play behaviors in cats, are available and can help to increase activity in a sedentary cat. Because cats enjoy novelty, owners are encouraged to purchase several types of toys that their cats enjoy and rotate the toys to maintain interest. Some cats also enjoy going for walks outdoors with their owners and can be trained to walk using a harness and leash. Finally, just as with dogs, a visual body score chart can be used to evaluate an adult cat's body condition (see Figure 23-2). If an adult cat cannot maintain normal body condition on a free-choice regimen, portion-controlled feeding should be used.

References

1. McGreevy PD, Thomson PC, Pride C, and others: Prevalence of obesity in dogs examined by Australian veterinary practices and the risk factors involved, *Vet Rec* 156:695–707, 2005.

2. Scarlett JM, Donoghue S, Saidla J, and others: Overweight cats: prevalence and risk factors, *Int J Obes* 18:S22–S28, 1994.

3. Colliard L, Paragon BM, Lemuet B, and others: Prevalence and risk factors of obesity in an urban population of healthy cats, *J Feline Med Surg* 11:135–140, 2009.

4. Laflamme D: Development and validation of a body condition score system for dogs, *Canine Pract* 22:10–15, 1997.

5. Laflamme DP, Schmidt DA, Deshmukh A: Correlation of body fat in cats using body condition score or DEXA, *J Vet Intern Med* 8:214, 1994.

24

Performance

Dogs work with people in a variety of capacities, including acting as aids for the blind and the physically disabled, herding and guarding sheep, hunting, pulling sleds on arctic expeditions and races, and performing protection and drug detection tasks for the police and military. In addition, many owners and their dogs participate in a variety of dog sports, including agility, Flyball, obedience trials, tracking tests, hunting trials, and lure-coursing tests. The type of training, level of exercise, and daily routine that a dog experiences vary with the type of work or sport. In general, all working dogs have higher energy requirements than adult dogs during periods of normal maintenance. Depending on the type and intensity of work, modifications in the nutrient composition of the diet and changes in the daily feeding regimen of a performance dog may be necessary.

ENDURANCE PERFORMANCE

Endurance performance in dogs, as in humans, involves prolonged periods of exercise at sub-maximal levels of exertion. Much of what we currently understand about the nutritional needs of hard-working endurance dogs comes from studies of Alaskan sled dogs. Sled dogs working in cold environments represent the ultimate canine endurance athletes. These dogs have been used as the accepted mode of transportation in Alaska and surrounding territories for many years. During the Gold Rush of the late 1800s, prospectors traveled to the Yukon Territory and used dogs to cross the northern tundra in search of gold. As mining camps and towns developed, sled dog trails were forged to connect coastal towns to interior camps. These trails provided the major transport routes for the provision of food and supplies to the camps. Although most of the mining camps are now mere ghost towns, dogs and dog sledding remain an integral part of the area's economy and culture. In addition to their importance in Alaska, sled dog teams have been used by explorers of the North and South Poles. Robert Perry reached the North Pole via dog sled in 1909, and Roald Amundsen reached the South Pole

with his team of dogs in 1911. Sled dog teams continue to provide transportation in certain areas of the world. In addition, mushing and sled dog racing have become popular outdoor sports for many dog enthusiasts. Today, sled dog races are held in many parts of the world, including Europe, Alaska, and several of the lower 48 states.

The Iditarod is one of the most well-known and publicized long-distance sled dog races. Informally called the "the last great race on earth," the Iditarod is run every March, beginning in Anchorage and ending in Nome. The trail that is followed is symbolically designated to be 1049 miles long (1000 miles because it is at least that long, and 49 miles because Alaska was the forty-ninth state to be admitted to the union). Officially, the race distance is 1158 miles by the northern route or 1163 miles by the southern route. Because of its great length and the difficult terrain, the Iditarod represents the ultimate endurance test for the canine athlete. Dog teams average up to 100 miles per day in subzero temperatures and over difficult snow-covered terrain. Nutritionists and exercise physiologists interested in the care and nutrition of these dogs have used this race and similar long-distance sled dog races to collect valuable information about the energy, nutrient, water, and electrolyte needs of working dogs. In addition, studies of certain types of hunting dogs, search and rescue dogs, and military dogs also provide information regarding the needs of dogs that work for long periods of time at sub-maximal levels of exertion. This research has provided information for the development of diets that provide optimal nutrition for working dogs; it has also contributed to improved information about the proper care and husbandry of dogs engaged in endurance exercise.

Physiology

The type of work that occurs during endurance competitions differs from that performed during short races or sprinting events, such as Greyhound racing or lure coursing. Greyhounds engage in brief, intense bouts of high-speed running, while sled dogs pull for several hours at a time at slower speeds. Dogs used for hunting typically engage in both types of exertion. These dogs often work for hours at a time over a period of several days (endurance), interspersed with occasional bouts of high-intensity sprinting. Metabolically, the energy necessary for short and intense sprints is obtained primarily through anaerobic pathways and secondarily through aerobic metabolism. In contrast, the energy that is needed for endurance work is predominantly derived from aerobic metabolism.

Greyhounds engage in brief, intense bouts of high-speed running, sled dogs pull for several hours at a time at slower speeds, and dogs used for hunting typically engage in both types of exertion. Metabolically, the energy necessary for short and intense sprints is obtained primarily through anaerobic pathways and secondarily through aerobic metabolism. In contrast, the energy that is needed for endurance work is predominantly derived from aerobic metabolism.

Fat and carbohydrate are the two principal fuels that supply energy to working muscle. During the low-intensity (aerobic) exercise associated with endurance, fat is the most important fuel used. This is supplied by free fatty acids (FFAs) derived from triglycerides of muscle and other tissues. As the intensity of exercise increases, a shift toward more anaerobic metabolism occurs, and carbohydrate becomes increasingly important as a source of energy. This carbohydrate is supplied by muscle glycogen and, as muscle glycogen becomes depleted, is supplemented by the production of glucose by the liver (gluconeogenesis). This metabolic response to different intensities of exercise and training has been observed in rats, humans, and dogs.[1-5] For example, the rate of muscle glycogen utilization in trained dogs completing a high-intensity anaerobic test is almost twenty-fold greater than the rate observed in dogs during a period of aerobic exercise.[6]

Fat is the most important fuel used during low-intensity, aerobic exercise. This is supplied by free fatty acids derived from triglycerides of muscle and other tissues.

As the intensity of exercise increases, a shift toward more anaerobic metabolism occurs, and carbohydrate becomes increasingly important as a source of energy. This carbohydrate is supplied by muscle glycogen and via gluconeogenesis.

An examination of the types of muscles that are involved in endurance exercise provides information about the types of energy sources needed. The skeletal muscles of dogs contain three main types of muscle fibers: type I (slow twitch) and types IIa and IIb (fast twitch). Slow-twitch fibers have a high capacity for aerobic metabolism, and fast-twitch fibers can use both oxidative (aerobic) and anaerobic pathways.[7] The slow-twitch fibers use fatty acids and glucose for fuel and are believed to be important for endurance events. Although these fibers are found in all skeletal muscles, their numbers predominate in antigravity muscles such as the dog's anconeus and the quadratus muscles.[8] In general, endurance athletes have higher numbers of well-developed, slow-twitch fibers, and athletes involved in high-speed sprinting events have a higher proportion of fast-twitch fibers. Athletic conditioning is important for conditioning muscles and building muscle mass. Athletic training for endurance events increases the body's reliance upon fatty acid oxidation during submaximal bouts of exercise. This adaptation has been demonstrated in rats, humans, and dogs.[1,2] Moreover, the type of diet that is fed affects the use of fatty acids by working muscles, independent of the effects of training.[6,9]

Glycogen Loading

Although it is generally accepted that energy is the nutrient of most concern for working dogs, there has been much debate about the best way to supply dietary energy to enhance endurance performance. Increasing stamina and strength are goals for the nutritional programs of many human athletes. As a result, a great deal of research has been conducted concerning ways to supply fuel to long-distance runners and cyclists.[1,10] An important limiting factor in prolonged exercise is the amount of glycogen present in the working muscles because the onset of fatigue is highly correlated with muscle glycogen depletion.[11,12] In addition, endurance for submaximal exercise can be increased by raising muscle glycogen stores and decreased by lowering muscle glycogen.[12,13] Therefore a major goal when feeding human endurance athletes is to either increase muscle glycogen stores or delay muscle glycogen depletion during periods of exercise.

The procedure of glycogen loading (also called *carbohydrate loading*) was developed for human athletes with the intent of increasing muscle glycogen stores before periods of prolonged exercise. Glycogen loading was initially accomplished by first depleting muscle glycogen through exhaustive exercise and/or consumption of a low-carbohydrate diet, followed by the consumption of a high-carbohydrate diet for 4 to 7 days.[14,15] The preliminary glycogen depletion phase presumably resulted in glycogen supercompensation when the subject consumed a diet that is high in starch for several subsequent days. The beneficial effects that higher initial glycogen stores have on endurance are believed to be the result of the availability of larger amounts of glycogen for anaerobic energy metabolism in the working muscles. However, controlled studies have shown that in the first stage, glycogen depletion is unnecessary and may even be detrimental to training performance and health.[16,12] Today, many endurance athletes regularly consume a high-carbohydrate diet and concentrate on carbohydrate loading for the last few days prior to an endurance event but do not engage in the preliminary depletion phase.

Providing Energy for Working Dogs: Fat or Carbohydrate?

There are important differences between human athletes and working dogs. In dogs, approximately 70% to 90% of the energy for sustained work is derived from fat metabolism, and only a small amount of energy is derived from carbohydrate metabolism.[17,18] Similarly, early field studies with sled dogs and laboratory studies with Beagles indicated that the ability to use fatty acids through aerobic pathways was more important than the use of muscle glycogen through anaerobic pathways during hard work.[1,19,20] In an often referenced study, a dog team that was fed a high-carbohydrate diet performed poorly and developed a stiff gait while racing.[21] When the dogs were changed to a diet containing increased levels of fat and protein, performance improved and the observed lameness resolved. The researchers suggested that feeding a high-carbohydrate diet to sled dogs may be responsible for the occurrence of a form of exertional rhabdomyolysis. Exertional rhabdomyolysis is a disorder caused by rapid anaerobic metabolism of muscle glycogen, resulting in an accumulation of lactic acid. Lactic acid accumulation can have several adverse side effects, including damage to muscle-tissue membranes, edema, and inhibition of lipolysis and glycolysis. These studies were the impetus for the theory that dietary fat is metabolically the preferred fuel for hard-working dogs.

Subsequent controlled studies with several types of working dogs have supported this hypothesis and have also provided important information regarding the feeding management and training for working dogs. Both the level of conditioning and the type of diet fed significantly affect energy use in working dogs. In a study with 16 Alaskan Huskies, one group of dogs was fed a high-fat diet containing 60% of calories as fat, while the second group was fed a high-carbohydrate diet, containing 60% of calories as carbohydrate.[22] The dogs completed standard aerobic and anaerobic tests on a treadmill prior to conditioning, after a 4-week aerobic training period, and again after a 4-week anaerobic training period. Results of the aerobic tests showed that both groups of dogs relied primarily upon FFAs and used little glycogen to complete the tests (Figures 24-1 and 24-2). Dogs that were fed the high-fat diet had significantly greater preexercise and postexercise FFA concentrations when compared with dogs fed the high-carbohydrate diet, even *before* they were conditioned through training. The concentration of FFAs in the blood is a major determinant of fatty acid utilization by muscle, and it is an accepted indicator of fatty acid metabolism. These results showed that feeding a high-fat diet to working dogs before and during athletic training enhances the dog's ability to mobilize and use fatty acids as fuel.

A second controlled study examined the effect of diet on oxygen consumption (Vo_2 max), mitochondrial volume, and maximal rates of fat oxidation in a group of endurance-trained Labrador Retrievers.[9] When dietary fat was increased from 15% to 60% of calories, dogs showed almost 50% increase in Vo_2 max and a 45% increase in maximal fat oxidation during aerobic exercise tests. These values indicate enhanced efficiency of fat utilization and capacity for aerobic work. Mitochondrial volume in muscles increased 50% in response to

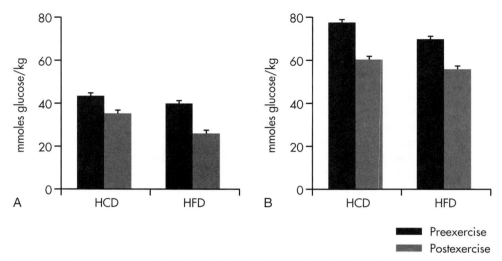

Figure 24-1　Muscle glycogen concentrations in trained and untrained dogs (aerobic tests). A, Untrained and, B, aerobically trained. *HCD,* High-carbohydrate diet; *HFD,* high-fat diet; *mmoles,* millimoles.

(From Reynolds AJ, Taylor CR, Hoeppler H, and others: The effect of diet on sled dog performance, oxidative capacity, skeletal muscle microstructure, and muscle glycogen metabolism. In Carey DP, Norton SA, Bolser SM, editors: *Recent advances in canine and feline nutritional research, Iams international nutritional symposium,* Wilmington, Ohio, 1996, Orange Frazer Press.)

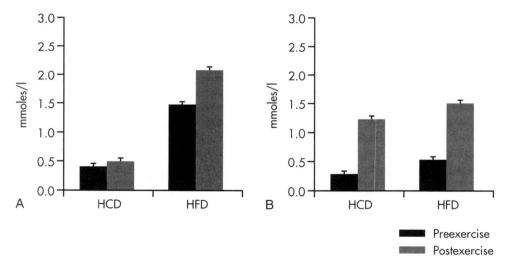

Figure 24-2　Serum free fatty acid concentrations in trained and untrained dogs (aerobic tests). A, Untrained and, B, aerobically trained. *HCD,* High-carbohydrate diet; *HFD,* high-fat diet; *mmoles,* millimoles.

(From Reynolds AJ, Taylor CR, Hoeppler H, and others: The effect of diet on sled dog performance, oxidative capacity, skeletal muscle microstructure, and muscle glycogen metabolism. In Carey DP, Norton SA, Bolser SM, editors: *Recent advances in canine and feline nutritional research, Iams international nutritional symposium,* Wilmington, Ohio, 1996, Orange Frazer Press.)

increasing fat in the diet. There is speculation that feeding a high-fat diet improves aerobic work capacity and efficiency in dogs by stimulating mitochondrial growth.

Although fat is the primary metabolic fuel for endurance dogs, and high-fat diets best supply this fuel,

adequate muscle glycogen stores are still important during exercise. As in other species, muscle glycogen depletion during prolonged exercise is associated with fatigue and a decline in performance in working dogs. The two factors that appear to have the greatest influence on muscle glycogen stores are athletic conditioning and diet (see Figure 24-1). In the study described previously, only small amounts of glycogen were used by dogs during the aerobic tests.[9] However, some glycogen metabolism is always necessary to permit the continuation of FFA metabolism during aerobic work. In addition to this need, racing sled dogs experience periods of intense running near the end of races or when covering difficult terrain. Similarly, hunting dogs and certain types of service and sports dogs work predominantly at low intensities, interspersed with occasional bouts of high-intensity physical exertion.

To learn more about the needs of dogs during these periods, researchers also examined energy metabolism in endurance-trained sled dogs during bouts of intense anaerobic activity.[6] Completion of an initial 4-week training period significantly increased the muscle glycogen levels in all of the dogs in the study, regardless of the type of diet that was fed. While dogs that were fed a high-carbohydrate diet stored more muscle glycogen than those fed a high-fat diet, the carbohydrate-fed dogs also metabolized more glycogen to complete the anaerobic test. As a result, muscle glycogen levels at the completion of the standard anaerobic test were depleted similarly in the groups of dogs fed the two different diets. As in other species, dogs performing anaerobic tests rely heavily upon muscle glycogen as an energy source. The researchers concluded that feeding high-fat diets to endurance-trained dogs not only prepares muscles to efficiently mobilize and use FFAs as an energy source, it also appears to have a glycogen-sparing effect that helps to prolong glycogen use.

Finally, although dogs react similarly to other species by showing rapid glycogen depletion following a single bout of strenuous exercise, there is recent evidence that trained sled dogs are resistant to prolonged glycogen depletion when subjected to repeated exercise episodes over multiple days. Early studies with human athletes suggested that completing consecutive days of prolonged running results in cumulative muscle glycogen depletion, and it is this depletion and the inability to completely replenish glycogen stores that is responsible for the onset of fatigue and loss of performance.[23,24] Continuing to exercise when muscle glycogen stores are low has also been associated with increased protein degradation in skeletal muscle, a potential risk factor for injury.[25] Recent studies with a group of trained

Alaskan sled dogs examined muscle glycogen levels during prolonged bouts of exercise. In the first study, 36 conditioned sled dogs consuming a high-fat, low-carbohydrate diet ran approximately 100 miles per day for up to 5 consecutive days.[26] Muscle glycogen was measured prior to the start of the exercise period and immediately following each day's run. The first day's workout caused a rapid depletion in glycogen levels to about 21% of preexercise levels. However, glycogen levels subsequently increased to 50% to 65% of initial stores after the second day of exercise and remained at that level for the remainder of the 5-day period. This change was especially remarkable since the dogs were consuming relatively little carbohydrate in their training diet. The underlying metabolic cause for muscle glycogen replenishment may have been enhanced use of noncarbohydrate fuel sources during subsequent days of exercising or to the rapid replenishment of glycogen stores during rest periods. Although the study was not designed to determine the underlying cause, serum ketones and glycerol concentrations increased over the 5-day period, suggesting that utilization of fat-based energy sources was at least partially responsible for the maintenance of muscle glycogen in the exercising dogs.[27]

A subsequent study was conducted to determine the underlying cause of glycogen replenishment in dogs during multiple days of endurance work.[28] Changes in muscle glycogen and muscle triglyceride concentrations were measured in a group of sled dogs over a 4-day period of 100-mile per day training runs. A group of six similarly trained dogs served as the nonexercising control group. All of the dogs were fed a high-fat training diet and muscle biopsies were performed immediately after each day's run and again following feeding and a period of rest. Following the first day's run, dogs had utilized more than 60% of the glycogen stored in skeletal muscle, corroborating the results of the previous study. However, running the same distance on each subsequent day resulted in only a 5% additional decrease in glycogen stores. This change diminished to almost negligible levels on the final day. In contrast, as the use of muscle glycogen decreased, the use of muscle triglyceride increased. These findings are supported by previous work showing that extramuscular fat and protein substrate play an important role in supporting work in sled dogs during periods of prolonged and submaximal exercise. It appears that plasma FFAs become the predominant energy substrate during this time. Because blood urea nitrogen (BUN) concentrations also increase during prolonged and submaximal exercise, protein substrates may also be important. Together the results of these studies suggest that the primary metabolic adaptation that occurs during prolonged and repeated bouts of exercise in dogs is a reduced rate of glycogen depletion caused most likely by increased reliance on fat-related energy substrates, most importantly plasma FFAs. Although there is some evidence that human athletes subjected to multiple days of endurance exercise also shift their metabolism away from muscle glycogen and toward fat-based substrates, the dog may be especially efficient at this type of shift given the dog's naturally high aerobic metabolic capacity and demonstrated response to training and to high-fat diets.[29-31]

Both the level of conditioning and the type of diet fed affect energy use in working dogs. Feeding a high-fat diet to working dogs before and during athletic training enhances the dog's ability to mobilize and use fatty acids as fuel during endurance exercise and may help to spare glycogen stores from depletion.

Protein for Working Dogs

Endurance training and racing result in increased protein needs for dogs.[32] Several physiological and metabolic changes contribute to an increased dietary requirement. Athletic conditioning results in adaptive anabolic changes that facilitate efficient delivery of oxygen and nutrients to working muscles. These changes include increases in blood volume, red blood cell mass, capillary density, mitochondrial volume, and the activity and total mass of metabolic enzymes.[33] The increased tissue mass associated with athletic training must be supplied by additional protein in the diet. In addition, there is a slight but significant increase in protein catabolism during endurance exercise associated with an increased rate of skeletal muscle turnover.[34,35] This occurs as a result of exercise-induced muscle damage and oxidation of protein. It is estimated that up to 10% of energy in exercising dogs can be derived from the metabolism of gluconeogenic amino acids.[36,37]

In a study of the protein needs of dogs during endurance training, diets supplying either 16%, 24%, 32%, or 40% of calories from protein were fed to sled dogs throughout a 12-week training period.[38] Dogs that were fed 40% protein maintained a larger plasma volume and red blood cell mass during training than dogs fed diets containing less than 40% protein. The amount of protein in the diet also appeared to influence susceptibility to injury. While there were no injuries in any of the dogs that consumed the 32% or 40% protein diets, all of the dogs fed the 16% diet were injured at some point during the 12-week period, which kept them out of training for 2 or more days. It appears that the proportion of energy that is supplied by protein should be increased in the diets of endurance dogs in training to ensure adequate tissue accretion, prevent tissue loss, and possibly aid in the prevention of injury. Optimal protein concentrations of between 30% and 40% of calories are recommended in foods formulated for endurance dogs (Box 24-1).

BOX 24-1   PRACTICAL FEEDING TIPS: ENDURANCE PERFORMANCE

Feed a highly digestible, energy- and nutrient-dense diet (4000 kcal of metabolizable energy/kg or greater).

Diet should contain:

Calories from protein: 30% to 35%; high-quality animal source proteins

Calories from fat: 50% to 65%

Calories from carbohydrate: 10% to 15%

Omega-6:omega-3 fatty acid ratio between 5:1 and 10:1

Moderately fermentable fiber: 3% to 7%

Provide continual access to clean, fresh water.

Feed two or more meals per day on a portion-controlled basis.

Feed the largest meal of the day after the day's training is complete.

Provide a meal 1.5 to 2 hours before training or an endurance event.

Feed a carbohydrate-containing supplement immediately after endurance exercise to promote glucose repletion.

While providing enough protein in the diet is important, feeding a diet that contains more protein than the dog needs is neither necessary nor beneficial. Protein consumed in excess of the needs of tissue replacement and growth will be used as an energy source. Protein is one of the least desirable muscle energy fuels because it is inefficiently metabolized and cannot be stored in the body like fat or glycogen. The diet should supply adequate calories as fat and carbohydrate so that the protein that is fed can be used primarily for tissue protein synthesis and spared for use as an energy source. For the canine athlete, the most efficiently used fuel appears to be fat, with carbohydrate supplying a smaller proportion of the calories in the diet.

Performance dogs have increased needs for dietary protein. Athletic conditioning leads to increases in blood volume, red blood cell mass, capillary density, and mitochondrial volume. The increased tissue mass associated with this training must be supplied by additional protein in the diet. In addition, there is a slight but significant increase in protein catabolism during endurance exercise associated with an increased rate of skeletal muscle turnover. Finally, it is estimated that up to 10% of energy in exercising dogs can be derived from the metabolism of gluconeogenic amino acids.

Caloric Requirement during Endurance Work

The total energy requirement of an endurance dog depends on the intensity and duration of the exercise and the environmental conditions in which the animal is working. Early research suggested that energy needs increase to between 1.5 and 2.5 times the normal maintenance requirements in dogs working in ambient temperatures.[39-41] Working in cold weather may further increase requirements by about 50%. Data for these estimates were collected from draft dogs that were covering relatively short distances and traveling at slower speeds than racing sled dogs. Typical dog teams used for hauling freight travel less than 20 miles per day at speeds of about 5 miles per hour. Energy needs for these dogs are estimated to be between 4000 and 8000 kilocalories (kcal)/day.[41,42]

In contrast, dogs trained for racing in long-distance sled races typically run 70 miles or more per day and travel at speeds of up to 9 miles per hour. Studies of these dogs found that racing sled dogs competing in a medium distance race (300 miles) expended an average of 11,200 kcal/day and consumed an average of 10,600 kcal/day (Figure 24-3).[43] These values are equivalent to burning 460 kcal/kilogram (kg) of body weight per day and consuming 440 kcal/kg of body weight per day. The researchers observed that the calculated values for

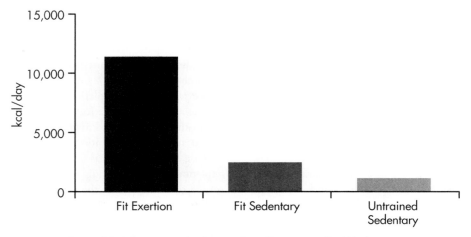

Figure 24-3   Energy expenditure of sled dogs competing in a medium distance race (kcal/day).

(From Hinchcliff KW, Reinhart GA, Burr JR, and others: Energy metabolism and water turnover in Alaskan sled dogs during running. In Carey DP, Norton SA, Bolser SM, editors: *Recent advances in canine and feline nutritional research, Iams international nutritional symposium,* Wilmington, Ohio, 1996, Orange Frazer Press.)

sustained metabolic rate for these dogs appears to exceed previously predicted maximal values for mammals of their size. These extraordinarily high energy requirements and expenditures predicate the need to provide a diet that is energy dense and highly digestible to allow the ingestion of needed calories in a volume of food that the dog's stomach and gastrointestinal system are capable of handling. However, the vast majority of working dogs do not work for the duration and at intensities that result in such dramatic increases. Although a limited number of studies have been conducted, measured estimates for hunting dogs fall between the earlier estimates provided of 1.5 and 2.5 times maintenance requirements (see p. 255).

Water and Electrolyte Requirements

The same researchers who measured caloric intake and expenditure in racing sled dogs also examined water intake, water turnover, and electrolyte balance during medium- and long-distance races.[44-46] Dogs competing in a 300-mile race had a measured water turnover rate of approximately 250 milliliters (ml)/kg of body weight per day. This is equal to about 5 liters (L) per day for an average-size sled dog. By comparison, sled dogs that were not racing had water turnovers of only 0.9 L per day. Dogs lose water primarily through respiration, urine, feces, and, to a very small degree, perspiration. The extremely high water loss in working sled dogs is primarily a result of increased urinary water loss. In all animals, urinary water loss is related to the obligatory urinary solute load, which in turn is affected by the quantity of food consumed and the composition of the diet.[47] Diets with a high protein concentration and/or large caloric intake result in higher obligatory solute loads. Because sled dogs consume up to 12,000 kcal/day when they are racing, they have extremely high solute loads and, as a result, very high obligatory urinary water losses. Dogs must be provided with fresh water frequently during racing to offset these losses and prevent dehydration.

Electrolyte balance is also an important consideration in exercising animals. Exercise-induced hyponatremia occurs in horses and humans and may be associated with clinical signs.[48,49] Decreases in serum sodium and potassium levels have also been observed in sled dogs during long-distance races.[44,46,50] A recent study that measured serum chemistry changes

in Alaskan sled dogs over a 5-day endurance test also reported progressive reductions in serum globulin (protein) concentrations and increased serum chloride, urea nitrogen, and creatine kinase (CK).[51] While only mild aberrations were observed and no clinical signs were reported, exercise-associated hyponatremia, cation depletion, and hypoproteinemia have been observed in some endurance-trained dogs during periods of prolonged racing.[44,46,52] These changes may be attributable to the solute diuresis and urine sodium losses mandated by the large energy intake (and resultant solute loads), and to mild exercise-induced damage to muscles.

Although reported in few studies, values for urine osmolality do not appear to change dramatically in response to exercise. However, there may be a shift in the type of solutes present in the urine.[46] Endurance exercise caused a decrease in urinary sodium, potassium, and chloride concentrations and an increase in urine urea concentration. Increased urinary urea will occur as a direct result of the higher energy and protein intake of racing dogs. This change imposes significant increases in obligatory urinary water and sodium loss, even in the face of renal cation conservation. Although decreases in serum cation concentration have not been associated with clinical signs in any of the dogs studied, these data indicate the importance of providing racing sled dogs a diet with an adequate level of sodium.

Glycogen Repletion after Endurance Exercise

As discussed previously, feeding dogs a diet that is formulated to spare glycogen is more successful than feeding a diet designed to increase muscle glycogen stores (i.e., glycogen loading) for endurance performance. However, glycogen depletion is still associated with fatigue and impaired performance in racing sled dogs, as in other species.[53-55] Providing various types of carbohydrate supplementation immediately following exercise has been used as a strategy for resolving this depletion and for providing an immediately available source of energy. Both the timing of the supplement and its nutrient composition are important.

The rate of muscle glycogen repletion following exhaustive exercise is substantially enhanced if a carbohydrate supplement is ingested immediately after exercise.[56,57] When a carbohydrate snack is ingested within 30 minutes of finishing an exhaustive training session, the rate of glycogen repletion during the following 2 hours is up to threefold greater than if carbohydrate had not been ingested. If ingestion of carbohydrate is delayed for 2 hours after exercise, the rate of glycogen repletion to working muscles is only half the rate observed when carbohydrate is consumed immediately after exercise. The mechanism believed to be responsible for this effect involves enhanced blood flow to muscles immediately following exercise. Exercise-induced blood flow to muscle results in increased glucose transport and, subsequently, enhanced glucose uptake and glycogen synthesis by the muscles. If carbohydrate intake is delayed, blood glucose level still increases, but the rate of muscle glycogen repletion is slowed. Because protein ingestion is associated with increased and prolonged insulin release, it has been theorized that including protein with a postexercise carbohydrate supplement may further enhance muscle glycogen repletion.[58,59] However, results of studies that examined the effectiveness of postexercise carbohydrate plus protein supplements with human athletes have reported inconsistent results, indicating that protein may not be needed for efficient replenishment of muscle glycogen stores.

Feeding a carbohydrate-containing supplement immediately after exercise has been shown to be an effective means of muscle glycogen repletion in sled dogs. In one study, sled dogs were fed either a water and glucose polymer solution, or water alone, immediately after an exhaustive training run.[60] Dogs that consumed the glucose polymer (1.5 grams [g]/kg of body weight) had significantly increased rates of muscle glycogen repletion when compared with dogs that were not supplemented (Figure 24-4). Plasma glucose levels increased significantly within 100 minutes of supplementation and were presumably responsible for enhanced delivery of glucose to muscles (Figure 24-5). A subsequent study examined the effects of feeding either water alone, water with a glucose polymer, or water with the glucose polymer and an added protein hydrolysate.[61] Postexercise supplementation was provided after each day's training run over a 2-month period. Both types of supplement enhanced glycogen repletion within 24 hours of exercise, but there was no difference in any biochemical measures of glucose metabolism (insulin, glucose, or glucagons levels) between the dogs fed the glucose polymer alone and those that were fed the glucose polymer plus a protein hydrolysate. Therefore

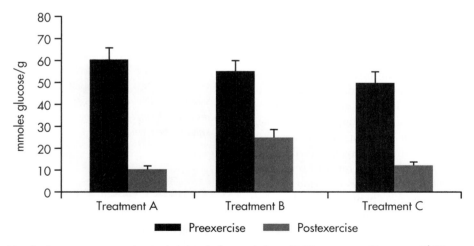

Figure 24-4   Muscle glycogen concentration in sled dogs before and after a 30-kilometer run. *Treatment A,** Water-only following exercise; *treatment B,†* water plus 1.5 g/kg glucose polymer after exercise; *treatment C,†* water-only following exercise.
*Biopsied 1 hour before and immediately after exercise.
†Biopsied 1 hour before and 4 hours after exercise.

(From Reynolds AJ, Taylor CR, Hoeppler H, and others: The effect of diet on sled dog performance, oxidative capacity, skeletal muscle microstructure, and muscle glycogen metabolism. In Carey DP, Norton SA, Bolser SM, editors: *Recent advances in canine and feline nutritional research, Iams international nutritional symposium,* Wilmington, Ohio, 1996, Orange Frazer Press.)

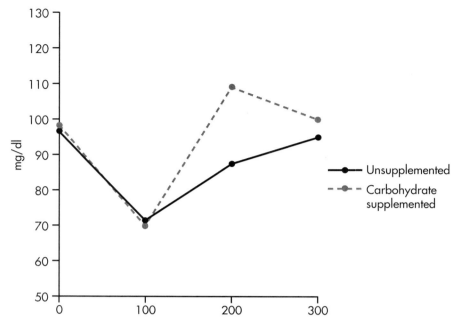

Figure 24-5   Blood glucose concentrations after exercise in sled dogs fed water or 1.5 g/kg glucose polymer. (From *Performance dog nutrition symposium*, Dayton, Ohio, 1995, The Iams Company. Used with permission.)

it appears that postexercise carbohydrate supplementation in endurance-trained dogs helps to enhance muscle glycogen repletion, but including protein with the supplement does not further enhance this effect.

The practice of providing a glucose polymer as a carbohydrate supplement immediately after exhaustive exercise or during multiple-day events may be especially helpful when sled dogs and other types of working dogs are fed diets that supply most of their calories as fat and when bouts of exercise are separated by only a few hours. In a typical medium- or long-distance race, sled dogs run for 4 to 6 hours at time, followed by a 2- to 4-hour rest period. During rest periods the dogs are usually provided with a small meal or snack and are fed their full meal once they have finished running for the day. Although it is now generally accepted that endurance-trained dogs perform best when fed a high-fat, low-carbohydrate food as the primary diet, providing a high-carbohydrate snack immediately following long bouts of exercise can dramatically influence glycogen replenishment and may enhance performance.

The practice of providing a carbohydrate supplement immediately after exhaustive exercise or during multiple-day athletic events is especially helpful when working dogs are fed diets that supply most of their calories as fat and when bouts of exercise are separated by only a few hours. The provision of a high carbohydrate snack immediately following long bouts of exercise can dramatically influence glycogen replenishment and may enhance performance.

Practical Feeding and Diets for Endurance Dogs

It is now evident that dietary fat is an important component in the diet of working dogs because of its ability to efficiently supply energy to working muscles. In addition to its beneficial effects upon aerobic metabolism, fat also has a significant influence upon a diet's energy density and digestibility. The most efficacious way to increase both energy density and diet digestibility is to supply energy in the form of high-quality fat. A classic study with Beagles demonstrated the importance of diet digestibility and fat content.[19] A group of dogs were fed either a commercial, dry diet formulated for maintenance or one of three highly digestible, high-fat diets. After a period of dietary adaptation, endurance was measured using a standard treadmill test. The dogs fed the maintenance diet experienced exhaustion after 103 minutes, but the dogs fed the more energy-dense, highly digestible diets did not experience exhaustion until they had run for a significantly longer period (137 minutes). Analysis of these data showed that performance level in the Beagles was positively correlated with diet digestibility and the intake of digestible fat.

An animal with increased energy needs must consume a great deal of food to meet those needs. During long-distance racing or other forms of endurance work, dogs' elevated energy needs require the intake of a large volume of food. If the food that is fed is low in digestibility, a large amount of dry matter (DM) must be ingested, and intake may be limited by the dog's gastric capacity and his or her ability to digest and assimilate large boluses of food. Therefore, in addition to the need for a high fat content as an energy source, high digestibility is necessary to limit the total volume of food that the dog must consume at each meal. Although some maintenance diets can supply enough energy if consumed in large enough quantities by working dogs, they may become bulk-limiting and thus limit performance in dogs with very high energy requirements. Foods formulated for working dogs should contain high-quality sources of protein, fat, and carbohydrate to ensure high digestibility and availability of nutrients and minimize the volume of food that must be fed to meet a dog's needs.

Feeding practices that are best suited for hard-working dogs are designed to minimize gastrointestinal expansion during bouts of work and maintain a high work capacity throughout the session of exercise. Dogs should be fed on a portion-controlled basis so that the trainer can strictly regulate the timing and the size of meals. The main meal of the day should be fed after the day's session of training to allow adequate digestion of food. If possible, at least two meals should be provided per day, and a small meal can be provided 1.5 to 2 hours before endurance activity. A carbohydrate-containing drink or food can be fed immediately following exhaustive periods of work.

Depending upon the type of work and the environmental conditions, water losses can increase by tenfold to twentyfold during exercise. Therefore it is important that dogs are provided with water at frequent intervals throughout a session of work. Even mild dehydration can lead to reduced work capacity, decreased strength, and hyperthermia.[62] Working dogs should be given frequent opportunities to drink small amounts of fresh water during periods of extended work. In addition, water can be added to meals as a method of increasing water intake during periods of heavy training or racing. This practice prevents the development of even mild dehydration. Cool water is preferable because it is more palatable to most dogs and is more effective in helping to cool the body.[63]

Working dogs should be fed on a portion-controlled basis so that the trainer can strictly regulate the timing and the size of meals. In general, hard-working dogs should be fed two to three meals per day, with a small meal fed 1.5 to 2 hours before long periods of submaximal exercise. Frequent access to cool water should be provided at regular intervals throughout a session of work.

SPRINT-RACING PERFORMANCE

The exercise that sprint-racing dogs engage in is substantially different from that required of endurance sled dogs. Greyhound races are extremely short, sprinting events. In the United States, racing takes place on an oval tract and involves distances between $5/16$ and $3/8$ of a mile. During a race, dogs reach speeds of 36 to 38 miles per hour, but they maintain this speed for only 30 to 40 seconds. Other types of sprint-racing activities include dogs that are trained for lure-coursing events, dogs engaged in Flyball, agility, and Frisbee competitions, and some types of hunting activities, such as retrieving on land or strenuous swimming.

It is known that brief, intense periods of exercise preclude the mobilization and delivery of fatty acids and the adequate oxygenation of tissue necessary for aerobic metabolism.[64] Thus the primary source of energy for this type of exercise is the anaerobic metabolism of carbohydrate. Both muscle glycogen and circulating blood glucose supply energy to muscles during brief bouts of intense work.[65] This process differs from endurance exercise, in which FFAs and a small amount of glycogen supply energy to the working muscles. Post-race biochemical data collected from racing Greyhounds indicate that the sprint-racing dogs rely primarily on anaerobic metabolism for energy.[66,67] Blood lactate levels increase up to fiftyfold from pre-race values to post-race values, which reflects the significant contribution of anaerobic metabolism of carbohydrate to the energy demands of the race.[66,68,69] It appears that the Greyhound is well adapted to this type of work because both lactate levels and blood pH return to normal values within 1 hour of the race. Training also increases the body's ability to metabolize accumulated lactic acid following an intense bout of exercise.[70]

Studies with human athletes indicate that dietary modification is more effective in influencing endurance athletes than sprinters. This may be a result of the fact that two factors that influence endurance during prolonged periods of exercise are the body's ability to use fat for energy and the quantity of glycogen stored in the working muscles. As discussed previously, both of these factors can be influenced by diet. Sprinters, on the other hand, rapidly use muscle glycogen and circulating glucose through anaerobic metabolism. A study with human runners showed that although the practice of glycogen loading increased the amount of exercise time until exhaustion, it did not appear to influence running speed at the beginning of the race.[10] Conversely, there is some evidence that feeding racing Greyhounds a food that is very high in protein and fat, and that has reduced carbohydrate, may have a moderately negative effect on racing performance.[71] In this study, the high-protein diet provided excess protein (37% of metabolizable energy [ME]) and was compared with a diet containing moderate and adequate levels of protein (24% of ME). Therefore it was speculated that the reduced performance was a result of reduced levels of carbohydrate needed for racing and the inefficient use of protein as an energy source.

Sprint-racing dogs should be fed a diet that is energy dense and highly digestible. Feeding a food that has been formulated for performance ensures that DM intake during racing or training is not excessive. Intake should be carefully monitored to ensure optimal body weight because slight restriction of food and the maintenance of a lean body condition are associated with improved performance in sprinting events.[72] The food fed to dogs involved in sprinting events should also contain moderate to high levels of digestible fat and protein and a moderate amount of highly digestible carbohydrate. Similar to endurance-trained dogs, carbohydrate supplementation after intense bouts of exercise for sprinting dogs may also be helpful in enhancing repletion of muscle glycogen stores.

> *In contrast to endurance dogs, sprint-racing dogs draw energy from the anaerobic metabolism of carbohydrates; muscle glycogen and circulating blood glucose fuel muscles during their brief periods of intense work. Many hunting dogs engage in short and intense periods of running periodically throughout the day. These dogs should be fed energy-dense, highly digestible diets that have been formulated for performance and should be fed to maintain a lean and well-muscled body condition.*

DOG SPORTS AND SERVICE DOGS

Most of the understanding of the nutritional needs of exercising dogs is based upon the previously reviewed studies of endurance sled dogs, racing Greyhounds, and dogs running in controlled settings on treadmills. However, most working dogs fall somewhere in between the extremes of submaximal endurance work (sled dogs) and the short bursts of intense exercise seen in sprint racing (Greyhounds). For example, dogs that work as hunting companions or in competitive field trials typically work for several hours at submaximal levels that are interrupted by short bursts of intense running when flushing or retrieving game. Conversely, most dogs used as service dogs that aid disabled owners work for long periods, but at relatively low levels of intensity. A wide range of dog-related activities and sports are also enjoyed today by both owners and their dogs. Dogs competing in agility or Flyball events can be compared most closely with sprint-racing dogs, while tracking dogs and obedience dogs are more similar to endurance-trained dogs, as they work at much lower levels of intensity and for longer periods. Although each of the many ways in which dogs work and compete in sports have not been studied, an understanding of the metabolic changes and nutrient needs associated with both submaximal endurance work and high-intensity exercise are helpful when making recommendations for these different types of canine athlete.

The goals for the nutrition and feeding of all working dogs are to maintain optimal body condition and weight, support performance, and prevent fatigue and injury. Of greatest concern is energy. All working dogs will have energy needs that are higher than comparable dogs living a sedentary lifestyle. However, the duration and the intensity of the work will determine the magnitude of this difference. Dogs working at low or moderate intensity for long periods of time (hunting dogs, service dogs, and military/police dogs) will require a consistent increase in caloric intake to maintain body weight. For hunting dogs, an increase is needed during the training period and hunting season, but not during times of the year when dogs are not working.[73] Although the energy needs of service dogs and of dogs competing in obedience or other dog sports have not been studied, it is expected that an increase is needed to maintain condition during prolonged periods of training and competing but not during off-season periods.

All working dogs will have energy needs that are higher than a comparable dog living a sedentary lifestyle. Dogs working at low or moderate intensity for long periods of time (hunting dogs, service dogs and military/police dogs) will require a consistent increase in caloric intake to maintain body weight. For hunting dogs, an increase is needed during the training period and hunting season, but not during times of the year when dogs are not working. It is expected that energy needs of service dogs and of dogs competing in obedience or other dog sports increase to maintain condition during prolonged periods of training and competing but are at maintenance during off-season periods.

As discussed previously, the best way to provide the extra energy needed by canine athlete is to increase dietary fat and feed a food that is both energy dense and highly digestible. If energy content of the food is too low, the quantity of food that must be consumed to meet increased caloric needs may exceed the physical capacity of the dog's stomach and intestinal tract. In practice, this leads to an increased rate of passage, decreased diet digestibility, and the production of increased volume and decreased quality of stools. For example, a year-long study of body condition and hunting performance in a group of Pointers reported that dogs fed a calorie-dense and highly digestible food maintained body condition and performed significantly better throughout the hunting season than did dogs fed a food that was lower in both energy density and digestibility.[74]

The source of dietary fat may also be important. Although there are limited studies available, there is evidence that foods containing predominantly saturated fatty acids may negatively affect olfactory acuity in working dogs.[75] This is an important consideration for hunting dogs, tracking dogs, and dogs used in the detection of narcotics and explosives. Although the underlying mechanism is not fully understood, it is theorized that altering the proportion of saturated and unsaturated fatty acids in a dog's diet modifies the fatty acid composition of cells of the nasal epithelium and affects a dog's ability to detect low concentrations of odorants. Specifically, the composition of cell membrane phospholipids influences fluidity and permeability of cell membranes, which might in turn affect response to odorants. Interestingly, the same study was the first to demonstrate that physical conditioning improves a dog's ability to maintain olfactory acuity following a bout of exercise. Dogs that were not conditioned showed a reduced ability to detect odors following a 1-hour period of running, and also showed reduced overall olfactory acuity over an 8-week period when fed a food that was high in saturated fat. Conversely, dogs that were well conditioned did not show a reduction in olfactory acuity in response to exercise and were not affected by the type of fat in the diet. Although additional work is needed, these results suggest that the source and type of fat included in the diet of working dogs should be considered along with the overall concentration of fat.

In recent years, the role that antioxidant nutrients play in reducing oxidative stress during exercise and other types of physiological stress has been studied.[76] Strenuous exercise imposes significant oxidative stress and can lead to oxidative damage of cells and tissues.

Canine athletes that are fed high-fat diets may be at increased risk because of an increased propensity of fatty acid oxidation associated with high-fat intake. The most frequently studied antioxidant nutrient is alpha-tocopherol (vitamin E). A study with racing sled dogs reported that the circulating lipoproteins of dogs supplemented with vitamin E, beta-carotene, and lutein showed increased resistance to in vitro oxidative damage, and a reduction in exercise-related deoxyribonucleic acid (DNA) damage when compared with lipoproteins of unsupplemented dogs.[77] However, a subsequent study failed to show any protective benefit when racing sled dogs were supplemented with a similar combination of vitamin E, beta-carotene, and lutein.[78] In this study, muscle damage was assessed using postexercise CK levels. More recently, the polyphenols and flavonoids that are present in certain fruits and vegetables, particularly in blueberries, have been studied. These compounds have strong antioxidant properties and exert their effects via several biochemical pathways. A group of unconditioned sled dogs were supplemented with approximately 20 g of wild blueberries per day for 2 months and were exercised for a distance of 7 miles on 2 consecutive days.[79] Plasma CK levels increased similarly in both the supplemented and the control groups of dogs, but levels were within a range that is considered normal for exercising dogs and not indicative of exercise-induced muscle damage. Although the addition of blueberries did not affect CK response to exercise, supplementation did cause an elevation in plasma total antioxidant potential (TAP), which is a measure of the body's antioxidant status. Although additional studies are needed, these preliminary results suggest that exercising dogs may benefit from a diet containing increased antioxidant nutrients.

WEATHER EXTREMES

Adverse weather conditions in the form of extreme cold or heat result in increased energy needs in dogs and cats. This increase can be quite substantial depending on the severity of the weather. A study of dogs living in an arctic environment showed that an increase in energy intake of 70% to 80% was necessary for the dogs to maintain normal body temperatures without experiencing weight loss.[80] Dogs are capable of a significant level of cold-induced thermogenesis, a mechanism involving an increase in metabolic rate during exposure to a cold environment. The increased metabolic rate produces additional body heat that is used to maintain body temperature. Although the increased energy needs of dogs in arctic environments are very great and result in large increases in daily energy intake, dogs housed outside during moderately cold weather also experience a degree of cold-induced thermogenesis.

A study with Labrador Retrievers and Beagles showed that as environmental temperatures decreased from 59° Fahrenheit (F) (thermal neutral zone) to 47° F, the dogs' ME intake increased and remained high until the ambient temperature was increased.[81] During the cold period, there was a slight decrease in mean body weight despite increased energy intake. Results from this study indicate that an average increase in ME intake of 25% is necessary to maintain body weight in dogs housed in cool conditions. This figure can be used as a general guide for increasing the ME intake of dogs that are housed outdoors during the winter months. However, factors such as the dog's size, its coat type and length, the type of shelter that is provided, and weather conditions such as wind and drifting snow significantly influence the amount of food needed by dogs housed in cold environments. For example, a study with Beagles, Labrador Retrievers, and Siberian Huskies found that the ME requirements of Siberian Huskies are less affected by fluctuations in environmental temperature than are the ME intakes of Beagles and Labrador Retrievers.[82] It appears that the double coats of Huskies act as a protective barrier to insulate them against large fluctuations in environmental temperature.

The energy needs of dogs and cats also increase with high environmental temperatures and humidity. The exposure to high ambient temperature causes an increase in the amount of energy that must be used to cool the body. Working dogs in humid environments experience slight increases in energy needs; at the same time they often exhibit a reduction in appetite.[74,83] Therefore it is important to provide dogs working in hot environments with a diet that is high in caloric and nutrient density so that nutritional needs may be met without the consumption of large quantities of food. It is also especially important that cool water be provided continuously in warm or humid environments.

References

1. Bergstrom J, Hermansen L, Hultman E, and others: Diet, muscle glycogen and physical performance, *Acta Physiol Scand* 71:140–150, 1967.

2. Issekutz BJR, Miller HI, Paul P: Aerobic work capacity and plasma FFA turnover, *J Appl Physiol* 20:293–296, 1965.

3. Miller H, Issekutz B, Rodahl K: Effect of exercise on the metabolism of fatty acids in the dog, *Am J Physiol* 205:167–172, 1963.

4. Paul P, Issekutz B, Miller HI: Interrelationship of free fatty acids and glucose metabolism in the dog, *Am J Physiol* 211:1313–1320, 1966.

5. Conlee RK, Hammer RL, Winder WW, and others: Glycogen repletion and exercise endurance in rats adapted to a high fat diet, *Metabolism* 39:289–294, 1990.

6. Reynolds AJ, Fuhrer L, Dunlap HL, and others: Effect of diet and training on muscle glycogen storage and utilization in sled dogs, *J Appl Physiol* 79:1601–1607, 1997.

7. Armstrong RB: Distribution of fiber types in locomotory muscles of dogs, *Am J Anat* 163:87–98, 1982.

8. Guy PS, Snow DH: Skeletal muscle fibre composition in the dog and its relationship to athletic ability, *Res Vet Sci* 31:244–248, 1981.

9. Reynolds A, Hoppeler H, Reinhart G, and others: Sled dog endurance: a result of high fat diet or selective breeding? *FASEB J* 9:A996, 1995.

10. Karlsson J, Saltin B: Diet, muscle glycogen and endurance performance, *J Appl Physiol* 31:203–206, 1971.

11. Green HJ: How important is endogenous muscle glycogen to fatigue in prolonged exercise? *Can J Physiol Pharmacol* 69:290–297, 1990.

12. Sherman WM, Costill DL, Fink WJ, and others: Effect of exercise-diet manipulation on muscle glycogen and its subsequent utilization during performance, *Int J Sports Med* 2:114–118, 1981.

13. Fielding RA, Costill DL, Fink WJ, and others: Effects of pre-exercise carbohydrate feedings on muscle glycogen use during exercise in well-trained runners, *Eur J Appl Physiol* 56:225–229, 1987.

14. Ahlborg BJ, Bergstrom J, Brohult J: Human muscle glycogen content and capacity for prolonged exercise after different diets, *Forvarsmedicin* 3:85–89, 1967.

15. Bergstrom J, Hultman E: A study of glycogen metabolism during exercise in man, *Scan J Clin Lab Invest* 19:218–228, 1967.

16. Blom PCS, Costill NK, Vollestad NK: Exhaustive running: inappropriate as a stimulus of muscle glycogen supercompensation, *Med Sci Sports Exerc* 19:398–403, 1987.

17. Therriault DG, Beller GA, Smoake JA, and others: Intramuscular energy sources in dogs during physical work, *J Lipid Res* 14:54–61, 1973.

18. Paul P, Issekutz B: Role of extramuscular energy sources in the metabolism of the exercising dog, *Am J Physiol* 22:615–622, 1976.

19. Downey RL, Kronfeld DS, Banta CA: Diet of Beagles affects stamina, *J Am Anim Hosp Assoc* 16:273–277, 1980.

20. Hammel EP, Kronfeld DS, Ganjam VK, and others: Metabolic responses to exhaustive exercise in racing sled dogs fed diets containing medium, low and zero carbohydrate, *Am J Clin Nutr* 30:409–418, 1977.

21. Kronfeld DS: Diet and the performance of racing sled dogs, *J Am Vet Med Assoc* 162:470–473, 1973.

22. Reynolds AJ, Fuhrer L, Dunlap HL, and others: Lipid metabolite responses to diet and training in sled dogs, *J Nutr* 124:2754S–2759S, 1994.

23. Costill DL, Bowers R, Branam G: Muscle glycogen utilization during prolonged exercise on successive days, *J Appl Physiol* 31:834–838, 1971.

24. Kirwan JP, Costill DL, Mitchell JB: Carbohydrate balance in competitive runners during successive days of intense training, *J Appl Physiol* 65:2601–2602, 1988.

25. Bloomstrand E, Stalin G: Effect of muscle glycogen on glucose, lactate and amino acid metabolism during exercise and recovery in human subjects, *J Physiol* 514:293–302, 1999.

26. McKenzie E, Holbrook T, Williamson K, and others: Recovery of muscle glycogen concentrations in sled dogs during prolonged exercise, *Med Sci Sports Exerc* 37:1307–1311, 2005.

27. Hinchcliff KW, Jose-Cunilleras E, Davis MS: Muscle triglyceride concentration and fat metabolism during endurance exercise by sled dogs, *Physiologist* 47:302, 2004.

28. McKenzie EC, Hinchcliff KW, Valbeerg SJ, and others: Assessment of alterations in triglyceride and glycogen concentrations in muscle tissue of Alaskan sled dogs during repetitive prolonged exercise, *Am J Vet Res* 69:1097–1103, 2008.

29. Brouns F, Saris WHM, Beckers SE: Metabolic changes induced by sustained exhaustive cycling and diet manipulation, *Int J Sports Med* 10:S49–S62, 1989.

30. McClelland G, Zwingelstein G, Taylor CR, Weber JM: Increased capacity for circulatory fatty acid transport in a highly aerobic mammal, *Am J Physiol* 266:R1280–R1286, 1994.

31. Issekutz B Jr, Issekutz AC, Nash D: Mobilization of energy sources in exercising dogs, *J Appl Physiol* 29:691–697, 1970.

32. Adkins TO, Kronfeld DS: Diet of racing sled dogs affects erythrocyte depression by stress, *Can Vet J* 23:260–263, 1982.

33. Querengaesser A, Iben C, Leibetseder J: Blood changes during training and racing in sled dogs, *J Nutr* 124:2760S-2764S, 1994.

34. Carter SL, Rennie CD, Hamilton SJ, Tarnopolsky MA: Changes in skeletal muscles in males and females following endurance training, *Can J Physiol Pharmacol* 79:386–392, 2001.

35. Wakshlag JJ, Kallfelz FA, Barr SC, and others: Effects of exercise on canine skeletal muscle proteolysis: an investigation of the ubiquitin-proteasome pathway and other metabolic markers, *Vet Ther* 3:215–225, 2002.

36. Hinchcliff KW, Olson J, Crusberg C, and others: Serum biochemical changes in dogs competing in a long distance sled race, *J Am Vet Med Assoc* 202:401–405, 1993.

37. Gollnick PD: Energy metabolism and prolonged exercise. In Lamb DR, Murray R, editors: *Perspectives in exercise science and sports medicine*, vol 1, Carmel, Ind, 1988, Benchmark Press.

38. Reynolds AJ: Effect of diet on performance. In *Proc Perform Dog Nutrition Symp*, Fort Collins, Colo, 1995, Colorado State University.

39. Orr NWM: The feeding of sledge dogs on Antarctic expeditions, *Br J Nutr* 20:1–11, 1966.

40. Gannon JR: Nutritional requirements of the working dog, *Vet Ann* 21:161–166, 1981.

41. Orr NWM: The food requirements of Antarctic sledge dogs. In Graham-Jones O, editor: *Canine and feline nutritional requirements*, Oxford, England, 1965, Pergamon Press.

42. Wyatt HT: Further experiments on the nutrition of sledge dogs, *Br J Nutr* 17:273–279, 1963.

43. Hinchcliff KW, Swenson RA, Schreier CJ, and others: Metabolizable energy intake and sustained energy expenditure of Alaskan sled dogs during heavy exertion in the cold, *Am J Vet Res* 58:1457–1462, 1997.

44. Hinchcliff KW, Swenson RA, Burr JR, and others: Exercise-associated hyponatremia in Alaskan sled dog: urinary and hormonal responses, *J Appl Physiol* 83:824–829, 1997.

45. Hinchcliff KW, Swenson RA, Schreier CJ, and others: Effect of racing on serum sodium and potassium concentrations and acid-base status of Alaskan sled dogs, *J Am Vet Med Assoc* 210:1615–1618, 1997.

46. Hinchcliff KW, Reinhart GA, Burr JR, and others: Effect of racing on water metabolism, serum sodium and potassium concentrations, renal hormones, and urine composition of Alaskan sled dogs. In Reinhart GA, Carey DP, editors: *Recent advances in canine and feline nutrition, Iams nutrition symposium proceedings,* vol 2, Wilmington, Ohio, 1998, Orange Frazer Press.

47. Kohn CW: Composition and distribution of body fluids in dogs and cats. In DiBartola S, editor: *Fluid therapy in small animal practice*, Philadelphia, 1992, Saunders.

48. Surgenor S, Uphold RE: Acute hyponatremia in ultra-endurance athletes, *Am J Emerg Med* 12:441–444, 1994.

49. Schott HC, McGlade KS, Molander HA, and others: Body weight, fluid, electrolyte, and hormonal changes in horses competing in 50- and 100-mile endurance rides, *Am J Vet Res* 58:303–309, 1997.

50. Burr JR, Bradley DM, Vaughn DM, and others: Serum biochemical values in dogs before and after competing in long-distance races, *J Am Vet Med Assoc* 211:175–179, 1997.

51. McKenzie EC, Conilleras EJ, Hinchcliff KW, and others: Serum chemistry alterations in Alaskan sled dogs during five successive days of prolonged endurance exercise, *J Am Vet Med Assoc* 230:1486–1492, 2007.

52. Kronfeld DS, Hammel EP, Ramberg CF: Hematological and metabolic responses to training in racing sled dogs fed diets containing medium, low or zero carbohydrate, *Am J Clin Nutr* 30:419–430, 1977.

53. Armstrong R, Saubert C, Sembrowich W: Glycogen depletion in rat skeletal muscle fibers at different intensities and duration of exercise, *Pflugers Arch* 352:243–256, 1974.

54. Bergstrom J, Hultman E, Roch-Norlund AE: Muscle glycogen synthetase in normal subjects: basal values, effect of glycogen depletion by exercise and of a carbohydrate rich diet following exercise, *Scand J Clin Lab Invest* 29:231–236, 1972.

55. Hodgson DR, Rose RJ, Allent JR, and others: Glycogen depletion patterns in horses competing in day two of a three day event, *Cornell Vet* 75:366–374, 1985.

56. Ivy JL, Miller W, Power V: Endurance improved by ingestion of a glucose polymer supplement, *Med Sci Sports Exerc* 15:466–471, 1983.

57. Ivy JL, Katz AL, Cutler CL, and others: Muscle glycogen synthesis after exercise: effect of time of carbohydrate ingestion, *J Appl Physiol* 64:1480–1485, 1988.

58. Van Loon LJ, Saris WH, Kruijshoop M, Wagenmakers AJ: Maximizing post-exercise muscle glycogen synthesis: carbohydrate supplementation and the application of amino acid or protein hydrolysate mixtures, *Am J Clin Nutr* 72:106–111, 2000.

59. Jentjens RI, van Loon LJ, Mann CH: Addition of protein and amino acids to carbohydrates does not enhance post-exercise muscle glycogen synthesis, *J Appl Physiol* 91:839–846, 2001.

60. Reynolds AJ, Carey DP, Reinhart GA, and others: The effect of post exercise carbohydrate supplementation on muscle glycogen synthesis in trained sled dogs, *Am J Vet Res* 58:1252–1256, 1997.

61. Wakshlag JJ, Snedden K, Otis AM, and others: Effects of post-exercise supplements on glycogen repletion in skeletal muscle, *Vet Ther* 3:226–234, 2002.

62. Gisolfi CV: Water and electrolyte metabolism in exercise. In Fox EL, editor: *Nutrient utilization during exercise*, Columbus, Ohio, 1983, Ross Laboratories.

63. Fink WJ, Greenleaf JE: Fluid intake and athletic performance. In Haskell W, Scala J, Whittam J, editors: *Nutrition and athletic performance: proceedings of a conference on nutritional determinants of athletic performance*, 1981.

64. Askew EW: Fat metabolism in exercise. In Fox EL, editor: *Nutrient utilization during exercise*, Columbus, Ohio, 1983, Ross Laboratories.

65. Saltin B, Karlsson J: Muscle glycogen utilization during work of different intensities. In Saltin B, Karlsson J, editors: *Muscle metabolism during exercise*, vol 2, New York, 1971, Plenum Press.

66. Rose RJ, Bloomberg MS: Responses to sprint exercise in the Greyhound: effects on hematology, plasma biochemistry and muscle metabolism, *International greyhound symposium*, Orlando, Fla, 1983.

67. Dobson GB, Parkhouse WS, Weber SW, and others: Metabolic changes in skeletal muscle and blood of Greyhounds during 800-m track sprint, *Am J Physiol* 255:R513–R519, 1988.

68. Ilkiw JE, Davis PE, Church DB: Hematologic, biochemical, blood-gas, and acid-base values in Greyhounds before and after exercise, *Am J Vet Res* 50:583–586, 1989.

69. Nold JL, Peterson LJ, Fedde MR: Physiological changes in the running Greyhound: influence of race length, *Comp Biochem Physiol* 100A:623–627, 1991.

70. Donovan DM, Brooks GA: Endurance training affects lactate clearance not lactate production, *Am J Physiol* 244:E83–E92, 1983.

71. Hill RC, Lewis DD, Scott KC, and others: Effect of increased dietary protein and decreased dietary carbohydrate on performance and body composition in racing Greyhounds, *Am J Vet Res* 62:440–447, 2001.

72. Hill RC, Lewis DD, Randell SC, and others: Effect of mild restriction of food intake on the speed of racing Greyhounds, *Am J Vet Res* 66:L1065–L1070, 2005.

73. Ahlstrom O, Skrede A, Speakman J, and others: Energy expenditure and water turnover in hunting dogs: a pilot study, *J Nutr* 136:2063S–2065S, 2006.

74. Lepine AJ, Altom EK, Davenport GM, Kelley RL: Effect of diet on hunting performance of English Pointers, *Vet Ther* 2:10–23, 2001.

75. Altom EK, Davenport GM, Myers LJ, Cummins KA: Effect of dietary fat source and exercise on odorant-detecting ability of canine athletes, *Res Vet Sci* 75:149–155, 2003.

76. McMichael MA: Oxidative stress, antioxidants, and assessment of oxidative stress in dogs and cats, *J Am Vet Med Assoc* 231:714–720, 2007.

77. Baskin CR, Hinchcliff KW, DiSilvestro RA, and others: Effects of dietary antioxidant supplementation on oxidative damage and resistance to oxidative damage during prolonged exercise in sled dogs, *Am J Vet Res* 61:886–891, 2000.

78. Piercy RJ, Hinchcliff KW, DiSilvestro RA, and others: Effect of dietary supplements containing antioxidants on attenuation of muscle damage in exercising sled dogs, *Am J Vet Res* 61:1438–1445, 2000.

79. Dunlap KL, Reynolds AJ, Duffy LK: Total antioxidant power in sled dogs supplemented with blueberries and the comparison of blood parameters associated with exercise, *Comp Biochem Physiol* 143:429–434, 2006.

80. Durrer JL, Hannon JP: Seasonal variations of intake of dogs living in an arctic environment, *Am J Physiol* 202:375–378, 1962.

81. Blaza SE: Energy requirements of dogs in cool conditions, *Can Pract* 9:10–15, 1982.

82. Finke MD: Evaluation of the energy requirements of adult kennel dogs, *J Nutr* 121:S22–S28, 1991.

83. McNamara JH: Nutrition for military working dogs under stress, *Vet Med Small Anim Clin* 67:615–623, 1972.

25

Geriatrics

Improvements in the control of infectious diseases and in the nutrition of dogs and cats have resulted in a gradual increase in the average lifespan of companion animals. While the maximum lifespan of a given species remains relatively fixed, the average lifespan within a population of domesticated animals can be significantly affected by health care, genetics, and nutrition. By 2002, it was estimated that 30% to 40% of dogs and cats in the United States were 7 years of age or older, and approximately ⅓ of these pets were older than 11 years.[1,2] The increased number of senior and geriatric pets and the understanding that most of these dogs and cats have been cherished family members for many years necessitates increased attention to the care and nutrition of this portion of our companion animal population. Nutritional goals for aging pets include supporting health and vitality, preventing the onset or slowing the progression of age-related health disorders, and enhancing the pet's quality of life and, if possible, life expectancy.

AGING VERSUS SENESCENCE

The *aging process* refers to the natural series of life stages, beginning with conception and continuing through development, adulthood and finally senescence (geriatric stage). Although it is often misconstrued as such, aging is not a pathological process, but rather comprises the normal time-dependent changes that occur during the life of every individual. As many pet owners who cherish their senior dog or cat will attest, living with a healthy older dog or cat can be a wonderful experience. For example, older pets are often well behaved, are enjoyable to live with, and have a well-established set of endearing habits. Other changes associated with older pets are neither positive nor negative, such as the development of a graying muzzle or a slightly reduced activity level. Undesirable age-related changes are those associated with illness, changes in mobility, changes in cognitive function and the development of behavior problems. The deteriorative changes that may negatively affect a senior pet's overall health and quality of life are referred to as *senescence*.[3]

A variety of theories have been proposed to explain the phenomena of aging and senescence.[4] Several of these focus on genetic controls, such as the somatic mutation and gene regulation theories. Others examine the impact of temporal changes in homeostatic mechanisms of different body systems or the accumulation of the damaging products of cellular aging. For example, the oxidative stress theory postulates that aging is linked to energy expenditure and the cumulative cellular damage caused by the free radicals that are the byproducts of oxidative metabolism.[5,6] None of these theories singularly explains all of the changes that are observed during aging; nor are they necessarily mutually exclusive. Most likely, aging and senescence are multifactorial processes influenced by genetics and a myriad of internal and external environmental factors.

LIFESPANS OF DOGS AND CATS

From an evolutionary perspective, domesticated dogs and cats present a unique example of two species that enjoy an extended life stage beyond successful maturation and reproduction. Natural selection works principally on survival and fitness up to and throughout an individual's reproductive age and this impact diminishes as an animal enters its postreproductive years. In the wild, nondomesticated species typically do not enjoy a long postreproductive life, and older animals rapidly experience increased vulnerability to predation, accidents, and disease. In contrast, companion dogs and cats are protected from the pressures that have historically impacted their progenitor species. Many live well into their geriatric years, a life phase that is accompanied by age-related degenerative diseases and increased incidence of various types of cancer.

Because genes that regulate late-life deterioration have not been subjected to the same pressures of natural selection as those that support reproductive success, it can be argued that seeing an increase in the diseases of senescence is a natural byproduct of domestication. Indeed, several of the theories of aging suggest that the same genes that confer early maturation and a high rate of reproductive success may, at the same time, contribute to illness or disease later in life.[7,8] Such genes would persist in a population because of their beneficial impact upon reproductive fitness. In the case of species that invariably die young because of extrinsic (environmental) factors, the negative effects of such genes upon senior fitness would be irrelevant and therefore would be maintained. Conversely, when extrinsic factors are naturally absent or are controlled by human intervention (i.e., the species enjoys a relatively low postreproductive mortality rate), genes that promote longevity may begin to confer a selective advantage. Although the relationship between extrinsic mortality and longevity has been shown to be complex and influenced by other factors, this theory helps to explain the influence of domestication on dog and cat longevity.

The maximum lifespan of the dog is estimated to be about 27 years, but few dogs live to be older than 18 years of age. When all breeds are considered, the average lifespan of the domestic dog is approximately 13 years.[9] Intraspecific variations in longevity are of special interest with dogs because of the wide range in body size and conformation between breeds. Many of the large and giant breeds have a significantly shorter lifespan than the average of 13 years, while small and toy breeds tend to live longer. Numerous studies have shown that when examined across breeds, there is a significant negative relationship between lifespan and mature body size in dogs.[10-12] The shortened lifespan of giant breeds appears to be a result of the artificial selection for extremely large dogs and accompanying rapid early growth rates. Developmental skeletal diseases related to higher growth rates are an important (but not the only) contributing factor to the shorter lifespan of these dogs. For example, a recent pilot study found that mature body weight was more strongly correlated (negatively) with lifespan in dogs than other measures of size, such as height at the withers.[13] Although this study did not find breed to be a significant factor, they reported that some heavy but short-in-stature breeds, such as the Bulldog, experienced a shorter lifespan due to the influence of inherited structural disorders. The construction of breed standards that enforce a closed studbook and require absolute reproductive isolation has led to inbreeding practices and the overuse of a small number of individuals (usually males) in an already limited gene pool. This has contributed to the propagation of the more than 500 identified inherited diseases of purebred

TABLE 25-1   SUGGESTED AGES FOR GERIATRIC DOGS AND CATS

Species/Size	Age considered geriatric
Dogs	
Toy/small breeds (5-20 lb)	11.5 years
Medium breeds (21-50 lb)	10.0 years
Large breeds (51-90 lb)	9.0 years
Giant breeds (>90 lb)	7.5 years
Cats	12.0 years

dogs, many of which may contribute to a shortened lifespan for the affected breed.[14,15] Although purebred breeding is less widespread in the domestic cat, inbreeding in purebred cats may eventually lead to similar negative effects upon health and longevity. (Recognizing these problems, reputable breeders use careful selection and screening practices to reduce the incidence of genetically influenced health problems in their breed.)

Because breeds of dogs differ in average lifespan and susceptibility to disease, an individual dog's breed, size, and current health must be considered when determining whether or not he/she should be considered geriatric. General guidelines divide dogs into four categories based upon their adult size, with smaller dogs considered elderly at a later age than larger dogs (Table 25-1).[16] However, the dog's body condition, activity level, overall health, and the presence of chronic or debilitating disease must always be considered.[17] In general, cats age more slowly than most dogs and do not tend to show breed differences in aging or longevity. The average lifespan of cats that are kept indoors is approximately 14 years, and the cat's maximum lifespan may be as high as 25 to 35 years. Healthy cats are considered to be geriatric when they are approximately 10 to 12 years old.

When all breeds are considered, the average lifespan of the domestic dog is approximately 13 years. However, many of the large and giant breeds have a significantly shorter lifespan than this average, while some small and toy breeds live much longer. In general, cats age more slowly than most dogs and do not tend to show breed differences in aging or longevity. The average lifespan of cats that are kept indoors is approximately 14 years.

BOX 25-1 AGE-RELATED CHANGES IN LABORATORY VALUES FOR DOGS*

Unchanged	Decreased	Increased
Alanine aminotransferase	Albumin	Globulin
Blood urea nitrogen (BUN)	Albumin:globulin ratio	Platelets
BUN:creatinine ratio	Creatinine	Neutrophils
Cholesterol	Hematocrit	Serum potassium
Creatine kinase	Hemoglobin	Serum sodium
Eosinophils	Lymphocytes	Serum triglycerides
Gamma-glutamyl-transferase	Red blood cells	
Lactate dehydrogenase	Serum calcium	
Magnesium		
Serum chloride		
Total bilirubin		

*Data collected from 36 young and old Fox Terriers (1.8 vs. 11.5 years) and Labrador Retrievers (1.5 vs. 9.6 years). (From Hayek MG: Age-related changes in physiological function in the dog and cat: nutritional implications. In Reinhart GA, Carey DP, editors: *Recent advances in canine and feline nutrition, Iams nutrition symposium proceedings,* vol 2, Wilmington, Ohio, 1998, Orange Frazer Press.)

BOX 25-2 AGE-RELATED CHANGES IN LABORATORY VALUES FOR CATS*

Unchanged	Decreased	Increased
Eosinophils	Alanine aminotransferase	Cholesterol
Hematocrit	Alkaline phosphatase	Globulin
Lymphocytes	Aspartate aminotransferase	Monocytes
Neutrophils	Albumin	
Serum potassium	Albumin:globulin ratio	
	Creatinine kinase	
	Hemoglobin	
	Serum calcium	
	Serum phosphorus	
	White blood cells	

*Data collected from 40 young and old cats (0.9 vs. 8.9 years). (From Hayek MG: Age-related changes in physiological function in the dog and cat: nutritional implications. In Reinhart GA, Carey DP, editors: *Recent advances in canine and feline nutrition, Iams nutrition symposium proceedings,* vol 2, Wilmington, Ohio, 1998, Orange Frazer Press.)

AGE-ASSOCIATED PHYSIOLOGICAL CHANGES

In all animals, the biological effects of aging include a gradual decline in the functional capacity of organs, beginning shortly after the animal has reached maturity. A set of preliminary studies reported age-related changes in laboratory values for the dog and cat (Boxes 25-1 and 25-2).[18,19] Although the limited number of animals that were examined preclude using these data to make generalized conclusions about age-related changes to blood chemistry and cell data, these data suggest that multiple physiological systems are affected during the normal aging process. However, the clinical significance of these changes is not known and may not be relevant in many cases. In addition, different systems of the body age at different rates, and the degree of compromised function that must occur before clinical signs are seen depends on many factors in a pet's life. Although one pet may exhibit severe pathological effects of aging by 7 years, another may exhibit no clinical signs even at 12 years. It is also not unusual for more than one chronic disease to be present in a single geriatric pet. This variability necessitates that older animals be assessed as individuals, using functional changes in body systems rather than chronological age to categorize them with the geriatric population.

Metabolic Effects and Changes in Body Composition

An animal's basal metabolic rate (BMR) naturally slows with aging. This decline is caused primarily by changes in body composition, specifically a loss of lean body tissue. Normal aging in all animals is associated with decreases in lean body tissue (muscle) and total body water and an increase in the proportion of body fat. A decline in body water accompanies the loss of lean body tissue because lean tissue contains 73% water, while adipose tissue contains only 15% water. Age-related changes in body composition may differ for dogs and cats. An early study comparing young and old dogs reported that the body fat content of young dogs was between 15% and 20%, while that of older dogs was between 25% and 30%.[20] In contrast, the body fat content of adult,

TABLE 25-2 BODY COMPOSITION IN YOUNG AND OLD CATS AND DOGS*			
	LEAN MASS (%)	FAT MASS (%)	BONE MASS (%)
Young cats	69	30	1
Old cats	64	35	1
Young dogs	79	18	3
Old dogs	70	27	3

*Data collected from 40 young (less than 1.5 years) and old (greater than 7 years) cats, and 36 young (less than 1.5 years) and old (greater than 7 years) Fox Terriers and Labrador Retrievers. (From Hayek MG, Davenport GM: Nutrition and aging in companion animals, *J Anti Aging Med* 1:117, 1998.)

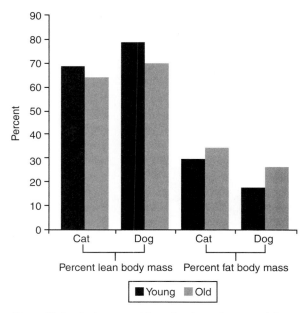

Figure 25-1 Body composition of senior and young-adult dogs and cats.

(From Hayek MG, Davenport GM: Nutrition and aging in companion animals, *J Anti Aging Med* 1:117, 1998.)

Normal aging in dogs and cats is associated with reduced resting metabolic rate, a decline in activity level, decreased lean body mass, and increased body fat. However, lifestyle factors can influence these changes. While some pets voluntarily reduce their physical activity as they become older, others remain active and athletic well into their senior years and maintain a lean and well-muscled body condition. Therefore each dog and cat must be assessed individually to determine the need for a change in daily caloric intake.

normal weight cats has been reported to be between 8% and 13%, but did not change significantly between the ages of 1 and 9 years.[21] Conversely, more recent data collected from a colony of young and old cats and dogs found that the body fat of young cats averaged 30% and increased to 35% in cats that were older than 7 years (Table 25-2, Figure 25-1).[22] The higher body fat in the more recent study may reflect the increased incidence of obesity among cats or a difference in feeding regimen and body weight in the different groups of cats studied. In dogs, fat body mass index increased from a mean of 18% in dogs less than 1.5 years to 27% in dogs older than 7 years of age. In both dogs and cats, the percentage of lean body mass declined with age (see Figure 25-1).

Lifestyle factors must be considered when assessing the metabolic rate and energy needs of older pets. While some pets voluntarily reduce their physical activity as they become older, others remain active and athletic well into their senior years. It is estimated that total daily energy requirements may decrease by as much as 30% to 40% during the last third of a pet's lifespan as a result of both reduced activity and decreased metabolic rate.[23] However, because physical activity helps to offset age-associated losses of lean body tissue, the BMR in older pets that are very active may not decrease significantly. Therefore, while BMR and energy needs generally decrease with aging, once again pets must be assessed individually to determine whether or not a decrease in daily caloric intake is warranted.

Changes in the Integumentary System

The skin loses elasticity and becomes less pliable with age as a result of increased pseudoelastin in the elastic fibers. This loss of elasticity is often accompanied by hyperkeratosis of both the skin and the follicles. Follicles may atrophy, resulting in areas of hair loss. The loss of melanocytes (pigment cells) in the hair follicles and reduced activity of the enzyme tyrosinase results in the production of white hairs, often observed around the muzzle and face of older dogs and cats. Changes in sebum production can result in scaly skin and cause an older animal's hair coat to become dry and dull. The incidence of skin neoplasia also increases with age. The median age for the development of skin tumors is about 10.5 years in dogs and 12 years in cats.[24]

Changes in the Gastrointestinal System

It has been suggested that a number of changes take place in the gastrointestinal tract as animals age. These include reduced salivary and gastric acid secretions and decreases in villi size, rate of cellular turnover, and colonic motility.[23] Although it has been theorized that the aging of the gastrointestinal tract leads to a decreased ability to digest and absorb nutrients, studies on healthy older dogs and cats show conflicting results. A study comparing the digestive efficiency of 1-year-old Beagles to elderly Beagles (10 to 12 years old) found no difference in the older dogs' ability to digest and absorb nutrients.[25] Similarly, a later study reported no significant difference in digestibility coefficients measured in young adult Beagles and very old Beagles (16 or 17 years old).[26] In contrast, while a more recent study found no significant differences in protein, fat, or energy digestibility between young (less than 6 years old) and old (greater than 8 years old) dogs, there was a trend toward reduced digestibility coefficients in the older group of dogs.[27]

Fewer studies have been conducted with geriatric cats. However, data that are available indicate that aging changes in the digestive capabilities of cats may be more significant than those observed in dogs. One study reported no significant differences in overall digestive efficiency between young adult cats and cats that were older than 10 years of age, but the older group of cats had a lower mean fat digestibility coefficient (0.80) than the young group (0.88).[28] This trend has been corroborated by subsequent studies.[27,29] When six different age groups of cats were studied, protein digestibility decreased slightly and fat digestibility decreased significantly as cats aged.[27] Together these two trends led to a highly significant linear relationship between age and a decline in diet energy digestibility. The oldest group of cats (12 to 14 years) had significantly lower digestibility coefficients for energy than all of the younger age categories. Interestingly, these older cats (12 to 14 years) were able to maintain normal weight by consuming more food than the younger cats. These results suggest that cats are capable of self-regulating their intake very precisely, even in the face of reduced digestive capacities. Although not determined in this study, possible underlying causes for age-related decreases in digestive capability include reductions in pancreatic enzyme secretion or bile acid secretion in elderly cats. These data indicate that a slight to moderate reduction in gastrointestinal functioning may occur in some healthy older pets. While these changes may not severely affect health, they should be considered when formulating and selecting diets for geriatric dogs and cats.

Changes in the Urinary System

Although a gradual decline in renal function is normal in older animals, a substantial loss of functioning nephrons must occur before changes in renal function are significant. Still, chronic renal failure is a major cause of illness and mortality in geriatric cats and is the third leading cause of death in old dogs. Therefore, age-related changes in renal health have been studied in detail in dogs and cats.[30-32] One of the first studies evaluated clinical changes in renal function in a colony of Beagles over a period of 13 years.[32] Results showed that nephrosclerosis was the most frequently diagnosed kidney lesion in older dogs. The data from this study also indicated that normal kidney aging may lead to nephron loss of up to 75% before clinical or biochemical signs occur in older dogs. Animals with less than 75% loss are usually clinically normal but may be more susceptible to renal insult than younger animals still possessing renal reserve capacity.

In contrast, another study that compared nutrient utilization and metabolism in young and old Beagles reported no loss of renal functioning associated with aging.[25] These results were supported by a subsequent study that examined the effects of aging and dietary protein intake on renal function and morphology in dogs.[33] All of the dogs were between 7 and 8 years old at the start of the study and were uninephrectomized to reduce renal mass by 50%. This procedure was included in the study design because a reduction of renal mass makes residual renal tissue more vulnerable to insult and would be expected to exacerbate any effects of aging or diet. Over a 4-year period, none of the dogs showed a decline in renal functioning. Age-related changes to the kidneys included the development of moderate renal lesions, but these were not affected by diet and did not significantly affect renal functioning. When the dogs in this study were compared with young dogs that had been uninephrectomized, the older dogs had compensatory responses to uninephrectomy that were indistinguishable from those of the young dogs. However, the older dogs did show a blunted renal response to a protein meal when compared with younger dogs. Results of these studies illustrate the importance of evaluating geriatric patients as individuals when assessing renal function. Aging alone is not associated with clinical signs of reduced renal functioning or chronic renal disease.

When renal disease does occur in older pets, it directly affects nutrition and dietary management because clinical kidney insufficiency is associated with weight loss, muscle wasting, altered plasma protein profiles, decreased caloric and nutrient intake, intestinal malabsorption, and reduced assimilation and use of nutrients. The accumulation of the metabolic end products of protein, of which urea is the most abundant, may further contribute to the development of the clinical and physiological abnormalities of renal failure. Dietary modification can be instituted to minimize the accumulation of these end products in the bloodstream and to slow progression of disease, while still supplying adequate energy and protein to maintain weight and minimize muscle wasting (see Section 5, pp. 417-425 for a complete discussion).

Changes in the Musculoskeletal System

As discussed previously, aging is associated with a decline in the percentage of lean body (muscle) mass. Bone mass also decreases slightly as animals age. Both the number and size of muscle cells decrease with age, and the cortices of the long bones become thinner, dense, and brittle. The composition of the articular cartilage matrix changes with age; specifically reduced number of chondrocytes leads to decreased production of glycosaminoglycans, type 1 collagen, and chondroitin sulfate. Aging cartilage becomes less resilient and has limited ability to regenerate in response to intense activity or

trauma. In some cases, the cumulative and pathological outcome of these changes is the development of osteoarthritis. Following an initial peak in incidence due to developmental bone diseases in young dogs, the risk of developing joint problems increases in dogs that are 5 to 7 years of age or older.[34] The presence of joint pain associated with osteoarthritis may also affect a pet's appetite and ability to eat. Along with medical therapy, there are several nutraceuticals that may aid in the management of arthritis in older pets (see Chapter 37, pp. 502-506 for a complete discussion).

Changes in the Immune System

Similar to humans and other animals, immunocompetence declines with age in dogs and cats.[35-37] Cell-mediated immunity (i.e., T-cell immunity) is the most severely affected component of the immune system. Reduced T-cell responsiveness is implicated as having a role in numerous degenerative diseases such as osteoarthritis, cancer, and increased susceptibility to infection. Studies with dogs have also demonstrated age-related declines in mitogen stimulation, chemotaxis, and phagocytosis.[36] Older dogs may have decreased white blood cell and immature neutrophil counts and increased mature neutrophils and circulating levels of immunoglobulin G.[38] Although only two breeds were compared, there is evidence that the rate of decline in the immune system may differ between breeds of dogs.[39] Older cats may exhibit reduced mitogen response, and delayed type 1 hypersensitivity and antibody responses.[40] Because the free radical theory of aging predicts that the cumulative effects of free radical reactions and their byproducts lead to cellular damage and death, the potential exists to ameliorate age-related dysregulation of the immune system through nutritional intervention (see pp. 270-271).

Changes in the Cardiovascular System

Heart-related disease is a common cause of morbidity in older pets and is estimated to occur in up to 30% of aged dogs.[41] The incidence in cats is not known, but it is thought to occur less frequently.[42] Cardiac output decreases by as much as 30% between midlife and old age. Maximal heart rate and oxygen consumption during exercise also decrease significantly. For example, a study comparing cardiovascular responses during exercise in young and old dogs found that aging led to a loss of cardiovascular reserve and adaptability, which was presumed to contribute to cardiovascular disease in some older dogs.[43] In animals with adult onset heart disease, fibrosis and myocardial necrosis eventually interfere with normal conduction pathways and result in arrhythmias. Normal vascular changes of aging include hyaline thickening of the media of the blood vessels and increased deposition of calcium in the intima of the aorta and the media of the peripheral arteries.[44] All of these changes contribute to a progressive increase in the workload of the heart, which can eventually lead to the development of congestive heart disease or heart failure.

Changes in the Special Senses

Old age may result in a general decline in an animal's ability to react to stimuli and changes in the sensations of vision, hearing, and taste. Nuclear sclerosis or cataracts of the lens are frequently seen in older dogs and cats and can lead to partial or complete blindness. Hearing impairment caused by cochlea degeneration is also common. Finally, a decrease in taste acuity may lead to decreased interest in food, reduced intake, and weight loss in some older pets.

Changes in Behavior

The most common behavioral problems that occur in old dogs and cats are secondary to degenerative disease and other geriatric changes.[45] Several of these behavioral changes may affect a pet's ability or desire to obtain adequate nutrition. For example, pets suffering from the chronic pain of arthritis may become increasingly irritable and reluctant to engage in any type of activity, including eating. On the other hand, the development of diabetes mellitus in dogs may be accompanied by a ravenous appetite. Depression or pathological mourning as a result of the loss of a beloved housemate or owner can result in severe anorexia in older pets. If prolonged, this can lead to weight loss and increased susceptibility to illness. Changes in the social structure of the family, usually because of the introduction of another pet, may also cause elderly dogs or cats to change their eating patterns. In some instances, social facilitation may cause an abrupt increase in intake,

predisposing the pet to obesity. In other cases, intimidation by the new pet may cause the older animal to suddenly decrease food intake.

One of the most noticeable changes in the behavior of geriatric pets is their resistance to a change in daily routine. A move to a new residence, the introduction of a new pet, or a change in the owner's work schedule may be met with depression, alterations in elimination patterns, and/or changes in eating habits. It is important to be aware that geriatric cats are particularly predisposed to behavior problems when their environment is altered.[46] Introducing changes gradually and allowing the elderly pet sufficient time to adapt is often effective in minimizing stress and preventing the occurrence of behavioral problems.

Changes in cognitive function in older dogs and cats may occur due to age-related functional changes in the central nervous system. *Cognitive dysfunction syndrome* (CDS) refers to a collection of geriatric behavior changes that have no organic cause and which may include disorientation, anxiety, memory loss, and reduced ability to learn or react to environmental changes.[45] Behavior changes reported by owners of affected dogs and cats include decreased interaction with the owner or other pets, increase in irritability or aggression, loss of house or litter box training, disruption of normal sleep patterns, and a drastic increase or decrease in activity level.[47] Although several categories of CDS in dogs and cats have been identified, it is generally accepted that the underlying causes involve progressive changes that are both neuropathological and neurochemical in nature. Neuropathological changes include neuronal loss, thickening of the meninges, and the formation of beta-amyloid deposits and plaques.[48,49] Neurochemical changes include alterations in neurotransmitter levels and receptors.[50] Studies of these changes have found a correlation between cognitive disorders in old animals and the accumulation of oxidative damage to brain cells.[51,52] The brain appears to be particularly susceptible to the damaging effects of oxygen free radicals because of its high lipid content, high rate of oxidative metabolic activity, and limited ability to regenerate.[51,53] In response to this knowledge, nutritional interventions, most commonly the provision of various antioxidant nutrients, have been studied for their efficacy in slowing progression or managing signs of CDS (see pp. 270-271).

NUTRIENT CONSIDERATIONS FOR OLDER PETS

When considering the nutrition and feeding practices that can support healthy aging in dogs and cats, beneficial interventions include those that provide optimal levels of essential nutrients while helping to delay age-related physiological changes and reduce accumulation of detrimental byproducts that contribute to cellular senescence. Senior and geriatric dogs and cats have a need for the same nutrients that were required during earlier physiological states. However, the quantities of nutrients required per unit of body weight may change, and the way in which nutrients are provided to the pet may require modification. Such changes usually depend on changes in energy requirements and the presence or degree of degenerative disease. Nutrients that may be of specific concern or of added benefit to senior dogs and cats are discussed in the following sections.

Energy

Most senior pets experience a slight to moderate reduction in daily energy needs. A controlled study of the energy needs in older dogs and cats found that as cats and dogs age, their requirement for energy progressively declines.[27] Dogs that were older than 8 years consumed approximately 18% fewer calories than breed-matched dogs less than 6 years of age. While the effect in cats was less pronounced, a decline in energy requirements with age was also seen. However, it is important to note that the oldest group of cats (12 to 15 years) actually consumed a greater quantity of food. It was theorized that this increase occurred to compensate for a slightly reduced capacity to digest dietary fat and protein in the oldest group of cats.

Elderly pets vary greatly in their energy needs, depending on individual temperament, presence of degenerative disease, ability to digest and assimilate nutrients, and amount of daily exercise. Caloric intake should be carefully monitored in older pets to ensure adequate intake of calories and nutrients while at the same time preventing the development of obesity. Dogs and cats that are between 7 and 9 years of age are beginning to age and are at the highest risk for obesity. Therefore pet owners and veterinarians should carefully monitor the dietary intake and weight status of these pets to ensure that their intake matches their energy needs as energy expenditure begins to decline. This is most easily accomplished by selecting a pet food that is formulated to be less energy dense, while still providing optimal levels of essential nutrients for senior pets.

Most dogs and cats experience slight to moderate reductions in daily energy needs as they age. Intake and body weight should be carefully monitored in older pets to ensure adequate consumption of calories and nutrients while at the same time preventing the development of obesity. Foods that are formulated for senior pets will be slightly lower in energy density while still providing optimal levels of essential nutrients.

Protein and Amino Acids

The decrease in lean body mass that occurs with aging results in a loss of the protein reserves that can normally be used by the body during reactions to stress and illness. Stress triggers nervous, metabolic, and hormonal adaptations that allow an animal to adapt to changes in the environment and aversive stimuli such as infectious agents or injury. The mobilization of body protein is a characteristic physiological response to stress. Older animals are subject to a high incidence of disease and physiological stress and are therefore especially vulnerable if their ability to react is compromised. It is important that geriatric pets be provided with high-quality protein at a level that is sufficient to supply the essential amino acids needed for body maintenance needs and to minimize losses of lean body tissue.

Studies conducted with human subjects have shown that the efficiency of protein use is slightly lower in the elderly than in young adults. The amount of available energy in the form of egg protein required for nitrogen balance was reported to be 4% in young men, but it increased to 6% in elderly men.[55] Similar results have been reported in dogs. An early study compared the protein requirements in young and old animals.[56] The ratio of liver and muscle protein to deoxyribonucleic acid (DNA) was measured and used as an estimate of body protein reserves. Protein:DNA ratios were maximized when young adult dogs were fed a semipurified diet containing 12.4% protein. Old dogs, on the other hand, required 18.8% protein to maximize body protein reserves. This increased need did not appear to be caused by reduced digestive capacity in the older dogs. A subsequent study compared the digestive capabilities of 12-year-old dogs to 1-year-old dogs and found no difference in the ability of old dogs to digest protein and other nutrients from four different diets when compared with young adult dogs.[57]

A more recent study examined the effects of feeding graded levels of dietary protein to groups of young and geriatric dogs.[58] The dogs were fed isocaloric diets containing either 16%, 24%, or 32% crude protein for a period of 8 weeks. At the end of the feeding period, whole body protein turnover and rates of protein synthesis and degradation were measured using administration of the tracer amino acid ^{15}N-glycine.[59] Results showed a positive correlation between whole body protein turnover and dietary protein level in both young-adult and geriatric Beagles. Regardless of age, the rates of whole body protein synthesis and degradation increased with increasing level of protein intake, while nitrogen balance did not change. Although the study showed that young and elderly dogs do not appear to have a protein requirement that is higher than 16% to maintain nitrogen balance, increased nitrogen flux through the body's metabolic pool that is associated with higher protein intake may be an important source of dietary amino acids needed for tissue repair, immune system support, and energy in older animals. This theory is supported by evidence from a study that fed young-adult and senior dogs foods that contained 16% or 32% protein, supplied as either chicken or chicken plus corn gluten meal.[60] After 7 weeks of feeding, the senior dogs that were fed the 32% protein diet had increased percent lean body mass compared with senior dogs that were fed the lower protein diet (Figure 25-2). The younger adults did not demonstrate a change in lean body tissue in response to increasing dietary protein.

Finally, there is some evidence of breed differences in the rate of whole-body protein turnover in senior dogs. When young-adult and senior Labrador Retrievers and Fox Terriers were fed diets containing 18%, 24%, or 30% protein, the young dogs had higher net protein (nitrogen) accretion when compared with the older dogs, regardless of breed.[61] This difference was due to

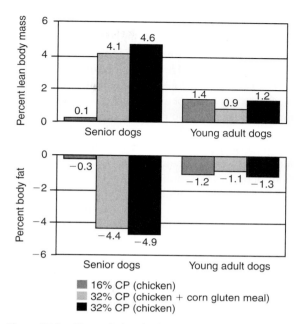

Figure 25-2 Change in lean body mass and body fat in young-adult and senior Beagles fed different levels and sources of protein. *CP*, Crude protein.

(From Davenport G, Gaasch S, Hayek MG, and others: Effect of dietary protein on body composition and metabolic responses of geriatric and young-adult dogs, *J Vet Intern Med* 15:306, 2001.)

increased rates of protein synthesis and lower rates of protein degradation in the younger dogs. Increasing dietary protein did not significantly affect nitrogen balance, but did tend to positively influence nitrogen retention. Senior dogs of both breeds also showed a decrease in whole body protein degradation when consuming the 30% protein diet. Breed differences were observed, and these effects differed with age group. Senior Fox Terriers showed a pronounced increase in body protein accretion in response to the higher protein diets, when compared with the 18% protein diet. However, this change did not lead to an increase in lean body mass. Conversely, both young and old Labrador Retrievers and young Fox Terriers showed increased lean body mass in response to increasing dietary protein.

When all data are considered, the minimum dietary protein requirement of geriatric dogs is probably between 16% and 24% when supplied as a high-quality protein source. However, additional benefits such as support of lean body mass may be provided to geriatric dogs if they are fed a diet containing more than 24%

protein. Providing higher protein may help to offset a loss of protein reserves and support an older animal's ability to respond to stress. In addition, the decreased total energy needs of older pets may result in the need to slightly increase the proportion of protein calories in the diet. Premium and superpremium pet foods formulated for senior and geriatric pets contain high-quality protein sources and therefore can provide an adequate level and quality of protein to older animals. However, pet food brands that contain minimal amounts of protein from poor-quality sources may not be capable of providing adequate protein nutrition to senior pets. Similarly, energy-dense foods with reduced levels of protein that are formulated for dogs and cats with existing kidney failure do not supply appropriate levels of protein for healthy elderly dogs and cats.

As discussed previously, decreased renal functioning is a normal occurrence with aging in humans, rats, and to some degree, dogs and cats. As a direct result of this knowledge, and because of a series of studies conducted on rats, some investigators once recommended that all elderly pets receive moderately reduced protein diets in an attempt to prevent or minimize the progression of kidney dysfunction.[62] However, it is essential that healthy, geriatric dogs and cats receive adequate amounts of high-quality protein to minimize losses of body protein reserves, satisfy maintenance protein needs, and support the ability to respond to stress. Although a reduction in protein intake affects the expression of clinical signs of chronic renal failure once a certain level of dysfunction has occurred, there is no evidence to support a systematically reduced protein level in the diets of healthy older pets. It is recommended that the protein in the diet of geriatric dogs and cats should not be restricted simply because of old age. Rather, elderly pets should receive foods containing optimal levels of high-quality protein. If chronic renal disease is diagnosed, moderate protein restriction and other dietary modifications are implemented as needed in response to an individual pet's clinical signs (see Section 5, pp. 417-425).

Older pets have slightly higher protein requirements than the maintenance needs of young adult animals. This is necessary to prevent or minimize age-associated losses in the body's protein reserves and to support the ability to respond to stress. The decreased daily energy needs of older pets also translate into an increased proportion of protein calories in foods formulated for seniors. Contrary to a common nutritional myth, dietary protein neither causes nor contributes to chronic renal disease in older pets. Therefore protein in the diets of healthy geriatric dogs and cats should never be restricted simply because of old age.

Fat

It has been theorized that the increase in the percentage of body fat that occurs with aging is partially a result of an increasing inability of the body to metabolize lipids.[25] Slightly decreasing the amount of fat in the diet may benefit geriatric dogs and cats, provided that the fat that remains in the diet is both highly digestible and rich in essential fatty acids (EFAs). A decrease in the proportion of calories contributed by fat also decreases the diet's energy density. This is an advantage for older pets that have reduced energy needs.

The type of fat that is included in foods for senior pets is also important. There is evidence suggesting that aging is associated with a gradual decline in the ability to desaturate EFAs.[63,64] This change appears to be due to decreased activity of desaturase enzymes, most specifically delta-6-desaturase.[65] Studies of old and young Beagles and Labrador Retrievers showed significant age-related differences in serum levels of arachidonic and eicosapentaenoic acid.[66] The data from this preliminary study indicated that there also may be breed-specific, age-related differences in the ability to elongate omega-3 and omega-6 fatty acids.

Antioxidant Nutrients

IMMUNOCOMPETENCE The free radical hypothesis of aging proposes that the accumulation of reactive oxygen byproducts over time leads to oxidative stress and damage to cells and tissues. The cells of the immune system are particularly vulnerable to oxidative stress because they contain high concentrations of polyunsaturated fatty acids (PUFAs) and because some of the immune system's mechanisms of action directly involve exposure to highly oxidizing environments. Therefore, nutrient interventions to slow some of the physiological signs of aging and to support a healthy immune system have focused on antioxidant nutrients. Supplementation with vitamin E and the carotenoids, beta-carotene and lutein, have been shown to maintain or even improve age-associated declines in immune function in several species, including dogs and cats.

A study examined the effects of beta-carotene supplementation on immune cell population and immune response in young and old Fox Terriers and Labrador Retrievers.[67] The results corroborated other work showing that both T-cell and B-cell populations in older dogs were reduced when compared with the populations of these cells in young adult dogs. Supplementation with a moderate level (20 milligrams [mg]/kilogram [kg]) of beta-carotene increased CD4+ T cells in the older dogs to levels not different from those of the young adults and increased in vitro T-cell response to concanavalin A (Con A). However, this effect was not seen when a high level of beta-carotene was fed (40 mg/kg). Older dogs supplemented with beta-carotene also tended to show an increase in their B-cell populations, but this trend was not statistically significant. There is also evidence that combined supplementation with antioxidant nutrients and mitochondrial cofactors (vitamin E, vitamin C, L-carnitine, dl-alpha-lipoic acid, and various sources of carotenoids) plus environmental enrichment (exercise and training/learning opportunities) significantly enhanced some measures of immunocompetence in older dogs.[68] While a modest effect was observed for supplementation and environmental enrichment individually in this study, the combination of these two factors was more effective than either factor alone. However, the inclusion of multiple nutrients and several forms of environmental enrichment precluded conclusions regarding the efficacy of particular nutrients or enrichment types.

The effect of supplemental vitamin E on immune function in older cats has also been studied. Young-adult and senior cats were fed either a control diet containing 60 international units (IU) vitamin E per kg or supplemented diets containing either 250 IU/kg or 500 IU/kg.[69] Similar to the response of the dog to beta-carotene, supplementation with moderate, but not high, levels of vitamin E resulted in improved T- and B-cell proliferation responses in old cats. Although the mechanisms underlying this phenomenon are not completely understood, the differing effects of moderate vs. high levels of vitamin E on immune function has also been demonstrated in other species.[70,71] Further research is needed to explore the potential efficacy of other antioxidant nutrients in supporting immunocompetence in older dogs and cats.

COGNITIVE DYSFUNCTION SYNDROME

Providing dietary antioxidants also has demonstrated efficacy in the treatment and management of signs of CDS in dogs and cats. In general, combinations of several antioxidant and mitochondrial cofactors (L-carnitine and dl-alpha-lipoic acid) have been studied (rather than inclusion of one or two individual nutrients).[72] (Note: Supplements for cats must exclude dl-alpha-lipoic acid as it is toxic to cats.) Recently, preliminary studies have been conducted to examine the neuroprotective effects of supplementation with the phospholipid phosphatidylserine in older dogs.[73] Collectively, studies of the effects of antioxidant and mitochondrial cofactor supplementation on cognitive dysfunction in dogs and cats suggest that this type of nutritional intervention may provide moderate benefit to some animals.[74-76] Specific improvements that have been reported in laboratory studies of dogs receiving the supplement include reduced number of errors when performing object or landmark discrimination tasks, or other tests of learning and cognitive function.[77,78] Interestingly, one study reported that although a combination of antioxidants were fed to aging Beagles, measured improvements in cognitive performance were positively correlated with blood concentrations of vitamin E.[79] Clinical trials with older dogs living in homes have reported significant reductions in disorientation, improved social interaction, and fewer house-soiling incidents in response to supplementation.[80,81] However, because no studies have examined the benefits of supplementation with a single nutrient, conclusions cannot currently be made regarding the respective influence of any particular nutrient or even class of nutrient.

FEEDING MANAGEMENT AND CARE OF OLDER PETS

Major objectives of the feeding and care of geriatric dogs and cats should be to maintain health and optimal body weight, slow or prevent the development of chronic illness, and minimize or improve clinical signs of diseases that may already be present. Routine care for geriatric pets should involve adherence to a consistent daily routine, regular attention to normal health care procedures, and periodic veterinary examinations to assess for the presence or progression of chronic disease. Stressful situations and abrupt changes in daily routines should be avoided. If a drastic change must be made in an older pet's routine, attempts should be made to minimize stress and accomplish the change in a gradual manner.

Optimal body weight can be maintained and obesity prevented through the judicious control of caloric intake and adherence to a regular exercise schedule. Although some adult dogs and cats are able to maintain normal body weights when fed free-choice, this may no longer be possible as the pet ages. Decreasing energy needs may lead to obesity in some older pets if a free-choice regimen is continued. It is recommended that senior and geriatric dogs and cats be fed at least two to three small meals per day, rather than one large meal. Feeding several small meals per day promotes improved nutrient use and may decrease feelings of hunger between meals. The timing and size of meals should also be strictly regulated. A regular schedule minimizes gastrointestinal stress and supports normal nutrient digestion and use. Fresh water should be available at all times to older dogs and cats.

Geriatric cats and some older dogs may become very particular about their eating habits. The pet's willingness to eat new foods may decrease. It may be necessary for owners to provide an especially strong-smelling or highly palatable food to their older cat. Other dogs and cats may accept only one particular brand or flavor of food. If possible, pet owners should accommodate these needs, provided that the preferred food can provide adequate nutrition to the pet.

If a chronic disease state that requires specific nutrient alterations is present (e.g., diabetes, renal disease, osteoarthritis, congestive heart failure), the pet should be fed a diet that is appropriate for the management of the disorder (see Section 5 for complete discussions). Healthy older pets can be fed a diet that contains high-quality ingredients, moderate to high levels of high-quality protein, and moderately reduced amounts of fat. Other nutrients that may be beneficial include increased levels of antioxidant nutrients, and the inclusion of mitochondrial cofactors such as L-carnitine and dl-alpha-lipoic acid. Premium and superpremium commercial pet foods that contain high-quality ingredients and targeted

nutrition for senior pets are suitable. Lower-quality pet foods are not generally recommended for elderly pets because some of these products provide poorly available nutrients.

Proper care of the teeth and gums is important for geriatric pets. If an owner is unable or unwilling to regularly examine and brush a pet's teeth, yearly dental prophylaxis by a veterinarian is necessary to decrease buildup of dental calculus and the development of periodontal disease. Dental problems can lead to decreased food intake, anorexia, and systemic disease if not treated promptly in older animals (see Chapter 34, pp. 437-441 for a complete discussion).

Regular and sustained periods of physical activity help to maintain muscle tone, enhance circulation, improve gastrointestinal function, and prevent excess weight gain. The level and intensity of exercise should be adjusted to an individual pet's physical and medical condition. Many dogs, if healthy and maintained in good condition, can enjoy walking, running, and playing active games with their owners well into old age. Almost all older dogs benefit from and enjoy two 15- to 30-minute walks per day. Although most cats do not readily accept walking on a lead, playing games with older cats can be an acceptable form of exercise (Box 25-3).

BOX 25-3 PRACTICAL FEEDING TIPS: ELDERLY COMPANION ANIMALS

Provide regular health checkups at least two times per year.

Avoid sudden changes in daily routine, environment, or diet.

Feed a diet that contains high-quality protein and is specifically formulated for geriatric pets.

Use portion-controlled feeding to prevent conditions of either obesity or weight loss; feed to maintain ideal body weight.

Provide a moderate level of regular exercise and regular opportunities for play and enjoyable interactions.

Maintain proper care of teeth and gums.

When necessary, provide a therapeutic diet to manage or treat disease.

References

1. American Veterinary Medical Association (AVMA): Total pet ownership and pet population. In *US pet ownership and demographics sourcebook*, Schaumburg, Ill, 2002, AVMA, pp 6–23.

2. Goldston RT, Notesworthy GD, Willard MD, and others: *Establishing a geriatrics management program*, St Louis, 1996, Ralston Purina.

3. Waters DJ: Aging well: how the science of aging informs the practice of wellness. In *Proc NAVC*, 2008, pp 4–7.

4. Sharma R: Theories of aging. In Timiras PS, editor: *Physiological basis of aging and geriatrics*, Boca Raton, Fla, 1994, CRC Press, pp 37–46.

5. Harman D: Aging, a theory based on free radical and radiation chemistry, *J Gerontol* 11:298–300, 1956.

6. Beckman KB, Ames BN: The free radical theory of aging matures, *Physiol Rev* 78:547–581, 1998.

7. Williams G: Pleiotropy, natural selection, and the evolution of senescence, *Evolution* 11:398-411, 1957.

8. Kirkwood TB: The disposable soma theory of aging. In Harrison DE, editor: *Genetic effects on aging*, vol 2, Caldwell, NJ, 1990, Telford Press, pp 9–19.

9. Brace JJ: Theories of aging, *Vet Clin North Am Small Anim Pract* 11:811–814, 1981.

10. Deeb BJ, Wolf NS: Studying longevity and morbidity in large and small breeds of dogs, *Vet Med* 89:702–713, 1994.

11. Patronek GJ, Waters DJ, Glickman LT: Comparative longevity of pet dogs and humans: implications for gerontology research, *J Gerontol Biol Sci Med Sci* 52:171–178, 1997.

12. Galis F, van der Sluijs I, van Dooren TJM, and others: Do large dogs die young? *J Exp Zool B Mol Dev Evol* 308:119–126, 2007.

13. Greer KA, Canterberry SC, Murphy KE: Statistical analysis regarding the effects of height and weight on life span of the domestic dog, *Res Vet Sci* 82:208–214, 2007.

14. Arman K: A new direction for kennel club regulations and breed standards, *Can Vet J* 48:47–58, 2007.

15. Ackerman L: *The genetic connection: a guide to health problems in purebred dogs*, Boulder, Colo, 1999, AAHA Press, pp 1–28.

16. Goldston RT: Introduction and overview of geriatrics. In Goldston RT, editor: *Geriatric and gerontology of the dog and cat*, Philadelphia, 1995, Saunders, pp 1–9.

17. Fortney WD: Clinical perspectives and issues related to senior companion animals. In *Proc WSAVA*, 2001, pp 48–52.

18. Strasser A, Niedmuller H, Hofecker G, and others: The effect of aging on laboratory values in the dog, *J Vet Med* 40:720–730, 1993.

19. Hayek MG: Age-related changes in physiological function in the dog and cat: nutritional implications. In Reinhart GA, Carey DP, editors: *Recent advances in canine and feline nutrition, Iams nutrition symposium proceedings*, vol 2, Wilmington, Ohio, 1998, Orange Frazer Press.

20. Meyer H, Stadfeld G: Investigation on the body and organ structures of dogs. In Anderson RS, editor: *Nutrition of the dog and cat*, Oxford, England, 1980, Pergamon Press.

21. Munday HS, Earle KE, Anderson P: Changes in body composition of the domestic shorthaired cat during growth and development, *J Nutr* 124:2622S, 1994.

22. Hayek MG, Davenport GM: Nutrition and aging in companion animals, *J Anti Aging Med* 1:117–123, 1998.

23. Mosier JE: Effect of aging on body systems of the dog, *Vet Clin North Am Small Anim Pract* 19:1–13, 1989.

24. MacDonald J: Neoplastic diseases of the integument, *Proc Am Anim Hosp Assoc* 17–20, 1987.

25. Sheffy BE, Williams AJ, Zimmer JF, and others: Nutrition and metabolism of the geriatric dog, *Cornell Vet* 75:324–347, 1985.

26. Buffington CA, Branham JE, Dunn GC: Lack of effect of age on digestibility of protein, fat and dry matter in Beagle dogs. In Burger IH, Rivers JPW, editors: *Nutrition of the dog and cat, Waltham symposium #7*, Cambridge, Mass, 1989, Cambridge University Press.

27. Taylor EJ, Adams C, Neville R: Some nutritional aspects of ageing in dogs and cats, *Proc Nutr Soc* 54:645–656, 1995.

28. Anantharaman-Barr HG, Gicquello P, Rabot R: The effect of age on the digestibility of macronutrients and energy in cats. In *Proc Brit Small Anim Vet Assoc Cong*, Birmingham, England, 1991, p 164.

29. Taylor EJ, Adams C, Coe S, and others: The effects of aging on the digestion of the cat. In *Proc First Cong Europ CNVSPA-FECAVA*, 1995, pp 309–310.

30. DiBartola SP, Rutgers HC, Zack PM, Tarr MJ: Clinicopathologic findings associated with chronic renal disease in cats: 74 cases (1973-1984), *J Am Vet Med Assoc* 190:1196–1202, 1987.

31. Cowgill LD, Spangler WL: Renal insufficiency in geriatric dogs, *Vet Clin North Am Small Anim Pract* 11:727–749, 1981.

32. Kaufman GM: Renal function in the geriatric dog, *Compend Contin Educ Pract Vet* 6:108–109, 1984.

33. Finco DR, Brown S, Crowell W, and others: Effects of aging and dietary protein intake on uninephrectomized geriatric dogs, *Am J Vet Res* 55:1282–1290, 1994.

34. Egenvall A, Bonnett BN, Olson P, Hedhammer G: Gender, age and breed pattern of diagnoses for veterinary care in insured dogs in Sweden during 1996, *Vet Rec* 146:551–557, 2000.

35. Meydani SM, Hayek MG: Vitamin E and aging immune response, *Clin Geriatr Med* 11:567–576, 1995.

36. HogenEsch H, Thompson S, Dunham A, and others: Effect of age on immune parameters and the immune response of dogs to vaccines: a cross-sectional study, *Vet Immunol Immunopathol* 97:77–85, 2004.

37. Strasser A, Teltscher A, May B, and others: Age-associated changes in the immune system of German Shepherd dogs, *J Vet Med Assoc* 47:181–192, 2000.

38. Strasser A, Niedermuller AJ, Zimmer JF, Ruan GD: The effect of aging on laboratory values in dogs, *J Vet Med* 40:720–730, 1993.

39. Kearns RJ, Hayek MG, Turek JJ, and others: Effect of age, breed and dietary omega-6 (n-6):omega 3 (n-3) fatty acid ratio on immune function, eicosanoid production, and lipid peroxidation in young and aged dogs, *Vet Immunol Immunopathol* 69:165–183, 1999.

40. Hayek MG, Massimino SP, Burr JR, Kearns RJ: Dietary vitamin E improves immune function in cats. In Reinhart GA, Carey DP, editors: *Recent advances in canine and feline nutrition, Iams nutrition symposium proceedings*, vol 2, Wilmington, Ohio, 1998, Orange Frazer Press, pp 555–563.

41. Hamlin RL: Managing cardiologic disorders in geriatric dogs. In *Proc Geriatr Med Symp*, 1987, pp 14–18.

42. Markham RW, Hodgkins EM: Geriatric nutrition, *Vet Clin North Am Small Anim Pract* 19:165–185, 1989.

43. Strasser A, Simunek M, Seiser M, and others: Age-dependent changes in cardiovascular and metabolic responses to exercise in Beagle dogs, *Zentralbl Veterinarmed A* 44:449–460, 1997.

44. Bright JM, Mears E: Chronic heart disease and its management, *Vet Clin North Am Small Anim Pract* 27:1305–1329, 1997.

45. Landsberg G, Araugo JA: Behavior problems in geriatric pets, *Vet Clin North Am Small Anim Pract* 35:675–698, 2005.

46. American Association of Feline Practitioners (AAFP): *Panel report on feline senior care*, 2005, AAFP/AFM, pp 15–17.

47. Neilson JC, Hart BL, Cliff KD: Prevalence of behavioral changes associated with age-related cognitive impairment in dogs, *J Am Vet Med Assoc* 218:1787–1791, 2001.

48. Dimakopoulos AC, Mayer RJ: Aspects of neurodegeneration in the canine brain, *J Nutr* 132:1579S–1582S, 2002.

49. Head E, Moffat K, Das P, and others: Beta-amyloid deposition and tau phosphorylation in clinically characterized aged cats, *Neurobiol Aging* 26:749–763, 2005.

50. Araujo JA, Studzinski CM, Milgram NW: Further evidence for the cholinergic hypothesis of aging and dementia from the canine model of aging, *Prog Neuropsychopharmacol Biol Psychiatry* 29:411–422, 2005.

51. Skoumalova A, Rofina J, Schwippelova Z, and others: The role of free radicals in canine counterpart of senile dementia of the Alzheimer type, *Exp Gerontol* 38:711–719, 2003.

52. Head E, Liu J, Hagen TM: Oxidative damage increases with age in a canine model of human brain aging, *J Neurochem* 82:375–381, 2002.

53. Rofina JE, Singh K, Skoumalova-Vesela A, and others: Histochemical accumulation of oxidative damage products is associated with Alzheimer-like pathology in the canine, *Amyloid* 11:90–100, 2004.

55. Zanni E, Calloway DH, Zezulka AY: Protein requirements of elderly men, *J Nutr* 109:513–524, 1979.

56. Wannemacher RW, McCoy JR: Determination of optimal dietary protein requirements of young and old dogs, *J Nutr* 88:66–74, 1966.

57. Sheffy BE, William AJ: Nutrition and the aging animal, *Vet Clin North Am Small Anim Pract* 11:669–675, 1981.

58. Williams CC, Cummins KA, Hayek MG, Davenport GM: Effects of dietary protein on whole-body protein turnover and endocrine function in young-adult and aging dogs, *J Anim Sci* 79:3128–3136, 2001.

59. Assimon S, Stein T: ^{15}N-glycine as a tracer to study protein metabolism in vivo. In Nissen S, editor: *Modern methods in protein nutrition and metabolism,* San Diego, 1992, Academic Press.

60. Davenport G, Gaasch S, Hayek MG, Cummins KA: Effect of dietary protein on body composition and metabolic responses of geriatric and young-adult dogs, *J Vet Intern Med* 15:306, 2001.

61. Davenport GM, Hayek MG, Flakoll PJ, Firkins JL: Protein and the aging animal. In *Proc WSAVA,* 2001, pp 39–44.

62. Branam JE: Dietary management of geriatric dogs and cats, *Vet Tech* 8:501–503, 1987.

63. Bolton-Smith C, Tavendale R, Woodward M: Evidence for age-related differences in the fatty acid composition of human adipose tissue, independent of diet, *Eur J Clin Nutr* 51:619–624, 1997.

64. Lorenzini A, Hrelia S, Biagi PL, and others: Age-related changes in essential fatty acid metabolism in cultured rat heart myocytes, *Prostaglandins Leukot Essent Fatty Acids* 57:143–147, 1997.

65. Biagi PL, Bordoni A, Hrelia S, and others: Gamma-linolenic acid dietary supplementation can reverse the aging influence on rat liver microsome delta-6-desaturase activity, *Biochem Biophys Acta* 1083:187, 1991.

66. Reinhart GA, Vaughn DM, Hayek MG, and others: Effect of age on canine hepatic delta-6 and delta-5 desaturase activity (abstract), *J Anim Sci* 75(Suppl):227, 1997.

67. Massimino S, Kearns RJ, Loos KM, and others: Effects of age and dietary beta-carotene on immunological variables in dogs, *J Vet Intern Med* 17:835–842, 2003.

68. Hall JA, Picton RA, Finneran PS, and others: Dietary antioxidants and behavioral enrichment enhance neutrophil phagocytosis in geriatric Beagles, *Vet Immunol Immunopathol* 113:224–233, 2006.

69. Hayek MG, Massimino ST, Ceddia MA: Interaction of nutrition and the aging immune system of the dog and cat. In *Proc WSAVA,* 2001, pp 22–28.

70. Leshchinsky TV, Klasing KC: Relationship between the level of dietary vitamin E and the immune response of broiler chickens, *Poultry Sci* 80:1590–1599, 2001.

71. Friedman A, Bartov I, Sklan D: Humoral immune response impairment following excess vitamin E nutrition in the chick and turkey, *Poultry Sci* 77:956–962, 1998.

72. Landsberg G: Therapeutic agents for the treatment of cognitive dysfunction syndrome in senior dogs, *Prog Neuropsychopharmacol Biol Psychiatry* 29:471–479, 2005.

73. Osella MC, Re G, Odore R, and others: Phosphatidylserine (PS) as a potential nutraceutical for canine brain aging: a review, *J Vet Behav* 3:41–51, 2008.

74. Landsberg G: Therapeutic options for cognitive decline in senior pets, *J Am Anim Hosp Assoc* 42:407–413, 2006.

75. Head E, Zicker SC: Nutraceuticals, aging and cognitive dysfunction, *Vet Clin North Am Small Anim Pract* 34:217–228, 2004.

76. Roudebush P, Zicker SC, Cotman CW, and others: Nutritional management of bran aging in dogs, *J Am Vet Med Assoc* 227:722–728, 2005.

77. Milgram NW, Head E, Zicker SC: Landmark discrimination learning in the dog: effects of age, an antioxidant fortified food and cognitive strategy, *Neurosci Biobehav Rev* 26:679–695, 2002.

78. Milgram NW, Head E, Zicker SC: Long-term treatment with antioxidants and a program of behavioral enrichment reduces age-dependent impairment in discrimination and reversal learning in beagle dogs, *Exp Gerontol* 39:753–765, 2004.

79. Ikeda-Douglas CJ, Zicker SC, Estrada J, and others: Prior experience, antioxidants and mitochondrial co-factors improve cognitive dysfunction in aged Beagles, *Vet Ther* 5:5–16, 2004.

80. Dodd CE, Zicker SC, Jewell DE, and others: Can a fortified food affect the behavioral manifestations of age-related cognitive decline in dogs? *Vet Med* 98:396–408, 2003.

81. Heath SE, Barabas S, Craze PG: Nutritional supplementation in cases of canine cognitive dysfunction—a clinical trial, *Appl Anim Behav Sci* 105:284–296, 2007.

26

Common Nutrition Myths and Feeding Practices

Like any science, nutrition has a number of myths and folklore about the feeding of dogs and cats. Some of these myths and feeding practices have their origins in scientific fact, but the facts have been exaggerated, obscured, or misapplied. Others are feeding practices that owners enjoy for emotional reasons but which have potential health risks for their pets. Some of these beliefs have arisen from nutritional misinformation perpetuated by a lack of scientific proof or disproof and by the pervasive desire to find easy solutions to medical or behavioral problems through diet. Although some of these practices and beliefs cause no harm to pets, others have the potential to adversely affect health or contribute to a dietary imbalance. A number of common feeding practices and nutritional myths are discussed in this chapter, as is the scientific research that addresses these beliefs.

FEEDING "HUMAN FOODS" TO DOGS AND CATS

Some owners enjoy feeding their dogs and cats "people foods" for the same reasons that they feed treats and snacks. Providing a special treat is a way of showing affection and love, and adding table scraps and other choice food items to a pet's food allows owners to express their affection for their pet and to feel that they are enhancing their pet's enjoyment of the meal. Although most of these foods become harmful only if they make up a high proportion of the pet's diet, some human foods are unsuitable for companion animals and should not be fed at all (Box 26-1).

Table Scraps

The table scraps that most owners select to feed to their dogs (and less frequently to cats) are the uneaten portions of meals that are highly palatable to dogs, such as fat trimmings and leftover meat. Vegetables and grains are less frequently fed. Therefore, while the leftovers that end up in the pet's bowl may be very tasty (and much appreciated), they usually do not provide balanced nutrition for a dog or cat. If table scraps are fed to pets, the amount should be carefully monitored. A good rule of thumb is that table scraps should never make up more than 5% to 10% of a pet's total daily caloric intake.

> *If table scraps are fed to dogs or cats, the amount should be carefully monitored, and the total amount should never make up more than 5% to 10% of a pet's total daily caloric intake.*

Meat and Poultry

Some owners believe that because cats and dogs are carnivorous in nature, they should be able to survive on an all-meat diet. However, the muscle tissue of meat and poultry alone cannot supply complete nutrition to companion animals. Although meat and poultry provide high-quality protein, as a single food source they are deficient in calcium, phosphorus, sodium, iron, copper, iodine, and several essential vitamins. It is true that, in the wild, the ancestors of dogs and cats survived on freshly killed meat. However, the fact that they consumed their entire prey, including bones, organs, and intestinal contents, is often overlooked. Just as with table scraps, the addition of meat and poultry to the diet should be strictly limited because of their potential to imbalance a pet's diet (Table 26-1).

Fish

Most cats and some dogs love the taste of fish. Interestingly, the cat food advertising campaigns used by some pet food companies have convinced people that cats prefer the taste of fish over many other food items. In reality, cats enjoy fish to about the same degree that they enjoy many other animal-source proteins. Although fish

BOX 26-1   PRACTICAL FEEDING TIPS: ADDING "PEOPLE FOODS" TO A PET'S DIET

The addition of extra foods should be limited to no more than 5% to 10% of the pet's daily caloric requirement.

Any meat, fish, or poultry that is fed should be well cooked, and all bones should be removed.

The use of milk and cheese should be strictly monitored. Some adult dogs and cats are lactose intolerant and cannot efficiently digest dairy products.

The exclusive use of any single food item should be avoided, even when adding it to the pet's diet in small amounts.

Correction of the nutrient imbalances of a poor diet by adding table scraps should not be attempted.

Vitamin and/or mineral supplements are unnecessary for healthy pets when a complete and balanced pet food is fed, and they can be detrimental to health.

Pet owners should be aware of the development of undesirable behaviors, such as begging during mealtimes and stealing food.

The addition of all extra foods should be discontinued if weight gain, gastrointestinal tract upset, or signs of nutrient imbalance are seen.

TABLE 26-1   NUTRIENT COMPOSITION OF A PERFORMANCE DRY DOG FOOD WITH ADDED PROPORTIONS OF BEEF (DRY-MATTER BASIS)*

Nutrient	Dry dog food	75% Dog food/25% Beef[†]	50% Dog food/50% Beef	25% Dog food/75% Beef
Protein	34%	39%	46%	55%
Fat	23%	24%	25%	26%
Carbohydrate	35%	30%	23%	14%
Crude fiber	1.9%	1.6%	1.3%	0.75%
Calcium	1.3%	1.1%	**0.87%**	**0.53%**
Phosphorus	1.0%	0.89%	**0.73%**	**0.53%**
Calcium:phosphorus ratio	1.3:1	1.2:1	1.2:1	1:1
Potassium	0.87%	0.89%	0.92%	**0.96%**
Sodium	0.60%	0.53%	0.44%	0.31%
Magnesium	0.11%	0.09%	0.08%	**0.06%**
Iron	215 mg/kg	183 mg/kg	142 mg/kg	**85 mg/kg**
Vitamin A	21,700 IU/kg	18,500 IU/kg	14,400 IU/kg	8600 IU/kg
Vitamin D	1950 IU/kg	1670 IU/kg	1290 IU/kg	**770 IU/kg**
Vitamin E	153 IU/kg	130 IU/kg	100 IU/kg	**60 IU/kg**
Thiamin	19.5 mg/kg	16.7 mg/kg	13 mg/kg	7.7 mg/kg
Riboflavin	25 mg/kg	21 mg/kg	16.5 mg/kg	10 mg/kg
Niacin	64 mg/kg	55 mg/kg	42 mg/kg	25 mg/kg
Metabolizable energy	4700 kcal/kg	4800 kcal/kg	5000 kcal/kg	5200 kcal/kg
Caloric distribution				
Protein	27%	31%	35%	41%
Fat	45%	45%	47%	48%
Carbohydrate	28%	24%	18%	10%

*Imbalanced nutrients are expressed in bold print. Nutrient levels were compared to the Association of American Feed Control Officials' *Nutrient Profiles* and corrected for differences in energy density.
[†]Beef = fresh ground round.

is a good source of protein for dogs and cats, similar to meat and poultry, it does not supply complete nutrition. In general, most types of deboned fish are deficient in calcium, sodium, iron, copper, and several vitamins. Some types of fish also contain small bones that are difficult to remove before cooking. Care should be taken if feeding fish because these bones may lodge in a pet's throat or gastrointestinal tract and cause perforation or obstruction.

FISH (TUNA) AND PANSTEATITIS   Tuna is commonly fed to cats because it is readily available and inexpensive, and because most cats love the taste. Although less available than tuna packed in water, canned tuna packed in oil is preferred by many cats, because of the enhanced flavor and texture provided by the oil. However, tuna (and several other types of fish, such as sardines) that is packed in oil also contains high levels of polyunsaturated fatty acids (PUFAs). If tuna is fed regularly, the excessive intake of PUFAs can result in a vitamin E deficiency. This risk occurs because an animal's vitamin E requirement is directly affected by the level of unsaturated fatty acids present in the diet. As the level of PUFAs increases, an animal's vitamin E requirement also increases. When cats are fed high amounts of PUFAs with no concomitant increase in vitamin E, their body fat is not sufficiently protected from oxidative degradation, resulting in oxidative stress and the formation of peroxides and hydroperoxides.[1] Over time, the accumulation of reactive peroxides in adipose tissue leads to a pathological condition called *pansteatitis,* which is characterized by chronic inflammation and yellow-brown discoloration of body fat.

Clinical signs of pansteatitis in cats include anorexia, depression, pyrexia, and hyperesthesia of the thorax and abdomen. The cat may demonstrate changes in behavior and agility and develop a poor or roughened hair coat.[2,3] Owners typically report that their cat has become intolerant of being picked up or held. Palpation of subcutaneous and intraabdominal fat deposits is painful to the cat and reveals the presence of granular or nodular fat deposits. Information concerning the cat's dietary history is needed for diagnosis, and confirmation is provided by histological examination of a fat biopsy sample. The fat of cats with pansteatitis is very firm and deep yellow to orange, with a diffuse inflammatory response.[3,4] The orange pigment (commonly referred to as *ceroid*) is believed to be

---

BOX 26-2   SIGNS OF PANSTEATITIS IN CATS

Depression and anorexia

Hyperesthesia (sensitivity to touch) of the chest and abdomen

Reluctance to move and decreased agility

Presence of abnormal fat deposits under the skin and in the abdomen

Dietary history that includes items that are high in unsaturated fats and low in vitamin E

---

an intermediate polymerization product of unsaturated fatty acids that have undergone peroxidation as a result of insufficient intracellular vitamin E (Box 26-2).

Some of the earliest published cases of pansteatitis occurred in cats that were fed canned, fish-based commercial cat foods comprised wholly or predominantly of red tuna and that were deficient in vitamin E.[4-6] Pansteatitis has also been described in cats that were fed unconventional or homemade diets consisting largely of tuna, sardines, or other oily fish.[7-9] Although reported infrequently, there is evidence that cats fed all-meat diets may be at increased risk of developing pansteatitis.[9]

Treatment of pansteatitis involves changing the cat's diet from one that is comprised primarily of fish and replacing it with a well-balanced cat food. Dietary changes may be difficult in cats that have become accustomed to eating only a single food item. This problem has been most commonly reported in cats receiving only red tuna as the principal component of their diet for an extended period of time. Along with correction of the diet, vitamin E (alpha-tocopherol) should be administered orally at a dose of 10 to 25 international units (IU) twice daily for several weeks, until all clinical signs have resolved and the cat is reliably consuming a balanced food.[9] Corticosteroid therapy may be used in severe cases to decrease inflammation and reduce pain. Prognosis for recovery from pansteatitis is usually very good, but may take several months in advanced cases.

RAW FISH AND THIAMINASE   Certain types of fish, such as carp and herring, contain a compound that destroys thiamin and may cause a thiamin deficiency.[10,11] Consumption of these types of fish has been shown to cause thiamin deficiency in a variety of species. For example, experimental studies with cats have produced signs of thiamin deficiency within 23 to 40 days of consuming diets composed solely of raw carp or raw salt-water herring.[10] The subcutaneous administration of thiamin resulted in recovery in all cases. Although both carp and herring can cause thiamin deficiency, perch, catfish, and butterfish do not show thiaminase activity. Other common types of fish that contain thiaminase include whitefish, pike, cod, goldfish, mullet, shark, and flounder. However, it is not known whether the thiaminase levels present in these fish are sufficient to produce deficiency in animals.[11] Thiaminase is a heat-labile enzyme and is denatured by normal cooking temperatures. As a result, the potential for thiamin deficiency exists only when uncooked fish is fed to pets.

Although naturally occurring thiamin deficiency is uncommon in dogs and cats, clinical cases have been reported. Cats appear to be more susceptible because of their high dietary requirement for thiamin and because of the tendency of owners to feed cats diets containing fish products.[12] Most clinical cases have involved cats fed diets that contained a large proportion of raw fish.[10,13] Similarly, a group of sled dogs that was fed a diet consisting of frozen, uncooked carp developed clinical signs of thiamin deficiency during a 6-month period.[14] The addition of oatmeal, a dry dog food, and 100 milligrams (mg) of thiamin per day to the diets of the affected dogs resulted in complete recovery within 2 months.

Because thiamin is essential for normal carbohydrate metabolism, the central nervous system is severely affected by a deficiency of this vitamin. Initial clinical signs of deficiency include anorexia, weight loss, and depression.[13,15] As the deficiency progresses, neurological signs of ataxia, paresis, and, eventually, convulsive seizures develop. The terminal stage is characterized by severe weakness and prostration and eventually leads to death. A diagnosis of thiamin deficiency in dogs and cats is made based on clinical signs and the dietary history of the animal. Elevated plasma pyruvate and lactate concentrations are also useful in confirming a diagnosis.

Treatment includes dietary correction that includes elimination of raw fish from the diet and its replacement with a well-balanced pet food and thiamin therapy. Thiamin should be administered intravenously or subcutaneously at a dose of 75 to 100 mg twice daily until neurological signs subside.[12] Oral thiamin supplementation should also be administered for several months following the initial clinical episode.[14] In most affected pets, these clinical signs will decrease within several days. However, if severe neurological damage has occurred, the pet may never make a full recovery. A permanent intolerance of physical exercise and some degree of persistent ataxia occasionally occurs in animals that have recovered from thiamin deficiency.

Because of the risk of inducing thiamin deficiency, raw fish should never be fed to dogs and cats. There is also the potential for parasite transmission when raw fish is fed. Therefore, if any type of fish is added to a pet's diet, it should always be well cooked, and only very small amounts should be fed.

Liver

Liver is an excellent source of iron, protein, copper, vitamin D, and several B vitamins. However, like other single food items, it is not a nutritionally complete food. Liver is severely deficient in calcium and excessively high in vitamin A (see below). Both of these nutritional imbalances can cause bone disorders. Vitamin A toxicosis has been shown to develop slowly over a period of years in cats that were regularly fed fresh liver as their primary dietary protein source (see below).[16,17] Although small amounts of liver added to a cat's diet are not harmful, liver as a primary component of the diet should be avoided.

VITAMIN A TOXICOSIS IN CATS: DEFORMING CERVICAL SPONDYLOSIS Cats that are fed diets composed exclusively of liver or other organ meats are at risk of developing vitamin A toxicosis. This practice is usually the result of well-meaning but poorly informed owners who believe that cats, being carnivores, will thrive on an all-meat or all-liver diet. The bone deformities of vitamin A toxicity develop very gradually and may go undetected for several years. However, over time severe and irreversible crippling occurs, and diagnosis is often too late to be of any help.[18,19]

The pathological result of vitamin A excess in cats is the development of a syndrome called *deforming cervical spondylosis*. The effects of excess vitamin A on bone growth and remodeling lead to the development of bony exostoses (outgrowths) along the muscular insertions of cervical vertebrae and the long bones of the forelimbs. Over time, these bony processes cause pain and impaired mobility.[20] Vitamin A–induced skeletal disease is not a practical problem in dogs, but it has been produced experimentally. Although uncommon in dogs, studies have shown that extremely high intakes of vitamin A during growth will result in decreased length and thickness of long bones, premature closure of epiphyseal growth plates, and the development of osteophytes.[21] However, dogs appear to be relatively resistant to vitamin A toxicosis because subsequent studies found that feeding up to 400,000 IU/kilogram (kg) of dry matter (DM) to puppies or 787,000 IU/kg of DM to adult dogs for periods of 6 months or 1 year caused no signs of toxicity and did not adversely affect bone density measurements.[22,23]

Initial clinical signs of deforming cervical spondylosis in cats include anorexia, weight loss, lethargy, and an increasing reluctance to move. Cats become unkempt in appearance, presumably because of an inability to self-groom. As the disease progresses, a very characteristic postural change is observed; cats adopt a marsupial-like sitting position, holding the front legs elevated off the ground. They also often walk with their hind limbs flexed, and ventriflexion of the head is decreased or altogether absent. A fixed-stare expression is often observed, probably as a result of reduced ability to move the neck and turn the head. Lameness in one or both of the front limbs is seen in the later stages.[24] Development of exostoses occurs primarily in the first three joints of the cervical vertebrae and joints of the forelegs. It has been theorized that the normal movements involved in a cat's regular licking and grooming practices result in these predilection sites. It appears that chronic intoxication with vitamin A increases the sensitivity of the periosteum to the effects of low levels of trauma and repetitive movements that would normally be insufficient to cause an inflammatory response (Box 26-3).[25]

Experimental studies show that the level of vitamin A required to produce skeletal lesions within only a few months' time in growing kittens is between 17 and 35 micrograms (µg)/gram (g) of body weight.[25] A 1-kg (2.2-pound [lb]) kitten would have to consume a minimum of 17,000 µg (~56,000 IU) of vitamin A per day to attain this level. According to the National Research

BOX 26-3 SIGNS OF DEFORMING CERVICAL SPONDYLOSIS IN CATS

Anorexia and weight loss

Increased lethargy and reluctance to move

Persistent lameness in one or both front legs

Decreased ability to self-groom

Decreased ventriflexion of the head

Posture changes by adopting a marsupial-like sitting position

Dietary history that includes items that contain a high concentration of vitamin A

Council's (NRC's) current *Nutrient Requirements,* a 1-kg kitten requires approximately 50 µg of vitamin A per day (1000 µg/kg of dry diet).[26] The safe upper limit for a kitten of this size is approximately 4000 µg per day. Using the previous study's data, the dose of vitamin A necessary to produce acute toxicity is therefore more than 300 times the recommended allowance. An adult cat weighing 5 kg (11 lb) would have to consume at least 85,000 µg of vitamin A daily to reach this toxic level. The daily vitamin A requirement for an active 5-kg adult cat is approximately 80 µg/day. Therefore an adult cat would have to consume 1000 times its daily requirement of vitamin A to achieve toxic levels. It is indisputable that a cat will never consume this level when being fed a nutritionally balanced pet food.

However, it would also be difficult for a cat to consume this high a level of vitamin A while being fed an all-liver diet. Beef liver contains approximately 160 µg (530 IU)/g.[27] An adult cat consuming 6 ounces (oz) of liver per day would be ingesting only 27,200 µg of vitamin A per day, quite a bit less than the levels described previously needed to create acute toxicity. However, all of the case studies reported in the literature found that deforming cervical spondylosis developed in cats that were fed liver diets. There are two possible explanations for this discrepancy. First, it is known that the livers of production animals vary greatly in vitamin A content.[27] The level of 160 µg of vitamin A per gram of beef liver is an average, not an absolute value. Second, and more importantly, all of the reported case studies occurred in adult cats that had been fed liver diets for a very long time.[28,29] The experimental work that has been conducted involved much higher levels of vitamin A and produced signs of toxicity in very short periods of time (i.e., months, rather than years). At lower doses of vitamin A, cervical spondylosis appears to develop slowly over the lifetime of the cat, and clinical signs of the disease do not become evident until much later in adult life. This conclusion is supported by the fact that the average age for the diagnosis of cervical spondylosis in pet cats is 4.25 years.[20] Therefore the reported level of vitamin A required to produce toxicity in the cat (17 to 35 µg/g of body weight) may reflect the experimental production of acute toxicity, but the level that can produce deforming cervical spondylosis, if excess vitamin A is consumed by pet cats for a long time, is probably significantly lower.

Regular supplementation of a cat's diet with liver, even if added to a balanced diet, has the potential to cause skeletal problems if the practice is continued for several years. When liver is fed exclusively, vitamin A toxicosis may occur concurrently with nutritional secondary hyperparathyroidism because of the low-calcium, high-phosphorus content of organ meats.[28] Cod liver oil fed as a supplement also has the potential to induce vitamin A toxicity. Adding 1 tablespoon (tbsp) of cod liver oil to a cat's food twice daily will result in an intake of approximately 10,000 µg of additional vitamin A per day. Fish liver oils are also excessively high in vitamin D, and excessive supplementation may result in the combined effects of vitamin A and vitamin D toxicosis.

The treatment of vitamin A toxicosis in cats includes removing the source of excessive vitamin A from the diet, replacing the source with a complete and balanced pet food, and providing supportive therapy. The prognosis is guarded because resolution of skeletal lesions may never be complete. In addition, if the cat has been fed a liver diet for a long time, the change to a balanced pet food may be difficult, if the cat has developed a fixed food preference.

Milk and Dairy Products

Almost all cats and dogs love the taste of milk. Although milk and dairy products are excellent sources of calcium, protein, phosphorus, and several vitamins, excessive intake may cause diarrhea in young and adult pets. Milk contains the simple sugar lactose. Lactose requires breakdown in the intestinal tract by the enzyme lactase.

Intestinal lactase activity declines as puppies and kittens reach adulthood. As a result, many adult cats and dogs do not produce sufficient amounts of lactase to handle the large quantity of lactose present in milk. Lack of sufficient lactase results in an inability to completely digest milk and subsequently causes digestive upsets and diarrhea. Dairy products such as cheese, buttermilk, and yogurt contain slightly lower levels of lactose. Even though these products may be better tolerated by some dogs and cats, they still have the potential for causing diarrhea and dietary imbalances if large quantities are fed. Most pets can tolerate and enjoy an occasional bowl of milk, but like all supplementation, the practice of feeding milk should be carefully limited.

Dairy products should not be used as a supplemental source of calcium or protein. Excess dietary calcium can contribute to the development of skeletal disorders in growing dogs and is not helpful in preventing eclampsia in lactating females (see Section 4, pp. 205-206 and Section 5, pp. 497-500). Although dairy products supply high-quality protein, they contain deficiencies and excesses of other nutrients and may contribute to a dietary imbalance if large amounts are added to an otherwise adequate diet.

Oils and Fats

Cod liver oil, vegetable oils, and animal fats are occasionally added to a pet's food to improve taste or to supply fat and additional vitamins. It is true that fish oils are excellent sources of vitamin A, vitamin D, and the omega-3 (n-3) fatty acids. However, both of these vitamins are toxic when consumed in excess. Because vitamins A and D are stored in the liver, the effects of excess intake are cumulative and develop over long periods. The daily addition of 1 or 2 tbsp of cod liver oil (or another vitamin A supplement) to a small pet's diet has the potential of eventually developing into a toxicity problem. In addition, oversupplementation with fat may result in either obesity or an eventual decrease in the quantity of food that is consumed. Food intake may decrease because energy needs will be met with a lower quantity of food. Deficiencies of other nutrients may then develop. Excessive intake of dietary fat may also cause digestive problems in some pets.

Some owners add fat to their pets' diets with the intention of improving coat quality. Dogs have a requirement for the essential fatty acid linoleic acid and possibly for alpha-linolenic acid, and cats require these fatty acids plus dietary arachidonic acid (see Section 2, pp. 81-86). Animals that are deficient in essential fatty acids will develop poor coat quality and skin problems. Poor quality or improperly stored pet foods may contain inadequate levels of these fatty acids. However, if a high-quality food is being fed, adding fat or oil should not be necessary. In most cases, diet is not the principal cause of skin problems or poor coat quality in companion animals. More probable causes of skin disorders include internal and external parasitic infections, allergies, and various hormonal imbalances. If a coat or skin problem persists in a dog or cat, even when a high-quality food is fed, a veterinarian should be consulted.

Eggs

Many dog owners are in the habit of regularly supplementing their dog's diet with eggs. The reasons for this practice are varied. Some owners believe that feeding eggs improves hair quality and adds luster and shine to their dog's coat. Others wish to increase or improve the protein in their dog's diet by adding egg protein. Eggs can also increase a food's palatability and acceptability for some dogs and cats.

It is true that egg protein has one of the highest biological values of common protein sources. Cooked egg protein is highly digestible and provides all of the necessary essential amino acids required by dogs for adequate growth and maintenance. Eggs are also a good source of iron, vitamin A, vitamin D, and several B vitamins. Eggs are also a source of essential fatty acids; approximately 4% of the fat in egg yolk is in the form of linoleic acid.

Although egg is a high-quality food ingredient, the white of the egg (albumen) contains several inhibitory substances that alter the metabolism of specific nutrients. The two most important are avidin, an inhibitor of biotin absorption, and a compound that interferes with the action of the pancreatic protease, trypsin (trypsin inhibitor). The antitryptic activity of egg white is a characteristic that is much less well documented in current literature than avidin, yet one that has the potential for causing severe nutritional imbalances.

AVIDIN AND BIOTIN   A syndrome termed "egg white injury" was first described in the 1920s. Animals fed raw egg whites as a component of their food developed a scaly skin rash, elevated blood cholesterol levels, and defects in nerve transmission. Eventually, the underlying cause was identified as a deficiency of biotin, brought about by an inhibitory substance in egg white that decreased availability of biotin. This factor was named "avid-albumin" or avidin. Avidin is a protein that is a secretory product of the hen's oviduct and is subsequently deposited in the albuminous portion of the egg. When consumed, avidin combines with dietary biotin in the intestine and prevents its absorption. The avidin in egg white is so effective in this capacity that raw egg white has been used to experimentally induce biotin deficiency in laboratory animals. Regardless, the danger of a pet owner inducing a biotin deficiency in a dog or cat by feeding supplemental eggs is slight because the yolk of the egg contains large quantities of biotin. In addition, cooking eggs denatures avidin and destroys its biotin binding ability. Practically speaking, potential risk for biotin deficiency will only occur if an owner supplements the pet's food with only the white of the raw egg. As in other species, signs of biotin deficiency in dogs and cats include dermatitis, loss of hair and poor growth rate.

EGG WHITE TRYPSIN INHIBITOR   The white of the egg also contains another potentially damaging inhibitory substance. This substance is actually a group of proteins that have antitryptic activity. The antitryptic effect of feeding raw egg white has received less attention than avidin, yet its capacity for causing nutritional problems in pets is potentially much greater. Early studies reported that dogs fed as little as two raw egg whites per day in their food exhibited loose stools, and when the amount was increased further, chronic diarrhea and weight loss developed.[30] Dried (uncooked) egg white was found to be just as active in causing diarrhea and weight loss as was fresh, raw egg white. The utilization of raw egg white protein (as determined by apparent digestibility) was reported to be only 58.6%. Subsequent feeding studies and in vitro tests of protein digestibility confirmed that the factor responsible for these effects was a group of trypsin inhibitor proteins found in the white of the egg.[31] Egg white trypsin inhibitor reduced a food's protein digestibility when included at just 7% of the diet, and a linear relationship was reported between the amount of egg white trypsin inhibitor and loss of protein digestibility.[32]

Similar to avidin, heat treatment denatures the trypsin inhibitor of egg white and allows utilization of the protein in the egg white and of other protein sources in the food. For example, the most recent study with dogs confirmed that the inclusion of raw (dried) egg in the diets of growing puppies impaired diet digestibility and caused chronic diarrhea and weight loss in all of the puppies during a 14-day feeding period.[33] However, when the same amount of heat-treated dried egg white was included in the food, stools were normal, the puppies showed healthy growth rates, and diet digestibility coefficients were improved. Laboratory analysis of each diet showed that trypsin inhibitor activity was significantly reduced in the heat-treated egg white, when compared with raw egg white.

Again, the practical relevance of this knowledge to the feeding of companion animals is that if an owner insists on adding egg products to a pet's food, the eggs should always be cooked thoroughly before feeding. This is necessary to denature both avidin and the trypsin inhibitors present in the egg white. In addition, feeding raw eggs is not recommended due to the risk of bacterial contamination. A general guideline is to limit eggs to just one or two cooked eggs per week for a medium or large dog. This level should not result in a dietary imbalance and will not affect energy consumption to the degree of causing weight problems.

If owners wish to add an occasional egg to their pet's food, eggs should always be cooked thoroughly to denature avidin and the trypsin inhibitors present in the egg white. Feeding raw eggs is also not advisable because of the risk of bacterial contamination. A general guideline is to limit eggs to just one or two cooked eggs per week for a medium or large dog.

Chocolate

Most dogs enjoy sweet flavors, including the taste of chocolate. Cats, on the other hand, are much less likely to find sweet foods palatable (see Section 1, pp. 46-48).[34] Chocolate contains a methylxanthine called *theobromine,* which is toxic to dogs when consumed in large quantities. Three methylxanthine compounds are commonly found in foods: caffeine, theophylline, and theobromine. Caffeine is most abundant in coffee, tea, and cola beverages, and theophylline is found primarily in tea. Theobromine is the most abundant methylxanthine that is contained in the cacao bean, which is the source of cocoa and chocolate products. The main sites of action of xanthine compounds in the body are the central nervous system, cardiovascular system, kidneys, smooth muscle, and skeletal musculature. Theobromine in particular acts as a smooth muscle relaxant, coronary artery dilatator, diuretic, and cardiac stimulant.

Although it is not a common clinical problem, theobromine toxicity in dogs can be life-threatening when it occurs. The dog is unusually sensitive to the physiological effects of theobromine, when compared with other species. This sensitivity appears to be the result of a lower rate of theobromine metabolism, resulting in a longer half-life in the bloodstream and tissues. After a single dose, the half-life of theobromine in the plasma of adult dogs is approximately 17.5 hours.[35] In comparison, theobromine's half-life in human subjects is 6 hours; in rats it is only 3 hours.[36,37] It has been theorized that the extended half-life in dogs may potentiate acute toxicity reactions to theobromine after the consumption of foods containing chocolate.[35]

Dogs having theobromine toxicity experience vomiting, diarrhea, panting, restlessness, increased urination or urinary incontinence, and muscle tremors. These signs usually occur about 4 to 5 hours after the dog has consumed the food containing chocolate. The onset of generalized motor seizures signifies a poor prognosis in most cases and often results in death.[38-40] Theobromine toxicity is treated by inducing vomiting as soon as possible. An activated charcoal "shake" given by gastric lavage may aid in decreasing the quantity of the drug that is absorbed into the bloodstream. Unfortunately, there is no specific systemic antidote for theobromine poisoning.

Although few controlled studies on the level of theobromine that constitutes a toxic dose have been conducted in dogs, data from long-term studies and case reports indicate that toxicity can occur when a dog consumes a dose of 90 to 100 mg/kg of body weight or more.[40] Factors such as individual sensitivity to theobromine, mode of theobromine administration, presence of other foods in the gastrointestinal tract at the time of ingestion, and variations in theobromine content between chocolate products cause wide variations in the susceptibility of individual dogs to chocolate poisoning. Chocolate products differ significantly in theobromine content and, therefore, in their ability to produce theobromine poisoning.

Chocolate liquor, commonly called *baking* or *cooking chocolate,* is the base substance from which all other chocolate products are produced. The average theobromine content of baking chocolate is about 1.22%.[41] A 1-oz square contains approximately 346 mg of theobromine. Therefore, if a medium-sized dog weighing 25 lb (11 kg) consumed 3 oz of baking chocolate, a potentially fatal dose of 94 mg of theobromine/kg would be ingested. Commercial cocoa powder (unsweetened) has an average theobromine content of 1.89%, which is the highest theobromine content of all commonly consumed chocolate products. However, dogs are less likely to consume baking chocolate or cocoa powder than other sweeter chocolate products. The addition of sugar, cocoa butter, and milk solids to baking chocolate, to produce sweet chocolates, results in a significant dilution of theobromine content. For example, the level of theobromine in semisweet chocolate pieces is 0.463%. A 25-lb dog would have to consume approximately ½ lb of semisweet chocolate to reach a potentially toxic level of 95 mg/kg. Similarly, milk chocolate contains 0.153% theobromine. The ingestion of approximately 1½ lb of milk chocolate would result in a potentially lethal dose for a 25-lb dog.

Dogs generally love the taste of chocolate, and owners occasionally give chocolate candy or foods containing chocolate to their dogs as a special treat. If a dog's intake of chocolate is strictly limited to occasional small treats, there is no danger of theobromine toxicity. All of the published case studies of theobromine toxicity in dogs have been the result of a pet accidentally ingesting a large amount of chocolate.[38-40] Still, if given the opportunity, many dogs readily overconsume chocolate-containing foods. Therefore all chocolate products should be stored in areas inaccessible to pets and large amounts of chocolate should never be fed to dogs.

Most dogs enjoy sweet flavors, including the taste of chocolate. However, chocolate contains theobromine, which is toxic to dogs when consumed in large quantities. If a dog's intake of chocolate is strictly limited to occasional small treats, there is no danger of theobromine toxicity. However, because many dogs will overconsume sweet foods if given the opportunity, all chocolate products should be stored in areas inaccessible to pets, and large amounts of chocolate should never be fed to dogs.

FEEDING BREWER'S YEAST OR THIAMIN REPELS FLEAS

The use of either brewer's yeast or the B-vitamin thiamin (one of the yeast's components) as a repellent for external parasites has a long history as a nutritional myth. This practice can be traced back to several studies with human subjects that were conducted during the 1940s. In one study, when subjects were given oral doses of 100 to 200 mg of thiamin per day, it was reported that they experienced lower numbers of mosquito bites and decreased severity of dermatological reactions.[42] Another early study reported that benefits were observed when infants and children with severe flea infestations were treated with 10 mg of thiamin per day.[43] However, neither of these studies were well controlled, and several subsequent studies with humans have failed to show any significant effect of thiamin supplementation on insect infestations.[44]

Companion animal owners and professionals, anxious to find safe and convenient means for controlling flea and mite infestations, quickly adopted this practice for use in dogs and cats. However, there is no evidence to indicate that feeding thiamin or brewer's yeast has a repellent effect on fleas or mites in these species. Two controlled studies have reported that neither brewer's yeast nor thiamin repelled fleas or mosquitoes in dogs. In the first study, dogs that were fed 14 g per day of active or inactive brewer's yeast had the same weekly flea counts as did a group of dogs that were not supplemented.[44] In the second study, neither flea counts nor the number of flea bites on dogs were affected by supplementation with 100 mg of thiamin per day.[45] Although supplementing pet's diets with brewer's yeast is probably not harmful, it is not effective in either repelling or controlling flea populations in homes or on the skin of companion animals.

FEEDING GARLIC OR ONIONS REPELS FLEAS

Feeding either of these two food items will certainly make a pet's breath smell, but it will not have any effect on fleas. Moreover, feeding large amounts of onion or garlic to dogs or cats can be toxic. Excess consumption of onions results in the formation of Heinz bodies on circulating red blood cells, which ultimately results in the development of hemolytic anemia. In severe cases, this anemia can be fatal.[46-48] The toxic compound in onions that is responsible for this effect is N-propyl disulfide. Signs of hemolytic anemia produced by onion toxicity include diarrhea, vomiting, depression, fever, and dark-colored urine. Although vomiting and diarrhea may be immediate, the remaining signs usually appear 1 to 4 days following the ingestion of the onion. Similarly, the ingestion of excessive amounts of garlic (*Allium sativum*) can cause oxidative damage to red blood cells, leading to both Heinz body formation and a condition called *eccentrocytosis*.[49,50] Eccentrocytes are red blood cells that contain abnormal hemoglobin and have been observed in cases of garlic and onion toxicity in dogs. When severe, eccentrocytosis can result in anemia. If onion or garlic toxicity is suspected, veterinary care should be sought immediately. Many dogs love the taste of onions and garlic and may overconsume if given the opportunity. Therefore onion- and garlic-containing foods should be fed only in small amounts to dogs and cats, and they certainly should not be expected to have an effect on flea infestations.

> *Contrary to popular belief, there is no evidence that feeding dogs and cats brewer's yeast, garlic, or onions effectively repels fleas or mites.*

DIET CAUSES ACUTE MOIST DERMATITIS ("HOT SPOTS")

Acute moist dermatitis is a condition that is commonly referred to as "hot spots" because it frequently occurs during warm months of the year and because the lesions that develop are inflamed and feel hot to the touch. This

skin disorder is most commonly seen in breeds of dogs that have very dense, heavy coats, and it may be related to poor ventilation of the skin or inadequate grooming to remove matted hair and debris. Hot-spot lesions can develop within just a few hours. The lesions are usually first noticed as a patch of missing hair. A round, red, moist area that is painful to touch rapidly develops. The area often has a yellowish center surrounded by a reddened ring of inflammation. Self-trauma occurs in the form of biting and scratching at the affected area because the lesions are usually intensely pruritic. If not treated, the spots may spread to other areas of the body.

Any factor that causes irritation, pruritus, or self-trauma can lead to acute moist dermatitis. Allergic reactions, external parasites, skin infections, an unhealed injury, or improper grooming can all initiate self-trauma and the development of a hot spot. It is believed by some pet owners that a diet that is too "rich" or too high in protein is the cause of hot spots. However, there is no evidence that a relationship exists between acute moist dermatitis and protein levels in the diet. Diet may play a role if the pet has an adverse reaction to food or an essential fatty acid deficiency. Adverse reactions to food may indirectly cause a hot spot to develop because allergies typically cause intense pruritus, which in turn may lead to self-trauma (see Section 5, pp. 396-402). Fatty acid deficiencies can occur when improperly formulated or improperly stored pet foods are fed and are characterized by a number of dermatological signs (see Section 2, pp. 85-86). However, both of these conditions occur infrequently and are not a primary underlying cause of hot spots.

THE OCCURRENCE OF "RED COAT" IN DOGS

The term "red coat" refers to a perceived change in coat color from almost any normal base color to a red or reddish brown. This change has been most frequently reported by individuals who exhibit and/or breed dogs. Among other factors, diet has been identified as a potential underlying cause of "red coat." The pet food ingredient beet pulp has been identified specifically, presumably because of the perception that this ingredient is red. However, the beet pulp that is included in pet foods is derived from sugar beets (not red beets) and is actually light brown. Moreover, there is no evidence suggesting a connection between the consumption of beet pulp and a change in coat color in dogs. Conversely, in addition to a number of environmental causes, there are several nutritional deficiencies that can affect coat texture and color in dogs and cats.

An understanding of normal coat color development is necessary to completely understand the potential causes of a change in coat color. In dogs and cats, an individual hair takes between 6 and 8 weeks to grow; this phase is called the *anagen phase of hair growth.* Once mature, the hair enters a resting period (telogen phase) and remains dormant for weeks or months before being shed to make room for a new hair. The color of a hair is determined by the type and amount of pigment that is deposited during the anagen phase while the hair is still in the hair follicle. Melanocytes, specialized pigment-producing cells within the follicle, secrete either yellow-red pheomelanin or black-brown eumelanin that is then deposited within the hair. Genetic factors affect the amount of each type of pigment that is produced, the distribution of pigment within the hair shaft, dilution or masking of color, and distribution of color in different areas of the body. These factors result in the wide variety of hair colors and coat patterns that are seen in different breeds of dogs. In addition to genetics, other factors that may affect the color of the hair during its growth or resting cycle include medications, topical substances, aging, environment, and diet.

A change in the color of a hair may be produced in one of two possible ways. A systemic factor can cause a change in the color of hairs as they develop in the hair follicle (e.g., a change in the pigment-producing cells). Because it occurs during pigment deposition, this type of color change extends from the skin surface outward toward the hair tip, and the portion of the hair that is affected depends on the length of time that the influencing factor was in effect. For example, if the change was only in effect for 2 weeks, the color change will appear as a horizontal band of color on the length of individual hair shafts. Because individual hairs within the entire coat are at different stages of development, the color change in the hair coat would be dispersed throughout the coat at different levels on each hair shaft. By definition, this type of change in coat color takes weeks to months to appear or disappear. Also,

because hair growth occurs randomly throughout the coat, it would be expected that any change in color would not be uniform, but would occur in only the hairs that were growing at the time that the influencing factor was present. Resting hairs would not be affected by any factor that affected a change in coat color in the growing hairs.

The second way that a change in coat color can occur is through the deposition of a substance on the outside of the hair shaft. This change could involve substances that are applied by the dog's owner, secreted by the dog's skin, or licked onto the hair by the dog. Environmental influences of this type include changes caused by sunlight exposure (ultraviolet [UV] irradiation), or by ambient temperature and humidity. This type of coat color change involves most or all of the hair shaft, and all of the hairs within a region of the body are typically affected. Therefore the appearance of this type of coat-color change is significantly different from the appearance of a coat color change that is seen when a systemic factor is the underlying cause.

There are several known factors that can affect hair coat color in dogs and that could be responsible for imbuing a red hue to the coat. Aging of hair naturally causes a change in color. As a hair approaches the end of its resting period and is ready to be shed, black hairs typically turn reddish to reddish brown. This change occurs primarily near the tip of the hair, with the base of the hair remaining black. However, in some cases, especially when hairs are retained for a long period without shedding, the entire hair may turn red. When the dog sheds his or her coat, these hairs are removed, and a return to normal color is seen. In addition to the age of the hair, exposure to sunlight can also cause black hairs to turn red. When this occurs, the change in color usually affects variable portions of the ends of the hairs. The color of the hair at the base (near the dog's skin) remains black. Topically applied dips or shampoos that contain insecticides can also turn hair a red hue. This effect can be seen with any natural coat color, but it will be most noticeable in white or light-colored dogs. When an applied agent is the cause, the change in color is uniform throughout the hair shaft. Similarly, frequent shampooing, use of certain types of rinses, and blow drying can all alter hair coat color.

A commonly observed cause of regional coat-color change in dogs is porphyrin staining. Porphyrin is a substance found in the tears and saliva of dogs that turns red upon exposure to sunlight. Porphyrin is a normal end product of hemoglobin metabolism and is the substance responsible for the reddish staining that is seen around the eyes of some breeds of dogs. Dogs that self-groom or lick excessively will also deposit porphyrins on their coat, causing these areas to stain red. Therefore licking that is associated with allergic reactions or other dermatological problems may cause reddening of the coat. In these cases, the entire length of the hair in certain regions of the body will be affected (see p. 287). However, there are no health risks associated with this phenomenon and it does not indicate a dietary deficiency or imbalance.

The frank deficiency of certain essential nutrients can adversely affect coat quality and color. A lack of copper in the diet and development of copper deficiency can lead to hypopigmentation of the coat that may manifest as a reddening or graying of the hairs. However, other clinical signs accompany copper deficiency, including anemia, skin lesions, and impaired growth in young animals. The anemia of copper deficiency eventually causes clinical illness in affected dogs, and in addition to color changes, the dog's coat will also become rough and coarse. Similarly, zinc deficiency causes changes to hair texture and color.[51] Dogs fed zinc-deficient foods develop a dry, harsh hair coat that fades in color. When a diet containing adequate zinc is provided, these clinical signs resolve. Although not common, naturally occurring zinc deficiency has been reported in dogs fed poorly formulated, inexpensive, dry dog foods.[52] However, attention by reputable manufacturers to both the concentration and the bioavailability of these minerals in pet foods minimizes the risk of deficiencies of copper or zinc as causes of coat color change in dogs.

Recent studies with growing kittens have shown that insufficient dietary levels of the aromatic amino acids phenylalanine and tyrosine cause a reduction in the total amount of melanin pigments deposited in hair; this manifests as black hairs changing to reddish-brown.[53,54] When kittens were fed foods containing less than 16 g total aromatic amino acids per kg of diet, they also developed several sensory neurological abnormalities.[55] Tyrosine is the precursor for both eumelanin and pheolmelanin, and plasma levels of tyrosine are positively correlated with the amount of pigment found in

hairs. Because the essential amino acid phenylalanine is the precursor for tyrosine, available tyrosine is expressed as the sum of these two amino acids. The authors of these studies concluded that a total aromatic amino acid content of 18 g/kg diet or more is needed by cats to prevent discoloration of black coats to reddish brown and possibly to prevent the development of deficiency-related neurological signs.

Because most of the red-coat problem claims had come from dog owners as opposed to cat owners, a pilot study with 12 black dogs (6 Labrador Retrievers and 6 Newfoundlands) was conducted to examine the potential role of tyrosine in the "red-coat" problem.[56] Adult dogs were fed a commercial large-breed dog food with or without supplemental phenylalanine and tyrosine included at ~2.0 and ~2.5 times the Association of American Feed Control Officials' (AAFCO's) minimum requirement. After 5 months of feeding, the coats of dogs fed supplemental phenylalanine and tyrosine were reported to be blacker than the coats of the nonsupplemented dogs. The nonsupplemented dogs had a red hue in their coats, suggesting that modestly reduced tyrosine levels in a food could explain the "red-coat" syndrome that has been reported by some pet owners. However, because only three dogs were fed each diet in this study and only a single base dog food was fed, additional studies with dogs are needed to fully examine this relationship. Regardless, many pet food manufacturers have subsequently increased the levels of phenylalanine and tyrosine in their foods to ensure that adequate tyrosine is available for optimal hair pigmentation in dark-colored breeds.

ETHOXYQUIN CAUSES HEALTH PROBLEMS IN DOGS AND CATS

Ethoxyquin is a synthetic antioxidant that is included in some animal and human foods as a preservative to protect fats and fat-soluble vitamins from oxidative degradation (see Section 3, pp. 155-158 for a complete discussion of antioxidant preservatives). Without the inclusion of antioxidants in pet foods, oxidative processes lead to rancidity of the food. Rancid fat is offensive in odor and flavor and includes compounds that are toxic when consumed. The inclusion of antioxidants in commercial pet foods ensures the food's safety, nutritional integrity, and flavor. Starting in the late 1980s ethoxyquin was identified by dog breeders and owners as a potentially dangerous synthetic preservative. Depending on the source of the information, ethoxyquin was believed to be responsible for reproductive problems, autoimmune disorders, behavior problems, and various types of cancers in dogs and cats.

Prior to approval by the Food and Drug Administration (FDA), ethoxyquin's safety in foods was studied in a variety of species, including rabbits, rats, poultry, and dogs. The original studies on which the FDA based approval for the inclusion of ethoxyquin in animal feeds included a 1-year chronic toxicity study in dogs. Data from this and other studies were used when ethoxyquin was first marketed to determine a "safe tolerance level" of 150 parts per million (150 mg/kg) of food.[57] Subsequent studies failed to show any adverse health or reproductive effects of ethoxyquin when it was fed to several generations of dogs and at levels of up to 360 mg/kg of the diet (the highest concentration that was tested).[58] However, data from another study showed that feeding high levels of ethoxyquin may result in pigment accumulation in the liver and an increase in serum levels of certain liver enzymes.[59] A series of in vitro studies also reported that ethoxyquin had both cytotoxic and genotoxic effects upon cultured human lymphocytes and that these effects were dose dependent.[60,61] Because there is also evidence that direct exposure to high levels of ethoxyquin cause health problems in human workers, a search for new types of antioxidants or improved forms of ethoxyquin has been undertaken in recent years.[62-64]

In response to the new data, pet food manufacturers have voluntarily limited ethoxyquin concentrations in pet foods to 75 parts per million or less in foods that use this preservative. No harmful effects of ethoxyquin have been demonstrated at these levels. Most manufacturers have also developed foods that contain no ethoxyquin. In addition, numerous foods are now available that are preserved entirely or primarily using naturally derived antioxidants (see Section 3, pp. 156-157). Consumers should always read labels to ensure that the product that they select includes ingredients that they feel confident about feeding to their dog or cat. As with other additives and ingredients, ethoxyquin must be included in the list of ingredients and should be identified as a preservative.

HIGH-FAT PET FOODS CAUSE HYPERLIPIDEMIA

Today, most people are aware of the relationship of dietary fat and cholesterol to the development of atherosclerosis and coronary artery disease in humans, and of the importance of limiting these nutrients in their diet. In recent years, this knowledge has led some pet owners to apply these same nutritional principles to the diet of their companion animals. However, there exist some very basic differences between these species in the ways in which dietary fat is assimilated and metabolized. Unlike humans, dogs and cats are capable of consuming a wide range of dietary fat while still maintaining normal blood lipid levels. This is presumably because dogs and cats first evolved as carnivorous predators with a diet that normally contained a high proportion of animal fat. The capability to consume, digest, and assimilate a high-fat diet has remained with these species throughout the domestication process.

Both hyperlipidemia and atherosclerosis are rare conditions in dogs and cats. When cases of these conditions do occur, they are either of genetic origin or develop secondary to other disease states. For example, an inherited defect in lipoprotein lipase activity in cats causes elevated triglyceride and cholesterol levels.[65] The disorder eventually leads to the development of severe peripheral nerve paralysis. It is proposed that an autosomal recessive mode of inheritance, similar to that of an analogous disease in humans, is responsible for this disorder. There is also some evidence for the existence of an inherited defect in lipid metabolism in Miniature Schnauzers, Beagles, and, possibly, Brittany Spaniels.[66-68] Abnormally elevated plasma cholesterol concentrations have also been identified in Briards, suggesting the existence of an inherited disorder of lipid metabolism in this breed (see Section 5, pp. 300-304).[69] A second cause of hyperlipidemia in companion animals is the presence of certain preexisting disorders. Diseases that may cause secondary hyperlipidemia include diabetes mellitus, hypothyroidism, pancreatitis, hyperadrenocorticism, nephrotic syndrome, and liver disease.[70] Certain medications such as glucocorticoids and immunosuppressant drugs may also result in transient increases in blood lipid levels in some pets.

When elevated triglyceride levels occur in dogs and cats, they may produce clinical signs of anorexia, lethargy, abdominal pain, seizures, vomiting, diarrhea, and development of a lipid-laden aqueous humor. Hypercholesterolemia, on the other hand, may be related to the development of atherosclerotic lesions, lipemia retinalis, and lipid opacification of the cornea.[67] Traditionally, the dietary treatment for hyperlipidemia in dogs and cats has been a low-fat diet.[70] Both primary and secondary hyperlipidemia appear to respond well to a strict adherence to low-fat, low-calorie diets in these species. However, feeding a low-fat diet to healthy pets with the intention of preventing hyperlipidemia and elevated cholesterol levels is unnecessary. Balanced, low-fat diets can be used for the treatment of obesity and for weight maintenance in adult pets that lead sedentary lifestyles. However, the concerns that humans have with dietary lipids and heart disease do not apply to companion animals, except in the specific circumstances discussed.

COPROPHAGY (STOOL EATING) IS CAUSED BY A NUTRIENT DEFICIENCY

Coprophagy (stool eating) is relatively common in dogs but rarely observed in cats. Contrary to popular belief, the majority of dogs that coprophagize are not consuming a diet that is deficient in one or more essential nutrients, nor do they have gastrointestinal disease.[71] Most dogs will consume the feces of ruminant or nonruminant herbivorous species such as horses, cattle, deer, or rabbits. In addition, many dogs that live with cats will eat cat feces if allowed access to the litter box. Although less common, some dogs also consume canine feces, including their own.

The dog's evolutionary history provides a reasonable explanation for this behavior. Although the dog's ancestor, the wolf, is considered to be a social predator, this species is also an adept food scavenger. Unlike the more carnivorous feline species, most canids will eat carcasses killed by natural causes or other predators; various types of vegetation and fruits; and even garbage. Eating feces is a manifestation of scavenging behavior and is observed both in pet dogs and in captive and wild wolves. Although ingestion of herbivorous species' feces may supplement the dog's diet with certain vitamins, there is no evidence that dogs (or wolves) selectively coprophagize in an attempt to obtain nutrients that are deficient in their diet. In addition, female dogs and wolves routinely consume the feces of their puppies. It has been theorized that this behavior may continue after puppies are whelped, or that it can be socially facilitated between dogs within the same household. The best way to prevent stool eating is to limit access to fecal matter by monitoring walks, restricting the dog's access to the feces of wild animals such as rabbits and deer, and keeping the yard free of feces. In addition, training techniques such as teaching dogs to "leave it" and to reliably come when called are helpful in deterring dogs from coprophagizing.

Contrary to popular belief, dogs that coprophagize are not attempting to balance a deficient diet, nor do they have gastrointestinal disease. Rather, eating feces is a common type of scavenging behavior and is also observed in female dogs that are caring for puppies. The best way to prevent stool eating is to limit access to fecal matter by monitoring walks, restricting the dog's access to the feces of wild animals such as rabbits and deer, and keeping the yard free of feces.

VITAMIN C SUPPLEMENTATION PREVENTS SKELETAL DISEASE IN GROWING DOGS

The practice of supplementing the diets of growing dogs with ascorbic acid can be traced back to a early report that compared the development of hypertrophic osteodystrophy (HOD) in young dogs with the bone abnormalities associated with scurvy (vitamin C deficiency) in humans.[72] Radiographic examinations of dogs with HOD and humans with scurvy both show radiotranslucent zones in affected metaphyses and eventual subperiosteal hemorrhages. Follow-up studies adding supportive evidence for a role of ascorbic acid in HOD reported decreased levels of ascorbic acid in the plasma and urine of dogs with HOD.[73-75] Because of these similarities, it was theorized that an endogenous deficiency of ascorbic acid in dogs was responsible for the development of HOD in growing dogs. HOD is characterized by excessive bone deposition and retarded bone resorption and occurs most often in the distal ulna, radius, and tibia (see

Section 5, pp. 493-494).[76] Affected dogs exhibit acute pain and swelling in the metaphyseal regions of the long bones, intermittent pyrexia, and, occasionally, anorexia.

Although these original studies enjoyed widespread interest, a series of later studies found that a very crucial difference between HOD in dogs and scurvy in humans had been overlooked by the early investigations.[77] HOD is characterized by osteopetrosis, involving excess bone deposition in the metaphysis and periosteum and retarded bone resorption. Scurvy, on the other hand, is an osteoporotic condition, involving the demineralization of bone caused by impaired collagen formation by osteoblasts in the developing skeleton. This major difference provides incontrovertible evidence that the two conditions are not the same disorder. Subsequent controlled studies of the efficacy of supplemental ascorbic acid as a therapeutic treatment for HOD found no benefit to bone health.[78] A study with growing Labrador Retrievers reported that supplementation with 500 mg of ascorbic acid per day from weaning to 4½ months of age had no effect on the development of skeletal disorders.[79] Both groups of dogs in the study were fed a highly palatable, energy-dense diet on a free-choice regimen. Dogs in both the supplemented and the nonsupplemented groups developed skeletal lesions indicative of HOD. In addition, supplemented dogs were found to have higher levels of circulating serum calcium. It was postulated that this "relative hypercalcemia" may have led to elevated calcitonin levels. Persistent hypercalcitoninism has the potential to contribute to the bone changes observed in many of the developmental skeletal disorders in young dogs (see Section 5, pp. 491-500). It was concluded that supplemental ascorbic acid has no preventive effect and may even exacerbate the development of certain skeletal lesions in growing dogs. Similar to other developmental skeletal diseases, HOD is more likely to be caused by overnutrition leading to a high rate of growth than to an endogenous lack of ascorbic acid (see Section 5, pp. 493-494).

Although the original attention awarded to ascorbic acid status in dogs pertained specifically to HOD, this association was expanded without scientific support to include several other developmental bone disorders such as canine hip dysplasia (CHD) and osteochondrosis. As a result, many breeders and professionals habitually began to supplement growing dogs' diets with ascorbic acid in the hope of preventing the onset of these diseases. However, there is no evidence to support the claim that supplemental ascorbic acid can prevent the development of either of these disorders in growing dogs.

In addition to being unwarranted, ascorbic acid supplementation in dogs and cats may be detrimental. Excess ascorbic acid is excreted in the urine as oxalate, and a high concentration of oxalate has the potential to contribute to the formation of calcium oxalate uroliths in the urinary tract. A more practical and scientifically supported route to preventing the development of skeletal diseases in dogs includes selective breeding practices that cull dogs with skeletal disease from the breeding pool of animals, the promotion of moderate growth rates in puppies, and feeding a high-quality, balanced, food that contain optimal amounts of protein, moderately reduced fat, and moderate amounts of calcium, without added supplements (see Section 5, pp. 494-500 for a complete discussion).

Studies show that supplemental ascorbic acid has no preventive effect and may even exacerbate the development of certain skeletal lesions in growing dogs. A more practical and scientifically supported route to preventing the development of skeletal diseases in dogs includes the use of careful breeding practices and feeding puppies to promote moderate, rather than rapid, rates of growth.

References

1. Momoi Y, Goto Y, Tanide K, and others: Increase in plasma lipid peroxide in cats fed a fish diet, *J Vet Med Sci* 63:1293–1296, 2001.

2. Gaskell CJ, Leedale AH, Douglas SW: Pansteatitis in the cat: a report of five cases, *J Small Anim Pract* 16:117–121, 1975.

3. Cordy DR: Experimental production of steatitis (yellow fat disease) in kittens fed a commercial canned cat food and prevention of the condition by vitamin E, *Cornell Vet* 44:310–318, 1954.

4. Munson TO, Holzworth J, Small E, and others: Steatitis ("yellow fat") in cats fed canned red tuna, *J Am Vet Med Assoc* 133:563–568, 1958.

5. Griffiths RC, Thornton GW, Willson JE: Pansteatitis (yellow fat) in cats, *J Am Vet Med Assoc* 137:126–128, 1960.

6. Cropper N: Pansteatitis in cats fed fish-based commercial foods, *Can Vet J* 21:192–193, 1980.

7. Watson ADJ, Porges WL, Huxtable CR, and others: Pansteatitis in a cat, *Aust Vet J* 49:388–392, 1973.

8. Summers BA, Sykes G: Pansteatitis mimicking infectious peritonitis in a cat, *J Am Vet Med Assoc* 180:546–549, 1982.

9. Niza MM, Vilela CL, Ferreirá LM: Feline pansteatitis revisited: hazards of unbalanced home-made diets, *J Feline Med Surg* 5:271–277, 2003.

10. Smith DC, Proutt LM: Development of thiamine deficiency in the cat on a diet of raw fish, *Pro Soc Exp Bio Med* 56:1–5, 1944.

11. Jubb KV, Saunders LZ, Coates HV: Thiamine deficiency encephalopathy in cats, *J Comp Pathol* 66:217–227, 1956.

12. Loew FM, Martin CL, Dunlop RH, and others: Naturally occurring and experimental thiamine deficiency in cats receiving commercial cat food, *Can Vet J* 11:109–113, 1970.

13. Jarrett J: Thiaminase-induced encephalopathy, *Vet Med Small Anim Clin* 65:705–708, 1970.

14. Houston D, Hulland TJ: Thiamine deficiency in a team of sled dogs, *Can Vet J* 29:383–385, 1988.

15. Everett GM: Observations on the behavior and neurophysiology of acute thiamin deficient cats, *Am J Physiol* 141:139–149, 1944.

16. Baker JR, Hughes IB: A case of deforming cervical spondylosis in a cat associated with a diet rich in liver, *Vet Rec* 83:44–45, 1968.

17. Seawright AA, Hrdlicka J: Severe retardation of growth with retention and displacement of incisors in young cats fed a diet of raw sheep liver high in vitamin A, *Aust Vet J* 50:306–315, 1974.

18. Clark L, Seawright AA, Hrdlicka J: Exostoses in hypervitaminotic A cats with optimal calcium-phosphorus intakes, *J Small Anim Pract* 11:553–561, 1970.

19. Fry PD: Cervical spondylosis in the cat, *J Small Anim Pract* 9:59–61, 1968.

20. English PB, Seawright AA: Deforming cervical spondylosis of the cat, *Aust Vet J* 40:376–381, 1964.

21. Cho DY, Frey RA, Guffy MM, and others: Hypervitaminosis A in the dog, *Am J Vet Res* 36:1597–1603, 1975.

22. Goldy GG, Burr JR, Longardner CN, and others: Effects of measured doses of vitamin A fed to healthy Beagle dogs for 26 weeks, *Vet Clin Nutr* 3:42–49, 1996.

23. Cline JL, Czarnecki-Maulden GL, Losonsky JM, and others: Effect of vitamin A on bone density and mucosal epithelium in dogs (abstract), *J Anim Sci* 73(Suppl):192, 1995.

24. Seawright AA, Steele DP, Clark L: Hypervitaminosis A of cats in Brisbane, *Aust Vet J* 44:203–206, 1968.

25. Seawright AA, English PB, Gartner RJW: Hypervitaminosis A and deforming cervical spondylosis of the cat, *J Comp Pathol* 77:29–38, 1967.

26. National Research Council: *Nutrient requirements of dogs and cats*, Washington, DC, 2006, National Academy Press.

27. United States Department of Agriculture: Nutritive value of foods, *Home and Garden Bulletin,* No. 72, Washington, DC, 1981, US Government Printing Office.

28. Riser WH, Brodey RS, Shirer JF: Osteodystrophy in mature cats: a nutritional disease, *J Am Radiol Soc* 9:37–46, 1968.

29. Lucke VM, Bardgett PL, Mann PGH, and others: Deforming cervical spondylosis in the cat associated with hypervitaminosis A, *Vet Rec* 82:141–142, 1968.

30. Bateman WG: The digestibility and utilization of egg whites, *J Biol Chem* 26:263–291, 1916.

31. Lineweaver H, Murray CW: Identification of the trypsin inhibitor of egg white with ovomucoid, *J Biol Chem* 171:565–581, 1947.

32. Mabee DA, Morgan AF: Evaluation of dog growth of egg yolk protein and six other partially purified proteins, some after heat treatment, *J Nutr* 43:261–279, 1951.

33. Czarnecki-Maulden GL, Rudnick RC: Development of a successful spray-dried egg white-based experimental diet for dogs: effect of heat treatment on diet utilization, *Nutr Res* 10:109–115, 1990.

34. Houpt KA, Smith SL: Taste preferences and their relation to obesity in dogs and cats, *Can Vet J* 22:77–81, 1981.

35. Gans JH, Korson R, Cater MR, and others: Effects of short-term and long-term theobromine administration to male dogs, *Toxicol Appl Pharmacol* 53:481–496, 1980.

36. Welch RM, Hsu SY, DeAngelis RL: Effect of arvelor 1254, phenobarbital and polycyclic aromatic hydrocarbons on the plasma clearance of caffeine in the rat, *Clin Pharmacol Ther* 22:791–798, 1977.

37. Drouillard DD, Vesell ES, Dvorchick BN: Studies on theobromine disposition in normal subjects, *Clin Pharmacol Ther* 23:296–302, 1978.

38. Hoskam EG, Haagsma J: Chocolate poisoning terminating in the death of two Dachshunds, *Tijdschr Diergeneesk* 99:523–525, 1974.

39. Decker RA, Meyers GH: Theobromine poisoning in a dog, *J Am Vet Med Assoc* 161:198–199, 1972.

40. Glauberg A, Blumenthal PH: Chocolate poisoning in the dog, *J Am Anim Hosp Assoc* 19:246–248, 1983.

41. Zoumas BL, Kreiser WR, Martin RA: Theobromine and caffeine content of chocolate products, *J Food Sci* 45:314–316, 1980.

42. Shannon WR: Thiamine chloride: an aid in the solution of the mosquito problem, *Minn Med* 26:799–803, 1943.

43. Eder HL: Flea bites: prevention and treatment with thiamine hydrochloride, *Arch Ped* 62:300, 1945.

44. Halliwell REW: Ineffectiveness of thiamine (vitamin B_1) as a flea-repellent in dogs, *J Am Anim Hosp Assoc* 18:423–426, 1982.

45. Baker NF, Farver TB: Failure of brewer's yeast as a repellent to fleas on dogs, *J Am Vet Med Assoc* 183:212–214, 1983.

46. Farkas MC, Farkas JN: Hemolytic anemia due to ingestion of onions in a dog, *J Am Anim Hosp Assoc* 10:65–66, 1974.

47. Spice RN: Hemolytic anemia associated with ingestion of onions in a dog, *Can Vet J* 17:181–183, 1976.

48. Kay JM: Onion toxicity in a dog, *Mod Vet Pract* 64:477–478, 1983.

49. Caldin M, Carli E, Furlanello T, and others: A retrospective study of 60 cases of eccentrocytotsis in the dog, *Vet Clin Pathol* 34:224–231, 2005.

50. Yamato O, Kasai E, Katsura T, and others: Heinz body hemolytic anemia with eccentrocytosis from ingestion of Chinese chive *(Allium tubersoum)* and garlic *(Allium sativum)* in a dog, *J Am Anim Hosp Assoc* 41:68–73, 2005.

51. Fadok VA: Zinc responsive dermatosis in a Great Dane: a case report, *J Am Anim Hosp Assoc* 18:409–414, 1982.

52. Sousa CA, Stannard AA, Ihrke PJ: Dermatosis associated with feeding generic dog food: 13 cases (1981-1982), *J Am Vet Med Assoc* 192:676–680, 1988.

53. Morris JG, Yu S, Rogers QR: Red hair in black cats is reversed by addition of tyrosine to the diet, *J Nutr* 132:1646S–1648S, 2002.

54. Anderson PJB, Rogers QR, Morris JG: Cats require more dietary phenylalanine or tyrosine for melanin deposition in hair than for maximal growth, *J Nutr* 132:2037–2042, 2002.

55. Dickinson PJ, Anderson PJB, Williams DC, and others: Assessment of the neurologic effects of dietary deficiencies of phenylalanine and tyrosine in cats, *Am J Vet Res* 65:671–680, 2004.

56. Biourge V, Sergheraert R: Red coat syndrome: a dietary cause. In *Proc WSAVA Cong*, 2001.

57. Monsanto Chemical Company: A five-year chronic toxicity study in dogs with santoquin. In *A report to the Food and Drug Administration*, 1964.

58. Dzanis DA: Safety of ethoxyquin in dog foods, *J Nutr* 121:S163–S164, 1991.

59. Dzanis DA: Ethoxyquin, product families and more. In *Proceedings of the petfood forum*, Chicago, 1998, Watts Publishing.

60. Blaszcyk A, Skolimowski J: Apoptosis and cytotoxicity caused by ethoxyquin and two of its salts, *Cell Mol Biol Lett* 10:15–21, 2005.

61. Blaszcyk A: DNA damage induced by ethoxyquin in human peripheral lymphocytes, *Toxicol Lett* 163:77–83, 2006.

62. Alanko K, Jolanki R, Estalander T, Kanerva L: Occupational 'multivitamin allergy' caused by the antioxidant ethoxyquin, *Contact Derm* 39:263–264, 1998.

63. Blaszczyk A, Skolimowski J: Apoptosis and cytotoxicity caused by ethoxyquin salts in human lymphocytes in vitro, *Food Chem* 105:1159–1163, 2007.

64. Dorey G, Lockhart B, Lestage P, Casara P: New quinolinic derivatives as centrally active antioxidants, *Bioorg Med Chem Lett* 10:935–939, 2000.

65. Jones BR, Johnstone AC, Cahill JI, and others: Peripheral neuropathy in cats with inherited primary hyperchylomicronaemia, *Vet Rec* 119:268–272, 1986.

66. Rogers WA, Donovan EF, Kociba GJ: Idiopathic hyperlipoproteinemia in dogs, *J Am Vet Med Assoc* 166:1087–1091, 1975.

67. Hubert B, Braun JP, La Farge F, and others: Hypertriglyceridemia in two related dogs, *Comp Anim Pract* 1:33–35, 1987.

68. Whitney MS, Boon GD, Rebar AH, and others: Ultracentrifugal and electrophoretic characterization of the plasma lipoproteins of Miniature Schnauzer dogs with idiopathic hyperlipoproteinemia, *J Vet Intern Med* 7:253–260, 1993.

69. Watson P, Simpson KW, Bedford PGC: Hypercholesterolemia in Briards in the United Kingdom, *Res Vet Sci* 54:80–85, 1993.

70. Bauer JE: Evaluation and dietary considerations in idiopathic hyperlipidemia in dogs, *J Am Vet Med Assoc* 206:1684–1687, 1995.

71. Overall KL: Coprophagia. In Overall KL, editor: *Clinical behavioral medicine for small animals*, St Louis, 1997, Mosby.

72. Gratzl E, Pommer A: Moller-Barlow's disease in the dog, *Wien Tierarztl Mschr* 28:481–492, 513–519, 531–537, 1941.

73. Meier H, Clark ST, Schnelle GB, and others: Hypertrophic osteodystrophy associated with disturbance of vitamin C synthesis in dogs, *J Am Vet Med Assoc* 130:483–491, 1957.

74. Grondalen J: Metaphyseal osteopathy (hypertrophic osteodystrophy) in growing dogs: a clinical study, *J Small Anim Pract* 17:721–735, 1976.

75. Holmes JR: Suspected skeletal scurvy in the dog, *Vet Rec* 74:801–813, 1962.

76. Alexander JW: Selected skeletal dysplasias: craniomandibular osteopathy, multiple cartilaginous exostoses, and hypertrophic osteodystrophy, *Vet Clin North Am Small Anim Pract* 13:55–70, 1983.

77. Woodard JC: Canine hypertrophic osteodystrophy, a study of the spontaneous disease in litter mates, *Vet Pathol* 19:337–354, 1982.

78. Muir P, Dubielzig RR, Johnson KA, and others: Hypertrophic osteodystrophy and calvarial hyperostosis, *Compend Contin Educ Pract Vet* 18:143–151, 1996.

79. Teare JA, Krook L, Kallfelz A, and others: Ascorbic acid deficiency and hypertrophic osteodystrophy in the dog: a rebuttal, *Cornell Vet* 69:384–401, 1979.

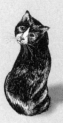

Section 5

Nutritionally Responsive Disorders

Nutrition is a vital component for the health of all companion animals. Section 4 presented information about the results of feeding imbalanced diets and inappropriate food items. Another way that nutrition affects the health of an animal is through inherited disorders of nutrient metabolism. There are several diseases in companion animals that are genetic in origin and affect an animal's ability to digest, absorb, or metabolize certain nutrients. These disorders are examined in Chapter 27. Dietary management, when effective, is also discussed.

Nutrition also affects health when diet is used to either manage or treat disease. Dietary therapy plays an important role in the treatment of a number of chronic diseases in dogs and cats, even though the underlying cause of the disease may be unrelated to diet. For example, dietary therapy has been proven to be efficacious in the management of obesity, diabetes mellitus, urolithiasis, chronic kidney failure, certain skin disorders, intestinal diseases, feline hepatic lipidosis, joint health disorders, and cardiovascular disease.

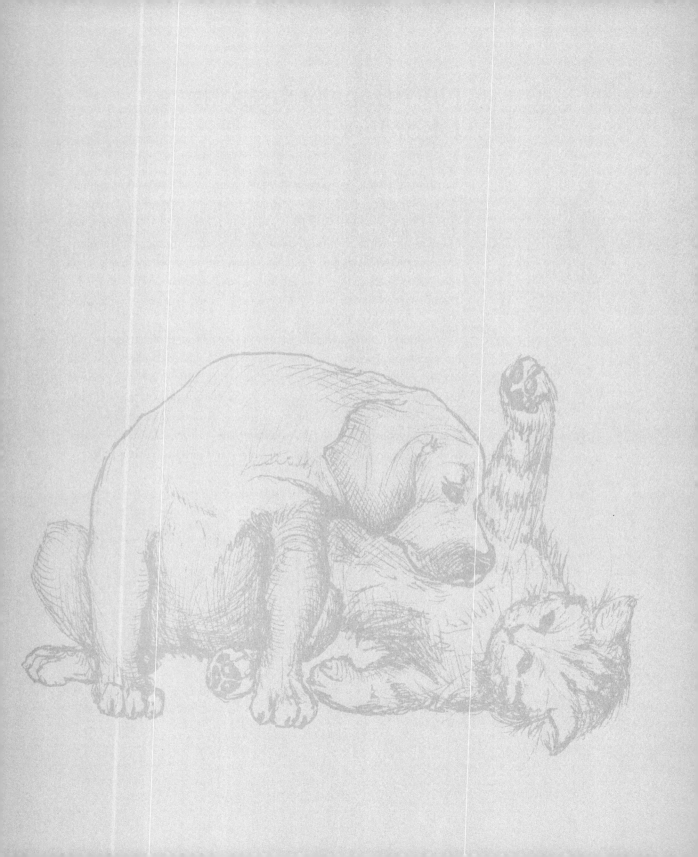

27

Inherited Disorders of Nutrient Metabolism

Clinical disease can occur in some companion animals as a result of the inability to absorb, assimilate, or metabolize specific nutrients. In some cases, breed predispositions can be found, and the disorder appears to have a genetic basis. Five specific examples in dogs involve lipid metabolism, purine metabolism, and the nutrients vitamin B_{12}, copper, and zinc. Although inherited disorders of metabolism are less well documented in cats, a familial hyperlipidemia has been reported in this species (Table 27-1).

MALABSORPTION OF VITAMIN B_{12}

Vitamin B_{12} (cobalamin) is required by the body as a coenzyme for several metabolic reactions and for normal deoxyribonucleic acid (DNA) synthesis and erythropoiesis. Vitamin B_{12} deficiency results in macrocytic anemia and neurological impairment. Absorption of B_{12} from the diet requires the presence of a compound called *intrinsic factor* (IF). In the dog, IF is produced by the gastric mucosa and the pancreas and binds to cobalamin as it passes through the gastrointestinal tract.[1] The IF-B_{12} complex attaches to specific receptor sites on cells lining the intestinal mucosa and is absorbed into the body. Without the presence of IF, cobalamin absorption is severely impaired.

Like other species, dogs require very small amounts of dietary vitamin B_{12} because of the body's ability to store adequate amounts of B_{12} in the liver for long periods of time. In addition, efficient reabsorption of excreted vitamin B_{12} through the enterohepatic circulation results in efficient conservation of this nutrient. As a result, naturally occurring deficiencies of vitamin B_{12} are not common in the canine species.

Inherited vitamin B_{12} malabsorption was first identified in Giant Schnauzers. Analysis of pedigrees and a series of breeding studies demonstrated a simple autosomal recessive mode of inheritance in this breed.[2] The disorder has since been reported in Border Collies,

Australian Shepherds, Beagles, Shar-Peis, and cats.[3-6] Studies of a human condition, Imerslund-Grasbeck syndrome (I-GS), characterized by B_{12} malabsorption and juvenile-onset megaloblastic anemia, revealed a similar mode of action to that of Giant Schnauzers and Australian Shepherds with B_{12} malabsorption.[7] Studies revealed that B_{12} malabsorption in dogs is most often due to mutation of the amnionless gene, whereas in humans I-GS is most often related to mutation of the cubilin gene, both of which are essential for proper IF function.[8]

Clinical signs develop when puppies are between 6 weeks and 5 months of age, and include lethargy, failure to thrive, loss of appetite, neutropenia (decreased white blood cell count), and nonregenerative anemia. Vitamin B_{12} deficiency can be diagnosed in affected puppies as early as 2 weeks of age by comparing their serum cobalamin concentration with that of normal littermates.[9] Other signs that have been reported include elevated plasma ammonia levels and hyperammonemic encephalopathy.[3,6,10] However, the underlying cause of these signs is not completely understood.[9]

Vitamin B_{12} malabsorption diagnosis can be confirmed through analysis of serum B_{12} levels, response to parenteral administration of the vitamin, the presence of elevated levels of methylmalonic acid in the urine, and genetic testing. For example, DNA genetic testing of Giant Schnauzers and Australian Shepherds is available at the University of Pennsylvania Metabolic Genetic Screening Laboratory.[10] Elevated urinary levels of methylmalonic acid can confirm the diagnosis because it is excreted only when the normal metabolism of certain amino acids, fatty acids, and cholesterol is blocked because of the lack of a necessary B_{12}-containing coenzyme. Normally, dogs excrete less than 10 milligrams (mg) of methylmalonic acid per gram (g) of creatinine in the urine. Giant Schnauzers with vitamin B_{12} malabsorption excrete between 4000 and 6000 mg/g of creatinine.[11]

Tests have shown that the intestinal absorption of nutrients in affected dogs is normal, with the exception

TABLE 27-1 SELECTED INHERITED DISORDERS OF NUTRITIONAL METABOLISM

DISORDER	BREEDS AFFECTED	TREATMENT
Malabsorption of vitamin B_{12}	Giant Schnauzer	Intramuscular injections of B_{12}
Copper-storage disease	Doberman Pinscher	Copper-restricted diet, zinc acetate supplementation
	Bedlington Terrier	
	West Highland White Terrier	
	Cocker Spaniel	
Lethal acrodermatitis	Bull Terrier	None
Zinc malabsorption	Siberian Husky	Zinc supplementation
	Alaskan Malamute	
	Great Dane	
	Doberman Pinscher	
Hyperlipidemia	Miniature Schnauzers, cats	Restricted-fat, restricted-calorie diet
Abnormal purine metabolism	Dalmatians	Reduced-purine diet, production of alkaline urine, adequate hydration, allopurinol

of vitamin B_{12}. Moreover, oral administration of vitamin B_{12}, with or without IF, is not effective in resolving clinical signs or in raising serum B_{12} levels. These results and immunoelectron microscopy studies of ileal morphology indicate the defect may be located at the level of the cell receptor in the small intestine. Specifically, affected dogs lack a receptor for the IF-cobalamin complex in their brush border microvilli.[2] Long-term treatment of this disorder involves the regular administration of intramuscular injections of vitamin B_{12}. This injection bypasses the intestine and provides tissues with the necessary vitamin. Complete resolution of clinical signs has been reported with a dosage as low as 1 mg every 4 to 5 months. In other cases, a weekly dosage of 0.5 mg has been used.[10]

COPPER-STORAGE DISEASE

Copper is an essential micronutrient, needed for iron absorption and transport, hemoglobin formation, electron transport proteins, various antioxidants, and normal functioning of the cytochrome oxidase enzyme system (see Section 1, p. 41 and Section 2, pp. 113-114).[12] The normal metabolism of copper in the body involves the passage of excess copper through the liver and excretion in bile. Disorders that affect bile excretion often result in an accumulation of copper in the liver, sometimes to toxic levels. In these cases, copper toxicosis in the liver is a secondary disorder that develops as an effect of the primary liver disease.[13] Hepatopathy (acute

hepatic necrosis, subacute hepatitis, chronic hepatitis, and cirrhosis) associated with increased liver copper concentration has been noted in many dog breeds including Cocker Spaniels, Dalmatians, German Shepherd Dogs, Keeshonds, Kerry Blue Terriers, Labrador Retrievers, Old English Sheepdogs, Poodles, Samoyeds, and rarely, even in cats.[14-18]

A primary, hepatic copper-storage disease, also known as *copper toxicosis,* has been conclusively identified in the Bedlington Terrier and may also occur in certain other breeds of dogs. Inherited canine copper-storage disease involves the impaired removal of copper from the liver, resulting in accumulation of the mineral as the dog ages. Its development is independent of diet and eventually will cause chronic, degenerative liver disease. The mode of inheritance in Bedlington Terriers is a simple, autosomal recessive gene that shows no sex predilection.[19-22] A variation of this disorder occurs in West Highland White and Skye Terriers.[21,23] The mode of inheritance in these breeds is not fully understood. The concentration of copper in the liver does not reach levels that are as high nor do the copper levels consistently increase with age as observed in Bedlington Terriers.[15,24] Other breeds that have been reported to be at risk for familial diseases of copper metabolism include Dalmatians, Cocker Spaniels, Labrador Retrievers, and Doberman Pinschers.[21,25] Because only female Doberman Pinschers appear to be affected, a sex-linked mode of inheritance is suspected in this breed.[26] In addition, affected Dobermans show reduced copper excretion and increased oxidative stress, which suggests this is a new variant of primary copper toxicosis.[27]

Inherited copper-storage disease in Bedlington Terriers is caused by impaired removal of copper from the liver, resulting in accumulation of the mineral as the dog ages. This eventually results in chronic, degenerative liver disease in most animals. Normal liver copper concentration in dogs ranges from 200 to 400 parts per million (ppm) of dry weight (dw), and this level remains constant throughout life.[28] Bedlington Terriers with copper-storage disease begin to accumulate the mineral shortly after birth. Biopsies of the livers of affected puppies show increased copper in the hepatocytes as early as 5½ months of age.[29] During the first few months of life, while copper is accumulating, there is no liver damage, and serum levels of liver enzymes remain within normal range. But when hepatic copper reaches a toxic level of approximately 2000 ppm, centrolobular hepatitis with concomitant elevation of liver enzymes develops. Individual dogs vary significantly regarding the age at which toxic levels are reached and in their susceptibility to clinical signs. Even after toxicity occurs, levels continue to accumulate, sometimes reaching as high as 10,000 ppm dw.[13]

The identification of a DNA marker for the copper toxicosis locus in Bedlington Terriers led to the ability to reliably diagnose individual cases and identify pedigrees and lineages in which the gene for this disorder is prevalent.[30,31] However, recently this diagnostic method has been complicated by the discovery of diverse haplotypes that lead to false negatives in some Bedlington terriers with copper toxicosis.[32,33] Therefore serum chemistry profiles continue to be useful as a preliminary screening tool for the onset of liver disease in young dogs. Liver biopsies should be considered if elevated levels of the liver enzyme alanine amino transaminase are observed. Clinical signs of disease do not usually manifest until the dog is between 4 and 8 years old, although some may show signs as early as 1 year or as late as 11 years of age.[21] Widespread liver necrosis and postnecrotic cirrhosis begin to cause clinical signs that are associated with liver disease. Lethargy, anorexia, vomiting, abdominal pain, and occasionally ascites and icterus are observed. Some dogs suffer acute tubular necrosis in the kidneys and show polyuria and polydipsia in addition to signs of liver disease.[21] Acute episodes of liver necrosis may cause sudden death in a small number of affected dogs.

Treatment involves lifelong feeding of a copper-restricted diet and the administration of medications that either decrease intestinal absorption or increase urinary excretion of copper.[21,34] Two chelating agents, penicillamine and trientine, have been used in dogs with copper-storage disease and act by increasing urinary excretion of copper.[35,36] However, despite the reported use of these drugs, controlled efficacy and treatment regimen studies have not been conducted in dogs, and penicillamine may be toxic in some animals.[21,34] Zinc acetate, which functions to block the intestinal absorption of copper, may be the treatment of choice for dogs with copper-storage disease.[34,37] Results of a study that examined the efficacy of zinc acetate in the treatment of copper-storage disease in Bedlington Terriers and West Highland White Terriers found that administration at dosages that resulted in plasma zinc concentrations of 200 to 500 micrograms (µg)/deciliter (dl) suppressed hepatic inflammatory disease and reduced hepatic copper concentrations. It appeared that hepatic function could be restored by the long-term administration of zinc acetate in affected dogs. The administration of 100 mg of zinc acetate twice daily is recommended for the first 3 months of treatment. After this period, the dosage can be reduced to 50 mg twice daily. For maximum effectiveness, the zinc should not be administered with the dog's food. Plasma zinc concentrations should be measured every 2 to 3 months to confirm that the level has increased appropriately and that the concentration does not exceed 1000 µg/dl. Affected dogs require lifelong therapy and their copper status must be monitored closely to guard against the potential for copper deficiency.

ZINC MALABSORPTION

Although zinc deficiency and zinc-responsive dermatosis can be caused by feeding an imbalanced diet, another potential cause involves an inherited predisposition for impaired zinc absorption. Several breeds of dogs appear to be affected by zinc malabsorption, and varying levels of severity for this disorder have been reported. The most severe zinc-related disorder is lethal acrodermatitis in Bull Terriers. This genetic disease is inherited as an autosomal recessive gene and results in an inability to absorb dietary zinc, even when high levels of the mineral are added to the diet.[38] At birth, affected puppies show lighter pigmentation than is normal for the breed.

Their growth is stunted, and severe skin lesions develop by 6 to 10 weeks of age.[39] Cell-mediated immunodeficiency, acquired T-cell deficiency, poor responsiveness of T lymphocytes to mitogen stimulation, and selective deficiency of immunoglobulin A (IgA) also occurs.[40,41] The immunodeficiency results in increased susceptibility to pyoderma and multiple infections throughout the body. There is also some evidence that the behavioral disorders of tail-chasing and idiopathic aggression in this breed may be related to zinc malabsorption.[42] This disorder is invariably fatal and has a median survival age of only 7 months. Nearly all affected dogs die before 15 months of age and there is currently no reliable test that can identify carriers of this disease.[38]

Less severe zinc-responsive disorders occur in Alaskan Malamutes, Siberian Huskies (Figure 27-1), and, occasionally, Great Danes and Doberman Pinschers.[43-47] Research has shown that Alaskan Malamutes afflicted with inherited chondrodysplastic dwarfism have an impaired ability to absorb intestinal zinc.[47] Dwarfism in this breed has a simple autosomal recessive inheritance, and zinc malabsorption appears to be a component of this disorder. However, impaired zinc absorption has also been described in Malamutes that are not afflicted with chondrodysplasia.[43] The mode of inheritance of the zinc-responsive dermatoses is currently unknown. The onset of this syndrome usually occurs at puberty, and some dogs show signs only during times of physiological stress, such as pregnancy or exposure to weather extremes. Dermatological signs include crusting, scaling, and underlying suppuration around the face, elbows, scrotum, prepuce, and vulva. In chronic cases, hyperpigmentation of the affected skin surface is seen. The dogs are usually nonpruritic until the lesions have become extensively crusted. Mild to moderate weight loss and a dull, dry coat are also observed. Histopathological examinations of skin biopsies show diffuse parakeratotic hyperkeratosis.

Another zinc-responsive disorder occurs in rapidly growing puppies of many breeds including Beagles, German Shorthaired Pointers, Great Danes, Standard Poodles, and many others.[44] The severity of signs is highly variable within a litter. Some puppies appear nearly normal and others are depressed, anorexic, and emaciated. Hyperkeratotic plaques may occur with thickened, fissured foot pads and planum nasale. In both of these syndromes, oral supplementation with zinc results in rapid resolution of the skin lesions. However, only Malamutes usually require supplementation throughout life to prevent a recurrence of clinical signs. A therapeutic dose of 10 mg/kilogram (kg)/day of zinc sulfate ($ZnSO_4$) usually suffices. Large dogs are often given 100 to 200 mg of $ZnSO_4$ twice daily.[44] $ZnSO_4$ can cause emesis in some dogs, but this can be prevented in most cases by giving the mineral with the dog's food. In a small proportion of cases, supplementation is necessary only during periods of stress.

DISORDERS OF LIPID METABOLISM

The term *hyperlipidemia* is sometimes used interchangeably with *hyperlipoproteinemia* when referring to elevated levels of triglycerides and/or cholesterol in

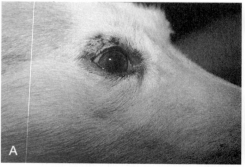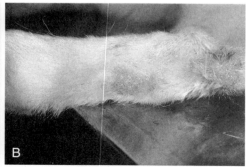

Figure 27-1 Inherited zinc malabsorption in a Siberian Husky. A, Face. B, Hock.
(Courtesy Candace Sousa, DVM, Animal Dermatology Clinic, Sacramento, Calif.)

animals that have been fasted for at least 12 hours.[48] However, the term *hyperlipoproteinemia* specifically refers to excessive circulating lipoproteins. *Hypercholesterolemia* describes excessive circulating cholesterol, while *hypertriglyceridemia* refers to elevated concentrations of triglycerides, either of which may occur alone or in combination with hyperlipoproteinemia.[49]

Most of the cases of hyperlipidemia seen in companion animals occur secondary to another underlying disorder that affects lipid metabolism. Diseases that may cause secondary hyperlipidemia include diabetes mellitus, hypothyroidism, pancreatitis, nephrotic syndrome, hyperadrenocorticism, cholestasis, hypercholesterolemia, and liver disease.[50-54] In addition, certain medications such as glucocorticoids and immunosuppressant drugs may cause transient increases in blood lipid levels. *Familial*, or *primary*, *hyperlipidemia* refers to cases in which a heritable basis for hyperlipidemia can be found. Two well-documented inherited disorders of lipid metabolism occur in dogs and cats: hyperlipidemia in Miniature Schnauzers and lipoprotein lipase (LPL) deficiency in cats. In addition, hypercholesterolemia has been reported in Miniature Schnauzers with hyperlipidemia, in Briards in the United Kingdom, in Shetland Sheepdogs in Japan, and in a family of Rough Collies.[53-56]

Lipoprotein Metabolism

A basic understanding of the mechanisms of lipid transport in the blood is necessary for an examination of hyperlipidemia. Because lipids are insoluble in water, transport in the blood requires complexing with more soluble molecules such as proteins and phospholipids. Free fatty acids (FFAs) are carried in the bloodstream by albumin, a serum protein. Triglycerides and cholesterol esters are carried by lipoproteins, which are spherical macromolecular complexes made up of a lipid core surrounded by a thin outer membrane. Apoproteins, the proteins that are present in the lipoprotein's outer membrane, are recognition sites for target tissues and act as enzyme cofactors in lipid metabolism reactions.[57]

Lipoproteins can be categorized according to their lipid components and resultant aqueous densities. Like humans, dogs have four major classes of lipoproteins, each of which has a principal lipid component and one or more transport functions.[51] Chylomicrons are synthesized in response to the absorption of fat from the intestine and function in the transport of dietary triglyceride to extrahepatic tissues and cholesterol to the liver. Chylomicrons appear in the blood approximately 2 hours postprandially, causing a transient increase in plasma triglyceride concentration. When they are delivered to tissues, the triglycerides are hydrolyzed to fatty acids and glycerol by the enzyme LPL. The second category of lipoproteins, called *very–low-density lipoproteins* (VLDLs), transport endogenous triglycerides from the liver to extrahepatic tissues for use as an energy source or for storage in adipose tissue. In contrast to chylomicrons, VLDLs are produced continuously, so that in the fasting state, VLDLs are the main carriers of endogenously produced triglyceride. Low-density lipoproteins (LDLs) transport cholesterol from the liver to extrahepatic tissues for incorporation into cell membranes and for steroid hormone synthesis. Finally, the high-density lipoproteins (HDLs) also transport cholesterol, but they are responsible for moving excess cholesterol out of extrahepatic cells back to the liver for excretion in bile, a process called "reverse cholesterol transport."

Postprandial hyperlipidemia is a natural occurrence that reflects a transient rise in chylomicrons; in dogs it normally resolves within 6 to 10 hours following consumption of a meal.[58,59] Hyperlipidemia that persists for 12 hours or more after food is withheld warrants investigation.[51] In dogs, fasting serum triglyceride concentrations greater than 150 mg/dl and/or total cholesterol concentration greater than 300 mg/dl are considered abnormally high. In cats, fasting triglyceride concentrations of greater than 100 mg/dl and/or cholesterol concentrations greater than 200 mg/dl should be investigated.[60]

A number of health problems may be caused by persistent hyperlipidemia in companion animals. Hypertriglyceridemia, especially when severe, is associated with abdominal pain, vomiting, diarrhea, anorexia, seizures, hepatomegaly, and the abnormal deposition of lipid in certain tissues.[58,60,61] Like some hereditary hypertriglyceridemias in humans, elevated triglyceride levels in dogs and cats may also increase the risk for development of acute pancreatitis.[57,62] Hypercholesterolemia is not common in dogs and cats, but has been reported in Shetland Sheepdogs, Beagles, Briards, Collies, and Miniature Schnauzers.[53-55,62,63] It is generally not associated with as many health risks as is hypertriglyceridemia.

Corneal lipid depositions have been reported in dogs with hyperlipidemia and may be the result of elevated blood cholesterol.[64,65] For example, a family of Collies was found to have familial idiopathic hypercholesterolemia, and most of the dogs developed corneal lipidosis.[56] In contrast to humans, dogs and cats rarely develop atherosclerosis in response to hypercholesterolemia, and when atherosclerosis is seen, it is usually the result of congenital or spontaneous hypothyroidism.[66]

Hyperlipidemia in Miniature Schnauzers

Hyperlipidemia in Miniature Schnauzers is a well-documented familial disorder.[62,67] It is reported that many clinically normal dogs of this breed are found to have persistent fasting hyperlipidemia during routine veterinary examinations.[62] There is no sex predilection, and the disorder is usually first seen in Schnauzers that are older than 4 years of age. The hyperlipidemia is associated with elevated triglycerides and is typically characterized by chylomicron excess. Serum cholesterol levels are either normal or slightly increased.[57] A recent investigation of the prevalence of hypertriglyceridemia in Miniature Schnauzers found that nearly a third (32.8%) had triglyceride concentrations that were higher than the reference range for healthy dogs. Only 5.4% of control dogs from the general population have hyperlipidemia, which does suggest a genetic predisposition in this breed.[68] Increased serum lipase and amylase activities have been recognized in hyperlipidemic Miniature Schnauzers that present with acute pancreatitis. In these cases, the pancreatitis is believed to be caused by the hypertriglyceridemia.

Affected dogs are either asymptomatic or have recurrent episodes of abdominal pain or distress, vomiting, and/or diarrhea. Seizures have also been associated with persistent hyperlipidemia in this breed.[67] Owners may report that episodes of abdominal distress last several days, followed by spontaneous recovery. In many cases, the clinical signs and history are similar to those of dogs with acute pancreatitis, but radiographic and laboratory evidence does not often support this diagnosis. This syndrome has been termed "pseudopancreatitis" by one investigator.[62] Hyperlipidemia in Miniature Schnauzers is believed to be hereditary because of the high breed predisposition and because most affected Miniature Schnauzers lack evidence of diseases that cause secondary hyperlipidemia.[57]

The underlying cause of primary hyperlipidemia in Miniature Schnauzers is not known, but is characterized by excessive VLDL particles with or without concurrent chylomicronemia, and mild hypercholesterolemia.[57] LPL activity was decreased in lipemic Miniature Schnauzers compared to LPL activity in nonlipemic Miniature Schnauzers and in other breeds.[69] It is theorized that either a familial deficiency of the enzyme LPL or the absence of an apoprotein that functions to activate LPL may be responsible. The enzyme LPL is located in capillary and endothelial tissue and hydrolyzes the triglycerides that are transported by chylomicrons and VLDLs for transport into cells. A defect in the synthesis or activity of this enzyme prevents the delivery of dietary triglycerides to tissues and leads to the retention of chylomicrons and impaired VLDL metabolism. The absence of an important apoprotein called *apolipoprotein C-II* (apo C-II) would have a similar effect. Apo C-II is normally a component of chylomicrons and VLDL and is a cofactor for LPL. In humans, individuals with an apo C-II deficiency have clinical symptoms similar to individuals with LPL deficiency.[70,71]

> *Hyperlipidemia in Miniature Schnauzers is a well-documented familial disorder. Although not all dogs show clinical signs, more than 30% of the breed may be affected. Because signs mimic those of acute pancreatitis, the disease has been termed "pseudopancreatitis."*

Feline Lipoprotein Lipase Deficiency

A well-recognized inherited deficiency of LPL in cats causes hyperchylomicronemia and has been shown to be inherited as an autosomal recessive trait.[72-75] The hyperlipidemia is caused by markedly elevated fasting triglyceride concentrations as a result of increased chylomicrons and, to a lesser extent, VLDLs.[76] Clinical signs may or may not be present, and the severity of clinical disease is not well correlated with the degree of hyperlipidemia. The age of onset of clinical signs varies from as young as 3 weeks to middle age.[76] Cats homozygous for LPL deficiency have a lower percentage of body fat compared to heterozygous carriers or normal cats, but lean body mass is not influenced.[77] Kittens suckling queens homozygous for LPL deficiency are at a distinct disadvantage and often must be hand reared or fostered.[78]

When cats present with clinical disease, the most common signs include the development of subcutaneous xanthomas (lipid deposits) and lipemia retinalis. The xanthomas occur most often in areas of the body where trauma caused damage to capillaries, leading to extravasation of lipids.[79] Variable peripheral neuropathies are seen in some cases. The signs of nerve damage develop slowly and are characterized by the loss of conscious proprioception and motor function, with retention of sensation of pain. These neuropathies are thought to be caused by compression of nerves by lipid granulomata at sites of trauma.[57] A study of a family of cats reported that LPL-deficient cats produced an abnormal LPL protein that failed to bind normally to vascular endothelium, rendering it inactive.[74] These results support the theory that an inherited disorder of lipid metabolism involving a deficiency of active LPL occurs in the cat.

A well-recognized inherited deficiency of lipoprotein lipase in cats causes hyperlipidemia and appears to be the result of an autosomal recessive trait. The most common clinical signs include subcutaneous xanthomas and lipemia retinalis. Some cats develop peripheral neuropathies that are slowly progressive and characterized by the loss of conscious proprioception and motor function.

Diagnosis of Primary Hyperlipidemias

The diagnosis of primary hyperlipidemia is one of exclusion, as all causes of secondary hyperlipidemia must be ruled out first. Primary hyperlipidemia is seen most frequently as a familial disorder in Miniature Schnauzers and Beagles, although other breeds may be affected.[80] The pet's breed, family lineage, age, and clinical history can be used to support a diagnosis. A 12- to 18-hour fasting blood sample should be taken and cholesterol and triglyceride concentrations should be measured.[48,81]

If there is a history of recurrent abdominal pain, vomiting, or diarrhea, serum amylase and lipase activities should be measured to monitor pancreatic pathology.

Quantification of the plasma concentrations of each lipoprotein class may assist in the differential diagnosis of hyperlipidemia. An estimate of the lipoprotein pattern can be obtained through electrophoresis, but major differences exist between dog, cat, and human plasma lipoproteins in circulation. Dogs and cats have HDL predominance and are more resistant to LDL and cholesterol elevations than humans.[82] A precipitation technique for canine plasma lipoprotein quantitation has been published, but has not been widely adapted for routine veterinary clinical use.[83] Some human commercial laboratories offer precipitation and electrophoresis studies to analyze and interpret dog and cat sera, but this approach should only be used if staff are specifically trained to interpret electrophoresis scans of canine lipoproteins.[82,49] Even with expert interpretation, electrophoretic separation of lipoproteins is not a disease-specific technique and cannot always differentiate between the functional classes of elevated lipoproteins.[58] Laboratory techniques that can accurately identify lipoproteins that are not adequately differentiated by electrophoresis are not used by most diagnostic laboratories, and so samples must be referred to research laboratories.[57]

If LPL deficiency is suspected in a cat, determination of plasma activity of this enzyme is suggested. LPL activity can be indirectly assayed by collecting plasma before and after the administration of heparin. Heparin administration stimulates the release of endothelial LPL and causes increased LPL activity.[81,84] Diagnosis of LPL inactivity can be made by collecting blood prior to and 10 minutes after intravenous administration of heparin and comparing plasma lipid concentrations.[85] In the normal cat, LPL activity increases following heparin administration, leading to increased hydrolysis of chylomicrons triglycerides and VLDL. In the LPL-deficient cat, plasma lipid concentrations remain unchanged following heparin administration.[86]

Dietary Treatment of Primary Hyperlipidemia

The aim of treatment for primary hyperlipidemia is to reduce and maintain plasma lipid concentrations at levels that no longer predispose the dog or cat to health risks. Dietary intervention is recommended in animals that have fasting hypertriglyceridemia of greater than 500 mg/dl or hypercholesterolemia greater than 750 mg/dl.[60,61] Miniature Schnauzers that have fasting hypertriglyceridemia but no clinical signs should be treated if the elevated concentration of triglycerides persists in two consecutive samples taken several weeks apart.[62]

In both dogs and cats, a diet that is restricted in fat and calories is recommended.[85] Feeding less fat decreases the influx of triglyceride-containing chylomicrons into the bloodstream, reduces the load on LPL, and promotes the clearance of chylomicrons and VLDLs. For successful dietary management, the diet should contain less than 20% fat, with an ideal level of between 8% and 12% (on a dry-matter basis [DMB]).[59,62] Follow-up blood samples should be taken several weeks after switching to the new diet. It is imperative that the restricted-fat diet is the animal's only source of food. All fatty table scraps and treats must be discontinued. Owners should be cautioned that dogs with hyperlipidemia may be susceptible to acute pancreatitis, and that a single high-fat meal may result in the onset of this disease. If a fat-restricted diet normalizes blood triglyceride levels, dietary management should be continued for the remainder of the pet's life.

Feeding a low-fat diet to cats with LPL deficiency has been shown to normalize blood lipid levels and cause a regression of xanthomas and peripheral neuropathies within 12 weeks of lowering plasma lipid concentrations.[72,87] Similarly, clinical signs in Miniature Schnauzers usually resolve when serum triglyceride levels are normalized.[67] Most Miniature Schnauzers with hyperlipidemia can be successfully managed by diet, but more drastic fat reduction may be necessary as the pet ages. If any clinical signs of acute pancreatitis develop, periodic follow-up examinations should be conducted and veterinary care should be sought immediately. In some cases, reducing the level of fat in the diet is not sufficient to reduce blood lipid levels. Cases of pure hyperchylomicronemias respond better to dietary fat restriction than cases of mixed hypertriglyceridemias.[86]

Several lipid-lowering drugs are approved for use in humans, but not in dogs or cats. Although there are some reports of success using drugs such as fibric acid derivatives (clofibrate, gemfibrozil, etc.) and pharmacological doses of niacin, the efficacy of these therapies has not been proven. Niacin reduces serum triglycerides, but adverse effects are frequent and include vomiting, diarrhea, erythema, pruritus, and abnormal liver function tests.[81] Although use of the fibrates in humans is generally associated with 20% to 40% reduction in serum triglyceride concentrations, reported adverse effects of gemfibrozil in the dog and cat include abdominal pain, vomiting, diarrhea, and abnormal liver function tests.[81]

Marine fish oils, which contain high amounts of omega-3 fatty acids such as eicosapentaenoic acid (EPA) and docosahexaenoic acid (DHA), have also been used as an adjunct therapy for hyperlipidemia in dogs.[48,72] Studies with humans and other animals have shown that these oils reduce plasma triglyceride and cholesterol concentrations by decreasing the production of VLDLs.[88,89] Improved triglyceride levels have been reported in hyperlipidemic dogs receiving supplemental marine oil at doses up to 30 to 60 mg/kg daily, with no clinical or biochemical side effects.[48,59,90] Although not effective for all dogs, marine oil supplementation may help to normalize blood lipid levels in animals that are not responding adequately to dietary fat restriction alone.

The amelioration of clinical signs is the best indicator of long-term prognosis in pets with primary hyperlipidemia. The animal's health is invariably improved if dietary fat restriction is strictly enforced and blood lipid levels can be lowered to normal or near-normal concentrations. Naturally, the presence of any secondary, underlying disorders that could contribute further to hyperlipidemia, such as insulin-dependent diabetes mellitus or hypothyroidism, increases the health risks and makes long-term management more difficult in these pets.

The goal of treatment for primary hyperlipidemia is to reduce and maintain plasma lipid concentrations at levels that no longer predispose the pet to health risks. A fat-restricted diet is recommended and is fed for the remainder of the pet's life and is often sufficient to control clinical signs. Although not effective for all dogs, supplementation with omega-3 fatty acids may help to normalize blood lipid levels in animals that are not responding adequately to dietary fat restriction alone.

PURINE METABOLISM IN DALMATIANS

Purines are components of the nucleic acids that are found in the nucleus of plant and animal cells. All mammals are capable of synthesizing purines for tissue growth and maintenance. Purines are also obtained through the reuse of dietary or endogenous nuclear material. Nuclear material that is ingested and hydrolyzed contains purine bases that can be converted back into nucleotides to be used for growth and maintenance by the body. Normal cellular turnover and tissue maintenance, along with the digestion of excess dietary purines, results in purine catabolism. A primary end product of purine catabolism is uric acid. If the liver enzyme urate oxidase is present, uric acid is further degraded to form the compound allantoin. Uric acid that is not converted to allantoin is present in body tissues as its salt, monosodium urate.

Most mammals, with the exception of humans, the higher apes, and Dalmatians, convert most uric acid to allantoin and as a result excrete very little urate in the urine. Dalmatians are unique in that they excrete both urate and allantoin in their urine as end products of purine metabolism.[91,92] Compared with other breeds of dogs, Dalmatians have increased levels of urate and decreased levels of allantoin in the bloodstream and urine.[93] Other breeds of dogs excrete 10 to 60 mg of urate per 24-hour period, and their serum urate concentration is approximately 0.25 mg/dl.[91,94,95] In contrast, Dalmatians excrete approximately 400 to 600 mg of urinary urate in a 24-hour period.[91,93,96] However, these values can range from less than 200 mg to greater than 1 g of uric acid. The mean serum urate concentration in Dalmatians is about 0.5 mg/dl, with a range of 0.3 to 4.0 mg/dl, approximately twofold to fourfold the values in other dog breeds.[91,95]

Dalmatians excrete both urate and allantoin in their urine as end products of purine metabolism. They have higher levels of urate in their blood and urine than other breeds of dogs, as well as reduced renal tubular reabsorption of urate. Excess urate in the urine can lead to the development of urate urolithiasis in some dogs.

There appear to be two separate underlying mechanisms that are responsible for the Dalmatian's high production of uric acid and low production of allantoin. A defective uric acid transport system in the liver results in decreased oxidation of uric acid to allantoin by urate oxidase.[97] The second problem involves the kidneys. Compared with other species and other breeds of dogs, Dalmatians have reduced renal tubular reabsorption of urate.[91] In other breeds, 98% of the uric acid in the glomerular filtrate is reabsorbed in the proximal tubules and returned to the liver for further oxidation to allantoin. Dalmatians have reduced ability to reabsorb uric acid in the proximal tubules, resulting in increased urinary excretion of urate. In humans and some other primates, loss of urate oxidase activity alone is the underlying cause of increased uric acid concentrations.[98] Evolutionary accumulation of several mutations to the urate oxidase gene is the cause of altered enzyme activity in humans, but this is not the case in Dalmatians.[94] Hyperuricosuria is found in all Dalmatians and is inherited as an autosomal recessive gene or genes.[99] Because of the prevalence of this disorder, a Dalmatian x Pointer outcross was used to introduce the normal allele into the Dalmatian gene pool. (Interestingly, the pigmented spots of the low-uric-acid backcross dogs are usually smaller and less well defined when compared with purebred Dalmatians.) This led to a theory that spot selection may have contributed to fixing the hyperuricosuria trait in the Dalmatian breed.[100] Further studies may identify the exact gene or genes that are responsible. Once identified, backcross dogs could be used for breeding purposes to attempt to eliminate the inherited disease from the Dalmatian breed.[101]

Altered purine metabolism in Dalmatians does have some medical significance. Although allantoin is highly soluble, urate has a low aqueous solubility. Its accumulation in the body can result in the precipitation of urate crystals in serum or urine. In humans, crystallization occurs in body tissues when serum urate values are greater than 6.5 mg/dl.[102] The presence of urate crystals causes the medical affliction that is commonly called "gout," which is characterized by inflammation, swelling, and painful joints. Interestingly, although Dalmatians do not convert uric acid to allantoin, their serum does not attain urate concentrations as high as those in humans with gout. Rather, because of the reduced reabsorption of urate in the renal tubules, Dalmatians excrete large amounts of urate in the urine, preventing buildup in the serum. Although this capability appears to protect Dalmatians from developing signs of gout, the shift of excess urate from the serum to the urine causes other problems.

The presence of a high concentration of urate in the urinary tract of Dalmatians appears to predispose dogs of this breed to the development of urate urolithiasis. In dogs, urate uroliths or calculi are composed primarily of ammonium urate. A sufficiently high concentration of both urate and ammonium in the urine is necessary for the formation of these uroliths. Studies show that although urate calculi account for only 5% of calculi found in dogs, 45% to 65% of those that are seen come from Dalmatians. Furthermore, 75% to 100% of calculi found in Dalmatians are composed completely or partially of urate.[103-107] Urate urolithiasis is significantly more common in male Dalmatians than in females.[96,105] A study of over 500 Dalmatian urate uroliths revealed a 50:1 ratio of males to females.[107] The anatomical differences between the urethras of males and females may partially explain this disparity.[108] The small, rounded urate crystals pass readily through the wider female urethra, but they may tend to lodge in the male urethra as it enters the narrow groove in the os penis. Conversely, others have reported that female dogs that are not Dalmatians are more likely to form urate-containing calculi than males.[96] Therefore it appears that additional factors may be responsible for the higher incidence or urate urolithiasis in male Dalmatians.

Clinical signs of urolithiasis in the dog, regardless of the type of urolith present, depend on the duration of the urolithiasis, the size of the uroliths, their location in the tract, and the presence or absence of a concomitant urinary tract infection. General signs include frequent urination and the voiding of small amounts of urine, the appearance of pain or straining during urination, and hematuria. Urethral obstruction is characterized by anuria, depression, anorexia, vomiting, and/or diarrhea. Complete obstruction always constitutes a medical emergency.

Although high urinary uric acid excretion is a major predisposing factor for the development of urate urolithiasis in Dalmatians, it is not the sole cause. Most Dalmatians excrete urate in the urine at a concentration above its solubility limits. However, not all Dalmatians develop urate uroliths, and urate excretion is not well correlated with the development of uroliths.[109] Other predisposing factors that may be involved include urinary ammonium concentration, urine pH, the presence of a urinary tract infection, and dietary purine intake. The incidence of urate urolithiasis in the Dalmatian breed is not known, but it has been suggested that the majority of dogs never experience clinical signs of this disease, and that the incidence rate may be as low as 1%.[110] Conversely, a recent study showed that prevalence in male Dalmatians may be as high as 34%.[111]

Treatment for urate urolithiasis in dogs usually requires surgical removal of the calculi.[112] Prophylactic measures for Dalmatians that are predisposed to urate urolithiasis include feeding a diet that promotes alkaline urine and is low in purines, as well as ensuring adequate hydration.[94] A reduced-purine diet decreases the amount of urate precursors present in the urine, and the production of an alkaline urine increases the solubility of urate uroliths.[113] The diet should provide moderate to low levels of high-quality protein. Moderate restriction of protein results in decreased ammonium ion production from the catabolism of excess protein. Ingredients that are high in protein also tend to be high in purines. The moderate restriction of protein therefore also reduces purine intake. Oral administration of sodium bicarbonate is effective in changing the alkalinity of the urine. It is hypothesized that control of any concomitant urinary tract infections may also aid in preventing recurrence.[109]

Daily administration of the drug allopurinol is often used as a prophylactic method in Dalmatians that are predisposed to urate urolithiasis.[114] Allopurinol is an inhibitor of the enzyme xanthine oxidase, which is necessary for the degradation of purines.[112] Administration of this drug results in a decrease in uric acid production. However, this can result in increased levels of xanthine in the urine and lead to urinary calculi that contain xanthine. An increased incidence of this type of calculi has been reported in Dalmatians that have received allopurinol.[105,115]

References

1. Batt RM, Horadagoda NU, Simpson KW: Role of the pancreas in the absorption and malabsorption of cobalamin (vitamin B-12) in dogs, *J Nutr* 121:S75–S76, 1991.

2. Fyfe JC, Giger U, Hall CA, and others: Inherited selective intestinal cobalamin malabsorption and cobalamin deficiency in dogs, *Pediatr Res* 29:24–31, 1991.

3. Vaden SL, Wood PA, Ledley FD, and others: Cobalamin deficiency associated with methylmalonic acidemia in a cat, *J Am Vet Med Assoc* 200:1101–1103, 1992.

4. Huff A, Seng A, Wang P, and others: Screening for hereditary diseases by the Josephine Deubler Genetic Disease Testing Laboratory (PennGen) at the University of Pennsylvania, *Tufts' canine and feline breeding and genetics conference*, 2005.

5. Fordyce HH, Callan MB, Giger U: Persistent cobalamin deficiency causing failure to thrive in a juvenile Beagle, *J Small Anim Pract* 41:407–410, 2000.

6. Battersby IA, Giger U, Hall EJ: Hyperammonaemic encephalopathy secondary to selective cobalamin deficiency in a juvenile Border Collie, *J Small Anim Pract* 46:339–344, 2005.

7. Xu D, Kozyraki R, Newman TC, and others: Genetic evidence of an accessory activity required specifically for cubilin brush-border expression and intrinsic factor-cobalamin absorption, *Blood* 94:3604–3606, 1999.

8. He Q, Madsen M, Kilkenney A, and others: Amnionless function is required for cubilin brush-border expression and intrinsic factor-cobalamin (vitamin B_{12}) absorption in vivo, *Blood* 106:1447–1453, 2005.

9. Fyfe JC: Haematology of selective intestinal cobalamin malabsorption. In Feldman BF, Zinkl JG, Jain N, editors: *Schalm's veterinary hematology*, ed 5, Philadelphia, 2000, Wiley-Blackwell.

10. Huff A, Seng A, Tuneva J, and others: Molecular, metabolic, and hematologic screening for hereditary diseases at the University of Pennsylvania (PennGen), *Tufts' canine and feline breeding and genetics conference*, 2007.

11. Fyfe J, Jexyk P, Giger U, and others: Inherited selective malabsorption of vitamin B_{12} in Giant Schnauzers, *J Am Anim Hosp Assoc* 25:533–539, 1989.

12. Linder MC, Hazegh-Azam M: Copper biochemistry and molecular biology, *Am J Clin Nutr* 63:797S–811S, 1996.

13. Thornburg LP: A perspective on copper and liver disease in the dog, *J Vet Diagn Invest* 12:101–110, 2000.

14. Cooper VL, Carlson MP, Jacobson J, and others: Hepatitis and increased copper levels in a Dalmatian, *J Vet Diagn Invest* 9:201–203, 1997.

15. Thornburg LP, Rottinghaus G, McGowan M, and others: Hepatic copper concentrations in purebred and mixed-breed dogs, *Vet Pathol* 27:81–88, 1990.

16. Haynes JS, Wade PR: Hepatopathy associated with excessive hepatic copper in a Siamese cat, *Vet Pathol* 32:427–429, 1995.

17. Meertens NM, Bokhove CA, van den Ingh TS: Copper-associated chronic hepatitis and cirrhosis in a European Shorthair cat, *Vet Pathol* 42:97–100, 2005.

18. Fuentealba IC, Aburto EM: Animal models of copper-associated liver disease, *Comp Hepatol* 2:5, 2003.

19. Brewer GJ: Wilson disease and canine copper toxicosis, *Am J Clin Nutr* 67:1087S–1090S, 1998.

20. Hyun C, Filippich LJ: Inherited canine copper toxicosis in Australian Bedlington Terriers, *J Vet Sci* 5:19–28, 2004.

21. Thornburg LP, Polley D, Dimmitt R: The diagnosis and treatment of copper toxicosis in dogs, *Can Pract* 11:36–39, 1984.

22. van De Sluis B, Rothuizen J, Pearson PL, and others: Identification of a new copper metabolism gene by positional cloning in a purebred dog population, *Hum Mol Genet* 11:165–173, 2002.

23. Ubbink GJ, van de Broek J, Hazewinkel HA, and others: Cluster analysis of the genetic heterogeneity and disease distributions in purebred dog populations, *Vet Rec* 142:209–213, 1998.

24. Haywood S, Rutgers HC, Christian MK: Hepatitis and copper accumulation in Skye Terriers, *Vet Pathol* 25:408–414, 1988.

25. Webb CB, Twedt DC, Meyer DJ: Copper-associated liver disease in Dalmatians: a review of 10 dogs (1998-2001), *J Vet Intern Med* 16:665–668, 2002.

26. Johnson GF, Zawie DA, Gilbertson SR, and others: Chronic active hepatitis in Doberman Pinschers, *J Am Vet Med Assoc* 180:1438–1442, 1982.

27. Spee B, Mandigers PJ, Arends B, and others: Differential expression of copper-associated and oxidative stress related proteins in a new variant of copper toxicosis in Doberman Pinschers, *Comp Hepatol* 4:3, 2005.

28. Keen CL, Lonnerdal B, Fisher GL: Age-related variations in hepatic iron, copper, zinc, and selenium concentrations in Beagles, *Am J Vet Res* 42:1884–1887, 1981.

29. Thornburg LP, McAllister D, Ebinger WL, and others: Copper toxicosis in dogs. I. Copper-associated liver disease in Bedlington Terriers. II. The pathogenesis of copper-associated liver disease in dogs, *Can Pract* 12(33-38):41–45, 1985.

30. Yuzbasiyan-Gurkan V, Blanton SH, Cao Y, and others: Linkage of a microsatellite marker to the canine copper toxicosis locus in Bedlington Terriers, *Am J Vet Res* 58:23–27, 1997.

31. Holmes NG, Herrtage ME, Ryder EJ, and others: DNA marker C04107 for copper toxicosis in a population of Bedlington Terriers in the United Kingdom, *Vet Rec* 142:351–352, 1998.

32. Hyun C, Lavulo LT, Filippich LJ: Evaluation of haplotypes associated with copper toxicosis in Bedlington Terriers in Australia, *Am J Vet Res* 65:1573–1579, 2004.

33. van de Sluis B, Peter AT, Wijmenga C: Indirect molecular diagnosis of copper toxicosis in Bedlington Terriers is complicated by haplotype diversity, *J Hered* 94:256–259, 2003.

34. Brewer GJ, Dick RD, Schall W, and others: Use of zinc acetate to treat copper toxicosis in dogs, *J Am Vet Med Assoc* 201:564–568, 1992.

35. Richter K: Common canine hepatopathies, *Tufts animal expo*, 2002.

36. Twedt DC, Sternlieb I, Gilbertson SR: Clinical, morphologic, and chemical studies on copper toxicosis of Bedlington Terriers, *J Am Vet Med Assoc* 175:269–275, 1979.

37. Schall WD: Use of zinc acetate for the treatment and prevention of canine copper hepatotoxicosis. In Bonnagura JD, Kirk RW, editors: *Kirk's current veterinary therapy XII*, Philadelphia, 1995, Saunders.

38. Jezyk PF, Haskins ME, MacKay-Smith WE, and others: Lethal acrodermatitis in Bull Terriers, *J Am Vet Med Assoc* 188:833–839, 1986.

39. Miller WH Jr: Nutritional considerations in small animal dermatology, *Vet Clin North Am Small Anim Pract* 19:497–511, 1989.

40. Felsberg PJ: Hereditary and acquired immunodeficiency diseases. In Bonagura JD, editor: *Kirk's curent veterinary therapy XIII: small animal practice*, St Louis, 2000, Saunders.

41. McEwan NA, Huang HP, Mellor DJ: Immunoglobulin levels in Bull Terriers suffering from lethal acrodermatitis, *Vet Immunol Immunopathol* 96:235–238, 2003.

42. Dodman NH, Bronson R, Gliatto J: Tail chasing in a Bull Terrier, *J Am Vet Med Assoc* 202:758–760, 1993.

43. Willemse T: Zinc-related cutaneous disorders of dogs. In Kirk RW, editor: *Current veterinary therapy XI*, Philadelphia, 1992, Saunders.

44. Scott DW, Miller WH Jr, Griffin CE: Zinc-responsive dermatosis. In Scott DW, Miller WH Jr, Griffin CE, editors: *Muller and Kirk's small animal dermatology*, ed 5, Philadelphia, 1995, Saunders.

45. Codner EC, Thatcher CD: The role of nutrition in the management of dermatoses, *Semin Vet Med Surg (Small Anim)* 5:167–177, 1990.

46. Fadok VA: Zinc responsive dermatosis in a Great Dane: a case report, *J Am Anim Hosp Assoc* 18:409–414, 1982.

47. Brown RG, Hoag GN, Smart ME, and others: Alaskan Malamute chondrodysplasia. V. Decreased gut zinc absorption, *Growth* 42:1–6, 1978.

48. Watson TDG, Barrie J: Lipoprotein metabolism and hyperlipoproteinemia in the dog and cat: a review, *J Small Anim Pract* 34:479–487, 1993.

49. Schenck PA: Canine hyperlipidemia: causes and nutritional management. In Pibot PP, Biourge V, Elliott DA, editors: *Encyclopedia of canine clinical nutrition*, Ithaca, NY, 2008, International Veterinary Information Service (www.ivis.org).

50. Barrie J, Watson TDG, Stear MJ, and others: Plasma cholesterol and lipoprotein concentrations in the dog: the effects of age, breed, gender and endocrine disease, *J Small Anim Pract* 34:507–512, 1993.

51. Bauer JE: Lipoprotein-mediated transport of dietary and synthesized lipids and lipid abnormalities of dogs and cats, *J Am Vet Med Assoc* 224:668–675, 2004.

52. Johnson MC: Hyperlipemia disorders in dogs, *Compend Contin Educ Pract Vet* 27:361–370, 2005.

53. Whitney MS, Boon GD, Rebar AH, and others: Ultracentrifugal and electrophoretic characteristics of the plasma lipoproteins of miniature schnauzer dogs with idiopathic hyperlipoproteinemia, *J Vet Intern Med* 7:253–260, 1993.

54. Watson P, Simpson KW, Bedford PG: Hypercholesterolaemia in Briards in the United Kingdom, *Res Vet Sci* 54:80–85, 1993.

55. Sato K, Agoh H, Kaneshige T, and others: Hypercholesterolemia in Shetland Sheepdogs, *J Vet Med Sci* 62:1297–1301, 2000.

56. Jeusette I, Grauwels M, Cuvelier C, and others: Hypercholesterolaemia in a family of rough collie dogs, *J Small Anim Pract* 45:319–324, 2004.

57. Whitney MS: Evaluation of hyperlipidemias in dogs and cats, *Semin Vet Med Surg (Small Anim)* 7:292–300, 1992.

58. Watson TD, Mackenzie JA, Stewart JP, and others: Use of oral and intravenous fat tolerance tests to assess plasma chylomicron clearance in dogs, *Res Vet Sci* 58:256–262, 1995.

59. Downs LG, Crispin SM, LeGrande-Defretin V, and others: The effect of dietary changes on plasma lipids and lipoproteins of six Labrador Retrievers, *Res Vet Sci* 63:175–181, 1997.

60. Armstrong PJ, Ford RB: Hyperlipidemia. In Kirk RW, editor: *Current veterinary therapy X: small animal practice*, Philadelphia, 1989, Saunders.

61. Barrie J: Hyperlipidemia. In Bonagura JD, editor: *Kirk's current veterinary therapy XII: small animal practice*, Philadelphia, 1995, Saunders.

62. Ford RB: Idiopathic hyperchylomicronemia in Miniature Schnauzers, *J Small Anim Pract* 34:488–492, 1993.

63. Manning PJ: Thyroid gland and arterial lesions of Beagles with familial hypothyroidism and hyperlipoproteinemia, *Am J Vet Res* 40:820–828, 1979.

64. Crispin S: Ocular lipid deposition and hyperlipoproteinaemia, *Prog Retin Eye Res* 21:169–224, 2002.

65. Zech LA Jr, Hoeg JM: Correlating corneal arcus with atherosclerosis in familial hypercholesterolemia, *Lipids Health Dis* 7:7, 2008.

66. Liu SK, Tilley LP, Tappe JP, and others: Clinical and pathologic findings in dogs with atherosclerosis: 21 cases (1970-1983), *J Am Vet Med Assoc* 189:227–232, 1986.

67. Bodkin K: Seizures associated with hyperlipoproteinemia in a Miniature Schnauzer, *Can Pract* 17:11–15, 1992.

68. Xenoulis PG, Suchodolski JS, Levinski MD, and others: Investigation of hypertriglyceridemia in healthy Miniature Schnauzers, *J Vet Intern Med* 21:1224–1230, 2007.

69. Jaeger JQ, Johnson S, Hinchcliff KW, and others: Characterization of biochemical abnormalities in idiopathic hyperlipidemia of Miniature Schnauzer dogs, *ACVIM*, Charlotte, NC, June 4-8, 2003.

70. Rader DJ, Hobbs HH: Disorders of lipoprotein metabolism. In Fauci AS, Braunwald E, Kasper DL, and others, editors: *Harrison's principles of internal medicine*, ed 17, New York, 2008, McGraw-Hill.

71. Connelly PW, Maguire GF, Little JA: Apolipoprotein CIISt. Michael. Familial apolipoprotein CII deficiency associated with premature vascular disease, *J Clin Invest* 80:1597–1606, 1987.

72. Jones BR, Johnstone AC, Cahill JI, and others: Peripheral neuropathy in cats with inherited primary hyperchylomicronaemia, *Vet Rec* 119:268–272, 1986.

73. Johnstone AC, Jones BR, Thompson JC, and others: The pathology of an inherited hyperlipoproteinaemia of cats, *J Comp Pathol* 102:125–137, 1990.

74. Peritz LN, Brunzell JD, Harvey-Clarke C, and others: Characterization of a lipoprotein lipase class III type defect in hypertriglyceridemic cats, *Clin Invest Med* 13:259–263, 1990.

75. Watson T, Gaffney D, Mooney C, and others: Inherited hyperchylomicronaemia in the cat: lipoprotein lipase function and gene structure, *J Small Anim Pract* 33:213–217, 1992.

76. Jones BR: Inherited hyperchylomicronaemia in the cat, *J Small Anim Pract* 34:493–499, 1993.

77. Backus RC, Ginzinger DG, Ashbourne Excoffon KJ, and others: Maternal expression of functional lipoprotein lipase and effects on body fat mass and body condition scores of mature cats with lipoprotein lipase deficiency, *Am J Vet Res* 62:264–269, 2001.

78. Reginato CF, Backus RC, Rogers QR: Improved growth of lipoprotein lipase deficient kittens by feeding a low-fat, highly digestible diet, *J Nutr Biochem* 13:149–156, 2002.

79. Chanut F, Colle MA, Deschamps JY, and others: Systemic xanthomatosis associated with hyperchylomicronaemia in a cat, *J Vet Med A Physiol Pathol Clin Med* 52:272–274, 2005.

80. Bauer JE: Evaluation and dietary considerations in idiopathic hyperlipidemia in dogs, *J Am Vet Med Assoc* 206:1684–1688, 1995.

81. Elliott DA: Dietary and medical considerations in hyperlipidemia. In Ettinger SJ, Feldman EC, editors: *Textbook of veterinary internal medicine*, ed 7, St Louis, 2010, Saunders.

82. Bauer JE: Comparative lipoprotein metabolism and lipid abnormalities in dogs and cats. Part II. Diagnostic approach to hyperlipemia and hyperlipoproteinemia, *21st annual forum of the American College of Veterinary Internal Medicine Conference*, 2003.

83. Barrie J, Nash AS, Watson TDG: Quantatative analysis of canine plasma lipoproteins, *J Small Anim Pract* 34:226–231, 1993.

84. Brunzell JD, Iverius PH, Scheibel MS, and others: Primary lipoprotein lipase deficiency, *Adv Exp Med Biol* 201:227–239, 1986.

85. Jones BR: Hyperlipidaemia in dogs and cats, *World Small Animal Veterinary Association world congress proceedings*, 2003.

86. Bauer JE: Hyperlipidemias. In Ettinger SJ, Feldman EC, editors: *Textbook of veterinary internal medicine*, ed 5, Philadelphia, 2000, Saunders.

87. Grieshaber T, McKeever P, Conroy J: Spontaneous cutaneous (eruptive) xanthomatosis in two cats, *J Am Anim Hosp Assoc* 27:509–512, 1991.

88. Kendrick JS, Higgins JA: Dietary fish oils inhibit early events in the assembly of very low density lipoproteins and target apoB for degradation within the rough endoplasmic reticulum of hamster hepatocytes, *J Lipid Res* 40:504–514, 1999.

89. Minihane AM, Khan S, Leigh-Firbank EC, and others: ApoE polymorphism and fish oil supplementation in subjects with an atherogenic lipoprotein phenotype, *Arterioscler Thromb Vasc Biol* 20:1990–1997, 2000.

90. Logas D, Beale KM, Bauer JE: Potential clinical benefits of dietary supplementation with marine-life oil, *J Am Vet Med Assoc* 199:1631–1636, 1991.

91. Duncan H, Curtiss AS: Observations on uric acid transport in man, the Dalmatian and the non-Dalmatian dog, *Henry Ford Hosp Med J* 19:105–114, 1971.

92. Kuster G, Shorter RG, Dawson B, and others: Uric acid metabolism in Dalmatians and other dogs. Role of the liver, *Arch Intern Med* 129:492–496, 1972.

93. Sorenson JL, Ling GV: Metabolic and genetic aspects of urate urolithiasis in Dalmatians, *J Am Vet Med Assoc* 203:857–862, 1993.

94. Duncan H, Wakim KG, Ward LE: The effects of intravenous administration of uric acid on its concentration in plasma and urine of Dalmatian and non-Dalmatian dogs, *J Lab Clin Med* 58:876–883, 1961.

95. Briggs OM, Harley EH: Serum urate concentrations in the Dalmatian Coach Hound, *J Comp Pathol* 95:301–304, 1985.

96. Case LC, Ling GV, Ruby AL, and others: Urolithiasis in Dalmatians: 275 cases (1981-1990), *J Am Vet Med Assoc* 203:96–100, 1993.

97. Giesecke D, Tiemeyer W: Defect of uric acid uptake in Dalmatian dog liver, *Experientia* 40:1415–1416, 1984.

98. Oda M, Satta Y, Takenaka O, and others: Loss of urate oxidase activity in hominoids and its evolutionary implications, *Mol Biol Evol* 19:640–653, 2002.

99. Trimble H, Keeler CE: The inheritance of "high uric acid excretion" in dogs, *J Hered* 29:280–289, 1938.

100. Safra N, Schaible RH, Bannasch DL: Linkage analysis with an interbreed backcross maps Dalmatian hyperuricosuria to CFA03, *Mamm Genome* 17:340–345, 2006.

101. Safra N, Ling GV, Schaible RH, and others: Exclusion of urate oxidase as a candidate gene for hyperuricosuria in the Dalmatian dog using an interbreed backcross, *J Hered* 96:750–754, 2005.

102. Yu TF, Gutman AB, Berger L, and others: Low uricase activity in the Dalmatian dog simulated in mongrels given oxonic acid, *Am J Physiol* 220:973–979, 1971.

103. White EG: Symposium on urolithiasis in the dog. I. Introduction and incidence, *J Small Anim Pract* 7:529–535, 1966.

104. Brown NO, Parks JL, Greene RW: Canine urolithiasis: retrospective analysis of 438 cases, *J Am Vet Med Assoc* 170:414–418, 1977.

105. Osborne CA, Clinton CW, Bamman LK, and others: Prevalence of canine uroliths. Minnesota Urolith Center, *Vet Clin North Am Small Anim Pract* 16:27–44, 1986.

106. Ling GV, Franti CE, Ruby AL, and others: Urolithiasis in dogs. II. Breed prevalence, and interrelations of breed, sex, age, and mineral composition, *Am J Vet Res* 59:630–642, 1998.

107. Houston DM, Moore AE, Favrin MG, and others: Canine urolithiasis: a look at over 16,000 urolith submissions to the Canadian Veterinary Urolith Centre from February 1998 to April 2003, *Can Vet J* 45:225–230, 2004.

108. Albasan H, Lulich JP, Osborne CA, and others: Evaluation of the association between sex and risk of forming urate uroliths in Dalmatians, *J Am Vet Med Assoc* 227:565–569, 2005.

109. Porter P: Urinary calculi in the dog. II. Urate stones and purine metabolism, *J Comp Pathol* 73:119–135, 1963.

110. Fetner PJ: Uric acid dermatitis, *Dalmatian Quarterly*, pp 11–13, 1991.

111. Bannasch DL, Ling GV, Bea J, and others: Inheritance of urinary calculi in the Dalmatian, *J Vet Intern Med* 18:483–487, 2004.

112. Collins RL, Birchard SJ, Chew DJ, and others: Surgical treatment of urate calculi in Dalmatians: 38 cases (1980-1995), *J Am Vet Med Assoc* 213:833–838, 1998.

113. Bartges JW, Osborne CA, Felice LJ: Canine xanthine uroliths: risk factor management. In Kirk RW, Bonagura JD, editors: *Current veterinary therapy XI: small animal practice*, Philadelphia, 1992, Saunders.

114. Ling GV, Case LC, Nelson H, and others: Pharmacokinetics of allopurinol in Dalmatian dogs, *J Vet Pharmacol Ther* 20:134–138, 1997.

115. Ling GV, Ruby AL, Harrold DR, and others: Xanthine-containing urinary calculi in dogs given allopurinol, *J Am Vet Med Assoc* 198:1935–1940, 1991.

28

Development and Treatment of Obesity

Obesity is the most common form of malnutrition seen in companion animals in the United States and other industrialized countries. Although incidence estimates vary depending upon the population that was surveyed and methodology used, there is consensus that between 20% and 50% of dogs living in homes are overweight or obese.[1-3] Using the lowest value of 20%, the translation of this figure into actual dog numbers is sobering. Of the 72 million dogs living in homes in the United States today, at least 14 million are obese.[4] Similarly, recent studies of house cats report that between 25% and 50% of the cats seen by veterinarians are overweight or obese.[5-7] This means that at least 21 million of the 82 million cats living in U.S. homes are overweight. Middle-aged adults (5 to 8 years) are most likely to be above their ideal body weight, while fewer young adults and geriatric pets are overweight.[8] Similar to humans, dogs that are overweight when they are adolescents are more likely to gain excessive amounts of weight as adults.[9] It is theorized that the incidence of obesity in companion animals has increased because a sedentary lifestyle has become the norm rather than the exception for many. In addition, the provision of highly palatable and energy-dense foods may further contribute to the energy imbalance that leads to obesity.

Unfortunately, like contemporary American humans, a large proportion of cats and dogs, between 25% and 50%, are overweight or obese. Living a sedentary lifestyle, along with overfeeding highly palatable and energy-dense foods, may be important contributing factors.

DEFINITION AND HEALTH RISKS

Obesity is defined as the excessive accumulation of fat in the adipose storage areas of the body, eventually contributing to adverse effects on health and mortality.[10] Dogs and cats that are 10% to 20% above their ideal body weight are generally classified as overweight, and those whose body weight is greater than 20% above normal are classified as obese.[6] This standard is corroborated by evidence in human subjects that health problems associated with overweight conditions begin to increase when weight is 15% or greater above ideal. Similar to humans, numerous health risks are associated with overweight conditions in dogs and cats.

Several metabolic aberrations are associated with obesity in dogs and cats. Obese dogs and cats frequently develop glucose intolerance and abnormal basal insulin and insulin response curves.[11,12] Persistent hyperinsulinemia is theorized to be an important factor in the eventual development of diabetes mellitus in overweight pets; overweight cats are more than three times more likely to develop diabetes mellitus than normal weight cats.[13] Recent research shows that these changes are influenced by the increased production of adipocyte cytokines by fat cells and associated chronic inflammatory responses.[14] When body weight is reduced in obese dogs, glucose intolerance often improves to near-normal values.[15] Obesity in dogs is also associated with alterations in blood lipids, including increased plasma cholesterol and triglyceride concentrations.[16,17] Although these values do not necessarily exceed the upper limit of the reference range for dogs, they may be associated with other obesity-related health problems.

Obesity may contribute to the development of pulmonary and cardiovascular disease in dogs.[18] Excess weight puts a strain on the circulatory system because increased cardiac workload is required to perfuse the increased tissue mass. This increased workload may cause additional stress to a heart that is already weakened by fatty infiltration. Changes in pulmonary health lead to difficulties breathing (airway dysfunction) both during and after exercise.[19] There is also some evidence suggesting that overweight conditions contribute to secondary hypertension in dogs, although there is controversy about this relationship.[20,21] Studies in cats have not been conducted, but it is theorized that a similar effect may be found in this species.

Physical effects of carrying excess weight contribute to exercise and heat intolerance, joint and locomotor problems, and the development of osteoarthritis and chronic lameness. In a long-term prospective study, both the frequency and severity of osteoarthritis were greater in Labrador Retrievers that were fed ad libitum during the first several years of life than in dogs that were fed 25% less food and that weighed significantly less.[22] Increased weight was significantly and positively correlated with increased incidence and severity of osteoarthritis. Osteoarthritic changes also developed earlier in life in dogs that were overweight than in lean dogs. Similarly, cats that are overweight are more likely to show reduced mobility and to develop lameness than cats that are in optimal condition.[13]

In cats, there is an association between overweight conditions and certain types of dermatoses, such as feline acne, alopecia, and scale formation. These changes are presumed to be related to a reduced ability to self-groom and in some cases to the development of pressure sores from reduced activity. Other potential health risks to cats include hepatic lipidosis (specifically in the event of rapid weight loss) and feline lower urinary tract disease (FLUTD).[6,23]

A link between obesity and certain types of cancer has been reported in both dogs and cats by some authors. For example, one study reported that female dogs that were obese prior to a diagnosis of mammary carcinoma experienced increased risk of death from the disease when compared with dogs that were not overweight at the time of diagnosis.[24] Another study reported that being obese early in life increased a dog's risk of developing mammary tumors.[25] Conversely other researchers failed to find an association between canine mammary carcinoma and body weight.[26] Additional prospective studies that include larger groups of animals are needed to better understand this relationship and to tease out possible differences between types of cancer and their relationship to body condition.

Finally, obese dogs and cats are difficult to thoroughly evaluate during veterinary examinations because of the presence of overlying layers of adipose tissue and difficulty obtaining blood. Diagnostic imaging such as ultrasonography is also impeded in overweight animals. Like humans, overweight animals have an increased

---

BOX 28-1   HEALTH PROBLEMS ASSOCIATED WITH OBESITY IN DOGS AND CATS

Glucose intolerance and abnormal insulin response

Alterations in blood lipids (elevated cholesterol and triglyceride concentrations)

Increased risk for pulmonary and cardiovascular disease

Reduced exercise and heat tolerance

Joint and locomotor (mobility) problems

Reduced ability to self-groom and increased risk for dermatoses in cats

Increased surgical and anesthetic risks for morbidity and mortality

Possible increased risk for certain forms of cancer

Reduced quality of life

---

surgical and anesthetic risk, and experience increased incidence of morbidity and mortality following surgical procedures. For example, surgical time to complete ovariohysterectomy is significantly longer in overweight females than in lean dogs.[27] It is without question that altogether the numerous health risks associated with overweight conditions in companion animals negatively affect a pet's quality of life and contribute to both morbidity and mortality (Box 28-1).[28]

Health risks associated with overweight conditions in dogs and cats include hyperinsulinemia, glucose intolerance, diabetes mellitus, pulmonary and cardiovascular disease, exercise and heat intolerance, and orthopedic problems. Surgical risk is higher, and the incidences of postoperative morbidity and mortality increase.

DEVELOPMENT OF OVERWEIGHT CONDITIONS

The fundamental underlying cause of obesity is an imbalance between energy intake and energy expenditure that results in a persistent energy surplus (positive energy balance). Over time, the energy surplus results in weight gain and a change in body composition. The increase in body fat occurs either by an enlargement of fat cell size alone (hypertrophic obesity) or by an increase in both fat cell size and fat cell number (hyperplastic obesity). Pets that develop hyperplastic obesity are generally believed to be difficult to treat and have a poor long-term prognosis. Normal adipocyte hyperplasia occurs during specific critical periods of development. In most species, these periods occur during early growth and occasionally during puberty.[29] Once adulthood is reached, the total number of fat cells does not normally increase further. Overfeeding during adulthood results in an increase in fat cell size, but little or no change in fat cell number. Although conditions of extreme and prolonged overfeeding can result in fat cell hyperplasia in some animals, the majority of cases of adult onset obesity are a result of fat cell hypertrophy alone.[30,31]

The body has the capacity to add new adipocytes, but is not able to reduce its existing adipocyte number. This phenomenon, called the "ratchet effect," indicates that body fat can always increase, but it cannot decrease below a minimum level that is set by the total number of adipocytes and their need to remain lipid-filled. This fact is of importance when considering growth rate and weight gain in young, developing dogs and cats. Data from several studies with laboratory animals show that overnutrition during growth results in increased numbers of fat cells and total body fatness during adulthood.[32,33] Superfluous fat cell hyperplasia during the critical periods of adipose tissue growth may produce a long-term stimulus to gain excess weight in the form of excess adipocytes. The greater number of fat cells results in both an increased predisposition toward obesity in adulthood and an increased difficulty in maintaining weight loss when it occurs. Although this effect has not been specifically demonstrated in dogs and cats, it is theorized that persistent overnutrition during development in growing pets may result in both adipocyte hypertrophy and hyperplasia, leading to overweight conditions that are particularly refractory to treatment. The potential for an animal to produce excess numbers of fat cells during specific critical periods illustrates the importance of proper weight control throughout growth.

Similar to humans, dogs and cats may develop overweight conditions gradually, over a period of months or years, in response to a relatively small but prolonged energy imbalance. Conversely, some pets gain weight rapidly, over a period of a few weeks or months. This may occur when energy expenditure decreases significantly following the combined effects of neutering, attainment of mature body size, and reduced activity level, and is not accompanied by a reduction in energy intake. Feeding dogs free choice (ad libitum) may also lead to rapid weight gain when a new food is introduced or when a new dog is added to the home. Both novelty and social facilitation can contribute to a sudden increase in food consumption.

Two stages occur during the development of obesity: the dynamic phase and the static phase. During the initial dynamic phase, an animal consumes more energy than is expended, and the surplus energy is deposited as body fat and, to a lesser degree, as lean body tissue. As the dog or cat gains weight, its resting metabolic rate (RMR) increases proportionately to the increase in lean body mass. Eventually the increased RMR, coupled with the increased energy expenditure that is needed to move a larger body size, offsets the caloric surplus. At this point, zero energy balance is achieved, and the animal stops gaining weight. The static phase of obesity occurs when the animal is no longer gaining weight but achieves energy balance and maintains its overweight condition for a prolonged period of time.

RISK FACTORS FOR OBESITY

Although the problem of obesity appears very simple in terms of energy balance, a multitude of underlying factors can contribute to an animal's propensity to gain weight and to maintain an overweight body condition. Moreover, the development of obesity in an individual dog or cat can be the result of several separate influencing factors occurring simultaneously (Box 28-2). Factors that may contribute to the development of obesity can be classified as having either an endogenous or an exogenous origin. Endogenous factors include the animal's age, sex, and reproductive status, hormonal abnormalities, hypothalamic lesions, and genetic predisposition (breed). Exogenous factors include social and environmental influences on food intake, diet composition and palatability, and the pet's lifestyle (amount and type of exercise). Although most cases of companion animal obesity are a result of overfeeding, underexercising, or a combination of the two, it is important to recognize that each of these two conditions are typically the result of a combination of external and internal influencing factors.

Inadequate Exercise

A sedentary lifestyle is an important contributor to decreased energy expenditure and to the development of overweight conditions in companion animals.[2,34] In today's society, most dogs are kept as companions and house pets rather than as active, working partners to their human owners. Cats are also experiencing decreased activity levels. A significant proportion of cats lead sedentary, indoor lives rather than having the run of farms and neighborhoods as in the past. Living indoors and apartment dwelling have been identified as risk factors for weight gain in both dogs and cats.[5,35] It is postulated that this effect is due to reduced opportunities for outdoor exercise. Additional factors that influence the daily activity level of dogs and cats are breed, temperament, age, reproductive status, and the presence of certain chronic illnesses or developmental disorders. Moreover, a vicious cycle can occur in which an overweight pet becomes increasingly sedentary and reluctant to exercise because of obesity-induced exercise intolerance and mobility problems.

In normal animals experiencing moderate levels of exercise, physical activity contributes about 30% of the body's total energy expenditure. Decreased voluntary activity results in a direct reduction of this energy expenditure and can also affect a pet's daily food intake.

Research studies have shown that completely sedentary animals actually consume more food and gain more weight than do animals that experience moderate activity levels.[36] It appears that inactivity below a certain level cannot be entirely compensated for by an adequate decrease in food intake. As a result, animals that are maintained at or below this minimum activity level will consume more than their energy needs and will inevitably gain weight.

Factors that influence the amount of energy that is expended for exercise include the type, duration, and frequency of the activity. Other factors that affect the activity level of dogs and cats include breed, temperament, age, reproductive status, and the presence of certain chronic illnesses or developmental disorders.

Increasing Age

Obesity is most common in middle-aged adult dogs and cats. In one study, only 6% of female dogs between 9 and 12 months of age were evaluated as overweight, compared with 40% of mature adults.[37] This same trend is observed in cats.[6,7] As an adult animal ages, lean body mass gradually declines, resulting in reduced basal metabolic rate (BMR) and total daily energy needs. The loss of lean body mass is exacerbated if aging is accompanied by a decrease in exercise. The total daily energy needs of an average-size, 7-year-old dog may decrease by as much as 20% when compared with its needs as a young adult. If food intake does not decrease proportionately with decreasing energy needs as an animal ages, weight gain results.

Neutering

The increased incidence of overweight conditions in neutered dogs and cats has been recognized for many years.[38] Recent studies support these observations, showing that neutered adult pets generally weigh more and maintain higher body fat than intact animals of the same breed and size.[39-41] The underlying cause of these differences is probably a combination of physiological and environmental factors. Veterinarians often encourage clients to castrate or spay their pets shortly before they become sexually mature. As a result, many dogs and cats are neutered between 6 months and 1 year of age. This period corresponds to a natural decrease in activity level and in the animal's energy needs for growth. If owners are not aware of this change and continue to feed their pet the same amount of food, excess weight gain will result. Because spaying and neutering often occur just before maturity, the change in sexual status may be erroneously blamed for a weight gain that was actually the result of diminished energy needs and excess food intake.

However, there is also a direct effect of reproductive status upon feeding behavior and food intake. Female dogs and cats typically decrease their food intake during estrus, and the cause of this change has been attributed to estrogen. For example, a study with dogs examined the influence of estrus on voluntary food intake in 12 Beagle bitches.[42] Results showed that there was a tendency for females to decrease food consumption during the week that they were in estrus. The authors then examined food intake patterns in ovariohysterectomized and control-operated bitches. Over a period of 90 days, the ovariohysterectomized bitches consumed 20% more food and gained significantly more weight than did the sham-operated controls. The authors attributed the difference in weight gain to an increase in food intake and a decrease in voluntary activity. More recently, a study of ovarioectomized dogs showed that maintenance energy needs decreased while voluntary food intake increased significantly after being spayed.[43] Similar results have been observed in cats.[44] Both male and female cats tend to increase voluntary food intake after neutering and consume more food than intact adults.[45,46] Although the exact metabolic mechanism for this change is not known, hormonal alterations following neutering in cats (in addition to the loss of estrogen in females) include increases in plasma concentrations of insulin-like growth factor-1 (IGF-1) and prolactin.[47] It is theorized that increased IGF-1 may stimulate adipocyte proliferation and that persistently high levels of prolactin contribute to the maintenance of adipose tissue and possibly to the dysregulation of glucose metabolism seen in overweight cats. The orexigenic (appetite-stimulating) hormone ghrelin may also be involved in regulation of energy intake in neutered animals.

Finally, an animal's BMR is affected by neutering. When RMR was measured using respiratory indirect calorimetry in neutered and intact cats, heat coefficients were greater in intact male and female cats than in neutered animals.[39] Intact males had heat coefficients that were 28% higher than those of neutered males, and intact females had heat coefficients that were 33% higher than those of neutered females. When RMR is expressed on the basis of lean body tissue, no difference is seen between intact and neutered animals, suggesting that these differences are caused by the body composition changes seen in neutered animals. Regardless, the dramatic change in BMR can be interpreted to mean that neutered male cats may require 28% fewer calories, and females 33% fewer calories, than their intact counterparts.

Many shelters and veterinarians have adopted the use of early-age neutering (at 8 to 16 weeks of age) because of the benefits to pet population control. Recognition of the safety of these procedures for puppies and kittens led the American Veterinary Medical Association to approve a 1993 resolution supporting the concept of early-age neutering. However, one concern has been the potential of early-age neutering to influence a pet's tendency to become obese. A study compared metabolic rates and development of obesity in cats that were surgically neutered at 7 weeks of age, surgically neutered at 7 months of age, or left intact.[39] All of the cats in the study were fed ad libitum until they were 2 years of age and were assessed regularly for body condition, metabolic rate, and glucose tolerance. Because body weight alone is not an accurate predictor of obesity, body condition scores were assigned and body mass index was calculated. The body condition scores and body mass indices of the neutered males and females were significantly higher than those in the intact animals, indicating that neutered animals were more obese than intact animals. However, no differences were observed between animals neutered at 7 weeks of age and those neutered at 7 months of age. More recently, an epidemiological study of dogs in the United States found that the frequency of obesity was slightly lower in dogs that were neutered before 5.5 months of age when compared with dogs neutered after 6 months.[48] Together, these results indicate that early-age neutering presents the same level of risk of weight gain as does neutering at the traditional age of 6 to 9 months.

Caloric intake should generally be reduced after neutering to prevent weight gain. Neutering increases a pet's risk for overweight conditions via several mechanisms. The age that the dog or cat is neutered often corresponds with a natural decrease in the pet's growth rate and energy needs, which may lead to weight gain. Neutered animals also tend to consume more food and to have a reduced basal metabolic rate, both of which can contribute to an energy surplus if food intake is not controlled.

Genetic Predisposition (Breed)

Certain breeds of dogs reportedly have a disproportionately high incidence of obesity, although the breeds that are identified tend to vary with both the time of the study and region of the world. Early studies in the United Kingdom identified Cocker Spaniels, Labrador Retrievers, Shetland Sheepdogs, and the small Terrier breeds as being predisposed to obesity, while Boxers, German Shepherd Dogs, Fox Terriers, and the sight-hound breeds had a relatively low incidence.[49] Conversely, a study in Germany just a few years earlier reported that German Shepherd Dogs, Boxers, and Poodles were *more* likely to be overweight.[50] These differences suggest that the popularity of a breed and regional differences in type may influence breed predispositions. A more recent report of dogs in the United States identified Labrador Retrievers and Shetland Sheepdogs, as well as Golden Retrievers, Cocker Spaniels, Dachshunds, Miniature Schnauzers, Springer Spaniels, Chihuahuas, Basset Hounds, and Pugs as most likely to be overweight or obese.[8]

Although several environmental factors are also involved, genetically influenced body composition differences may partially explain the higher frequencies of overweight conditions in certain breeds of dogs. For example, it can be theorized that breeds that were developed for physical work and that naturally possess a higher muscle mass to body fat ratio will have a higher BMR than dogs of similar size that have a lower proportion of lean tissue and a higher proportion of body fat. One example is a comparison of Great Danes, bred for protection, with Newfoundlands, bred for cold-water rescue work. Adult Newfoundlands have lower energy requirements than adult Great Danes of similar weight;

this difference is speculated to be due to the higher proportion of lean body tissue seen in Great Danes.[51] More research that examines energy differences among dog breeds is necessary to increase understanding of possible predispositions to obesity. Few data are available concerning breed predilections to obesity in pet cats, but two studies have suggested that mixed-breed cats are more likely to be overweight than purebred cats, while another suggests that Manx cats show a higher frequency.[5,6,52] As purebred cats become increasingly popular and more breeds are developed, such predilections may become more evident in this species.

Endocrine Disorders

Two endocrine disorders that may influence body weight in companion animals are hypothyroidism and hyperadrenocorticism. Hypothyroidism results in a decreased BMR, which may in turn cause a predisposition for obesity. This disorder is diagnosed when clinical signs are observed and plasma levels of one or both of the thyroid hormone variants thyroxine (T_4) and triiodothyronine (T_3) are found to be below normal. Idiopathic atrophy of the thyroid gland is the most common cause of hypothyroidism in dogs. This disorder occurs most frequently in middle-aged and older dogs, and certain breeds show a higher incidence than the general population. These breeds include Golden Retrievers, Doberman Pinschers, Irish Setters, Boxers, Old English Sheepdogs, Miniature Schnauzers, Airedale Terriers, and some Spaniel breeds.[53] Spayed females are also more likely to develop the disorder than other dogs.[54] Hypothyroidism can occur in cats, but it is much less common and has not been well documented.

Clinical signs of hypothyroidism include lethargy, a dulled mental attitude, and exercise intolerance.[55] Common skin changes include alopecia; the development of a dry, coarse coat; and skin hyperpigmentation. Cold sensitivity and weight gain are clinical signs that result directly from the decreased BMR associated with hypothyroidism. However, only a small percentage of dogs exhibit all of these signs, and when obesity is seen, it is usually moderate. Regardless, an assessment of thyroid hormone levels should always be included in the differential diagnosis of obesity.

Hyperadrenocorticism (Cushing's syndrome) can also result in increased body size. This disorder is caused by the production of excess corticosteroids by the adrenal cortex, which may be caused by either an adrenal gland or a pituitary gland tumor. It is most common in middle-aged and older dogs, and breed predilections have been observed in Poodles, Dachshunds, Boxers, Brussels Griffons, and Boston Terriers.[56] Cushing's syndrome can occur in cats, but it is quite rare. The primary clinical signs of this disorder include polyuria, polydipsia, lethargy, hair loss, and the development of a pendulous abdomen. True obesity occurs in approximately 50% of the cases, although the presence of an enlarged abdomen may be perceived to be obesity by some pet owners. Diagnosis is based on adrenal function tests, which will differentiate between Cushing's-induced obesity and obesity as a result of other causes.

Alterations in Food Intake

Food intake is regulated in all animals by a complex system involving both internal physiological controls and external cues. Internal signals that affect appetite, hunger, and satiety include mechanical stimulation from the gastrointestinal tract; physiological responses to the sight, sound, and smell of food; and changes in plasma concentrations of specific nutrients, hormones, and peptides. External stimuli include factors such as food availability; the presence of other animals; the timing and size of meals; a food's composition, texture, and palatability; and the pet owner's beliefs and perceptions. Because owners exert complete control over the feeding of their dogs and cats, external cues that affect food intake are probably most important influences upon intake and the development of obesity in companion animals.

A well-researched external factor is feeding highly palatable foods that induce animals to overconsume. Studies with laboratory animals have shown that when rats are offered a highly palatable diet, they overeat and become obese.[57] This effect has been observed with high-fat diets, calorically dense diets, and "cafeteria" diets, which provide a variety of highly palatable food items.[58] Long-term exposure to highly palatable foods in human subjects also leads to permanent increases in body weight, fat cell size, and fat cell number. Although an endogenous predisposition to obesity and increased efficiency of weight gain may occur in some animals, the largest portion of weight gain observed when animals

are fed highly palatable diets is a direct result of overconsumption. Similarly, studies with human subjects have demonstrated that the quantity of food consumed varies directly with its palatability, and palatability does not appear to interact with levels of food deprivation. In other words, if food is perceived to be highly appealing, an individual tends to eat more of it, regardless of his or her initial level of hunger.[59]

Palatability is an important diet characteristic that is heavily promoted in the marketing of pet foods. Many owners select a product based upon their perceptions of the food's appeal and their pet's acceptance of the diet, rather than on indicators of nutritional adequacy. Semi-moist dog foods and treats contain variable amounts of simple sugars and other humectants that contribute to palatability. Wet foods and some premium dry foods are high in fat content. Fat contributes to both the palatability and caloric density of the food. Feeding pets highly palatable foods on an ad libitum basis may contribute to both the development and the maintenance of obesity because many dogs and cats readily overconsume these foods. Similarly, the common practice of feeding a variety of table scraps and other appealing treats to dogs and cats can induce many pets to overeat and gain excessive amounts of weight. For example, a retrospective study of dietary patterns in adult female dogs found that up to 50% of calories supplied to some dogs came from table scraps, particularly for the toy breed dogs.[60] Recent studies report that dogs fed many treats and table scraps or that are fed canned or homemade foods as their primary diet are more likely to be overweight.[8,61] Table scraps and some homemade diets that are fed to pets can also contain a high proportion of their calories from fat and thus contribute to a caloric imbalance.

The social setting of meals and pet owners' behavior and beliefs also influence eating behavior. Many animals increase food intake when consuming food in the presence of other pets. This process is called *social facilitation* and is usually more pronounced in dogs than in cats. In most dogs, social facilitation causes a moderate increase in food intake and an increased rate of eating. In some, the increase in food intake in response to another animal's presence can be extreme enough to cause weight gain. The owner's perceptions can also influence food intake. For example, results of a recent survey of cat owners reported that owners of overweight cats were more likely to interpret their cat's affiliative behaviors as requests for food than were owners of normal weight cats.[62] Similar results with dog owners have been reported; owners of overweight dogs tended to use food as a way to pacify all types of attention-seeking behaviors, thus using food to reinforce undesirable behaviors and as a "pet baby sitter" to induce the dog to be calm and quiet.

Similarly, meal frequency affects both food intake and metabolic efficiency. An increase in the number of meals per day results in increased energy loss to meal-induced thermogenesis (see Section 2, p. 60). There is also evidence in humans indicating that a decrease in lipogenesis (fat tissue synthesis) occurs when multiple meals are fed, as compared with consuming the same number of calories in only one or two meals.[63] However, if several meals are provided per day, portions must be strictly controlled. Increased feeding frequency often causes increased voluntary intake, thereby offsetting any metabolic benefits of multiple meals.

A final external factor that may be a contributing cause of obesity in companion animals is the nutrient composition of the diet. Nutrient composition affects both the efficiency of nutrient metabolism and the amount of food that is voluntarily consumed. Dietary fat is the primary nutritional factor influencing the development of obesity in humans. When fed ad libitum, high-fat diets lead to weight gain and obesity.[64] Although most animals decrease the volume of intake of a high-fat diet in an attempt to balance energy needs, the greater caloric density of the diet and its increased palatability usually offset this adjustment and result in an overall increase in energy intake. Additionally, the metabolic efficiency of converting dietary fat to body fat for storage is higher than is the efficiency of converting dietary carbohydrate or protein to body fat. For example, a recent study with dogs showed that modifying the diet's nutrient composition by increasing the proportion of fat by 8% caused a significant increase in abdominal fat deposition in the dogs, even though total caloric intake did not change.[65] Because dietary fat is more efficiently converted to body fat than protein or carbohydrate, if an animal is consuming more than its caloric requirement and if the excess calories are provided by fat, more weight will be gained than if the excess calories are coming from either carbohydrate or protein.

The caloric distribution of fat, carbohydrate, and protein is very important in determining a diet's potential contribution to weight imbalance in dogs and cats. As the percentage of metabolizable energy (ME) calories from fat increases in a pet food, the ability of the diet to meet the high energy demands of a hard-working dog also increases. However, if this diet is fed to a dog that does not need it, weight gain may occur if intake is not strictly monitored. Likewise, a food that contains a lower percentage of ME from fat will aid in weight loss or in the maintenance of normal body weight in a sedentary animal. The selection of a pet food should therefore always match the proportion of ME contributed by fat to the animal's lifestyle and activity level (Figure 28-1).

Important factors that can contribute to the development of obesity in dogs and cats include diet palatability, food composition and texture, and the timing and environment of meals. Just like their human counterparts, animals (especially dogs) tend to eat more, regardless of their initial level of hunger, when the food is highly palatable and presented in a social setting. More weight is gained when excess calories come from dietary fat than from protein or carbohydrate.

In recent years, the internal controls of hunger and satiety and their roles in obesity have received a great deal of attention (see Chapter 9, pp. 61-63). A wide range of neuroendocrine factors are involved in hunger and satiety. The functions and interactions of these compounds are complex and are influenced by numerous internal and external controls. Two peptides that may be important in the control of food intake in overweight animals are ghrelin and leptin. Ghrelin (i.e., growth hormone–releasing factor) is an enteric, orexigenic (appetite-stimulating) peptide. It stimulates the secretion of growth hormone and has been shown to increase appetite and food intake in human subjects and rats.[66] Plasma concentrations of ghrelin increase during the fasting state and decease postprandially. Recent studies have shown that obese dogs, like overweight human subjects, have lower circulating plasma ghrelin concentrations than do nonobese animals.[67] There is also evidence that obese subjects that have lost weight have higher plasma ghrelin levels.[68] It is postulated that this increase may

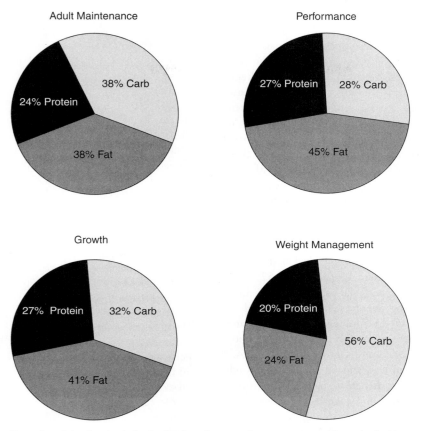

Figure 28-1   Examples of dog food caloric distributions (expressed as a percentage of metabolizable energy calories).

affect appetite and may be an important factor in the common tendency for previously overweight individuals to regain some or all of their lost weight.

Leptin is a cytokine produced by adipocytes that acts as a regulator of energy balance in the body. Its secretion is regulated by a variety of neuroendocrine factors, including insulin, glucocorticoids, and catecholamines. Circulating levels of leptin are directly proportional to the quantity of fat cells in the body; obese animals have chronically elevated plasma leptin.[69] Recent studies with dogs show that plasma leptin concentrations are highly correlated with body fat and its measure can be used as a quantitative marker for adiposity.[70] This relationship has also been demonstrated in cats, as well as a relationship between plasma leptin concentrations and insulin resistance, a finding that may be important for understanding factors that affect the development

of diabetes in overweight cats. While leptin appears to increase energy expenditure in normal weight individuals and reduces appetite when injected, its effects in obese dogs and cats and its relationship to the development and maintenance of overweight conditions are not completely clear. There is some research suggesting that vitamin A intake influences leptin by normalizing serum leptin levels during weight gain, which may contribute to reduced adiposity.[71] Other internal regulators of food intake that require more study include adiponectin, a cytokine that acts in synergy with leptin; tumor necrosis factor-alpha (TNF-α), a proinflammatory molecule that may be involved in insulin resistance; and a variety of uncoupling proteins (UCPs) that are located in the mitochondrial membrane and function to uncouple the respiration of adenosine triphosphate (ATP) synthesis and which may be involved in dietary thermogenesis.[72]

DIAGNOSIS

The diagnosis of obesity in companion animals should always include a veterinary examination for the presence of edema, ascites, hypothyroidism, hyperadrenocorticism, and diabetes mellitus. After these diseases have been ruled out, a comparison of the pet's current body weight with previous weight measurements or with the pet's weight shortly after reaching adulthood may be indicative of abnormal weight gain. Body weight in dogs and cats correlates moderately with body fat mass. Therefore recording a pet's body weight regularly provides a sensitive indicator of changes in body condition.[73] In some cases involving purebred dogs and cats, a comparison of the pet's body weight with the weights suggested by the breed's standard may also be a useful guideline for determining ideal body weight (Tables 28-1 and 28-2; also see Appendix 3, pp. 525-528).

Estimating percent body fat is the most accurate method of diagnosing obesity. Ultrasound provides a noninvasive, rapid method for estimating subcutaneous fat, but it is does not provide an estimate of whole body fat and is not practical in most clinical settings.[74] Likewise, estimates of lean and fat tissue in the body using the heavy isotope deuterium oxide is noninvasive and accurate, but requires sequential blood sampling and access to mass spectrometry equipment.[75] Dual energy x-ray absorptiometry (DEXA) has been shown to provide a very accurate measurement of total body fat and lean body mass and is frequently the method of choice in clinical trials.[76] This procedure has been used extensively in research settings to determine the body composition of many species, including dogs and cats.[77] However, DEXA is neither practical nor economical for use by most practicing veterinarians. Finally, bioelectrical impedance analysis (BIA) has been examined as a rapid and noninvasive clinical method for determining quantity of lean and fat tissue in pets.[78,79] BIA involves applying a series of electrodes to the surface of the animal's body and measuring degree of conductance and capacitrance when a low-level electrical current is applied. Because the body's fat free mass (FFM) contains more water than does its adipose tissue, lean tissue has a higher conducting volume than fat tissue. Conversely, fat cells cause greater impedance to the passage of current. BIA provides a comparative ratio of these two properties, and allows calculation of a value of FFM

TABLE 28-1 TYPICAL BODY WEIGHTS OF POPULAR BREEDS OF DOGS

Breed	Male (lb)	Female (lb)
Basset Hound	65-75	50-65
Beagle (13")	13-18	13-16
Beagle (15")	17-22	15-20
Boxer	55-70	50-60
Chihuahua	2-6	2-6
Chow Chow	45-50	40-50
Cocker Spaniel	25-30	20-25
Collie	65-75	50-65
Dachshund, Miniature	8-10	8-10
Dachshund, Standard	16-22	16-22
Dalmatian	50-65	45-55
Doberman Pinscher	65-80	55-70
English Springer Spaniel	49-55	40-45
German Shepherd	75-90	65-80
Golden Retriever	65-75	55-65
Labrador Retriever	65-80	55-70
Maltese	4-6	4-6
Miniature Schnauzer	16-18	12-16
Pekingese	10-14	10-14
Pomeranian	4-7	3-5
Poodle, Standard	50-60	45-55
Poodle, Miniature	17-20	15-20
Poodle, Toy	7-10	7-10
Rottweiler	80-95	70-85
Shetland Sheepdog	16-22	14-18
Shih Tzu	12-17	10-15
Siberian Husky	45-60	35-50
Yorkshire Terrier	4-7	3-6

and fat mass. Although commercially available BIA systems are available to practitioners, the recorded values are influenced by a number of factors, including but not limited to the pet's size, age, posture, hydration status, and fed or fasted state. Although BIA has been shown to be a reliable measure of body composition when all of these influencing factors are controlled, its sensitivity to environmental conditions and need for standardization make it currently impractical for most veterinary clinic settings.[80]

The most practical method for assessing excess body fat and obesity in dogs and cats is the use of morphometric techniques that combine the measurement and evaluation of visible body features and palpation of

TABLE 28-2 TYPICAL BODY WEIGHTS OF POPULAR BREEDS OF CATS

Breed	Male (lb)	Female (lb)
Abyssinian	7-10	6-8
American Shorthair	10-15	8-12
Birman	9-15	6-10
British Shorthair	12-18	9-15
Burmese	8-12	6-10
Cornish Rex	6-9	5-7
Devon Rex	8-10	5-8
Egyptian Mau	10-14	6-10
Exotic	7-14	6-10
Maine Coon	14-20	9-12
Norwegian Forest Cat	10-16	8-12
Ocicat	10-15	7-12
Persian	9-14	7-11
Ragdoll	12-20	8-15
Russian Blue	7-11	5-8
Scottish Fold	9-13	6-9
Siamese	11-15	8-12
Sphynx	8-12	6-9
Tonkinese	8-12	6-8

regions of the body that correspond to major adipose deposits. For dogs and cats, visual assessment is followed by palpation of the thickness of tissue overlying the rib cage, lumbar area, and tail base, and the thickness along the ventral abdomen. If a dog or cat is too thin, the ribs will be easily seen. An animal of normal weight will have barely visible ribs that can be easily felt when palpated. An overweight animal's ribs will not be visible and an overlying layer of fat can be felt. The pet is diagnosed as grossly obese if the ribs cannot be felt at all.

For practicing veterinarians and pet owners, visual assessment of dogs and cats can be standardized by using a body condition scoring (BCS) system. Several systems are available to practitioners and pet owners, all of which involve subjective ranking of body composition based upon visual assessment and palpation (Figures 28-2 and 28-3). The two most common systems use either five points (a score of 3 corresponds to ideal body condition) or nine points (a score of 5 corresponds to ideal body condition). Because the five-point system typically includes half-point assessments, the two scales are in practice very similar. Clinical trials have shown that body scoring systems provide a highly reliable method

for the diagnosis of obesity and are predictive of percent body fat.[81-83] Comparisons of body composition data collected using DEXA with assessments of body condition using a nine-point BCS revealed significant and positive correlations between body condition scores and percent body fat in both dogs and cats. Interestingly, although the predictive value of the scoring system was the same for both male and female pets, females of both species had a higher percentage of body fat than males that were assigned the same body condition score.[82,83] Two limitations of BCS systems are that their subjectivity can lead to wide interobserver variation and that some training in morphometric assessments may be needed. Recently, a seven-point system has been developed that provides an easy-to-use flow-chart and set of diagrams for pet owners.[84] However, this system still requires validation studies to determine if it effectively identifies overweight and obese pets.

BCS involves the assessment of several different areas of the body. Dogs and cats that are at their ideal body weight should have an hourglass shape when viewed from above, showing an observable waist behind the ribs (see Figures 28-2 and 28-3). In heavily coated animals, the waist should be easily palpated beneath the pet's hair coat. The loss of a waist as a result of excess fat between the muscles of the abdominal wall and the presence of a pendulous abdomen as a result of fat accumulation in intraabdominal sites are both indicative of excess body fat. Dogs have a tendency to develop fat deposits over the thorax and spine and around the base of the tail, while cats often accumulate fat just anterior to the inguinal region. In addition, overweight cats develop folds of skin and underlying fat in the flank area. Subjective evaluation of the animal's gait, exercise tolerance, and overall appearance can also be used to support a diagnosis of obesity.

The development of visual body condition assessment tools is also of benefit to pet owners. Veterinary practitioners can use illustrative charts to teach clients to monitor their pets' weights and body conditions. Standardized visual aids are helpful because an owner's perception of his pet's weight is often inaccurate. A survey of dog owners found that when clients were asked to identify whether their dog was overweight, underweight, or at an appropriate body weight, approximately 30% to 40% of owners of overweight dogs felt their dog was at an appropriate body weight.[83] Similarly, owners

Body Condition Scores

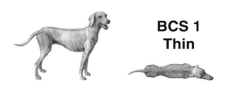

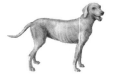

BCS 1
Thin

- Ribs, lumbar vertebrae, and pelvic bones visible at a distance and felt without pressure
- No palpable fat over tail base, spine, or ribs
- Diminished muscle mass
- Extreme concave abdominal tuck when viewed from side
- Severe hourglass shape when viewed from above

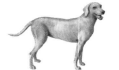

BCS 2
Underweight

- Ribs palpable with little pressure; may be visible
- Minimal palpable fat over ribs, spine, tail base
- Increased concave abdominal tuck when viewed from side
- Marked hourglass shape to waist when viewed from above

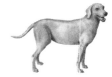

BCS 3
IDEAL

- Ribs and spine palpable with slight pressure but not visible; no excess fat covering
- Ribs can be seen with motion of dog
- Good muscle tone apparent
- Concave abdominal tuck when viewed from side
- Hourglass shape to waist when viewed from above

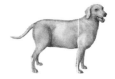

BCS 4
Overweight

- Ribs palpable with increased pressure; not visible and have excess fat covering
- Ribs not seen with motion of the dog
- General hefty appearance
- Abdominal concave tuck is reduced or absent when viewed from the side
- Loss of hourglass shape to waist with back slightly broadened when viewed from above

---

BCS 5
Obese

- Ribs and spine not palpable under a heavy fat covering
- Fat deposits visible over lumbar area, tail base, and spine
- Loss of hourglass shape to waist
- Complete loss of abdominal tuck with rounded abdomen
- Back is markedly broadened

Figure 28-2 Assessment of body conditions in the dog.

(Copyright © Procter & Gamble Co., Cincinnati, Ohio, 2009.)

Body Condition Scores

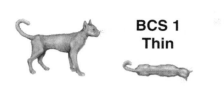
BCS 1
Thin

- Ribs, lumbar vertebrae, and pelvic bones visible at a distance and felt without pressure
- No palpable fat over tail base, spine, or ribs
- Diminished muscle mass
- Extreme concave abdominal tuck when viewed from side
- Extreme hourglass shape when viewed from above

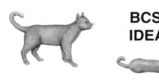
BCS 2
Underweight

- Ribs palpable with little pressure; may be visible
- Minimal palpable fat over ribs, spine, tail base
- Increased concave abdominal tuck when viewed from side
- Marked hourglass shape to waist when viewed from above
- No visible ventral fat pad

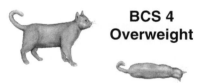
BCS 3
IDEAL

- Ribs and spine palpable with slight pressure but not visible; no excess fat covering
- Good muscle tone apparent
- Concave abdominal tuck when viewed from side
- Hourglass shape to waist when viewed from above
- Minimal ventral fat pad palpable

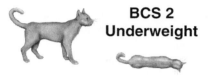
BCS 4
Overweight

- Ribs palpable with increased pressure; not visible and have excess fat covering
- General hefty appearance
- Abdominal concave tuck is reduced or absent when viewed from the side
- Loss of hourglass shape to waist with back slightly widened when viewed from above
- Visible ventral fat pad

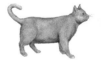

BCS 5
Obese

- Ribs and spine not palpable under a heavy fat covering
- Fat deposits visible over lumbar area, tail base, and spine
- Loss of hourglass shape to waist
- Complete loss of abdominal tuck
- Back is markedly widened
- Prominent ventral fat pad, which may sway from side to side when walking

Figure 28-3   Assessment of body conditions in the cat.
(Copyright © Procter & Gamble Co., Cincinnati, Ohio, 2009.)

of overweight cats tended to underestimate their cat's score on a standard body condition scale.[85] Interestingly, when cat owners and veterinarians were asked to select overweight cats from a series of illustrations of cats' silhouettes, owners and veterinarians were in close agreement as to which animals were overweight. Because some owners may be unable or reluctant to recognize weight gain or obesity in their own pet, the use of body condition charts may be helpful to veterinarians as a tool to teach about ideal body weight and to convince some owners of their pet's overweight condition.

Comparison of a pet's current body weight to an estimated ideal body weight, visual assessment and the use of body condition scoring are the most practical and reliable means of diagnosing obesity. Dogs and cats at ideal body weight should have an hourglass shape when viewed from above, showing an observable and easily palpable waist. Dogs have a tendency to develop fat deposits over the thorax and spine and around the base of the tail, while cats often accumulate fat just anterior to the inguinal region. Subjective evaluation gait, exercise tolerance, and overall appearance can also be used to support a diagnosis of obesity.

TREATMENT OF OBESITY

The short-term goal of the treatment of obesity is to reduce body fat stores. Although there are a variety of ways to attain this goal, it ultimately relies on the induction of a negative energy balance. Most simply, negative energy balance can be accomplished by restricting dietary intake, stimulating total energy expenditure, or a combination of the two. The long-term goal of treatment is for the pet to attain ideal body weight and condition and to maintain this weight for the remainder of his or her life. Three important components must be included in all weight-reduction programs for companion animals: pet owner education, exercise, and dietary modification. Dietary modification and exercise create an energy deficit that will result in weight loss. Behavior modification can be helpful in changing the owner's and the pet's behaviors, which will aid in weight loss and the prevention of weight regain.

Pet Owner Education and Commitment

Successful treatment of obesity in pets relies entirely upon the pet owner's understanding of and commitment to the weight-loss plan. Similar to human weight-loss programs, lack of compliance or long-term commitment by the owner can lead a pet to fail to lose weight or rapidly regain weight that is lost in the early stage of the program. Some owners are reluctant to admit that their pet is overweight, while others find it difficult to change many of the habits that contributed to their pet's weight gain. There is also evidence that owners tend to overreport the amount of exercise that they provide to their dogs, suggesting that misperceptions about a pet's activity needs may be an important contributor to overweight conditions.[86] Owner education should therefore include a candid discussion of the serious health risks and reduced quality of life associated with overweight conditions in dogs and cats. Once a program has been developed for a pet, including biweekly or monthly check-ups and evaluations of body weight encourage compliance and increase the chance of success.[87]

Identifying and changing habits of the owner that may have contributed to the pet's initial weight gain is essential. Such habits may include providing the pet with high-calorie table scraps, feeding a palatable and energy-dense food free-choice, encouraging or allowing begging, and frequently feeding dog biscuits and treats. Some alternative behaviors that can be practiced include keeping the pet out of the kitchen while meals are being prepared, decreasing the number of treats given per day or feeding only treats formulated for weight control, and breaking treats into small pieces and giving the pet only a small piece at a time. Owners can also be encouraged to provide attention, play, and exercise instead of food treats, especially in response to attention-seeking behaviors. Careful attention to daily activity patterns and the gradual introduction of increased duration and in some cases, intensity, of exercise is an important component of all weight-loss programs (see p. 327). Some owners may need to keep their dog or cat out of the dining area during mealtimes and to eliminate all "people foods" from their pet's diet. If the owner is in the habit of providing food ad libitum, they must be instructed to gradually switch the pet to a portion-controlled feeding regimen (see p. 335). Establishing a strictly regulated schedule so that all meals are provided at the same time each day can help to eliminate begging.

Identifying and changing habits of the owner that may have contributed to their pet's weight gain is essential for successful weight loss. Behaviors that can be practiced include keeping the pet out of the kitchen while meals are being prepared, decreasing the number and size of treats that are fed, and substituting play and attention for food reinforcers. In addition, portion-controlled meal feeding must be used during weight loss programs and a regular daily feeding schedule should be established.

Exercise

The inclusion of moderate, regular exercise in the treatment of obese pets affects body weight in several ways. Increased activity has the direct benefit of raising daily energy expenditure and thus contributing to the energy deficit that is necessary for weight loss. An increase in exercise also aids in the regulation of food intake. Studies with animals and humans have shown that caloric intake varies proportionally with energy expenditure during moderate to high levels of exercise. However, reduction of activity to a completely sedentary level results in increased food intake and eventual weight gain.[88,89] It appears that the normal physiological regulators of caloric intake do not function properly below a certain minimum level of physical activity, and an uncoupling of the relationship between energy expenditure and energy intake occurs. Even a small change in an overweight pet's activity level may be beneficial because of the possibility that normal physiological controls of food intake may be restored when activity increases.

Exercise also causes desirable changes in body composition. Regular and continued exercise results in a higher proportion of lean tissue to fat tissue. Because lean tissue is more metabolically active than fat tissue, increasing lean tissue contributes to the maintenance of a higher BMR during weight loss. Even during moderate weight-loss programs, between 10% and 25% of weight loss will be contributed by lean tissue.[90,91] As a result, a decline in metabolic rate naturally occurs in response to caloric restriction, resulting in a decreased rate of weight loss over time. The inclusion of regular exercise along with caloric restriction minimizes or completely eliminates this decline, allowing continued weight loss throughout the program.[92] Because regular physical activity helps to maintain lean body mass and elevated BMR, exercise is also an important factor in preventing weight regain following a successful weight-loss program.

Although not yet demonstrated in dogs and cats, some of the benefits of exercise to obese human subjects occur even in the absence of significant weight loss. For example, exercise contributes to the amelioration of the metabolic abnormalities associated with overweight conditions. These include improved glucose tolerance and insulin sensitivity, and reduced leptin insensitivity and adipocyte-induced inflammatory responses.[93-95] While weight loss improves glucose homeostasis and insulin sensitivity in overweight pets, it is not known if some of the metabolic benefits of exercise occur in dogs and cats independently of changes in body weight. Finally, improved mobility and a reduction in signs of pain and lameness associated with weight loss can contribute to a pet's interest in and enjoyment of exercise and to long-term improvements in activity.[96]

Physical activity should always be initiated at a low level with animals that are accustomed to a completely sedentary lifestyle. Recommendations for exercise should consider the pet's age, degree of obesity, and the presence of chronic health problems that may impact exercise tolerance. A general guideline of 15 to 30 minutes of moderate activity per day, provided at least 5 days per week, is usually a safe starting point. Daily exercise is ideal. Both the duration and the intensity of the exercise can be increased as the animal begins to lose weight and increases its exercise tolerance. Outdoor walking, running, swimming, or playing fetch and other games are recommended forms of exercise for dogs. Although it is sometimes difficult to induce an increase in physical activity in cats, many will enjoy walking outside on a harness or chasing and playing with toys inside. Other approaches include using treat balls that require batting and chasing to obtain food, and placing the cat's food bowls in areas of the home that require climbing stairs or jumping up. Whatever the chosen activity, it is important that the exercise program is regular and continues even after the weight-loss program has been completed.

Regular exercise contributes to the energy deficit during a weight-loss program, positively affects an animal's normal physiological control of food intake and helps to reduce the loss of lean tissue, which contributes to maintaining a normal resting metabolic rate during weight loss.

Dietary Management: Caloric Restriction

The first step to be taken when planning a diet is to weigh the pet and set a goal for weight reduction (Table 28-3 and Box 28-3). The degree of caloric restriction needed for weight loss is then estimated, and an appropriate food is selected. A final component of dietary management is the type of feeding regimen and schedule that is use.

WEIGHT-LOSS GOALS   Dogs and cats that are 15% or more above their ideal body weight should be placed on a weight-loss program. When initiating such a program, the determined rate of weight loss should be high enough to ensure a noticeable change within several weeks, yet low enough to minimize excessive hunger and the loss of lean body tissue. Because of the large variation in size and degree of obesity in individual animals, a recommended percentage of body weight loss per week should be used rather than a set quantity of weight loss. Studies with humans have shown that weekly rates of loss that are greater than 2% to 3% of body weight are unhealthy because lean body tissue losses are too great.[97] Similarly, excessively rapid weight loss in obese dogs and cats increases the risk of health problems and the development of undesirable behavior changes (see p. 331). Rapid weight loss is specifically contraindicated in cats because of the risk of developing hepatic lipidosis. Alternatively, if the rate of loss is too low (0.5% or less), owners may lose interest and motivation because results will not be observed for several weeks. Therefore a goal of 1% to 2% per week is recommended for dogs and a rate of 1% to 1.5% is recommended for cats.[98] Depending on the degree of obesity, this translates to a program that lasts from a few months to as long as 1 year. For example, an adult dog with an ideal body weight of 25 kilograms (kg) (55 pounds [lb]) that actually weighs 30 kg (66 lb) should lose between 0.3 and 0.6 kg (0.7 to 1.3 lb) per week. A starting point of about 1 lb of weight loss per week can be used as a target loss when calculating this dog's energy needs for the weight-loss program; this can be adjusted as needed based upon the dog's current intake and response to the caloric restriction (see Table 28-3 and Box 28-3). If this dog loses an average of 0.7 lb per week, ideal body weight will be attained within 4 months.

RECOMMENDED LEVEL OF CALORIC RESTRICTION   When determining the number of calories needed for weight loss, an estimate of the pet's caloric needs based upon current body weight must first be calculated. Although some nutritionists recommend using a pet's ideal body weight for this calculation, the accurate determination of ideal weight can be difficult for the practitioner and owner if the pet was overweight throughout development or has been overweight for a long period of time. Using current body weight provides a slightly higher initial caloric estimate for weight loss, but this value can be reduced gradually based upon the pet's response to feeding. Because most overweight pets are relatively inactive, equations that are formulated for inactive adults should be used for these calculations (Box 28-4; see Box 28-3).

A reasonable guideline for the initial caloric restriction for dogs is 60% of calories needed to maintain current body weight (see Table 28-3 and Box 28-3).[96,99] A slightly higher intake (70%) will result in a slower rate of loss, while reducing to 50% will lead to a more rapid rate of loss. Because of the health risks associated with rapid weight loss in cats, a more conservative initial restriction of 90% is recommended for cats. As with dogs, severe caloric restriction in cats results in increased losses of lean body tissue and lower losses of body fat. In addition, rapid weight loss increases the risk of developing idiopathic hepatic lipidosis, a serious and life-threatening disorder in cats (see Section 5, pp. 431-434). A useful approach with cats is to begin the weight-loss program by feeding 90% of maintenance energy requirement (MER) and evaluate weight and body condition for 2 weeks.[100] If rate of weight loss is not adequate, restriction can be gradually reduced to 60% of MER, again monitoring for 2 weeks. If the cat still does not lose weight, intake can be restricted further, but reductions should be gradual and closely supervised by the cat's veterinarian.

TABLE 28-3 ENERGY REQUIREMENTS FOR WEIGHT LOSS IN DOGS AND CATS

Dogs

Current weight (lb)	Current weight (kg)	ME* (kcal/day)	60% of ME (kcal/day)	Amount† (cups/day)
5	2.3	177	106	0.42
10	4.5	294	176	0.70
15	6.8	400	240	0.96
20	9.1	497	298	1.19
25	11.4	589	353	1.41
30	13.6	673	404	1.62
35	15.9	756	454	1.82
40	18.2	837	502	2.00
45	20.5	915	549	2.20
50	22.7	988	593	2.37
55	25.0	1062	637	2.55
60	27.3	1135	681	2.72
65	29.5	1202	721	2.88
70	31.8	1272	763	3.05
75	34.1	1340	804	3.22
80	36.4	1408	845	3.38
85	38.6	1471	883	3.53
90	40.9	1536	922	3.68
95	43.2	1600	960	3.84
100	45.5	1664	998	4.00
105	47.7	1724	1034	4.14
110	50.0	1786	1072	4.29
115	52.3	1847	1108	4.43
120	54.5	1905	1143	4.57

Cats

Current weight (lb)	Current weight (kg)	ME* (kcal/day)	60% of ME (kcal/day)	Amount‡ (cups/day)
4	1.8	164	98.4	0.33
5	2.3	181	109	0.36
6	2.7	193	116	0.39
7	3.2	207	124	0.41
8	3.6	217	130	0.43
9	4.1	228	137	0.46
10	4.5	237	142	0.47
11	5.0	247	148	0.49
12	5.4	255	153	0.51
13	5.9	264	158	0.53
14	6.4	273	164	0.55
15	6.8	280	168	0.56
16	7.3	288	173	0.58
17	7.7	294	176	0.59
18	8.2	302	181	0.60

Continued

TABLE 28-3　ENERGY REQUIREMENTS FOR WEIGHT LOSS IN DOGS AND CATS—cont'd

		CATS		
CURRENT WEIGHT (LB)	CURRENT WEIGHT (KG)	ME* (KCAL/DAY)	60% OF ME (KCAL/DAY)	AMOUNT‡ (CUPS/DAY)
19	8.6	307	184	0.61
20	9.1	314	188	0.63

ME, Metabolizable energy.

*Dogs: ME (inactive adult) = $95 \times W_{kg}^{0.75}$; cats (overweight): ME = $130 \times W_{kg}^{0.40}$.

†Calculated for a weight-control dog food that provides 250 kcal/cup. Adjustments must be made for foods with higher or lower caloric densities.

‡Calculated for a weight-control cat food that provides 300 kcal/cup. Adjustments must be made for foods with higher or lower caloric densities.

BOX 28-3　CALCULATION OF ENERGY NEEDS FOR A WEIGHT-LOSS PROGRAM (DOG)

TARGET WEIGHT LOSS PER WEEK

Ideal body weight = 25 kg (55 lb)

Actual body weight = 30 kg (66 lb)

Target weight loss per week =
30 kg × 2% = 0.6 kg/week (1.3 lb)

This dog should lose up to 1.3 lb per week when placed on a weight-loss program.

CALORIC REQUIREMENT FOR WEIGHT LOSS

Metabolizable energy requirement (inactive adult) =
$95 \times W_{kg}^{0.75}$

$(30 \text{ kg})^{0.75} \times 95 = 1217.8$ (approximately 1218 kcal/day)

Caloric restriction for weight loss =
1218 × 0.60 = 730.8 kcal/day

Volume of food to feed

　Diet A (400 kcal/cup) = 731/400 = 1.8 cups per day

　Diet B (250 kcal/cup) = 731/250 = 2.9 cups per day

BOX 28-4　CALCULATION OF ENERGY NEEDS FOR A WEIGHT-LOSS PROGRAM (CAT)

TARGET WEIGHT LOSS PER WEEK

Ideal body weight = 4.5 kg (10 lb)

Actual body weight = 6.5 kg (14.3 lb)

Target weight loss per week =
6.5 × 1.5% = 0.1 kg/week (0.2 lb)

This cat should lose approximately 0.2 lb per week when placed on a weight-loss program.

CALORIC REQUIREMENT FOR WEIGHT LOSS

Metabolizable energy requirement (overweight adult) =
$130 \times W_{kg}^{0.40}$

$(6.5 \text{ kg})^{0.40} \times 130 = 275$ kcal/day

Caloric restriction for weight loss =
275 × 0.60 = 160 kcal/day

Volume of food to feed

　Diet A (400 kcal/cup) = 160/400 = 0.40 cups per day

　Diet B (300 kcal/cup) = 160/300 = 0.53 cups per day

Once the initial daily caloric value for weight loss has been calculated, this value can be compared to the number of calories that the pet is currently consuming. This information can be obtained by requiring the owner to record all of the pet's food intake for several days, including brand names and label information, to allow an estimation of total calories. If the caloric value for weight reduction is not sufficiently lower than the estimated number of calories that the pet is reportedly consuming each day, adjustments should be made to ensure that the initial caloric deficit is lower than the pet's current intake. Finally, because there is some evidence that female dogs require greater reductions in daily energy intake than male dogs to achieve a similar degree of weight loss, the sex of the dog should be considered when estimating a starting energy deficit and making adjustments.[101]

RISKS OF SEVERE CALORIC RESTRICTION

Severe caloric deficits will naturally result in more rapid rates of weight loss. However, as stated previously, rapid weight loss causes greater losses of lean body tissue.

Although dogs can lose weight and maintain health on energy deficits as low as 40% of maintenance requirements, the long-term use of this level of restriction leads to reduced BMR and other indicators of slowed metabolic rate, such as reduced serum T_3 levels.[102] There is also evidence that, similar to human subjects, dogs react to rapid weight loss with an increased tendency for a rebound effect, meaning that they regain all of the lost weight shortly after finishing the weight-loss program.[103] The underlying cause for this is presumed to be the reduction in metabolic rate and possibly in voluntary activity that accompany excessive and rapid losses of lean body mass.[104] Severely restricted diets also exacerbate feelings of hunger, leading to undesirable behaviors such as begging for food, raiding garbage, or stealing food. Pet owners can be especially sensitive to these changes and may not continue with a program that appears to cause their pet distress or that induces behavior problems.

Examples The estimated daily caloric requirement of an overweight 66-lb dog is 1218 kilocalories (kcal) (see Box 28-3). Caloric restriction to 60% of this requirement equals 731 kcal/day. If a food that contains 400 kcal per 8-ounce (oz) cup is fed, this dog should receive about 1.8 cups of food per day. Conversely, if a weight-reduction food containing 250 kcal/cup is fed, the dog should receive about 3 cups of food per day. A caloric deficit of 3500 kcal is necessary to lose 1 lb of body fat. The daily calorie deficit provided by this regimen is 487 kcal. Therefore this amount of food should result in a loss of approximately 1 lb per week (7 × 487 = 3409 kcal). If exercise is included in the program, the additional energy deficit will be accounted for by increased energy expenditure, and a slightly greater weight loss will be seen. An example of caloric estimates for an overweight cat is provided in Box 28-4.

MONITORING WEIGHT LOSS During the weight-loss program, the pet should be weighed once each week, and a record or graph of weight loss should be kept. Caloric intake can be adjusted as the pet loses weight (see Table 28-3). If possible, follow-up veterinarian visits should be made every 2 to 3 weeks to record progress. Portion-controlled feeding should be used, even if a commercially prepared, reducing diet is fed. Portion-controlled feeding allows strict monitoring of a pet's total food intake and removes the opportunity for the pet to spontaneously increase its intake of

a reduced-energy food. It may also be helpful to feed several small meals per day rather than one or two large meals. This practice may decrease signs of hunger and increase the energy losses of meal-induced thermogenesis.[86] Once the target weight has been reached, the daily volume of food can be slowly increased until an amount that maintains ideal body weight is provided.

A weight-loss goal of 1% to 2% per week is recommended for dogs and 1% to 1.5% is recommended for cats. A reasonable guideline for initial caloric restriction is 60% of calories needed to maintain current body weight in dogs and 90% in cats. Although more severe caloric deficits will result in more rapid rates of loss, it also leads to increased loss of lean body tissue, excessive hunger and related behavior problems, and increased health risks.

Dietary Management: Types of Foods for Weight Loss

Some pet owners regularly feed their pets table scraps and a large number of treats. When this is the case, simply eliminating all of the extra tidbits and restricting the pet's intake to 70% to 90% of its body weight requirement may lead to adequate weight loss. This is the preferred method to use with pets that are only slightly overweight, are exercised regularly, and have well-motivated owners. When this type of caloric restriction is instituted, pets will naturally be hungrier than usual, and begging behaviors may increase proportionately. In addition, weight loss may be relatively slow due to the smaller caloric deficit. This may lead to poor compliance as owners will fail to see an appreciative weight change within several weeks. The lower limit of this type of dietary regimen, in terms of the caloric deficit, is set by the nutrient requirements of the dog or cat. Because a normal maintenance diet is being fed, it is imperative that the quantity provided is still sufficient to meet the pet's total nutrient requirements. Commercial pet foods that are formulated for adult maintenance contain adequate amounts of protein, fat, vitamins, and minerals to meet the needs of an animal at normal weight that is consuming adequate calories. If the volume of a maintenance diet is reduced too drastically in an effort to limit calories, nutrient deficiencies may develop.

Commercially prepared foods with reduced energy densities are formulated to contain adequate levels of nutrients while supplying fewer calories. Therefore, in cases of moderate to severe obesity or when owners are not strongly motivated to change their habits, a change of diet to a commercially prepared food with a reduced energy density is recommended for weight reduction.

DIETARY FAT The most efficient way to reduce the energy density of a food is to reduce its proportion of fat. On a weight basis, fat provides more than twice the calories of carbohydrate or protein and is also highly palatable to most dogs and cats. Therefore decreasing the fat content of a pet food reduces the food's caloric density and may also slightly decrease palatability. The type of fat included in the food is also an important consideration. As discussed previously, adipose tissue is metabolically active; fat cells produce proinflammatory cytokines that may play a role in some of the chronic diseases that are associated with obesity. Therefore, including a source of n-3 fatty acids at levels that shift the body's response away from proinflammatory substances may contribute to a reduction in chronic inflammation as the pet loses weight. Although there is some support for a beneficial antiinflammatory effect of n-3 fatty acids during weight loss in human subjects, not all studies have shown a benefit and studies that specifically target dogs and cats are needed.[105,106] Other potential benefits of including n-3 fatty acids to weight-loss diets include a reduction in plasma insulin and improved glucose tolerance during weight loss.[107]

A form of linoleic acid called *conjugated linoleic acid* (CLA) has also been studied for its effects during weight loss. CLA is comprised of a mixture of linoleic acid isomers that are produced by rumen and colonic bacteria. Including CLA in the diets of mice and pigs has been shown to reduce body fat and increase lean tissue, even when fed ad libitum.[108,109] Some of the theorized mechanisms underlying these benefits include inhibition of lipogenesis and increased lipolysis via competitive inhibition of enzyme systems involved in lipid metabolism. However, although CLA has been beneficial in other species, studies of CLA in dogs and cats report conflicting results. While some have reported mild improvements in body composition, others have failed to find a benefit.[110-112]

Almost all pet foods that are formulated for weight loss contain lower concentrations of fat than typical adult maintenance foods. Commercial, low-fat (lite) dry foods contain between 6% and 11% fat on a dry-matter basis (DMB). This percentage is equivalent to 15% to 26% of the calories in a diet that has an energy density of 3500 kcal/kg. The lower limit of fat content for a food is dictated by the need to provide essential fatty acids, fat that is needed for the transport of fat-soluble vitamins, and for sufficient palatability to ensure the food is accepted by the pet. While almost all of the pet foods that are marketed for weight reduction contain decreased levels of fat, significant differences occur in their levels of protein, digestible carbohydrate, and indigestible fiber.

PROTEIN Protein level in reducing diets is an important consideration with both dogs and cats to ensure that adequate essential amino acids are still provided as the pet is fed restricted calories. Studies with both dogs and cats have shown that increasing protein in weight-loss diets improves body composition; increased body fat is lost while loss of lean body tissue is minimized.[101,113,114] For example, overweight cats fed restricted amounts of a food containing 46% of ME as protein lost more body fat and retained more lean body tissue than did cats fed the same amount (calories) of a food containing 36% protein, even though overall weight change was the same between the two groups.[114] Similarly, when overweight dogs were fed restricted levels of diets containing either 20%, 30%, or 39% of ME from protein, all of the dogs lost weight, but those that were fed the 39% protein diet had the greater loss of body fat and the smallest loss of lean mass.[115]

Another benefit to increasing the proportion of protein in a weight-loss food is that protein has a higher dietary thermogenic response than fat. In other words, a high proportion of dietary protein increases the animal's net energy expenditure by increasing the amount of heat lost in response to meal ingestion. In addition, although not yet demonstrated in dogs or cats, there is evidence that high-protein diets may contribute to satiety.[116] This may occur because the conversion of excess amino acids to glucose via gluconeogenesis induces less insulin secretion and subsequently delays the onset of postprandial hypoglycemia, which is a potent signal of hunger. The type of protein and the proportions of its composite amino acids may influence satiety to differing degrees. A recent study with

TABLE 28-4 LOW-FAT/HIGH-FIBER VS. LOW-FAT/HIGH-CARBOHYDRATE REDUCING DIETS

	FAT (%)	CRUDE FIBER (%)	ENERGY DENSITY (KCAL/CUP)	ME ENERGY (% OF GROSS ENERGY)	FECAL SCORE (1-5)*	FECAL VOLUME (G/DAY)
Diet A	7.0	14.2	250	67.3	3.9	162.4
Diet B	9.7	3.0	270	87.8	4.5	46.5

Data on file at Procter & Gamble Pet Health and Nutrition Center, Lewisburg, Ohio.
ME, Metabolizable energy.
*Fecal score: 1 = watery, diarrhea; 5 = firm, compact.

dogs showed that six adult, normal weight dogs demonstrated increased satiety when fed ad libitum in response to a food that was high in both protein and fiber, but this response was not seen when fed increased protein alone.[117] Finally, providing adequate protein in the weight reduction foods for cat is especially important because of the cat's higher protein requirement and inability to adjust to drastic reductions in protein intake.[118] The risk of developing hepatic lipidosis during weight loss is positively correlated with the level of protein included in the reducing diet in cats.[119] Therefore weight reduction foods for cats should contain at least 30% of calories from high-quality protein.

Increasing the proportion of protein calories in a weight-loss food is necessary to ensure that adequate essential amino acids are still provided as the pet is fed restricted calories. Increasing protein in weight-loss diets also improves body composition; increased body fat is lost while loss of lean body tissue is minimized. Providing adequate protein in weight reduction foods for cats is especially important because of the cat's higher protein requirement, inability to adjust to drastic reductions in protein intake, and risk for developing hepatic lipidosis during weight loss.

CARBOHYDRATE When reduced energy foods are formulated for weight loss, part of the fat can be replaced by protein, and part can be replaced by digestible carbohydrate. Carbohydrate has less than half of the caloric density of fat and, similar to protein, produces a higher dietary thermogenic response than fat.[120] Foods that replace fat with complex carbohydrate without adding excessive levels of indigestible fiber retain the level of digestibility of higher-fat foods, but contain less

total calories (see Figure 28-1). An added advantage is that, unlike reducing diets that are high in fiber, this approach does not result in increased fecal volume or defecation frequency or have a negative impact upon stool quality (see Table 28-4, *diet B*). Because many overweight pets are glucose intolerant, carbohydrates that contribute to a relatively slow increase in blood glucose levels and modulate insulin response are the best choice.[121] Examples include corn, sorghum, and barley. Conversely, because rice is highly digestible and rapidly absorbed, it is not a good choice for inclusion in weight-loss foods (see Chapter 29, pp. 348-350).

Several studies have evaluated the efficacy of feeding low-fat, normal-fiber diets to overweight and obese cats for the purpose of weight reduction.[122,123] When pet cats that were up to 40% overweight were fed a low-fiber, moderate-fat, reducing diet to provide 60% of their calculated MER, all of the cats lost significant amounts of weight, and more than half reached close to their ideal body weight within 18 weeks.[122] Cats that were more than 30% above their ideal body weight at the start of the study took longer than 4 months to achieve targets weights, but they still lost weight consistently throughout the study.

In a subsequent study, a group of obese cats were fed a low-fat, low-fiber diet restricted to intakes that were calculated to achieve 1.5% body weight loss for a 16-week period.[123] The diet contained 9.2% fat, 1.9% fiber, and 33.5% high-quality protein. Fat contributed 23% of the ME calories in the diet. Cats lost an average of 21% of their body weight and 49% of their body fat. DEXA body composition analysis showed that lean body mass decreased only slightly, leading to a mean final body condition that was lower in fat and higher in lean tissue. Ultrasound-guided liver biopsies were obtained at the start and periodically throughout the study to monitor the effect of caloric restriction upon the development of hepatic lipidosis. Liver histology showed no lipid infiltration, indicating that the weight-loss program did not present a risk for the development of hepatic lipidosis. Results of these studies indicate that a low-fiber, low-calorie diet for cats can effectively and safely result in weight losses in overweight pets.

Most commercial pet foods formulated for weight loss or for consumption by sedentary pets have decreased levels of fat. Part of the fat can be replaced by protein, and part can be replaced with digestible carbohydrates, such as corn, barley, or sorghum. Replacing fat with digestible carbohydrate maintains a food's level of digestibility and does not negatively impact fecal volume, defecation frequency, or stool quality.

FIBER   An alternative way that the caloric density of a diet can be decreased is by diluting calories through the addition of indigestible fiber. The rationale is that in addition to reducing the food's caloric density, the increased bulk will contribute to satiety and decrease voluntary energy consumption. However, while dietary fiber does effectively dilute caloric density (see pp. 334-335), effects upon satiety in dogs and cats have not been consistently demonstrated, and the interpretation of results of published studies is controversial. One approach to examine satiety in dogs and cats is by measuring intake of a challenge meal. This procedure involves providing animals with a high-fiber food that is periodically followed by the offer of an additional meal later in the day. The premise is that if satiety is induced by increased fiber, dogs will consume less of the challenge meal, compared with dogs that are fed a normal maintenance diet. Although variable results are reported, in most cases feeding pets a high-fiber diet has not significantly influenced the volume of food that was ingested in the challenge meal.[124,125] Interpretation of results from this type of study are easily confounded by factors such as other nutrient alterations in addition to increased fiber, the amount of food fed prior to the challenge meal, the time that the animals are allowed access to food, and the interval after the last feeding. In addition, results may differ depending upon whether the animals are overweight and if they are limit-fed versus allowed to eat free-choice.

In one study, dogs fed a diet containing 10% crude fiber, 2.7% soluble fiber, and reduced fat consumed fewer total calories per day than dogs fed a lower-fiber food.[126] However, this difference was due to a dilution effect of the daily diet that was fed on a portion-controlled basis, not to reduced consumption of the challenge meal. When offered the challenge meal, dogs fed the high-fiber diet consumed the same volume of food as control dogs that were not fed the high-fiber, low-fat diet. As a result, when total calories consumed were calculated, the dogs fed the high-fiber, low-fat diet consumed fewer calories, principally because the energy density of the diet that was fed was significantly lower. The differences were due to portion-controlled feeding of a diluted diet, and it is questionable whether any significant effect upon satiety was induced. Similar results were reported in a more recent study.[112] While dogs fed a high-fiber food (22% crude fiber) consumed fewer total calories per day than dogs fed a normal-fiber food, they consumed a significantly higher volume of food per day, suggesting an attempt to balance energy needs by increasing (not decreasing) food intake. Although the authors interpreted this as a satiating effect of fiber, it is likely that the dogs consuming the high-fiber food were attempting to consume adequate calories but were limited by gut fill rather than internal signals of satiety.

Optimal levels of dietary fiber are necessary in the diets of all pets, regardless of weight. Fiber is needed for proper functioning of the gastrointestinal tract and as a source of short-chain fatty acids (SCFAs) for intestinal cells. However, the weight-reducing effect of high levels of indigestible fiber in the diet is questionable, and excessive fiber intake can produce a number of adverse side effects. High intakes of dietary fiber cause decreases in nutrient digestion and availability through interference with absorption of lipids, calcium, zinc, and iron, and increased losses of fecal energy and nitrogen.[127,128] Increasing the fiber in foods that are formulated for weight loss in dogs has also been shown to reduce the food's protein digestibility.[117] If a diet is simultaneously high in indigestible fiber and low in fat or other nutrients, it is possible that long-term feeding may result in nutrient deficiencies. Feeding restricted amounts for the purpose of weight loss increases this risk.

Increasing nonfermentable (insoluble) fiber also affects fecal production and defecation frequency. Results of studies with dogs have shown that providing more than 10% of dietary dry matter (DM) as fiber causes increased fecal production.[129] Fecal quality is also affected by the type of fiber that is used.[130,131] When high amounts of nonfermentable fiber are included in the diet, feces are dry and hard, which may lead to constipation. In contrast, if too much fermentable fiber is fed, this can lead to loose, watery stools, or diarrhea. Excess fiber consumption also causes increased gas production and defecation frequency. Although not usually a health risk, these latter side effects are certainly disagreeable to most pet owners (see Table 28-4). In addition, some high-fiber diets appear to have reduced palatability, especially for cats. This may induce further reductions in intake, leading to nutrient deficiencies or weight loss that is too rapid.

Although it is without question that fiber dilutes calories in a food, the lack of conclusive evidence for benefits to satiety in dogs and cats coupled with associated risks of reduced nutrient digestibility and negative effects upon defecation frequency and stool quality make the use of excessively high levels of indigestible fiber in weight-loss foods a poor choice for most weight-loss programs for dogs and cats.

L-CARNITINE   L-carnitine is an amino acid derivative (from the amino acids lysine and methionine) that is produced endogenously in the liver of most mammals. The cat is unique in that L-carnitine is synthesized in the kidney.[132] A primary function of carnitine is to facilitate the transport of long-chain fatty acids (as acyl-carnitine) across the inner mitochondrial membrane for beta-oxidation. Because L-carnitine is essential for the metabolism of fatty acids for energy, a deficiency results in reduced oxidation of fat for energy and affects both fat metabolism and energy production in the body. Carnitine is classified as a conditionally essential nutrient because even though it is well conserved via renal reabsorption, its synthesis may not be adequate in conditions during which energy production relies largely on beta-oxidation. In dogs, carnitine-responsive dilated cardiomyopathy has been described and carnitine deficiency may play a role in hepatic lipidosis in cats.[133] There is also evidence that supplemental carnitine enhances overall weight loss and reductions in body fat in overweight animals. For example, dogs fed a reduced calorie food that was supplemented with L-carnitine lost more body fat and total body weight over a 7-week period when compared with dogs fed the same food without added L-carnitine.[134] There is also some evidence that including L-carnitine in a reduced calorie food for cats accelerated the rate of weight loss and helped to preserve lean body mass.[135]

Feeding Regimen

When any type of reduced-calorie food is used for weight loss in dogs and cats, strict portion-controlled feeding should always be used. Most dogs and cats, given the opportunity, merely increase the volume of food that they eat in an effort to keep energy intake the same. The advantage of feeding a reducing diet is that fewer calories can be consumed in a larger volume of food and there is less risk of causing a nutrient imbalance during restricted feeding of the diet. For example, if a reducing pet food that contains 300 kcal/cup is fed, the dog used in the previous example would receive about 2½ cups of food a day rather than slightly less than 2 cups (see Box 28-3). This larger volume of food may result in a greater feeling of satiety and less tendency to beg or steal food. Moreover, these pet foods are specifically formulated by pet food manufacturers to provide balanced nutrition while lowering the amount of calories being consumed.

MAINTAINING WEIGHT LOSS

The dietary and exercise habits established during the treatment of obesity must be maintained for dogs and cats even after caloric restriction for weight loss has ended. The pet should be fed a well-balanced, complete food designed for adult maintenance and should continue with the level of daily exercise that was included in the weight-loss program. Pet owners should avoid reverting to old habits such as feeding table scraps, providing a large number of treats, or allowing begging behaviors. Some pets can be fed a normal adult maintenance pet food once they have reached ideal body weight. However, others easily gain weight when fed these foods. A reduced-calorie (weight control) food that is formulated for less-active adult pets is appropriate for weight maintenance in most animals following successful weight loss. In all cases, portion-controlled feeding two or more times per day is the feeding schedule that should be used.

PREVENTING OVERWEIGHT CONDITIONS IN DOGS AND CATS

Although a variety of different factors may contribute to the development of obesity, the two most important causes are overfeeding and underexercising. Obesity in pets can be successfully treated. However, the ideal situation is to prevent its occurrence in the first place. Veterinarians, veterinary staff, shelter staff, and breeders can have a large influence on the prevention of obesity in dogs and cats. Opportunities to advise clients and pet adopters regarding appropriate feeding management for new puppies and kittens occur during routine visits and when owners are first deciding upon a particular pet.

In human subjects, hyperplastic obesity, signified by the presence of an abnormally high number of adipose cells, is difficult to treat and has a poor long-term prognosis. The development of hyperplastic obesity usually takes place during growth and often leads to obesity in adult life. Although hyperplastic obesity has not been extensively studied in dogs and cats, it is assumed that the prognosis is similar to that in other species. It is possible that overnutrition in a young dog or cat sets the stage for a lifelong battle with obesity. It is imperative that adequate nutrients and calories for optimal growth be provided to young dogs and cats. However, feeding excess amounts of a calorically dense food may stimulate adipocyte hyperplasia and lead to an abnormally high rate of growth and weight gain. Growing pets should be fed an amount of food that promotes a normal growth rate and a lean body condition. Some pets are able to self-regulate and will not overeat. However, many young dogs and cats overeat as a result of boredom, competition with other animals, or the availability of a highly palatable food. In the majority of cases, portion-controlled feeding should be used, and the pet's weight and rate of gain should be strictly monitored. Daily exercise should be started when pets are young, and it should be continued throughout life.

During adulthood, portion-controlled feeding, regular exercise, and avoidance of the development of bad habits are the conditions necessary to prevent obesity. As pets age, their energy requirements naturally decrease. Exercise tolerance also decreases as pets get older, and these changes may predispose older pets to weight gain. Maintaining moderate levels of exercise and possibly changing the pet's diet to a ration that is low in energy density can help to prevent obesity in later years (Box 28-5).

BOX 28-5 PRACTICAL FEEDING TIPS: MANAGEMENT OF OBESITY IN DOGS AND CATS

Develop a program that will produce a target weight loss of 1% to 2% of total body weight per week (1% to 1.5% for cats).

Select an appropriate food for weight loss.

Restrict caloric intake to 60% to 70% of metabolizable energy for current body weight.

Eliminate all table scraps and treats; change feeding habits that contribute to overeating and obesity.

Include a program of moderate, daily exercise.

After desired weight loss has been achieved, adjust intake to maintain ideal body weight.

Prevent weight regain by continuing regular exercise and strictly monitoring caloric intake.

Tip: Many of the preventive and causative factors for obesity are the same for humans and animals. Lowering both your own and your pet's intake of fat and increasing the amount of exercise performed will benefit you both. People and their pets should take more walks, and people can even team up with their pets to improve health and maintain ideal weight.

References

1. Colliard L, Paragon BM, Lemuet B, and others: Prevalcne and risk factors of obesity in an urban population of healthy cats, *J Feline Med Surg* 11:135–140, 2008.

2. Robertson ID: The association of exercise, diet and other factors with owner-perceived obesity in privately owned dogs from metropolitan Perth, WA, *Prev Vet Med* 58:75–83, 2003.

3. Holmes KL, Morris PJ, Abdulla Z: Risk factors associated with excess body weight in dogs in the UK, *J Anim Physiol Anim Nutr* 91:166–167, 2007.

4. American Veterinary Medical Association (AVMA): *US pet ownership and demographics sourcebook* (2007 edition), Schaumburg, Ill, 2007, AVMA.

5. Scarlett JM, Donoghue S, Siadla J, Wills J: Overweight cats: prevalence and risk factors, *Int J Obes Relat Metab Disord* 18:S22–S28, 1994.

6. Lund EM, Armstrong PJ, Kirk CA: Prevalence and risk factors for obesity in adult cats from private US veterinary practices, *Intern J Appl Res Vet Med* 3:88–96, 2005.

7. Russell K, Sabin R, Holt S: Influence of feeding regimen on body condition in the cat, *J Small Anim Pract* 41:12–17, 2000.

8. Armstrong J, Lund EM: Obesity: research update. In *Proc Petfood Forum*, Chicago, Ill, 1997, Watts Publishing.

9. Glickman LT, Sonnenschein EG, Glickman NW, and others: Pattern of diet and obesity in female adult pet dogs, *Vet Clin Nutr* 2:6–13, 1995.

10. German AJ: The growing problem of obesity in dogs and cats, *J Nutr* 136:1940S–1946S, 2006.

11. Feldhahn JR, Rand JA, Martin G: Insulin sensitivity in normal and diabetic cats, *J Feline Med Surg* 1:107–115, 1999.

12. Mattheeuws D, Rottiers R, Kaneko JJ, and others: Diabetes mellitus in dogs: relationship of obesity to glucose tolerance and insulin response, *Am J Vet Res* 45:98–103, 1984.

13. Scarlett JM, Donoghue S: Association between body condition and disease in cats, *J Am Vet Med Assoc* 212:1725–1731, 1998.

14. Gayet C, Bailhache E, Dumon H: Insulin resistance and changes in plasma concentration of TNF-alpha, IGF1 and NEFA in dogs during weight gain and obesity, *J Anim Physiol Anim Nutr* 88:157–165, 2004.

15. Mattheeuws D, Rottiers R, Baeyens D, and others: Glucose tolerance and insulin response in obese dogs, *J Am Anim Hosp Assoc* 20:287–290, 1984.

16. Pena C, Suarez L, Bautista I, and others: Relationship between analytic values and canine obesity, *J Anim Phys Anim Nutr* 92:324–325, 2008.

17. Jeusette IC, Lhoest ET, Istasse LP, Eiez MO: Influence of obesity on plasma lipid and lipoprotein concentrations in dogs, *Am J Vet Res* 66:81–86, 2005.

18. Mizelle HL, Edwards TC, Montani JP: Abnormal cardiovascular responses to exercise during the development of obesity in dogs, *Am J Hypertens* 7:374–378, 1994.

19. Bach JF, Rozanski EA, Bedenice D, and others: Association of expiratory airway dysfunction with marked obesity in healthy adult dogs, *Am J Vet Res* 68:670–675, 2007.

20. Bodey AR, Michell AR: Epidemiological study of blood pressure in domestic dogs, *J Small Anim Pract* 37:116–125, 1996.

21. Montoya JA, Morris PF, Bautisa I: Hypertension: a risk factor associated with weight status in dogs, *J Nutr* 136:2011S–2013S, 2006.

22. Kealy RD, Lawler DF, Ballam JM, and others: Five-year longitudinal study on limited food consumption and development of osteoarthritis in coxofemoral joints of dogs, *J Am Vet Med Assoc* 210:222–225, 1997.

23. Biourge V, Massat B, Roff JM: Effects of protein, lipid or carbohydrate supplementation on hepatic lipid accumulation during weight loss in obese cats, *Am J Vet Res* 55:1406–1415, 1994.

24. Shofer FS, Sonnenschein EG, Goldschmidt NM, and others: Histopathologic and dietary prognostic factors for canine mammary carcinoma, *Breast Canc Res Treat* 13:49–60, 1989.

25. Alenza P, Pena L, Del Castillo N, Nieto AI: Factors influencing the incidence and prognosis of canine mammary tumours, *J Small Anim Pract* 41:287–291, 2000.

26. Philibert JC, Snyder PW, Glickman N: Influence of host factors on survival in dogs with malignant mammary gland tumors, *J Vet Intern Med* 17:102–106, 2003.

27. Van Goethem BEBJ, Rosenveldt KW, Kirpensteijn J: Monopolar versus bipolar electrocoagulation in canine laparoscopic ovariectomy: a nonrandomized prospective, clinical trial, *Vet Surg* 32:464–470, 2003.

28. Kealy RD, Lawler DF, Ballam JM: Effects of diet restriction on lifespan and age-related changes in dogs, *J Am Vet Med Assoc* 220:1315–1320, 2002.

29. Knittle JL, Fellner FG, Brown RE: Adipose tissue development in man, *Am J Clin Nutr* 30:762–766, 1977.

30. Bjorntorp P: The role of adipose tissue in human obesity. In Greenwood MRC, editor: *Obesity—contemporary issues in clinical nutrition*, New York, 1983, Churchill Livingstone.

31. Lemonnier D: Effect of age, sex and site of cellularity of the adipose tissue in mice and rats rendered obese by a high fat diet, *J Clin Invest* 51:2907, 1972.

32. Faust IM, Johnson PR, Hirsch J: Long-term effects of early nutritional experience on the development of obesity in the rat, *J Nutr* 110:2027–2034, 1980.

33. Johnson PR, Stern JS, Greenwood MRC, and others: Effect of early nutrition on adipose cellularity and pancreatic insulin release in the Zucker rat, *J Nutr* 103:738–743, 1973.

34. Allan FJ, Pfeiffer DU, Jones BR: A cross-sectional study of risk factors for obesity in cats in New Zealand, *Prev Vet Med* 46:183–196, 2000.

35. McGreevy PD, Thomson PC, Pride C, and others: Prevalence of obesity in dogs examined by Australian veterinary practices and the risk factors involved, *Vet Rec* 156:695–707, 2005.

36. Applegate EA, Upton DE, Stern JS: Food intake, body composition and blood lipids following treadmill exercise in male and female rats, *Physiol Behav* 28:917–920, 1982.

37. Glickman LT, Sonnerschein EG, Glickman NW: Pattern of diet and obesity in female adult pet dogs, *Vet Clin Nutr* 2:6–13, 1995.

38. Anderson RS: Obesity in the dog and cat, *Vet Ann* 14:182–186, 1975.

39. Root M: Early spay-neuter in the cat: effect on development of obesity and metabolic rate, *Vet Clin Nutr* 2:132–134, 1995.

40. Fettman MJ, Stanton CA, Banks LL, and others: Effects of neutering on body weight, metabolic rate and glucose tolerance of domestic cats, *Res Vet Sci* 62:131–136, 1997.

41. Martin L, Siliart B, Dumon H: Hormonal disturbances associated with obesity in dogs, *J Anim Physiol Anim Nutr* 90:355–360, 2006.

42. Houpt KA, Coren B, Hintz HF: Effect of sex and reproductive status on sucrose preference food intake and body weight of dogs, *J Am Vet Med Assoc* 174:1083–1085, 1979.

43. Jeusette I, Detilleus J, Cuvelier C, and others: Ad libitum feeding following ovariectomy in female Beagle dogs: effect on maintenance energy requirement and on blood metabolites, *J Anim Phys Anim Nutr* 88:117–121, 2004.

44. Armstrong PJ: Effect of ovariohysterectomy on maintenance energy requirement in cats, *J Am Vet Med Assoc* 209:1572–1581, 1996.

45. Martin L, Siliart B, Dumon H, and others: Leptin, body fat content and energy expenditure in intact and gonadectomized adult cats: a preliminary study, *J Anim Physiol Anim Nutr* 815:195–199, 2001.

46. Nguyen PG, Dumon HJ, Silart BS, and others: Effects of dietary fat and energy on body weight and composition after gonadectomy in cats, *Am J Vet Res* 65:1708–1713, 2004.

47. Martin L, Siliart B, Dumon H: Spontaneous hormonal variations in male cats following gonadectomy, *J Feline Med Surg* 8:309–314, 2006.

48. Spain CV, Scarlett JM, Houpt KA: Long-term risks and benefits of early-age gonadectomy in dogs, *J Am Vet Med Assoc* 224:380–387, 2004.

49. Edney ATB, Smith PM: Study of obesity in dogs visiting veterinary practices in the United Kingdom, *Vet Rec* 118:391–396, 1986.

50. Meyer HL, Drochner W, Weidenhaupt C: Ein Beitrag zum Vorkommen und zur Behandlung der Adipositas des Hundes, *Deutsche Tierärztliche Wochenschrift* 85:133–136, 1978.

51. Kienzle E, Rainbird A: Maintenance energy requirement of dogs: what is the correct value for the calculation of metabolic body weight in dogs? *Am J Clin Nutr* 121:S39–S40, 1991.

52. Robertson ID: The influence of diet and other factors on owner-perceived obesity in privately owned cats from metropolitan Perth, Western Australia, *Prev Vet Med* 40:75–85, 1999.

53. Milne KL, Hayes HM Jr: Epidemiologic features of canine hypothyroidism, *Cornell Vet* 71:3–14, 1981.

54. Panciera DL: A retrospective study of 66 cases of canine hypothyroidism, *J Am Vet Med Assoc* 204:761–767, 1994.

55. Panciera DL: Conditions associated with canine hypothyroidism, *Vet Clin North Am Small Anim Pract* 31:935–950, 2001.

56. Meyer DJ: Clinical manifestations associated with endocrine disorders, *Vet Clin North Am Small Anim Pract* 7:433–441, 1977.

57. Scalafani A, Springer O: Dietary obesity in adult rats: similarities to hypothalamic and human obesity syndromes, *Physiol Behav* 17:461–471, 1976.

58. Slattery JM, Potter RM: Hyperphagia: a necessary precondition to obesity? *Appetite* 6:133–142, 1985.

59. Hill SW: Eating responses of humans during meals, *J Comp Physiol Psych* 86:652–657, 1974.

60. Sloth C: Practical management of obesity in dogs and cats, *J Small Anim Pract* 33:178–182, 1992.

61. Kienzle E, Bergler R, Mandernach A: Comparison of the feeding behavior and the man-animal relationship in owners of normal and obese dogs, *J Nutr* 128:2779S–2782S, 1998.

62. Kienzle E, Bergler R: Human-animal relationship of owners of normal and overweight cats, *J Nutr* 136:1947S–1950S, 2006.

63. Fabry P, Tepperman J: Meal frequency—a possible factor in human pathology, *Am J Clin Nutr* 23:1059, 1970.

64. Blundell JE: Nutritional manipulation for altering food intake. In Wurtman RJ, Wurtman JJ, editors: *Human obesity*, New York, 1987, Academy of Sciences.

65. Kim Sl, Ellmerer M, Van Citters GW: Primacy of hepatic insulin resistance in the development of the metabolic syndrome induced by an isocaloric moderate-fat diet in the dog, *Diabetes* 52:2453–2460, 2003.

66. Cummings DE, Overduin J: Gastrointestinal regulation of food intake, *J Clin Invest* 117:13–23, 2007.

67. Jeusette I, Detilleux J, Shibata H: Effects of chronic obesity and weight loss on plasma ghrelin and leptin concentrations in dogs, *Res Vet Sci* 79:169–175, 2005.

68. Cummings DE, Weigle DS, Faayo RS: Plasma ghrelin levels after diet-induced weight loss or gastric bypass surgery, *N Engl J Med* 346:1623–1630, 2002.

69. Ishioka K, Soliman MM, Sagawa M: Experimental and clinical studies on plasma leptin in obese dogs, *J Vet Med Sci* 64:349–353, 2002.

70. Sagawa MM, Nakadomo F, Honjoh T, and others: Correlation between plasma leptin concentration and body fat content in dogs, *Am J Vet Res* 63:7–10, 2002.

71. Scarpace PJ, Sunvold GD, Bouchard GF: Vitamin A supplementation in cats abolishes the relationship between adiposity and leptin, *FASEB J* 14:A215, 2000.

72. Gayet C, Bailhache E, Martin L: Changes in plasma tumor necrosis factor (TNF-α), insulin-like growth factor (IGF1), non-esterified fatty acids (NEFA) and insulin sensitivity in overfed and food restricted dogs, *J Vet Intern Med* 17:417–418, 2003.

73. Burkholder WJ: Precision and practicality of methods assessing body composition of dogs and cats, *Compend Contin Educ Pract Vet* 23:1–15, 2001.

74. Morooka T, Niyama M, Uchida E: Measurement of the back fat layer in Beagles for estimation of obesity using two-dimensional ultrasonography, *J Small Anim Pract* 42:56–59, 2001.

75. Son HR, d'Avignon DA, Laflamme DP: Comparison of dual x-ray absorptiometry and measurement of total body water content by deuterium oxide dilution for estimating body composition in dogs, *Am J Vet Res* 59:529–532, 1998.

76. Toll PW, Gross KL, Berryhill SA, Jewell DE: Usefulness of dual energy x-ray absorptiometry for body composition measurement in adult dogs, *J Nutr* 124(Suppl):2601S–2603S, 1994.

77. Munday HS, Booles D, Anderson P, and others: The repeatability of body composition measurements in dogs and cats using dual energy x-ray absorptiometry, *J Nutr* 124(Suppl):2619S–2621S, 1994.

78. Scheltinga MR, Helton WE, Rounds J, and others: Impedance electrodes positioned on proximal portions of limbs quantify fluid compartments in dogs, *J Appl Physiol* 70:2039–2044, 1991.

79. Stanton Ca, Hamar DW, Johnson DE: Bioelctrical impedance and zoometry for body composition analysis in domestic cats, *Am J Vet Res* 53:251–257, 1992.

80. Elliott DA: Evaluation of multi-frequency bioelectrical impedance analysis for the assessment of extracellular and total body water in healthy cats, *J Nutr* 132:1757S–1759S, 2002.

81. Mawby DI, Bartges JW, d'Avignon A, and others: Comparison of various methods for estimating body fat in dogs, *J Am Anim Hosp Assoc* 40:109–114, 2004.

82. Laflamme D: Development and validation of a body condition score system for cats: a clinical tool, *Feline Pract* 25:13–18, 1997.

83. Laflamme D: Development and validation of a body condition score system for dogs, *Canine Pract* 22:10–15, 1997.

84. German AJ, Holden SL, Moxham G: A simple, reliable tool for owners to assess the body condition of their dog or cat, *J Nutr* 136:2021S–2022S, 2006.

85. Colliard L, Paragon BM, Lemuet B, and others: Prevalence and risk factors of obesity in an urban population of healthy cats, *J Feline Med Surg* 11:135–140, 2009.

86. Slater MR, Robinson LE, Zoran DL: Diet and exercise patterns in pet dogs, *J Vet Med Assoc* 207:186–190, 1995.

87. Yaissle JE, Holloway C, Buffington T: Evaluation of owner education as a component of obesity treatment programs for dogs, *J Am Vet Med Assoc* 224:1932–1935, 2004.

88. Melzer K, Kayser B, Saris WHM, and others: Effects of physical activity on food intake, *Clin Nutr* 24:885–895, 2005.

89. Pi-Sunyer FX: Exercise effects on calorie intake. In Wurtman RJ, Wurtman JJ, editors: *Human obesity*, New York, 1987, New York Academy of Sciences.

90. Butterwick F, Markwell PJ: Changes in the body composition of cats during weight reduction by controlled dietary energy restriction, *Vet Rec* 138:354–357, 1996.

91. Banning M: Obesity: pathophysiology and treatment, *J R Soc Health* 125:163–167, 2005.

92. Schultz CK, Bernauer E, Mole PA: Effects of severe caloric restriction and moderate exercise on basal metabolic rate and hormonal status in adult humans (abstract), *Fed Proc* 39:783, 1980.

93. Berggren JR, Jluver MW, Houmard JA: Fat as an endocrine organ: influence of exercise, *J Appl Physiol* 99:757–764, 2005.

94. Nassis GP, Papantakou K, Skendrei K, and others: Aerobic exercise training improves insulin sensitivity without changes in body weight, body fat, adiponectin and inflammatory markers in overweight and obese girls, *Metabolism* 54:1472–1479, 2005.

95. Dyck DJ: Leptin sensitivity in skeletal muscle is modulated by diet and exercise, *Exerc Sport Sci Rev* 33:189–194, 2005.

96. Impellizeri JA, Tetrick MA, Muir P: Effect of weight reduction on clinical signs of lameness in dogs with hip osteoarthritis, *J Am Vet Med Assoc* 216:1089–1091, 2000.

97. Weinsier RL, Wilson LJ, Lee J: Medically safe rate of weight loss for the treatment of obesity: a guideline based on risk of gallstone formation, *Am J Med* 98:115–117, 1995.

98. Burkholder WJ, Bauer JE: Foods and techniques for managing obesity in companion animals, *J Am Vet Med Assoc* 212:658–662, 1998.

99. Laflamme DP, Kuhlman G, Lawler DF: Evaluation of weight loss protocols for dogs, *J Am Anim Hosp Assoc* 33:252–259, 1997.

100. Center SA: Clinical weight management for dogs and cats. In *Proc WSAVA*, 2001, pp 56–69.

101. Diez M, Nguyen P, Jeusett I: Weight loss in obese dogs: evaluation of a high protein and low carbohydrate diet, *J Nutr* 132:1685S–1687S, 2002.

102. Brown RC, Ambrose J: The effect of weight loss on the resting metabolic rate in the obese dog (abstract), *Fed Am Soc Exp Biol* 5:A961, 1991.

103. Laflamme DP, Kuhlman G: The effect of weight loss regimen on subsequent weight maintenance in dogs, *Nutr Res* 15:1019–1028, 1995.

104. Crowell-Davis SL, Barry K, Ballam JM, and others: The effect of caloric restriction on the behavior of pen housed dogs: transition from unrestricted to restricted diet, *Appl Anim Behav Sci* 43:27–41, 1995.

105. Krebs JD, Browning LM, McLean NK, and others: Additive benefits of long-chain n-3 polyunsaturated fatty acids and weight-loss in the management of cardiovascular disease risk in overweight hyperinsulinaemic women, *Int J Obes* 30:1535–1544, 2006.

106. Devaraj S, Kasim-Karakas S, Jialal I: The effect of weight loss and dietary fatty acids on inflammation, *Curr Atheroscler Rep* 8:477–486, 2006.

107. Wilkins C, Long RC Jr, Waldron M, and others: Assessment of the influence of fatty acids on indices of insulin sensitivity and myocellular lipid content by use of magnetic resonance spectroscopy in cats, *Am J Vet Res* 65:1090–1099, 2004.

108. Park Y, Albright KJ, Liu W: Effect of conjugated linoleic acid on body composition in mice, *Lipids* 32:853–858, 1997.

109. Dugan MER, Aalhus JL, Schaefer AL: The effect of conjugated linoleic acid on fat to lean repartitioning and feed conversion in pigs, *Can J Anim Sci* 77:723–725, 1997.

110. Azain MJ: Conjugated linoleic acid and its effects on animal products and health in single-stomach animals, *Proc Nutr Soc* 62:319–328, 2003.

111. Leray V, Dumon H, Martin L: No effect of conjugated linoleic acid or garcinia cambogia on body composition and energy expenditure in non-obese cats, *J Nutr* 136:1982S–1984S, 2006.

112. Jewell DE, Edwards GL, Azain MJ, and others: Fiber but not conjugated linoleic acid influences adiposity in dogs, *Vet Ther* 7:78–85, 2006.

113. Bierer TL, Bui LM: High-protein low-carbohydrate diets enhance weight loss in dogs, *J Nutr* 134:2087S–2089S, 2004.

114. Laflamme DP, Hannah SS: Increased dietary protein promotes fat loss and reduces loss of lean body mass during weight loss in cats, *Int J Appl Res Vet Med* 3:62–68, 2005.

115. Hannah S: Role of dietary protein in weight management, *Compend Contin Educ Pract Vet* 21:32–33, 1999.

116. Veldhorst M, Smeets A, Soenen S, and others: Protein-induced satiety: effects and mechanisms of different proteins, *Physiol Behav* 94:300–307, 2008.

117. Weber M, Bissot T, Servet E, and others: A high-protein, high-fiber diet designed for weight loss improves satiety in dogs, *J Vet Intern Med* 21:1203–1208, 2007.

118. Center SA: Safe weight loss in cats. In Reinhart GA, Carey DP, editors: *Recent advances in canine and feline nutrition, Iams nutrition symposium proceedings*, vol 2, Wilmington, Ohio, 1998, Orange Frazer Press.

119. Biourge VC, Massat B, Groff JM, and others: Effects of protein, lipid or carbohydrate supplementation on hepatic lipid accumulation during rapid weight loss in obese cats, *Am J Vet Res* 55:1406–1415, 1994.

120. Schwartz RS, Ravussin E, Massari M, and others: The thermic effect of carbohydrate versus fat feeding in man, *Metabolism* 34:285–293, 1985.

121. Sunvold GD, Bouchard GF: The glycemic response to dietary starch. In *Recent advances in canine and feline nutrition, Iams nutrition symposium proceedings*, vol 2, Wilmington, Ohio, 1998, Orange Frazer Press, pp 123–131.

122. Center SA, Reynolds AP, Harte J, and others: Clinical effects of rapid weight loss in obese pet cats with and without supplemental L-carnitine, *J Vet Intern Med* 11:118, 1997.

123. Bouchard GF, Sunvold GD: Dietary modification of feline obesity with a low fat, low fiber diet. In Reinhart GA, Carey DP, editors: *Recent advances in canine and feline nutrition, Iams nutrition symposium proceedings*, vol 2, Wilmington, Ohio, 1998, Orange Frazer Press.

124. Butterwick RF, Markwell PJ: Effect of amount and type of dietary fiber on food intake in energy-restricted dogs, *Am J Vet Res* 58:272–276, 1997.

125. Butterwick RF, Markwell PJ: Effect of level and source of dietary fibre on food intake in the dog (abstract), *Proc Waltham Int Symp Pet Nutr Health*, 1993.

126. Jackson JR, Laflamme DP, Owens SF: Effects of dietary fiber content on satiety in dogs, *Vet Clin Nutr* 4:130–134, 1997.

127. Vahouny GV, Cassidy MM: Dietary fibers and absorption of nutrients (review), *Proc Soc Exp Biol Med* 180:432–446, 1985.

128. Fernandez R, Phillips SF: Components of fiber impair iron absorption in the dog, *Am J Clin Nutr* 35:107–112, 1982.

129. Fahey GC Jr, Merchen NR, Corbin JE, and others: Dietary fiber for dogs. Part I. Effects of graded levels of dietary beet pulp on nutrient intake, digestibility, metabolizable energy and digesta mean retention time, *J Anim Sci* 68:4229–4235, 1990.

130. Sunvold GD, Fahey CG Jr, Merchen NR, and others: Dietary fiber for dogs. IV. In vitro fermentation of selected fiber sources by dog fecal inoculum and in vivo digestion and metabolism of fiber-supplemented diets, *J Anim Sci* 73:1099–1119, 1995.

131. Sunvold GD, Fahey CG Jr, Merchen NR, and others: Dietary fiber for cats: in vitro fermentation of selected fiber sources by cat fecal inoculum and in vivo utilization of diets containing selected fiber sources and their blends, *J Anim Sci* 73:2329–2339, 1995.

132. Bremer J: Carnitine—metabolism and functions, *Physiol Rev* 63:1420–1480, 1983.

133. Carroll MC, Cote E: Carnitine: a review, *Compend Contin Educ Pract Vet* 23:45–52, 2001.

134. Sunvold GD: Carnitine supplementation promotes weight loss and decreased adiposity in the canine. In *Proc XXIII WSAVA*, 1998, p 746.

135. Center SA, Reynolds AP, Harte J: Clinical effects of rapid weight loss in obese cats with and without supplemental L-carnitine (abstract). In *Proc 15th ACVIM Forum*, 1997, p 665.

29

Diabetes Mellitus

Diabetes mellitus (DM) is an endocrine disorder that occurs in both dogs and cats. It is caused by the relative or absolute deficiency of the hormone insulin, which is produced by the beta cells of the pancreas. Insulin stimulates the transport of glucose and other nutrients across cell membranes for cellular use and is involved in a number of anabolic processes within the body. A lack of insulin activity leads to elevated blood glucose levels (hyperglycemia) and an inability of tissues to receive the glucose that they need (glucoprivation). Primary clinical signs include polyuria, polydipsia, polyphagia, and, in some cases, weight loss. Diagnosis is usually made using the initial signs of the disorder, which include the presence of a persistent hyperglycemia and a persistent or concurrent glucosuria.[1]

INCIDENCE AND RISK FACTORS

DM is currently one of the most frequently diagnosed endocrine disorders in companion dogs and cats. Depending upon the group studied, DM has an incidence ranging between 0.13% and 2% of the population of dogs and cats living in homes.[1] A recent study of an insured population of Swedish dogs estimated that 1.2% of dogs would develop DM before 12 years of age.[2] This prevalence has increased dramatically over the last 30 years.[3] Similarly, there is evidence that the incidence of DM in cats has been steadily increasing. In 1970, DM incidence in cats was reported to be less than 0.1%; this increased by more than tenfold by 1999.[4] Although other factors may be involved, increases in both obesity and the frequency of sedentary lifestyles in pet cats have probably contributed to this change. More recently, a study of pet cats in the United Kingdom reported the incidence of DM in an insured population of adult cats to be 0.4%.[5]

Risk factors for the development of DM in dogs include previous or concurrent hyperadrenocorticism, recurrent episodes of pancreatitis (estimated to cause 28% of cases), stress, and the presence of a genetic (breed) predisposition.[3,6,7] Intact females are more likely to be affected than males and may also develop an insulin-resistant type of DM during diestrus and pregnancy.[3] The increased incidence of DM in reproducing females may be explained by the insulin-antagonistic effects of progesterone and mammary tissue–derived growth hormone.[8] Increasing age is an important and consistently identified risk factor; most dogs with DM are older than 7 years at the time of diagnosis.[1,9] Many dogs diagnosed with DM are at normal body weight or even underweight at the time of diagnosis, and obesity has not been identified as a consistent risk factor for DM in dogs. Although there is some evidence from a small pilot study suggesting that dogs diagnosed with DM are more likely to have been chronically overweight when compared with healthy matched controls, other studies have not found this association.[10] Although it is well documented that obesity in dogs leads to insulin resistance and impaired glucose tolerance, these changes resolve with weight loss and do not typically lead to the development of overt diabetes.[11] This is an important way in which the pathogenesis of DM differs between dogs and cats.

Finally, recent studies suggest a strong genetic component for DM among certain dog breeds.[2,12] In the United States, breeds that experience significantly increased risk include Samoyeds, Siberian Huskies, Keeshonds, Finnish Spitz, Miniature Schnauzers, and Miniature Poodles.[3,12] A study of insured dogs in Sweden showed similar results and noted the prevalence of northern breeds in these groupings.[2] It was hypothesized that metabolic changes that favor adaptation to a cold environment may also increase susceptibility to DM. The Swedish study also reported a breed-sex interaction for susceptibility to DM. Female dogs were affected almost exclusively in some breeds, such as Border Collies, Norwegian Elkhounds, and Beagles. However, other breeds did not show a sex predilection. Dog breeds that have a low risk for developing DM include the Golden Retriever, Boxer, Papillion, and Tibetan Spaniel.

Although there are several important differences between DM in dogs and cats, cats experience many of the same risk factors as those reported in dogs. The chance of developing DM increases as cats age; between 70% and 90% of diabetic cats are 7 years or older, and more than 65% are 10 years or older at time of diagnosis.[13] Obesity is well documented as an important risk factor for DM in cats. Up to 80% of cats are overweight at the time of diagnosis, and overweight cats have an almost fivefold increased risk of developing DM compared with cats that are at their optimal weight.[14] One difference between dogs and cats is that neutered male cats have a higher risk of developing DM than do intact cats of either sex or spayed females. Other predisposing factors for cats include neutered status, indoor confinement and, related to living indoors, having a low level of physical inactivity.[1,4,15] Cats with complicating diseases such as pancreatitis, pancreatic neoplasia, acromegaly, hyperadrenocorticism, hyperthyroidism, and dental disease are also at increased risk.[16-19] The administration of medications such as progestagens and glucocorticoids has been associated with DM in cats.[20] Just as in dogs, there is evidence for a breed-specific predisposition in cats. Family lines of Burmese cats in Australia, New Zealand, and the United Kingdom show a higher frequency of DM when compared with other breeds and mixed-breed cats.[5,21] In some lines, more than 10% of the individuals are affected.[22]

Finally, there is evidence of a genetic component to DM in cats that is not breed specific. Some cats appear to be predisposed to developing glucose intolerance because of naturally occurring low insulin sensitivity. While these cats show no signs of DM when they are maintained at optimal body condition, they are more likely than other cats to develop DM if they gain weight and become obese.[1,23] For example, fasting hyperinsulinemia prior to weight gain was found to be the strongest risk factor for development of impaired glucose tolerance in a group of cats that were fed to induce weight gain.[23] This effect is theorized to be similar to the genetic component of type II DM that has been reported in human subjects. Insulin resistance is largely determined by genetics in humans, but its phenotypic expression and the development of DM is influenced by environmental factors, most notably obesity.[24]

Risk factors for the development of diabetes mellitus (DM) in dogs and cats include increasing age, sex (intact females

in dogs; neutered males in cats); previous or concurrent hyperadrenocorticism, pancreatitis, or acromegaly; and the presence of a genetic (breed) predisposition. Although many dogs diagnosed with DM are at normal body weight, or even underweight at the time of diagnosis, obesity is an important risk factor for DM in cats.

CLASSIFICATION OF DIABETES MELLITUS

DM is considered a heterogeneous syndrome, with its primary characteristic being a persistent and detrimental hyperglycemia. In humans, diabetes is typically classified as either type I or type II. The classification of diabetes in dogs and cats is generally patterned after the human classification, with some modification.

Type I Diabetes Mellitus

Type I diabetes (formerly referred to as insulin-dependent diabetes mellitus [IDDM]) is identified by an absolute lack of endogenous insulin and a resultant dependence upon exogenous insulin for survival. This form of the disease is often caused by the immune-mediated destruction of the pancreatic beta cells by T cells and antibodies. It is estimated that at least 50% of diabetic dogs have immune-mediated type 1 diabetes as indicated by the presence of islet cell antibodies.[25] Evidence in human subjects with type I DM suggests that there may be an immune-mediated component involving the gut immune system, but this has not been studied yet in dogs.[26] The majority of diabetic dogs also have an absolute insulin deficiency, although the underlying cause is not always known. As discussed previously, there is a strong association between DM and pancreatitis in dogs. It is theorized that extensive pancreatic damage and the loss of beta cells in dogs with recurrent or chronic pancreatitis may lead to the development of DM. In human patients with type I DM, the rate of progression to absolute insulin deficiency is highly variable and can occur rapidly (childhood onset) or very gradually (latent autoimmune diabetes of adults [LADA]). Because DM is typically diagnosed in dogs that are 7 years of age or older, it is theorized that the form of DM observed in dogs may be similar to LADA in human subjects. Type I diabetes is not well documented in cats, and the prevalence of islet cell antibodies in this species has not been reported.[27,28] Although many cats with diabetes will require insulin therapy at some point during their disease, the proportion of cats that have type I diabetes (i.e., an absolute lack of endogenous insulin production) is very low.

Type II Diabetes Mellitus

Type II diabetes is characterized by impaired insulin secretion; insulin resistance; and the deposition of amyloid in the islets of the pancreas. (In humans, type II diabetes was previously referred to as non–insulin-dependent diabetes mellitus [NIDDM].) Human subjects with type II DM do not usually require exogenous insulin therapy for survival, although insulin or oral hypoglycemic agents may be administered to better manage blood glucose levels. With this form of DM, the total amount of insulin secreted after a meal may be increased, normal, or decreased, and the pattern of insulin secretion is usually abnormal.[29] Insulin resistance occurs when an elevated concentration of circulating hormone is needed to adequately maintain blood glucose levels. Based upon glucose tolerance tests and measured levels of serum insulin, it appears that insulin resistance is a common feature of both canine and feline diabetes.[30,31] The persistent hyperglycemia that results from insulin resistance and abnormal insulin secretion results in glucose toxicity. Glucose toxicity exacerbates the metabolic abnormalities of diabetes and leads to impaired insulin secretion and to the destruction and loss of beta cells.

More than 80% of cats with DM have type II DM; the remaining cases are usually secondary to other conditions such as acromegaly, pancreatitis, or neoplasia. Amyloid deposition in pancreatic islets is a consistent histological finding in cats with diabetes. Amyloid is a precipitation product of a pancreatic compound called *amylin*. Amylin is cosecreted with insulin and helps to maintain normal blood glucose levels by stimulating the breakdown of muscle glycogen. Amyloid deposition contributes to a loss of the insulin-secreting beta cells of the pancreas, eventually causing decreased or insufficient insulin secretion. Although most diabetic cats are identified as having type II diabetes, more of these cats require insulin therapy than do humans with type II diabetes, probably because of the deposition

of amylin and the greater loss of beta cells in this species.[27,32,33] Because the effects of glucose toxicity are initially reversible, a substantial number of cats with type II diabetes that are promptly treated with diet and insulin therapy may revert to a state that does not require insulin weeks to months after hyperglycemia has been controlled.[34,35]

Peripheral insulin resistance primarily manifests itself after insulin binds to its cellular receptors, resulting in a decreased conversion of circulating glucose to glycogen or fat. In addition to being a characteristic of type II diabetes, insulin resistance also occurs as an adaptive response to low carbohydrate intake, allowing blood glucose levels to be conserved and maintained immediately after eating a low-carbohydrate meal.[36] It has been hypothesized that, as a species, the domestic cat is naturally insulin resistant when compared with other more omnivorous or herbivorous species. Insulin resistance would be expected to confer an adaptive advantage for a species that evolved as an obligate carnivore, consuming a diet that was high in protein but low in carbohydrate (see Section 2, pp. 76-77). A degree of peripheral resistance to insulin promotes the delivery of protein and fat to tissues while conserving blood glucose levels. If this theory is correct, it would follow that the consumption of a diet that is high in carbohydrate (such as some commercially available dry cat foods) would require cats to secrete much higher levels of insulin after eating than would be secreted after eating a high-protein, high-fat meal. Over time, the beta cells of the pancreas may no longer be able to meet this enhanced need, resulting in an abnormal or impaired insulin response. This hypothesis has been referred to as the "carnivore connection" and has been examined in humans and cats.[37]

However, as discussed previously, the presence of innate insulin resistance alone does not appear to lead to DM. The development of obesity, plus a sedentary lifestyle, increasing age, and neuter status are factors that contribute to the exacerbation of insulin resistance in cats and may lead to development of type II DM. Although more study of this hypothesis is needed, a recent survey study of 96 diabetic cats and 192 matched control cats found no association between the amount of dry cat food that was fed to cats and DM, but did corroborate both a sedentary lifestyle and indoor confinement as risk factors for DM.[15] Table 29-1 summarizes the classification of DM in dogs and cats.

TABLE 29-1 FORMS OF DIABETES MELLITUS (DM)

Form	Major underlying cause	Incidence (% of DM cases)	Treatment
Type I	Inability of beta cells to synthesize or secrete insulin	Dogs: >95% Cats: 20% or less	Exogenous insulin and dietary management
Type II	Insensitivity of peripheral tissues to insulin; impaired insulin secretion	Dogs: Rarely reported Cats: >80%	Weight loss, dietary management and/or hypoglycemic agents; insulin therapy (in some cases)

Type I diabetes is characterized by an absolute lack of endogenous insulin and dependence upon exogenous insulin. This form of the disease is often immune-mediated and is responsible for the majority of cases of diabetes mellitus (DM) in dogs. Type II diabetes is characterized by peripheral insulin resistance and in cats, the deposition of amyloid in the islets of the pancreas. More than 80% of cats with DM have type II DM; the remaining cases are usually secondary to other conditions such as acromegaly, pancreatitis, or neoplasia.

CLINICAL SIGNS AND PHYSICAL CHANGES

All of the clinical signs observed in pets with DM are associated with the short- or long-term effects of hyperglycemia and aberrations in carbohydrate, fat, and protein metabolism. Polydipsia, polyuria, polyphagia, and/or weight loss are usually the first signs observed. Cataracts are a consistent long-term complication of DM in dogs.[38] Many cats also develop evidence of lens opacification as well.[39] The microvascular effects of diabetes can contribute to the development of renal disease in some animals. Polyneuropathy develops in some cases and can present as weakness, depression, or urinary and bowel incontinence. In cats, this is often seen clinically as a plantigrade stance.[40] Bacterial infections, especially of the bladder, are common in animals with poor glycemic control.[41,42] Recently, a small case-controlled study with 20 diabetic cats reported that diabetic cats had a significantly increased risk of heart disease–related death when compared with their matched cohorts.[43] Because only a small number of cats were examined, additional studies are needed to explore this relationship.

Many of the health complications of DM can be minimized or prevented through stringent control of blood glucose levels. The general therapeutic goals in diabetes management are to minimize postprandial (after-meal) hyperglycemia, prevent hypoglycemia when insulin is being administered, resolve and minimize clinical signs, prevent or delay long-term complications, and improve overall health. For some cats, management goals can also include achieving remission (transient diabetes). Successful diabetic management can be achieved through exogenous insulin administration, administration of oral hypoglycemic agents, diet, weight loss (if indicated), exercise, and the control of concurrent illness. Oral hypoglycemic drugs may increase the deposition of amyloid in the pancreas in cats and so are not often prescribed for cats. The remainder of this chapter focuses primarily on the role of diet and weight control in managing DM in dogs and cats.

DIETARY TREATMENT

Dietary goals for dogs and cats with type I DM are to improve regulation of blood glucose by delivering nutrients to the body during periods when exogenous insulin is active and to minimize postprandial fluctuations in blood glucose levels. Dietary management does not eliminate the need for insulin replacement therapy, but it can be used to improve glycemic control. Dietary treatment for pets with type II DM can be instrumental in improving glycemic control and making the need for lifelong exogenous insulin therapy less likely. Factors that must be considered when developing an appropriate diet for a diabetic pet include the consistency and type of diet, its nutritional adequacy and nutrient composition, the pet's caloric intake and feeding schedule, and the presence of any other diseases.

Consistency and Type of Diet

Dogs and cats with diabetes should be fed a food that contains consistent amounts and sources of nutrients. Specifically, the type and quantity of nutrients that are delivered to the body should remain constant from day to day, and the proportions of calories in the diet that are supplied by carbohydrate, protein, and fat should stay the same. For pets with type I diabetes, the provision of a consistent diet allows the insulin dosage to be adjusted to closely fit the needs of the animal. Similarly, if pets with type II diabetes are being treated with oral hypoglycemic agents, the provision of a consistent diet is helpful in maintaining normal blood glucose levels. Changes in the ingredients or nutrient composition of a diet can disrupt the tight coupling of blood glucose levels with insulin activity that is needed for proper glycemic control. Therefore only pet foods that are guaranteed to use a fixed formulation should be selected for diabetic pets (see Section 3, p. 168). Manufacturers that use fixed formulations ensure that the nutrient composition and ingredients of a food remain consistent between batches. In contrast, manufacturers that use variable formulations may change ingredients depending on the availability and market prices. If information about the formulation type is not readily available, it can be obtained by contacting the manufacturer directly. In most circumstances, homemade diets should also be avoided with diabetic pets because of difficulties with maintaining nutrient consistency.

The type of commercial product that is fed is also of importance. Semimoist pet foods or snacks should not be fed to diabetic pets. Postprandial blood glucose and insulin responses have been shown to be highest when dogs are fed semimoist foods, compared with when they are fed either canned or dry pet foods.[44] This increase appears to be caused by the high level of simple carbohydrate found in semimoist products. These nutrients require minimal digestion in the small intestine and are rapidly absorbed following a meal. In contrast, the digestible carbohydrates found in dry and canned foods are made up primarily of complex carbohydrates (starch). Starches require enzymatic digestion to simple sugars before they can be absorbed into the body. This process slows the rate of delivery of glucose to the bloodstream. Complex carbohydrates and certain types of fiber also affect the rate of food passage through the gastrointestinal tract and the absorption of other nutrients in the diet. Dry pet foods generally contain higher levels of both complex carbohydrates and plant fiber than semimoist or canned foods do.

Foods selected for diabetic dogs and cats should contain consistent amounts and sources of nutrients. The type and quantity of nutrients that are delivered to the body should remain constant from day to day, and the proportions of calories in the diet that are supplied by carbohydrate, protein, and fat should stay the same. In addition, because of their high simple carbohydrate content, semimoist foods should not be fed to diabetic pets, even as treats.

Nutritional Adequacy and Nutrient Composition

The first consideration when identifying a food for a diabetic pet is the nutritional adequacy of the diet. Because long-term management is involved, the food must be nutritionally complete and balanced and must supply optimum levels of all the essential nutrients required by the pet. The methods discussed in Section 3 can be used to determine the nutritional adequacy of a commercial product. As discussed previously, the labels of over-the-counter pet foods will indicate if feeding trials have been conducted or if the food has been formulated to meet the Association of American Feed Control Officials' (AAFCO's) *Nutrient Profiles*. A food that has been tested using the AAFCO's animal feeding test protocols or that has been formulated to meet AAFCO's *Nutrient Profiles* should be selected. If a veterinary diet is prescribed, the label may not show this information, but the veterinarian should have literature available that fully describes the selected product.

Energy-Containing Nutrients

Diabetes is a disorder that affects the body's ability to metabolize carbohydrate, protein, and fat. Therefore the proportion of these nutrients in foods designed for managing DM is an important consideration. Overall energy content of the food must also be considered, especially in cases of underweight or overweight animals. Overweight animals with DM should be fed a food that is formulated for both weight and glycemic control.[45] Conversely, underweight animals should be fed foods with higher energy density to maintain or improve body condition.

PROTEIN   In human diabetics, high-protein diets are not recommended because of the incidence of diabetic nephropathy, a condition that may be exacerbated by the intake of large amounts of protein. However, this complication of diabetes is uncommon in dogs and cats, and protein restriction for diabetic dogs and cats is neither necessary nor recommended. Rather, diabetic dogs should be fed high-quality protein in amounts that meet their daily requirements. The protein content in foods for diabetic cats should be moderate or higher (≥30%, dry-matter basis), replacing digestible carbohydrate. Protein rather than fat is used to replace carbohydrate because dietary fat increases insulin resistance and decreases glucose tolerance. When dogs or cats are supplied with a reduced carbohydrate diet, increased protein is theorized to support hepatic gluconeogenesis and promote normalized blood glucose concentrations in diabetic cats. Large postprandial fluctuations in blood glucose concentrations are avoided because glucose produced via hepatic gluconeogenesis is released into the circulation at a slow and steady rate. In addition, reduced carbohydrate is believed to shift metabolism from glucose oxidation toward fat metabolism as the body's primary energy source. Benefits of this shift for diabetic animals include reduced insulin secretion, a shift from lipogenesis to lipolysis, and increased use of free fatty acids as a preferred energy source. In cats, increased fat metabolism leads to an increase in the ketone body beta-hydroxybutyrate. However, the levels observed in cats fed a high-protein, low-carbohydrate food are moderate and reportedly do not approach the dangerous levels seen during metabolic acidosis associated with uncontrolled DM.[45]

It is important to correctly diagnose the presence of concurrent illnesses when considering a food with increased protein and decreased carbohydrate for diabetic cats. Cats with concurrent renal disease may experience increased blood urea nitrogen when fed a food containing even moderately increased protein. In these cases, moderate protein restriction may be needed to control azotemia and clinical signs (see Chapter 32, pp. 417-419). Similarly, foods containing reduced protein and fat are often recommended for cats with pancreatitis as an approach to reducing cholecystokinin release. Increased protein diets are always contraindicated for animals with severe liver disease.

Diabetic dogs should be fed high-quality protein in amounts that meet their daily requirements and the protein content in foods for most diabetic cats should be modestly increased. In cases when increased protein is contraindicated because of concurrent renal or liver disease, moderate protein restriction may be needed, and a food containing moderately increased fiber should be fed to control glycemia.

FAT   Fat intake by diabetic dogs and cats should be moderately restricted if the pet is overweight. Alterations in lipid metabolism can cause the development of hypercholesterolemia and hepatic lipidosis in some diabetic animals. Restricted fat intake helps to prevent or minimize these changes and facilitates weight loss or weight management when it is needed. One potential advantage of dietary fat in the nutritional management of diabetes is its effects upon gastric motility. High levels of dietary fat delay gastric emptying and consequently may modulate the postprandial glycemic response.[46] In humans, diets containing monounsaturated fats have been shown to decrease serum total cholesterol, very–low-density lipoproteins (VLDLs), and triglycerides without increasing blood glucose levels. However, this advantage is offset by the potentiating effect of dietary fat upon insulin resistance and its potential to exacerbate the blood lipid abnormalities that occur as complications of diabetes. Because of these discrepant effects and because of the contribution of dietary fat to energy density, the diet for many diabetic pets should be relatively low in fat while still containing adequate levels of essential fatty acids (EFAs) (Boxes 29-1 and 29-2).

CARBOHYDRATE   The carbohydrate content of diets for diabetic dogs and cats is an important consideration because this nutrient has the greatest influence upon postprandial blood glucose levels. A pet food that

BOX 29-1 DIETARY MANAGEMENT OF DIABETES MELLITUS IN DOGS: DIET CHARACTERISTICS

Nutritionally complete and balanced

Consistent proportion of carbohydrate, fat, and protein

Consistency of ingredients (fixed formulation)

Greater than 40% of calories supplied by complex carbohydrate

Carbohydrate includes starch sources that minimize glycemic response

Moderate fiber level

High-quality protein source

Moderately restricted in fat (≤20% of total calories)

BOX 29-2 DIETARY MANAGEMENT OF DIABETES MELLITUS IN CATS: DIET CHARACTERISTICS

Nutritionally complete and balanced

Consistent proportion of carbohydrate, fat, and protein

Consistency of ingredients (fixed formulation)

Carbohydrate includes starch sources that minimize glycemic response

Moderately restricted in fat (≤20% of total calories)

Increased protein and decreased carbohydrate (if not contraindicated) *OR*

Optimal protein and selected carbohydrate/fiber blend, and reduced caloric content (if weight loss is needed)

example, whole-grain starches have a lower glycemic index than highly refined starches.[48] Human subjects demonstrate higher blood glucose and insulin responses when refined forms of wheat starch are consumed, compared with the response to potato or barley starches.[49,50] Barley in particular has been identified as a starch source that may be well-suited for diabetic diets.[50]

Similar variations in glycemic response have been observed in dogs and cats. In one study, diets containing 30% starch from corn, wheat, barley, rice, or sorghum were fed to healthy adult dogs for a minimum of 2 weeks.[51] Feeding rice resulted in the highest postprandial glycemic and insulin responses of the five starches that were studied. In comparison, feeding sorghum resulted in a comparatively lower glycemic response, and feeding barley resulted in a moderate glucose response and a reduced insulin response. Wheat and corn generally resulted in intermediate glycemic and insulin responses. In a study with cats, two diets formulated to contain a similar starch content (33%) from different sources (sorghum and corn versus rice) were fed free-choice to overweight cats.[52] Cats fed the food containing rice consumed more food and gained more weight than cats fed the sorghum and corn diet. The cats fed the rice-containing food were also more likely to experience higher blood glucose and insulin levels following a meal.

Several factors may be responsible for these differences. The proportion of amylose and the amount of dietary fiber that are associated with a starch source both affect the glycemic response.[53] Different types of rice contain varying amounts of amylose. Those with a high amylose content result in a higher glycemic response.[48] The relatively low glycemic index of barley has been attributed to its high amount of associated fiber and beta-glucan.[54] Because glycemic response is an important consideration when selecting foods for diabetic pets, these results indicate that both the amount and the source of the starch in the diet must be considered. While feeding rice may increase postprandial hyperglycemia, feeding barley or sorghum modulates the glucose and insulin response and therefore may be a better choice for diabetic pets.

Currently, a food that is low in simple carbohydrates, contains predominantly complex carbohydrates (starch), and has moderately increased fiber is recommended for diabetic dogs (see the next section). As a general rule, complex carbohydrate should provide 40% or more of the calories in foods for diabetic dogs. Diabetic cats may

minimizes the glycemic response is desirable because lessening fluctuations in blood glucose contributes to better control of diabetes and its associated complications. The term *glycemic index* refers to a ranking system that categorizes foods based upon their effects on blood glucose levels. In general, complex carbohydrates (starches) have a lower glycemic index than simple carbohydrates because they are more slowly digested and absorbed.[47] Types of starch also differ in their glycemic effects depending upon the plant source, its physical form, and the type of cooking and processing used. For benefit from a food that contains increased protein, moderate levels of fat, and reduced carbohydrate and fiber. As discussed previously, increasing protein and decreasing carbohydrate in diets formulated for diabetic cats leads to improved glycemic control, modulation of the hyperglycemic states, and improved insulin sensitivity.[55] One study showed that when used in combination with insulin injections, feeding this type of food increased the likelihood for transient DM in recently diagnosed cats, when compared with diabetic cats that were fed a high-fiber diet.[56] An alternative approach for cats is feeding a food containing an appropriate level of protein and a blend of complex carbohydrates and dietary fibers that are formulated to aid in glycemic control (see discussion of carbohydrate sources, pp. 348-350 and discussion of fiber blends, pp. 350-352).[57,58] When this type of food has been formulated for weight control (i.e., reduced fat and decreased caloric density), this approach can effectively reduce body weight in overweight diabetic cats, further contributing to normalizing glycemic control. Both dietary approaches have been shown to be efficacious for managing long-term glycemic control in diabetic cats.[45,55,59]

A food that is low in simple carbohydrates and contains predominantly complex carbohydrates (starch) as its carbohydrate source is recommended for diabetic dogs. The type of starch that is fed is also an important consideration. Rice-containing diets result in high postprandial glycemic response, while sorghum and barley have lower glycemic responses, and so are more appropriate. Diabetic cats can be fed a food that contains increased protein and reduced carbohydrate or a food that includes optimal protein, moderately increased fiber, and, if needed, reduced calories for weight control.

Dietary Fiber

The role of dietary fiber in the management of diabetic pets has been studied extensively. Both the amount and the type of fiber have been considered. One type of classification scheme divides fiber into two broad categories: soluble fiber or insoluble fiber. Soluble fibers include pectin, gums, mucilages, a few of the hemicelluloses, and fructooligosaccharides (FOS). These fibers have high water-holding capacities, delay gastric emptying, and are believed to slow the rate of nutrient absorption across the intestinal surface. Most soluble fibers are also highly fermentable by bacteria in the large intestine. Insoluble fibers include cellulose, lignin, and most of the hemicelluloses. These fibers have less initial water-holding capacity, cause a decrease in gastrointestinal transit time, and are less efficiently fermented by gastrointestinal bacteria.[60]

Research with human subjects has shown that a diet containing a high proportion of complex carbohydrate and soluble fiber dampens the postprandial glycemic response and aids in glycemic control.[61,62] Fiber promotes the slowed digestion and absorption of dietary carbohydrate, which results in a flattening of the glucose response curve after meals. Postprandial hyperglycemia is reduced when both soluble and insoluble fibers are fed, but soluble fibers have the most pronounced effect.[63,64] Soluble fiber also has the added benefit of causing a decrease in the low-density lipoprotein fraction of blood cholesterol in human subjects.[65] The proposed mechanism of action for soluble fiber is the ability of this type of fiber to form a gel in aqueous solutions, which results in an impairment of the convective transfer of glucose and water to the absorptive surface of the intestine. These "gel-forming" fibers are referred to as *viscous fibers.* As fiber viscosity increases, so does the fiber's ability to slow glucose diffusion, resulting in pronounced flattening of the glycemic response curve and improved control of glycemia in diabetic subjects.[66,67]

Studies with dogs demonstrate similar effects of dietary fiber. When groups of dogs with DM were fed diets containing 15% fiber, significant reductions in 24-hour blood glucose fluctuations and urinary glucose excretion were reported.[68] Slight reductions in monthly insulin requirements and blood glycosylated hemoglobin concentration were also observed. These effects occurred when either insoluble fibers (cellulose) or soluble fibers (pectin) were included as the food's primary fiber source. However, it is important to note that the experimental diets used in this study were created by adding supplemental fiber or carbohydrate to a balanced food, resulting in the dilution of calories and nutrients. These diets were compared with a high-carbohydrate, low-fat control diet that was not diluted. As a result, the control diet differed from the experimental diets not only in its fiber content, but also in fat content, caloric density, and nutrient density. As a result, dogs consuming the high-fiber diets were also consuming fewer calories per meal than dogs fed the control diet. Therefore it cannot be determined if the dampening effects of the fiber-containing diets in this study were due to slowed absorption of glucose, ingestion of fewer calories, or a combination of these two factors.

In a second study, dogs with type I diabetes were fed a commercial, canned diet that was diluted by the addition of either 20 grams (g) of wheat bran (insoluble fiber) or 20 g of guar (soluble fiber).[69] When the dogs consumed the canned food without added fiber, they all developed hyperglycemia within 60 minutes of eating, followed by development of a relative hypoglycemia between 90 and 240 minutes. The addition of guar to the food abolished the postprandial hyperglycemia in four of six dogs and significantly reduced it in the remaining two dogs. The addition of wheat bran also reduced the maximal postprandial peak in blood glucose, but to a lesser extent. These effects were observed in both diabetic dogs and healthy control dogs.

Although the effect upon daily postprandial fluctuations in blood glucose is an important criterion for a diabetic diet, an equally important criterion is the diet's long-term influence upon glycemic control and health. The effects of feeding increased amounts of insoluble fiber to dogs with naturally occurring type I diabetes were examined during two 8-month periods.[70] Canned diets containing either 11% or 23% total dietary fiber, supplied primarily by insoluble fiber (cellulose), were fed to 11 dogs. Caloric intake was controlled to provide an amount of food that maintained each dog's initial body weight. The dogs accepted both diets equally and maintained body weight with only slight fluctuations. Daily caloric intake was slightly less when dogs consumed the high-fiber diet versus the low-fiber diet, but this difference was not significant. Although there were no significant differences between the two treatment groups, when evaluated individually, glycemic control improved in 9 of the 11 dogs when they were consuming the high-fiber diet, compared with when they were consuming the low-fiber diet. Significant reductions in daily insulin requirements, fasting blood glucose, 24-hour mean blood glucose, urinary glucose excretion, glycosylated hemoglobin concentrations, and serum cholesterol were observed during the high-fiber period. In contrast, 2 of the 11 dogs demonstrated better glycemic control while consuming the low-fiber

diet. It was noted that although there were no significant differences, daily caloric intakes were lower for the nine dogs while consuming the high-fiber diets, and for the two dogs while consuming the low-fiber diets. These results suggest that caloric intake may have at least partially influenced glycemic control in the dogs in this study, despite attempts to provide consistent daily caloric intake.

These results suggest that feeding a diet containing increased amounts of insoluble fiber may improve control of glycemia in some dogs with naturally occurring DM but may not be appropriate for all dogs. It is also important to note that during the course of this long-term study, 4 dogs (from an original group of 15) died or were euthanized because of diabetic complications, and 9 of the 11 remaining dogs developed concurrent disorders that are commonly associated with diabetes. These disorders developed with approximately equal frequency when dogs were fed the low- or high-fiber diets and were controlled with appropriate treatment. However, this observation raises the question of whether or not the degree of glycemic control that is reported when a high-fiber diet is fed has long-term clinical benefits. Although improved glycemic control was observed in 9 of 11 dogs, overall health and quality of life were not evaluated. Long-term studies of fiber-containing diets that include a larger number of dogs and examine the effects of fiber-containing diets on the incidence and management of associated diabetic disorders are needed.

Feeding different types of soluble fibers and fiber blends has also been studied in dogs.[71-73] One group of researchers examined the effect of feeding a blend of FOS and beet fiber on diet digestibility and glycemic response in healthy adult dogs.[71] FOS are natural polymers of fructose that are found in various plants such as bananas, onions, and barley. This fiber (also referred to as a "prebiotic") is resistant to hydrolysis in the small intestine but is highly fermented in the large intestine (see Chapter 35, pp. 467-470). Sugar beet fiber is a moderately fermentable fiber that is frequently included in commercial pet foods. When healthy adult dogs were fed diets containing either 0%, 5%, or 10% of an FOS and beet-fiber blend, the highest fiber diet caused significant decreases in postprandial glucose concentration and preprandial (fasting) serum cholesterol concentration. Increases in fiber intake were associated with increased fecal output and water content and slightly decreased protein digestibility. However, the fiber blend had no effect on fasting blood glucose concentration or postprandial insulin response. Because daily caloric intake was kept constant in this study, the glycemic and cholesterol effects were not attributable to decreased energy intake. It was postulated that the influence of soluble fiber on serum metabolites may have been due to the effects of its fermentation products on nutrient and lipid metabolism in the liver or upon secretion of gastrointestinal tract hormones that control nutrient metabolism.

The effects of increasing soluble fiber viscosity on flattening of the postprandial glycemic response curve have also been studied in dogs.[72,74,75] Dog foods containing either 1% or 3% carboxymethylcellulose (CMC) of either high or low viscosity were fed to healthy dogs, and postprandial serum glucose and insulin concentrations were measured.[72] Dogs fed the high-CMC diets developed soft feces or diarrhea, while dogs fed the low-CMC diets had normal stools. The production of soft feces or diarrhea in dogs consuming diets containing soluble fiber has been reported previously and is considered to be a common side effect of feeding this type of fiber.[76] As with insoluble fiber, dogs had widely divergent responses to the consumption of CMC. Because of these variations, no statistically significant effects of CMC or viscosity were found. However, dogs fed diets containing 1% high-viscosity CMC showed the lowest mean values for postprandial glucose and insulin and had the longest time for postprandial blood glucose to return to the normal fasting range. In addition, serum glucose concentrations consistently decreased below the normal fasting range by 30 minutes after eating in dogs fed CMC-containing diets. This was not observed in dogs fed the control diet. These results suggest that the CMC may delay gastric emptying or slow nutrient absorption. In contrast, dogs fed the 3% CMC diet had the highest postprandial increases, indicating enhanced glucose absorption. These inconsistent results suggest that high amounts of CMC may actually enhance glucose absorption, although a specific mechanism for this response is not known.

Research examining the efficacy of high-fiber diets for the management of diabetic pets may have raised more questions than it has answered. While increased amounts of insoluble fiber have been shown to dampen the postprandial glycemic curve, it is possible that this is an effect of decreased energy intake caused by dilution of the diet, rather than a direct effect of fiber. Moreover, fiber's ability to provide long-term health benefits or improved quality of life or to prevent or ameliorate diabetic complications has not been thoroughly evaluated. The use of soluble fiber may have efficacy in delaying gastric emptying and slowing glucose absorption in the intestine. However, high amounts of soluble fiber are not well tolerated by dogs and can cause increased fecal water, loose stools, and diarrhea. Moreover, dogs appear to have highly variable responses to the inclusion of both types of fiber in their diets. Currently, the best solution appears to be through creation of fiber blends that function to slow gastric emptying time, modulate glucose absorption, and dampen the postprandial glycemic curve in diabetic pets. Several foods that meet these criteria are currently available as veterinary therapeutic diets for dogs and cats with DM.

Increasing dietary fiber can help to dampen the postprandial glycemic curve in diabetic dogs and cats. However, there is a great deal of individual variability among animals and different fiber types produce different results. The use of fiber blends that include both soluble and insoluble fiber types in foods for diabetic pets appear to be the most effective approach to modulate glucose absorption, and dampen the postprandial glycemic curve.

Chromium

The trace mineral chromium has been recognized as an essential nutrient needed for glucose metabolism since the late 1950s.[77] The biologically active form of chromium functions as a potentiator of insulin action and is called *glucose tolerance factor.* The precise composition of this factor is not known, but it appears that nicotinic acid is an essential component.[78,79] Theories for the mechanism of action of glucose tolerance factor include direct interaction with insulin, effect on the production of insulin receptors, and a postreceptor metabolic interaction.[80,81]

Chromium deficiency in humans is associated with abnormal glucose utilization and insulin resistance and has been hypothesized to be a factor in the development of adult-onset diabetes. Although variable results are reported, improved glucose tolerance is seen in some human diabetics when their diets are supplemented with this mineral.[82,83] Chromium supplementation has also been shown to increase glucose uptake by tissues in swine and cattle.[84,85] These results suggest that chromium supplementation may have a role in improving glycemic control in diabetic pets.

A set of experiments examined the effect of chromium supplementation on glucose metabolism and insulin sensitivity in healthy adult dogs.[86] In two experiments, groups of 24 Beagles were fed diets containing either 0, 0.15, 0.3, or 0.6 parts per million (ppm) of supplemental chromium tripicolinate. Dogs that received supplemental chromium had lower plasma glucose concentrations for 30 minutes and slightly higher glucose clearance rates for between 10 and 30 minutes following intravenous glucose administration when compared with the values for dogs that did not receive supplemental chromium. Chromium supplementation was associated with lower fasting blood glucose levels, but it did not affect the serum insulin response to glucose infusion. These results are consistent with those reported in humans and other species and suggest that chromium supplementation in dogs increases tissue sensitivity to the effects of insulin. Conversely, another study reported no beneficial effects when 13 insulin-treated diabetic dogs were supplemented with 20 to 60 micrograms (μg)/kilogram (kg)/day of chromium picolinate.[87] It is possible that benefits were not seen in this study because the dogs' diabetes was well controlled and the dogs were chromium replete.

Chromium supplementation has been studied in cats as well. One study in healthy, normal weight cats showed that the addition of chromium tripicolinate at 300 and 600 parts per billion (ppb) to the food produced improvement in glucose tolerance as measured by glucose half-life, area under the glucose curve, and absolute glucose concentrations.[88] Results of this study indicated that chromium supplementation improved tissue sensitivity to insulin in cats. Although the effects observed in these studies were relatively small, these data indicate that increasing the level of chromium in diets formulated for pets with risk factors for diabetes and for diabetic pets may improve glucose tolerance and aid in glycemic control. Cats with naturally occurring glucose intolerance and insulin resistance, that are genetically predisposed to glucose tolerance (i.e., Burmese cats), or animals that are marginally deficient in chromium are most likely to benefit from chromium supplementation.

Caloric Intake and Weight Control

The relationship between obesity and type II diabetes in humans and cats is well documented.[89] The relationship is not as well documented in dogs, but obesity does negatively affect glucose tolerance in dogs. The baseline plasma insulin level and insulin response to a glucose load increase linearly in dogs as a function of their degree of obesity, but these changes do not always result in DM and often resolve with weight loss.[11] Similarly, healthy but obese cats with normal fasting plasma glucose concentrations showed abnormal results on glucose tolerance tests and slightly elevated baseline serum insulin concentrations.[89] Significant delays in initial insulin response and substantially increased insulin responses at a later phase of the glucose tolerance test were found in the overweight cats. Decreased tissue sensitivity to insulin (insulin resistance) and impaired beta-cell responsiveness to stimuli are believed to be the cause of these changes. There may be several underlying causes of insulin resistance. The tissue of obese animals experience a down-regulation of cellular insulin receptors, and the receptors that are present may have reduced binding affinity for insulin.[90-92] In some cases, a postreceptor, intracellular defect in insulin action also occurs.[93] Ultimately, these changes decrease target tissues' ability to respond to insulin. Over time, beta-cell hyperresponsiveness develops, baseline insulin and insulin secretion increase in an attempt to compensate for the cellular resistance to insulin, and chronic hyperglycemia develops.

Weight reduction is an important aspect of the dietary management of diabetic animals that are overweight. When obesity is reduced in dogs and cats with abnormal insulin-secretory responses, glucose tolerance often improves.[11] In addition, weight loss in dogs with type I diabetes can result in enhanced tissue sensitivity to insulin, resulting in lowered daily insulin requirements. When a diabetic pet is overweight, caloric intake should be designed for weight loss and the eventual maintenance of ideal body weight. A food that is formulated to be complete and balanced—while containing moderately increased fiber, increased complex carbo-hydrates, and reduced fat—is recommended for most diabetic dogs. (Note: Adding complex carbohydrates or fiber to a normal diet in an attempt to decrease energy density is contraindicated because this practice may cause increased stool volume, loose stools, or diarrhea and can lead to nutrient imbalances.) Overweight dia-betic cats benefit from either a low-carbohydrate/high-protein or an increased-fiber food (see p. 350). In all cases that animals with DM are fed to promote weight loss, the pet's blood glucose should be carefully moni-tored and adjustments of insulin can be made as glucose tolerance improves.

> *Weight reduction is an important component of the dietary management of overweight diabetic pets. When obesity is reduced in animals with abnormal insulin-secretory responses, glucose tolerance usually improves. Weight loss in dogs with type I diabetes can result in enhanced tissue sensitivity to insulin, resulting in lowered daily insulin requirements. When a diabetic pet is overweight, caloric intake should be designed for weight loss and the eventual maintenance of ideal body weight.*

Timing of Meals

The feeding schedule for insulin-dependent animals should be planned so that nutrients are delivered to the body during peak periods of exogenous insulin activ-ity. This span will be determined by the type of insu-lin used and the time of day it is administered. Several small meals should be provided throughout the period of insulin activity, as opposed to feeding a single large meal. Feeding several small meals helps minimize postprandial fluctuations in blood glucose levels. Other factors that affect the degree of hyperglycemia that occurs following a meal include the composition of the food and the type of insulin administered.

If insulin is administered early in the morning, the first meal should be given immediately before the insu-lin injection. If the pet refuses to eat on any occasion, the insulin injection can be withheld. This approach protects against the risk of insulin-induced hypoglyce-mia, which can be life threatening. The remaining three or four meals in the day can be given at equally spaced intervals, depending on the action of the insulin used. Taking blood samples and measuring blood glucose lev-els every 1 to 2 hours throughout a 24-hour period will indicate if the feeding schedule coincides adequately with insulin activity. If postprandial blood glucose levels rise above 180 milligrams (mg)/deciliter (dl), the inter-val between feeding and insulin administration should be decreased. If hyperglycemia still occurs, the size of the meal should be decreased and/or the number of meals provided per day should be increased. Likewise, a meal should always be provided within 1 to 2 hours following the lowest blood glucose level.

Once an appropriate pet food and feeding schedule have been selected, the management program should be adhered to strictly. Pets that have previously been fed free choice should be gradually switched to the new regimen. Although most dogs will adapt quickly, cats can be very resistant to changes in their feeding routine and in the type of food that is fed. This resis-tance can make dietary management of a diabetic cat difficult for some owners. Mixing the new food into the cat's previous food and changing to a meal-feeding regimen over a period of several weeks can help decrease these problems. Allowing cats to nibble over the period of insulin activity is also effective in some cases.[94] Supplemental foods should not be given, and feeding times should vary as little as possible. Home monitor-ing of clinical signs and periodic monitoring of blood glucose curves and serum fructosamine levels and/or glycosylated hemoglobin concentrations (GHb) can be used to adjust the diet as the pet loses weight, has alter-ations in exercise, or requires adjustments in insulin dosage.[95]

References

1. Rand JS, Fleeman LM, Farrow HA, and others: Canine and feline diabetes mellitus: nature or nurture? *J Nutr* 134:2072S–2080S, 2004.

2. Fall T, Hamlin HH, Hedhammer A, and others: Diabetes mellitus in a population of 180,000 insured dogs: incidence, survival and breed distribution, *J Vet Intern Med* 21:1209–1216, 2007.

3. Guptill L, Glickman L, Glickman N: Time trends and risk factors for diabetes mellitus in dogs: analysis of veterinary medical data base records (1970-1999), *Vet J* 165:240–247, 2003.

4. Prahl A, Guptill L, Glickman NW, and others: Time trends and risk factors for diabetes mellitus in cats presented to veterinary teaching hospitals, *J Feline Med Surg* 9:351–358, 2007.

5. McCann TM, Simpson KE, Shaw DJ: Feline diabetes mellitus in the UK: the prevalence within an insured cat population and a question-based putative risk factor analysis, *J Feline Med Surg* 9:289–299, 2007.

6. Davison LJ, Herrtage ME, Steiner JM, and others: Evidence of anti-insulin autoreactivity and pancreatic inflammation in newly diagnosed diabetic dogs (abstract), *J Vet Intern Med* 17:395, 2003.

7. Catchpole B, Ristic JM, Fleeman LM, Davison LJ: Canine diabetes mellitus: can old dogs teach us new tricks? *Diabetologia* 48:1948–1956, 2005.

8. Eigenmann JE, Eigenmann RY, Rijnberk A: Progesterone-controlled growth hormone overproduction and naturally occurring canine diabetes and acromegaly, *Acta Endocrinol* 104:167–176, 1983.

9. Doxey DL, Milne EM, Mackenzie CP: Canine diabetes mellitus: a retrospective survey, *J Small Anim Pract* 26:555–561, 1985.

10. Klinkenberg H, Sallander MH, Hedhammar A: Feeding, exercise, and weight identified as risk factors in canine diabetes mellitus, *J Nutr* 136:1985S–1987S, 2006.

11. Mattheeuws D, Rottiers R, Baeyens D, and others: Glucose tolerance and insulin response in obese dogs, *J Am Anim Hosp Assoc* 20:287–290, 1984.

12. Hess RS, Kass PH, Ward CR: Breed distribution of dogs with diabetes mellitus admitted to a tertiary care facility, *J Am Vet Med Assoc* 216:1414–1417, 2000.

13. Panciera DL, Thomas CB, Eicker SW, and others: Epizootiologic patterns of diabetes mellitus in cats: 333 cases (1980-1986), *J Am Vet Med Assoc* 197:1504–1508, 1990.

14. Scarlett JM, Donoghue S: Associations between body condition and disease I cats, *J Am Vet Med Assoc* 212:1725–1731, 1998.

15. Slingerland LI, Fazilova VV, Plantiga EA, and others: Indoor confinement and physical inactivity rather than the proportion of dry food are risk factors in the development of feline type 2 diabetes mellitus, *Vet J* 179:247–253, 2009.

16. Buscher H, Jacobs M, Ong G, and others: Beta-cell function of the pancreas after necrotizing pancreatitis, *Dig Surg* 16:496–500, 1999.

17. Petersen ME, Taylor RS, Greco DS, and others: Acromegaly in 14 cats, *J Vet Med* 4:192–201, 1990.

18. Elliott DA, Feldman EC, Koblik PD, and others: Prevalence of pituitary tumors among diabetic cats with insulin resistance, *J Am Vet Med Assoc* 216:1765–1768, 2000.

19. Berg RI, Nelson RW, Feldman EC, and others: Serum insulin-like growth factor-1 concentration in cats with diabetes mellitus and acromegaly, *J Vet Intern Med* 21:892–898, 2007.

20. Peterson ME: Effects of megestrol acetate on glucose tolerance and growth hormone secretion in the cat, *Res Vet Sci* 42:354–357, 1987.

21. Lederer R, Rand J, Hughes IP, Fleeman LM: Chronic of recurring medical problems, dental disease, repeated corticosteroid treatment, and lower physical activity are associated with diabetes in Burmese cats (abstract), *J Vet Intern Med* 17:433, 2003.

22. Wade C, Gething M, Rand JS: Evidence of a genetic basis for diabetes mellitus in Burmese cats, *J Vet Intern Med* 13:269, 1999.

23. Appleton DJ, Rand JS, Sunvold GD: Insulin sensitivity decreases with obesity, and lean cats with low insulin sensitivity are at greatest risk of glucose intolerance with weight gain, *J. Feline Med Surg* 3:211–228, 2001.

24. Harris MI: Epidemiological studies on the pathogenesis of non-insulin dependent diabetes mellitus (NIDDM), *Clin Invest Med* 18:231–239, 1995.

25. Hoenig M: Pathophysiology of canine diabetes, *Vet Clin North Am Small Anim Pract* 25:253–256, 1995.

26. Akerblom HK, Vaarala O, Hyoty H: Environmental factors in the etiology of type I diabetes, *Am J Med Genet* 115:18–29, 2002.

27. Rand JS: Current understanding of feline diabetes mellitus: part 1, pathogenesis, *J Feline Med Surg* 1:143–153, 1999.

28. Lutz TA, Rand JS: Plasma inulin and insulin concentrations in normo- and hyperglycemic cats, *Can Vet J* 37:27–34, 1996.

29. Struble AL, Nelson RW: Non–insulin-dependent diabetes mellitus in cats and humans, *Compend Contin Educ Pract Vet* 19:935–945, 1997.

30. O'Brien TD, Hayden DW, Johnson EH, and others: High dose intravenous glucose tolerance test and serum insulin and glucagon levels in diabetic and non-diabetic cats: relationships to insular amyloidosis, *Vet Pathol* 22:250–261, 1985.

31. Mattheeuws D, Rottiers R, Kaneko JJ, and others: Diabetes mellitus in dogs: relationship of obesity to glucose tolerance and insulin response, *Am J Vet Res* 45:98–103, 1984.

32. O'Brien TD, Butler PC, Westermark P, Johnson KH: Islet amyloid polypeptide: a review of its biology and potential roles in the pathogenesis of diabetes mellitus, *Vet Pathol* 30:317–332, 1993.

33. Link KRJ, Rand JS: Glucose toxicity in cats, *J Vet Intern Med* 10:185, 1996.

34. Nelson RW, Feldman EC, Ford SL, and others: Transient diabetes mellitus in the cat. In *Proc Ann Conf Vet Intern Med Forum*, 1992, p 794.

35. Bennett N, Greco DS, Peterson ME, and others: Comparison of a low carbohydrate-low fiber diet and a moderate carbohydrate-high fiber diet in the management of feline diabetes mellitus, *J Feline Med Surg* 8:73–84, 2006.

36. Brand Miller JC, Colagiuri S: The carnivore connection: dietary carbohydrate in the evolution of NIDDM, *Diabetologia* 37:1280–1286, 1994.

37. Zoran DL: The carnivore connection to nutrition in cats, *J Am Vet Med Assoc* 221:1559–1567, 2002.

38. Beam S, Correa MT, Davidson MG: A retrospective-cohort study on the development of cataracts in dogs with diabetes mellitus: 200 cases, *Vet Ophthalmol* 2:169–172, 1999.

39. Williams DL, Heath MF: Prevalence of feline cataract: results of a cross-sectional study of 2,000 normal animals, 50 cats with diabetes mellitus and one hundred cats following dehydrated crises, *Vet Ophthalmol* 9:341–349, 2006.

40. Mizisin AP, Shelton GD, Burges ML, and others: Neurological complications associated with spontaneously occurring feline diabetes mellitus, *J Neuropathol Exp Neurol* 61:872–884, 2002.

41. Forrester SD, Troy GC, Dalton MN, and others: Retrospective evaluation of urinary tract infection in 42 dogs with hyperadrenocorticism or diabetes mellitus or both, *J Vet Intern Med* 13:557–560, 1999.

42. Bailiff NL, Nelson RW, Feldman EC, and others: Frequency and risk factors for urinary tract infection in cats with diabetes mellitus, *J Vet Intern Med* 20:850–855, 2006.

43. Litle CJL, Gettinby G: Heart failure is common in diabetic cats: findings from a retrospective case-controlled study in first-opinion practice, *J Small Anim Pract* 49:17–25, 2008.

44. Holste LC, Nelson RW, Feldman EC, and others: Effect of dry, soft moist, and canned dog foods on postprandial blood glucose and insulin concentrations in healthy dogs, *Am J Vet Res* 50:984–989, 1989.

45. Kirk CA: Feline diabetes mellitus: low carbohydrates versus high fiber? *Vet Clin North Am Small Anim Pract* 36:1297–1306, 2006.

46. El-Berheri Burgess BRB: Rationale for changes in the dietary management of diabetes, *J Am Diet Assoc* 81:258–270, 1982.

47. Jenkins DJA, Wolever TMS, Taylor RH, and others: Glycemic index of foods: a physiological basis for carbohydrate exchange, *Am J Clin Nutr* 34:362–366, 1981.

48. Jarvi AE, Karlstrom YE, Garnfeldt YE, and others: The influence of food structure on postprandial metabolism in patients with non–insulin-dependent diabetes mellitus, *Am J Clin Nutr* 61:837–842, 1995.

49. Bantle JP, Laine DC, Castle GW, and others: Postprandial glucose and insulin responses to meals containing different carbohydrate in normal and diabetic subjects, *N Engl J Med* 309:712, 1983.

50. Wolever TMS, Bolonesi C: Source and amount of carbohydrate affect postprandial glucose and insulin in normal subjects, *J Nutr* 126:2798–2806, 1996.

51. Sunvold GD, Bouchard GF: The glycemic response to dietary starch. In Reinhart GA, Carey DP, editors: *Recent advances in canine and feline nutrition, Iams nutrition symposium proceedings*, vol 2, Wilmington, Ohio, 1998, Orange Frazer Press.

52. Appleton DJ, Rand JS, Priest J, and others: Dietary carbohydrate source affects glucose concentrations, insulin secretion and food intake in overweight cats, *Nutr Res* 24:447–467, 2004.

53. Goddard MS, Young G, Marcus R: The effect of amylose content on insulin and glucose responses to ingested rice, *Am J Clin Nutr* 39:388–392, 1984.

54. Liljeberg HGM, Granfeldt YE, Bjorck IME: Products based on a high fiber barley genotype, but not on common barley or oats, lower postprandial glucose and insulin responses in healthy humans, *J Nutr* 126:458–466, 1996.

55. Bennett N, Greco DS, Peterson ME, and others: Comparison of a low carbohydrate-low fiber diet and a moderate carbohydrate-high fiber diet in the management of feline diabetes mellitus, *J Feline Med Surg* 8:73–84, 2006.

56. Mazzaferro EM, Greco DS, Turner AS: Treatment of feline diabetes mellitus using an alpha-glucosidase inhibitor and a low-carbohydrate diet, *J Feline Med Surg* 5:183–189, 2003.

57. Nelson RW, Scott-Moncrieff JC, Feldman EC: Effect of dietary insoluble fiber on control of glycemia in cats with naturally acquired diabetes mellitus, *J Am Vet Med Assoc* 216:1082–1088, 2000.

58. Frank G, Anderson W, Pazak H: Use of a high-protein diet in the management of feline diabetes mellitus, *Vet Ther* 2:238–246, 2001.

59. Rand JS, Marshall RD: Diabetes mellitus in cats, *Vet Clin North Am Small Anim Pract* 35:211–234, 2005.

60. Anderson JW: Physiological and metabolic effects of dietary fiber, *Fed Proc* 44:2902–2906, 1985.

61. Crapo PA: Carbohydrate in the diabetic diet, *J Am Coll Nutr* 5:31–43, 1986.

62. Riccardi G, Rivellese A, Pacioni D, and others: Separate influence of dietary carbohydrate and fiber on the metabolic control of diabetes, *Diabetologia* 26:116–121, 1984.

63. Nuttal FQ: Dietary fiber in the management of diabetes, *Diabetes* 42:503–508, 1993.

64. Vaaler S: Diabetic control is improved by guar gum and wheat bran supplementation, *Diabetic Med* 3:230–233, 1986.

65. Kay RM, Truswell AS: Effect of citrus pectin on blood lipids and fecal steroid excretion in man, *Am J Clin Nutr* 30:171–175, 1977.

66. O'Connor N, Tredger J, Morgan L: Viscosity differences between various guar gums, *Diabetologia* 20:612–615, 1981.

67. Holt S, Heading RC, Carter DC, and others: Effect of gel fiber on gastric emptying and absorption of glucose and paracetamol, *Lancet* 1:636–639, 1979.

68. Nelson RW, Ihle SL, Lewis LD, and others: Effects of dietary fiber supplementation on glycemic control in dogs with alloxan-induced diabetes mellitus, *Am J Vet Res* 52:2060–2066, 1991.

69. Blaxter AC, Cripps RJ, Gruffyd-Jones TJ: Dietary fibre and postprandial hyperglycemia in normal and diabetic dogs, *J Small Anim Pract* 31:229–233, 1990.

70. Nelson RW, Duesberg CA, Ford SL, and others: Effect of dietary insoluble fiber on control of glycemia in dogs with naturally acquired diabetes mellitus, *J Am Vet Med Assoc* 212:380–386, 1998.

71. Diez M, Hornick JL, Baldwin P, and others: Influence of a blend of fructo-oligosaccharides and sugar beet fiber on nutrient digestibility and plasma metabolite concentrations in healthy Beagles, *Am J Vet Res* 58:1238–1242, 1997.

72. Nelson RW, Sunvold GD: Effect of carboxymethylcellulose on postprandial glycemic response in healthy dogs. In Reinhart GA, Carey DP, editors: *Recent advances in canine and feline nutrition, Iams nutrition symposium proceedings*, vol 2, Wilmington, Ohio, 1998, Orange Frazer Press.

73. Burney MI, Massimino SF, Field CJ, and others: Modulation of intestinal function and glucose homeostasis in dogs by the ingestion of fermentable dietary fibers. In Reinhart GA, Carey DP, editors: *Recent advances in canine and feline nutrition, Iams nutrition symposium proceedings*, vol 2, Wilmington, Ohio, 1998, Orange Frazer Press.

74. Reppas C, Meyer JH, Sirois J, Dressman JB: Effect of hydroxyproplymethylcellulose on gastrointestinal transit and luminal viscosity in dogs, *Gastroenterology* 100:1217–1223, 1991.

75. Reppas C, Dressman JB: Viscosity modulates blood glucose response to nutrient solutions in dogs, *Diabetes Res Clin Pract* 17:81–88, 1992.

76. Nelson RW: Dietary management of diabetes mellitus, *J Small Anim Pract* 33:213–217, 1992.

77. Schwarz K, Mertz W: Chromium (III) and the glucose tolerance factor, *Arch Biochem Biophys* 85:292–295, 1959.

78. Urberg M, Zemel MB: Evidence for synergism between chromium and nicotinic acid in the control of glucose tolerance in elderly humans, *Metabolism* 36:896–899, 1987.

79. Olin KL, Stearns DM, Armstrong WH, and others: Comparative retention/absorption of [51]chromium from [51]chromium chloride, [51]chromium nicotinate and [51]chromium picolinate in a rat model, *Trace Elements Electrolytes* 11:182–186, 1994.

80. Evans GW: The effect of chromium picolinate on insulin controlled parameters in humans, *Int J Biosoc Med Res* 11:163–180, 1989.

81. Anderson RA, Polansky MM, Bryden NA, and others: Effects of supplemental chromium on patients with symptoms of reactive hypoglycemia, *Metabolism* 36:351–355, 1987.

82. Mossop RT: Effects of chromium (III) on fasting glucose, cholesterol, and cholesterol HDL levels in diabetics, *Cent Afr J Med* 29:80–82, 1983.

83. Glinsmann WH, Mertz W: Effect of trivalent chromium on glucose tolerance, *Metabolism* 15:510–520, 1966.

84. Bunting LD, Fernandez JM, Thompson DL, and others: Influence of chromium picolinate on glucose usage and metabolic criteria in growing Holstein calves, *J Anim Sci* 72:1591–1599, 1994.

85. Amoikon EF, Fernandez JM, Southern LL, and others: Effect of chromium tripicolinate on growth, glucose tolerance, insulin sensitivity, plasma metabolites and growth hormone in pigs, *J Anim Sci* 73:1123–1130, 1995.

86. Spears JW, Brown TT, Sunvold GD, and others: Influence of chromium on glucose metabolism and insulin sensitivity. In Reinhart GA, Carey DP, editors: *Recent advances in canine and feline nutrition, Iams nutrition symposium proceedings*, vol 2, Wilmington, Ohio, 1998, Orange Frazer Press.

87. Schachter S, Nelson RW, Kirk CA: Oral chromium picolinate and control of glycemia in insulin-treated diabetic dogs, *J Vet Intern Med* 15:379–384, 2001.

88. Appleton DJ, Rand JS, Sunvold GD, Priest J: Dietary chromium tripicolinate supplementation reduces glucose concentrations and improves glucose tolerance in normal-weight cats, *J Feline Med Surg* 4:13–25, 2002.

89. Nelson RW, Himsel CA, Feldman EC, and others: Glucose tolerance and insulin response in normal-weight and obese cats, *Am J Vet Res* 51:1357–1362, 1990.

90. Brennan CL, Hoenig M, Ferguson DC: GLUT4 but not GLUT 1 expression decreases early in the development of feline obesity, *Domest Anim Endocrinol* 26:291–301, 2004.

91. Bar RS, Gordon P, Roth J, and others: Fluctuations in the affinity and concentration of insulin receptors on circulating monocytes of obese patients: effects of starvation, refeeding and dieting, *J Clin Invest* 58:1123–1135, 1976.

92. Lockwood DH, Hamilton CL, Livingston JN: The influence of obesity and diabetes in the monkey on insulin and glucagon binding to liver membranes, *Endocrinology* 104:76–81, 1979.

93. Olefsky JM, Ciaraldi TP, Kolterman OG: Mechanisms of insulin resistance in noninsulin-dependent (type II) diabetes, *Am J Med* 79:12–21, 1985.

94. Martin GJW, Rand JS: Food intake and blood glucose in normal and diabetic cats fed ad libitum, *J Feline Med Surg* 1:241–251, 1999.

95. Bennett N: Monitoring techniques for diabetes mellitus in the dog and the cat, *Clin Tech Small Anim Pract* 17:65–69, 2002.

30

Dietary Management of Urolithiasis in Cats and Dogs

Lower urinary tract disease is a common disorder in dogs and cats. It is estimated to occur in approximately 0.6% of the owned cat population and is diagnosed in between 3% and 13% of cats presented for veterinary care.[1] In dogs, lower urinary tract disease is diagnosed in approximately 3% of dogs admitted to veterinary colleges in North America.[2] Urolithiasis is a specific type of lower urinary tract disease characterized by the presence of urinary crystals (crystalluria) or macroscopic concretions (uroliths or calculi) within the bladder or lower urinary tract, as well as associated clinical signs. Urethral plugs often contain varying proportions of mineral matter and so are classified with urolithiasis. In cats, urolithiasis is now considered to be one manifestation of a collection of lower urinary tract disorders collectively referred to as FLUTD (feline lower urinary tract disease).

Urolithiasis is associated with a set of diverse risk factors and can be caused by several different types of mineral aggregates. Dogs show breed predilections for certain types of urolith formation and are more susceptible to infection-induced urolithiasis than cats are.[3] In both species, identification of the mineral composition of uroliths is important because dietary treatment or management must be directed toward the specific type of urolith present. This chapter reviews the types of uroliths found in dogs and cats, historical shifts in canine and feline urolith composition and location, risk factors for their development, and dietary management to treat urolithiasis and to prevent recurrence.

INCIDENCE

Urolithiasis is typically a disease of adult animals. In cats, it is rarely seen in animals younger than 1 year old, and the majority of cats are first diagnosed when they are between 2 and 6 years old.[4] In dogs, the mean age at time of diagnosis is between 6 and 7 years.[5] More than 80% of uroliths in both dogs and cats are composed of

magnesium ammonium phosphate (struvite) or calcium oxalate. However, a major difference between struvite urolithiasis in cats and dogs is that most struvite uroliths in cats are not associated with urinary tract infection (sterile struvite), while urinary tract infection is common in dogs with struvite urolithiasis. Other, less frequently seen mineral composites include ammonium urate, xanthine, cystine, calcium phosphate, silica, and dried, solidified blood (cats).

More than 80% of uroliths in both dogs and cats are composed of magnesium ammonium phosphate (struvite) or calcium oxalate. However, a major difference between struvite urolithiasis in cats and dogs is that most struvite uroliths in cats are not associated with urinary tract infection (sterile struvite), while urinary tract infection is common in dogs with struvite urolithiasis.

Urolithiasis is typically a disease of adult animals. In cats, it is rarely seen in animals younger than 1 year old, and the majority of cats are first diagnosed when they are between 2 and 6 years old. Cats less than 4 years old are more likely to develop struvite uroliths, while cats older than 7 years old are at greater risk for developing calcium oxalate uroliths. In dogs, the mean age at time of diagnosis is between 6 and 7 years. Struvite, urate, and cystine calculi are associated with younger adults, and oxalate calculi are associated with older adults.

Initial studies of urolithiasis in cats found that the majority of cases were caused by struvite and a very small percentage was caused by calcium oxalate. However, by the early 1990s the percentages of struvite- and calcium oxalate–containing calculi observed in cats were approximately equal, and the prevalence of calcium oxalate uroliths continued to gradually increase as the prevalence of struvite uroliths decreased.[6] This reciprocal trend continued until 2002, after which the proportions of the two types of calculi again became approximately equal. A similar trend has been reported in dogs.[7,8] During the period that the incidence of feline calcium oxalate urolithiasis increased, there was a concomitant increase in cat foods formulated to decrease urine pH with the intention of preventing struvite urolithiasis. This change in formulation presumably reduced the risk of struvite urolithiasis in the subpopulation of cats that were susceptible to this type of urolith. Conversely, feeding an acidifying diet to healthy cats may have increased the risk for developing calcium oxalate calculi. As recognition of this trend became widespread, foods were formulated to produce more moderate changes in urine pH, correcting the shift that may have temporarily favored calcium oxalate formation.[6]

In both species, age of onset of urolithiasis is related to the type of urolith present. For example, struvite, urate, and cystine calculi are associated with younger dogs (mean age 4.25 to 5.92 years), and oxalate, silica, and brushite calculi are associated with older dogs (mean age 7.04 to 8.71 years).[5] In dogs younger than 1 year old, the most common urolith is infection-induced struvite.[9] Similarly, cats less than 4 years old are more likely to develop struvite uroliths, while cats older than 7 years are at greater risk for developing calcium oxalate uroliths.[6] Sex predispositions are also observed. Female cats have a higher prevalence of struvite urolithiasis than male cats, and more than 70% of cases of calcium oxalate urolithiasis are seen in male cats.[10,11] Studies with dogs have shown a similar relationship between sex and mineral prevalence.[12] Struvite-, urate-, or calcium phosphorus (apatite)–containing calculi are more common in female dogs, while oxalate-, cystine-, and silica-containing stones are seen more often in males.

There is a clear genetic influence on the development of urolithiasis in both dogs and cats. Early studies reported that, compared with domestic shorthair cats, Siamese had a decreased risk and Persians had an increased risk of developing FLUTD.[10,13] More recently, studies of calcium oxalate and struvite uroliths in cats revealed that British shorthair, exotic shorthair, foreign shorthair, Havana Brown, Himalayan, Persian, Ragdoll, and Scottish Fold cat breeds show a higher risk of calcium oxalate uroliths and that Chartreux,

domestic shorthair, foreign shorthair, Himalayan, oriental shorthair, and Ragdoll cat breeds have a higher risk for struvite uroliths.[11] It has been speculated that breed characteristics such as low activity and a tendency toward obesity may be influential factors. Breed predilections for urolithiasis in dogs may be more pronounced, but there is variability among study results. Calcium oxalate uroliths are reportedly more common in the Pomeranian, Miniature and Toy Poodle, Miniature and Standard Schnauzer, Lhasa Apso, Maltese, Yorkshire Terrier, Cairn Terrier, Shih Tzu, Bichon Frise, and Samoyed breeds.[5,7,14] Struvite uroliths are reported in the Bichon Frise, Shih Tzu, Lhaso Apso, Yorkshire Terrier, Dachshund, Miniature Schnauzer, Poodle, Pekingese, Pug, Welsh Corgi, Beagle, Cocker Spaniel, Springer Spaniel, and Labrador Retriever.[5,14,15] Conversely, Dachshunds, English Bulldogs, Newfoundland, Scottish Deerhound, Rottweiler, and Chihuahuas appear to be at increased risk for the development of cystine-containing calculi.[5,14] Finally, urate-containing calculi are most often seen in Dalmatians, English Bulldogs, and Miniature Schnauzers. Further complicating the situation, some canine urinary calculi have multiple layers composed of a variety of elements.[5]

Uroliths in dogs and cats have historically been located almost exclusively in the bladder and urethra. However a recent study reported a 10-fold increase in feline kidney and ureter uroliths (nephroliths and ureteroliths, respectively) during the 20-year period between 1980 and 1999.[16] Another study reported that only 10 feline uroliths submitted to the Minnesota Urolith Center for analysis were from the upper urinary tract in 1990, while 139 cases submitted in the year 2000 were located in the upper urinary tract.[17] The authors noted that this change occurred during a period in which the prevalence of chronic renal failure in cats was also increasing. Survey radiographic evaluation of the cats in this study revealed that 41% of the cats with chronic renal failure had evidence of nephroliths or ureteroliths.[17] However, none of the cats had shown clinical signs attributable to upper urinary tract stones, suggesting that these stones are often not detected. Acute ureteral obstruction by uroliths is an emerging clinical syndrome in cats that is not completely understood and warrants additional study.[18] The majority of upper urinary tract uroliths contain calcium in cats.[17] In contrast, in dogs, nephroliths and ureteroliths may contain struvite, calcium oxalate, or other urolith types.[19] Traditionally, many theories to explain calculi formation have focused on the urinary environment and saturation with particular components such as calcium and oxalate. However, the increased prevalence of upper urinary tract stones suggests that other factors may be involved. One theory proposed in humans, but not yet investigated in pets, is that an initial, primary calcium stone-forming event begins with injury in the vascular bed at the tip of the renal papilla, which subsequently leads to the formation of calcium oxalate–containing uroliths in the kidneys.[20,21]

CLINICAL SIGNS

Clinical signs of urolithiasis in dogs and cats are non-specific and depend on the location, size, and number of crystals or uroliths present within the urinary tract. Uroliths may be found in the bladder, urethra, kidneys, or ureters. Although uroliths can be up to several millimeters in diameter or even larger, most range in size from microscopic to the size of a grain of sand.

Initial clinical signs of lower urinary tract disease include frequent urination, dribbling of urine, and urination in inappropriate places (Box 30-1). Hematuria and a strong odor of ammonia in the urine are often observed. Pet owners may report additional signs of dysuria, such as prolonged squatting or straining following urination (often confused with constipation)

and frequent licking of the urogenital region. These signs are frequently the only signs that owners report to veterinarians. The most accurate method of diagnosis is double-contrast cystography, although survey radiography and ultrasonography are also useful.[22] Urinalysis is an important component in the diagnosis of all urinary disorders and provides additional information. However, because urinary crystals (crystalluria) may be present or absent in animals with urolithiasis, and because uroliths can be present without crystals, crystalluria by itself is not diagnostic.[23] In addition, normal urine can contain crystals, especially if it is concentrated or has been refrigerated prior to analysis. When uroliths are found and removed, definitive diagnosis is made by chemical analysis of the type of urolith that is present.

In some cases, partial or total urethral obstruction may develop. When obstruction occurs, a variable mixture of mineral components and a proteinaceous colloidal matrix forms a plug that molds itself to the shape of the urethral lumen.[24] Although this can occur in any dog or cat, it is most commonly reported in male cats, presumably because they have a longer and narrower urethra with a sudden narrowing at the bulbourethral glands as the urethra enters the penis.[25,26] If obstruction is complete, uremia develops rapidly and is characterized by abdominal pain, depression, anorexia, dehydration, vomiting, and diarrhea. Increased pressure in the urinary tract can cause renal ischemia, ultimately resulting in permanent renal damage. In severe cases the distended bladder may rupture, causing a transitory relief of signs, followed rapidly by the development of peritonitis and death. Uremia alone leads to coma and death within 2 to 4 days, so partial or total obstruction is always a medical emergency (see Box 30-1).

STRUVITE UROLITHIASIS IN CATS

Early studies reported that more than 95% of uroliths in cats were composed of struvite.[27,28] Because struvite crystals were found to be the most prevalent cause of urolithiasis in cats, research during the early 1980s focused on preventing these crystals from forming in the urine and on the development of effective dietary management for cats with struvite urolithiasis. Although it now appears that a substantial proportion of cases may

---

BOX 30-1   CLINICAL SIGNS OF UROLITHIASIS IN DOGS AND CATS

Frequent urination

Urination in inappropriate places

Prolonged squatting or straining following urination

Hematuria

Licking of urogenital region

Dribbling of urine

Depression

Anorexia

Vomiting and diarrhea

Dehydration

have other causes, prevention of the formation of struvite crystals is still an important and effective protocol for the management of urolithiasis in many cats.

Evidence indicates that three distinct types of struvite urolithiasis occur in cats. These are: (1) sterile struvite uroliths, (2) infection-induced struvite uroliths, and (3) urethral plugs containing a variable quantity of struvite crystals. Treatment and dietary management is directed at promoting the dissolution of struvite uroliths and treating urinary tract infection and inflammation if these are involved.

Struvite Formation

Several conditions are necessary for the formation of struvite crystals or uroliths in the urinary tract.[29] First, a sufficient concentration of the composite minerals magnesium, ammonium, and phosphate must be present. In addition, these minerals must remain in the tract for an adequate period to allow crystallization to occur. Therefore the production of concentrated urine and small volumes of urine are important contributing factors. Finally, a pH that is favorable for crystal precipitation must exist within the urinary tract environment. Struvite is soluble when urine pH is below 6.6, and struvite crystals form when urine pH is 7.0 and above.[30] The solubility of struvite crystals also depends on the products of Mg^{2+}, NH_4^+, and PO_4^{3-}, called the *struvite activity product* (SAP) as described by the following: SAP = $([Mg^{2+}] \times [NH_4^+] \times [PO_4^{3-}])$.[31] The SAP also increases concomitantly with urine pH. As urine pH increases above 6.8, the SAP begins to increase exponentially.

Sterile struvite urolithiasis in cats is associated with the previous factors and the absence of a detectable urinary tract infection. However, while the presence of alkaline urine is necessary for the initial formation of struvite crystals, studies of cats with sterile struvite urolithiasis have found that the urine of affected cats is not consistently alkaline. For example, a group of 20 cats with naturally occurring sterile struvite uroliths had a mean urine pH of 6.9 ± 0.4 at the time of diagnosis.[32] Practitioners must be cautioned that the production of neutral or acidic urine upon presentation should not be interpreted as precluding struvite as the underlying cause of urolithiasis.

Infection-induced struvite urolithiasis is less common in cats than dogs, but it still represents an important

form of disease, occurring most commonly in cats <1 year of age and >10 years of age.[33] Infection with urease-producing bacterial species (especially *Staphylococcus*) accompanied by signs of urolithiasis and the presence of struvite in the urinary tract are necessary for diagnosis. These microbes release the enzyme urease. Urease hydrolyzes urea to ammonia, causing increased concentrations of ammonia and phosphate ion, two components of struvite. The increased ammonia ion further contributes to urine alkalinization. Abnormalities in local host defense mechanisms, such as a perineal urethrostomy, and the quantity of urea that is found in the cat's urine, may predispose a cat to infection-induced urolithiasis.[34,35] However, because most cats are innately resistant to bacterial urinary tract infection, infection-induced struvite urolithiasis is encountered less commonly than sterile struvite. Antimicrobial therapy, preferably based on culture and sensitivity, is essential when treating cats with infection-induced struvite to prevent recurrence.

Several conditions are necessary for the formation of struvite uroliths in cats. These include a sufficient concentration of the composite minerals magnesium, ammonium, and phosphate, the production of concentrated urine, and urine pH that is 7.0 or greater. However, while the presence of alkaline urine is necessary for the initial formation of struvite crystals, not all cats will present with urine that is consistently alkaline.

Dietary Risk Factors

Diet and feeding practices represent important risk factors for struvite urolithiasis in cats (Box 30-2). These include the food's urine-acidifying and urine-protein-excretion properties, level of magnesium and sodium, digestibility, caloric density, and water content.[36] The cat's feeding schedule may also be important. More than any of the other risk factors involved, these are elements of a cat's life over which pet owners have some control and that can be modified during the treatment and long-term management of struvite urolithiasis.

As discussed previously, one of the factors necessary for the formation of struvite in urine is the presence of sufficient concentrations of its three composite minerals,

BOX 30-2   DIETARY RISK FACTORS FOR STRUVITE UROLITHIASIS IN CATS

Urine-acidifying properties (production of an alkaline urine)

Urine-protein-excretion properties

High magnesium content

High phosphorous content

High chloride content

High calcium content

Low moisture content

Low digestibility and caloric density

Feeding regimen (meal-feeding)

Low water intake and balance

magnesium, ammonium, and phosphate. Feline urine always contains high amounts of ammonium because of the cat's high protein requirement and intake. Urine phosphate in healthy cats is also usually high enough for struvite formation, regardless of dietary phosphorus intake. The concentration of urine magnesium, on the other hand, is normally quite low and is directly affected by diet.[37] Thus, early investigations of feline struvite urolithiasis focused on dietary magnesium as a potential causal agent. The manipulation of dietary magnesium levels to produce or prevent phosphate urolithiasis had previously been well documented in rats and sheep.[38,39] This work was used to suggest a role of this mineral in the etiology of urolithiasis in domestic cats. One of the first studies showed that urethral obstruction and cystoliths could be induced in adult male cats when they were fed a diet containing either 0.75% or 1.0% magnesium and 1.6% phosphate.[40] In this study, the obstructing uroliths were composed primarily of magnesium and phosphate. Subsequent work showed that high levels of dietary phosphorus were not necessary for urolith development, but they did increase the risk for urolith formation when dietary magnesium was also high.[41] However, if magnesium intake was low, the incidence of urolith formation was low, regardless of the level of phosphorus. In a later study by the same group, cats were fed diets containing 0.75%, 0.38%, or 0.08% magnesium on a dry-matter basis (DMB). Seventy-six

percent of the cats that were fed 0.75% magnesium and 70% of the cats that were fed 0.38% magnesium developed urolithiasis and obstructed within 1 year or less, whereas none of the cats fed 0.08% magnesium obstructed.[37] Similarly, when random-source and specific–pathogen-free cats were fed diets containing either high magnesium or high magnesium and high phosphorus levels, urethral obstruction was induced.[42] The obstructing material was identifiable as struvite by radiographic crystallography in one of the seven cats.

These studies demonstrated the relationship between increasing magnesium in the diet and an increased rate of urolith formation and urethral obstruction in cats. However, the significance of these data to the role of dietary magnesium in naturally occurring feline struvite urolithiasis is questionable because the levels of dietary magnesium used in these studies were all substantially higher than those normally found in commercial cat foods. The domestic cat requires only 0.016% available magnesium for growth and maintenance.[43] The Association of American Feed Control Officials' (AAF-CO's) Nutrient Profiles requires cat foods to contain a minimum of 0.04% magnesium.[44] Most commercial cat foods contain slightly higher than this amount but still less than 0.1%. Although the magnesium in naturally occurring ingredients is not 100% available, these levels supply cats with their magnesium requirement. The amount of magnesium in cat foods is higher than the cat's minimum requirement for magnesium, but it is still substantially lower than the levels used in the early experimental studies to induce struvite formation (0.4% to 1.0%).

A second problem with data from early studies involved the composition of experimentally produced uroliths. The struvite found in naturally occurring cases is composed of three minerals: magnesium, ammonium, and phosphate. However, experimentally induced uroliths in some studies were actually made up of magnesium phosphate, with no detectable ammonium.[40,41] The composition of urethral plugs that caused obstruction in cats fed experimental diets was also different from the composition of urethral plugs of cats with spontaneous disease. Although the experimentally induced plugs were composed almost exclusively of struvite crystal aggregations, urethral plugs found in spontaneous disease are most often composed of a mucogelatinous protein matrix that contains varying amounts of minerals (usually struvite), sloughed tissue, blood, and inflammatory cells.[45-47]

The most important confounding factor of these studies involved the form of magnesium added to the experimental diets. A group of investigators examined the effects of two different forms of supplemental dietary magnesium on the urine pH of adult cats.[48] The data showed that the addition of 0.45% magnesium chloride to a basal diet resulted in a significant lowering of urine pH. In contrast, when the cats were fed the same basal diet supplemented with 0.45% magnesium oxide, a significantly higher pH was produced. In a free-choice feeding regimen, mean urine pH in cats fed the basal diet was 6.9, and urine pH values in cats fed the magnesium chloride– and magnesium oxide–supplemented diets were 5.7 and 7.7, respectively. When urine samples were examined microscopically, crystal formation was observed in cats fed the basal diet and the magnesium oxide–containing diet, but not in cats fed the magnesium chloride–containing diet. Therefore the form of magnesium included in the diet influenced urine pH and the formation of crystals. The observation that high levels of magnesium result in increased struvite formation may have been confounded by the effect of magnesium chloride versus magnesium oxide on urine pH. It can be concluded that similarities exist between early studies of experimentally induced struvite urolithiasis and naturally occurring disease, but the presence of significant differences and confounding factors show that magnesium intake is not singularly responsible for the natural development of struvite urolithiasis. Subsequent studies showed that dietary magnesium is less significant as a dietary risk factor for struvite urolithiasis than are urine pH, urine volume, and water balance.

As discussed previously, struvite crystals form in feline urine with a pH of 7.0 or greater and are soluble at a pH of 6.6 or less. Normal, healthy cats typically have acidic urine with a pH between 6.0 and 6.5, except after meals.[37] In all animals, the consumption of a meal results in a rise in urine pH within 4 hours. This effect, called the *postprandial alkaline tide,* is caused by renal compensation for the loss of gastric acids that are secreted during digestion of the meal. To compensate for the loss of acid and to maintain normal pH in body fluids, the kidneys excrete alkaline ions, resulting in an increased urine pH. The magnitude of the alkaline tide is directly proportional to the size of the meal and to the acidifying or alkalinizing components within the meal. Depending on the nature of the diet and the size of the meal, the postprandial alkaline tide in cats can result in a urine pH as high as 8.0.[49]

Many studies have demonstrated the importance of urine pH in the formation of struvite crystals in cats.[48-52] One study examined the effects of feeding a canned diet, a dry diet, or a dry diet supplemented with a urine acidifier (1.6% ammonium chloride) on urine pH and struvite formation in adult male cats.[50] Urine pH was highest in cats fed the dry diet (mean = 7.55). The addition of ammonium chloride reduced urine pH to 5.97. The canned diet resulted in urine with a mean pH of 5.82. The most significant findings of this study concerned urine struvite formation. Struvite crystals were present in 78% of the cats fed the dry diet but only 9% of the cats fed the dry diet plus ammonium chloride. Intakes of dry matter (DM), magnesium, and other minerals were the same for cats fed each of the dry diets. None of the cats fed the canned diet developed urinary struvite crystals. In addition, when urine samples from all cats were adjusted to a pH of 7.0 using 0.5 molar (M) sodium hydroxide, 46% of the cats fed the canned diet and all of the cats fed the ammonium chloride–supplemented dry diet showed typical struvite formation. These results show that at similar levels of energy, DM, and magnesium intake, the most important factor affecting feline struvite formation is urine pH.

Regardless of the level of magnesium intake by a cat, the dietary manipulation of urine pH consistently affects struvite formation. When a dry diet containing a high level of magnesium (0.37%) was fed to adult male cats, the addition of 1.5% ammonium chloride resulted in a urine pH of 6.0 or less.[51] Cats fed the diet without supplemental ammonium chloride produced urine with a pH of 7.3. Of the nonsupplemented cats, 7 of the 12 formed struvite uroliths and obstructed on two occasions, while only 2 of the cats fed the acidifying diet obstructed on a single occasion. When the diets of the seven obstructed cats were supplemented with ammonium chloride, they experienced no further episodes of struvite urolith formation or obstruction. Radiographic examination prior to supplementation revealed visible uroliths, which dissolved after 3 months of consuming the acidifying diet. Similar results have been reported when diets containing levels of magnesium commonly found in commercial pet foods were fed. When adult cats were fed a purified diet containing only 0.045% magnesium, struvite formed, and the cats showed clinical signs of urolithiasis when the diet produced an alkaline urine.[47] However, if ammonium chloride was added as an acidifying agent, clinical signs disappeared within 4 days and did not recur while the acidifying diet was fed.

The domestic cat is a carnivorous mammal. Compared with an omnivorous or herbivorous diet, a carnivorous diet has the effect of increasing net acid excretion and decreasing urine pH.[53,54] This urine-acidifying effect is primarily a result of the high level of sulfur-containing amino acids found in meats. Oxidation of these amino acids results in the excretion of sulfate in the urine and a concomitant decrease in urine pH.[55] In addition, a diet that contains a high proportion of meat is lower in potassium salts than a diet containing high levels of cereal grains, which have been shown to produce an alkaline urine when metabolized.[56,57] Similarly, foods that contain high levels of digestible carbohydrate have been shown to increase urinary pH.[58] Therefore the inclusion of high levels of cereal grains and low levels of meat products in some commercial cat foods may be a contributing factor to the development of struvite urolithiasis. For example, the struvite-producing, commercial dry diet that was used in one of the previously discussed studies contained 46% cereal grains, primarily in the form of wheat meal.[50]

Although a certain amount of cereal is necessary for the extrusion and expansion process of dry foods, high levels of these ingredients may contribute to the production of alkaline urine. Conversely, the inclusion of large amounts of meat products in cat foods usually contributes to the production of more acidic urine. Furthermore, increasing meat-source protein may be preferable to using ammonium chloride supplementation to reduce urine pH.[59] Although supplementation with urine acidifiers such as DL-methionine and ammonium chloride decreased urine pH, supplementation did not reduce the concentration of urine organic fraction, which may serve as the matrix for struvite urolith formation.[60] Increasing dietary protein also increases urea diuresis, which can contribute favorably to increased urine volume.[61] However, increased protein may not be needed provided a food already promotes acidic urine. A case-control study designed to identify dietary factors associated with decreased risk of struvite uroliths

reported that foods formulated to include higher fat, lower protein, lower potassium, and increased urine-acidifying potential could potentially minimize formation of struvite uroliths in cats.[36]

As pet food manufacturers search for ingredients to include in cat foods that will naturally produce acidic urine, each ingredient must be separately evaluated for its effect on urine pH. For example, one study compared the urine-acidifying effects of corn gluten meal, poultry meal, and meat and bone meal when diets containing these ingredients were fed to cats.[62] Of the ingredients tested, corn gluten meal had the strongest acidifying effect on urine. Unlike most plant protein sources, corn gluten meal contains higher concentrations of sulfur-containing amino acids than either poultry meal or meat and bone meal. Corn gluten meal is unusual in that it is a cereal protein that produces acidic urine when fed to cats. A study comparing meat meal with corn gluten meal as a protein source for dry cat food found that meat meal was similar to corn gluten meal in its effects upon urinary pH, SAP, number of struvite crystals in urine, and other measures of struvite urolith risk.[63] In addition, DM digestibility and nitrogen utilization of the meat meal was significantly higher when compared with DM digestibility and nitrogen utilization of corn gluten meal. Another study by the same group compared fish meal with corn gluten meal as protein sources in cat foods and reported that the two protein sources did not differ significantly in either dry-matter digestibility or nitrogen utilization.[64] However, the fish meal protein source contributed to lower urine pH and SAP values. Conversely, when meat meal, chicken meal and corn gluten meal were compared, chicken meal had moderate digestibility and nitrogen utilization, but its relatively high calcium and phosphorous content led to increased urinary pH.[65]

Water Balance and Urine Volume

Decreased urine volume may be an important risk factor for the development of urolithiasis in cats. Diets that cause a decrease in total fluid turnover can result in decreased urine volume and increased urine concentration, both of which may contribute to struvite formation. It has been suggested that dry cat foods contribute to decreased fluid intake and urine volume. An early study showed that cats fed a dry cat food had decreased total water intakes when compared with cats consuming similar energy levels from canned food.[66] Cats did increase voluntary water intake when fed the dry food but not in sufficient amounts to fully compensate for the lower moisture content of the food. In another experiment, adult cats were fed a semipurified, basal diet containing varying levels of moisture.[67] The cats consuming a diet containing 10% moisture had an average daily urine volume of 63 milliliters (ml). This volume increased to 112 ml/day when the moisture content of the diet was increased to 75%. Urine specific gravity was also slightly higher in cats that were fed the low-moisture food. In both of these studies, the differences in urine volume were attributed to lower total water intake in the cats that were consuming low-moisture foods.

However, in contrast to these studies, two other groups of investigators found no difference in water consumption between cats fed dry diets and those fed canned diets. It appears that diet composition, especially fat content and caloric density, influences water turnover in cats fed different types of commercial diets. In a study examining the effects of diet type, composition, and digestibility on water-excretory patterns in cats, a comparison of three canned diets showed that when cats were fed diets containing high levels of fat (34% and 28% of DM), significantly less DM was consumed than when cats were fed a canned diet containing a relatively low level of fat (14%).[68] Fecal DM and fecal water content were lower in cats fed the high-fat diets. Because total water intake was the same for all cats, the cats consuming the high-fat diets excreted significantly higher volumes of water in their urine to achieve water balance. Further evidence supporting the importance of caloric density and fat content is demonstrated by a comparison of a low-fat canned food to three dry cat foods in the same study. Water volume in urine and feces was similar between cats fed the low-fat, canned ration and cats fed the three dry diets. Other than the large difference in water content, the nutrient content of the low-fat, canned food was very similar to that of the dry diets. Energy digestibility of the canned diet was also equivalent to that of the dry diets (79.3% and 78.7%, respectively) and was significantly lower than the mean digestibility of the high-fat, canned diets (90.3%). Statistical analysis of these data revealed that the percentage of water excreted in the urine of cats

is directly related to the fat and energy content of the diet, with correlation coefficients of 0.96 and 0.94, respectively.

Some investigators have advocated feeding only canned cat food to cats with a history of urolithiasis.[69,70] The intent is to increase water intake and cause a resultant increase in urine volume and decrease in urine specific gravity. However, the water content of the diet is probably not as important as are caloric density, fat content, and digestibility of the food. As was evident in the previously mentioned study, a poorly digestible canned cat food may not contribute to increased urine volume if large amounts of water are excreted in the feces. Conversely, the consumption of a cat food (canned or dry) that is energy dense and highly digestible will result in lower total DM intake. This decrease will be accompanied by decreased fecal volume and fecal water and increased urine volume. These effects may be beneficial in preventing urolithiasis in cats because urine will contain a lower concentration of the mineral components that lead to urolith formation. In addition, an increase in urine volume stimulates an increased frequency of urination, thus decreasing the time available for struvite formation.

In addition to urine pH, decreased urine volume and the production of highly concentrated urine are important risk factors for the development of urolithiasis in cats. Diets that cause a decrease in total fluid turnover can result in decreased urine volume and increased urine concentration, both of which may contribute to struvite formation. Dietary factors that contribute to water turnover include the amount of water included in the food, and the food's caloric density, fat content, and digestibility.

Feeding Method

The postprandial alkaline tide occurs as a result of meal ingestion and the subsequent excretion and loss of gastric acids.[71] Many factors affect its duration and magnitude. Domestic cats are nibblers by nature. When fed free-choice, most cats eat small meals every few hours throughout the day.[72,73] In general, this feeding regimen has the effect of reducing the magnitude of the alkaline tide but prolonging its duration. In contrast, depending on the alkalinizing effects of the diet, meal-feeding may cause greater fluctuations of shorter duration. The effects of a feeding regimen are further complicated by the type of diet fed, the eating patterns of the cat, and various dietary components.

In one study, cats were fed a dry, commercial food, either on a free-choice basis or once daily. The urine pH of cats fed ad libitum was maintained between 6.5 and 6.9 throughout the day. In cats fed the same diet once daily, urine pH increased 2 hours after the meal to 7.7 and then gradually decreased for the remainder of the day.[51] Another group of researchers fed cats two dry foods and three canned foods on an ad libitum basis and recorded urine pH throughout a 24-hour period.[37] One of the dry foods and two of the canned foods resulted in constant urine pH values of less than 6.3. However, the other dry and canned foods produced pH values that ranged from 6.5 to higher than 7.0. When the same foods were meal-fed once daily, all of the foods except one dry and one canned product resulted in peak urine pH values of greater than 7.0 within 4 hours after the start of the meal. These values all declined to less than 6.5 by approximately 16 hours after the meal. One dry and one canned food maintained pH values of 6.6 or less, even when meal-fed. These differences were attributed to different urine-acidifying components/ingredients present in the foods. More recently, a study that examined the long-term effects of acidifying diets found that ad libitum feeding was essential to maintain a mean urine pH of less than 6.5, even when an acidifying diet was fed.[27] The lower urine pH in cats fed ad libitum was attributed to the consumption of numerous small meals throughout the day, which minimized the amount of gastric acid secreted for each meal and subsequently decreased the postprandial alkaline tide.

In addition to urine pH, the effects of feeding regimen on urine volume and composition are important considerations. In a study that examined the relationship between method of feeding, food and water intake, urine volume, and urine composition, the period of highest urinary excretion of magnesium and phosphorus occurred preprandially and therefore did not coincide with the daily alkaline tide.[74] This study also found that ad libitum–fed cats had increased frequency of urination and greater total urine volume when compared with meal-fed cats. These effects may be beneficial in

minimizing urolith formation. Although these results indicate that the highest concentration of composite minerals does not occur during the time they would be most likely to precipitate, this may not be a necessary condition for struvite formation. Research has shown that urine pH is directly related to the size of the meal, and this relationship can be described by a simple linear model.[75] In other words, as the size of the meal increases, so does postprandial urine pH. These data also showed that as postprandial urine pH increased, the presence of struvite crystals increased accordingly. Struvite did not form when urine pH was maintained at less than 6.6.

Dietary Management

In clinical cases in which obstruction has occurred, immediate care involves stabilization of the cat's condition, fluid replacement therapy, and relief of bladder distention and urethral obstruction. Removal of the obstruction can usually be accomplished by either flushing the urolith or urethral plug out of the urethra or by cystocentesis. However, while cystocentesis immediately relieves the distended bladder, it usually does not remove the obstructing uroliths. When a bacterial urinary tract infection is present, appropriate antimicrobial therapy should be initiated. Long-term dietary management involves the removal or dissolution of any remaining struvite uroliths and the feeding of an appropriate food to minimize the likelihood of recurrence.

Remaining struvite uroliths that are present in the urinary tract can be removed either through surgical means or via diet-induced dissolution. Surgical intervention provides immediate relief to the animal, followed by recovery within 3 to 7 days. On the other hand, dietary dissolution is a noninvasive procedure but can take several weeks to months to be effective. When dietary intervention is used to dissolve existing struvite uroliths, a food that produces an acidic urine with a pH of 6.3 or lower and contains reduced magnesium should be selected.[76] Adding sodium chloride to the diet has been suggested as an agent to induce polydipsia and resultant polyuria with the intent of producing a more dilute urine and increasing the frequency of urination.[77] However, feeding increased amounts of sodium to cats increases renal excretion of calcium and so may contribute to the formation of calcium oxalate uroliths.[76]

For this reason, supplementing a cat's normal food with sodium chloride is not recommended.

Depending on the size and number of the uroliths present, complete dietary dissolution usually takes between 5 and 7 weeks.[78] There is also evidence suggesting that infection-induced struvite uroliths may take longer for dissolution than sterile struvite uroliths.[32] Regardless of the difference in time for dissolution, the eradication of infection caused by urease-producing bacteria is the most important factor in cats with infection-induced struvite urolithiasis.

A urine pH between 6.0 and 6.3 is desirable during the struvite dissolution phase of treatment.[30,76] Once a food has been selected, urine pH should be monitored 4 to 8 hours after initial consumption to ensure that adequate (but not excessive) acidification is occurring. Only the prescribed food should be fed, with no additional supplements or other cat foods. During the dissolution phase, cats should be monitored for struvite dissolution at 2- to 4-week intervals, using either palpation or radiography. Periodic evaluation of urine sediment for crystalluria may be helpful in assessing progress, but because many healthy, normal cats develop urine struvite crystals, the presence of crystalluria should not be interpreted as evidence of persistent urolithiasis.[62,79] The therapeutic food should be continued for at least 1 month following complete dissolution of struvite.[30,80,81] After this period, the diet can be changed to a maintenance product demonstrated to be effective in the management of struvite urolithiasis.

A maintenance food that is fed to prevent the recurrence of struvite urolithiasis should produce a slightly acidified urine, be moderate in caloric density and high in digestibility, and contain a relatively low level of magnesium. A urine pH of 6.6 or less prevents the formation of struvite crystals. Therefore a pH range between 6.0 and 6.5 is desirable for long-term maintenance. Dietary ingredients that have the effect of increasing urinary acid excretion include proteins of animal origin (because of their high sulfur–amino acid content) and compounds that result in an elevated absorption of chloride, phosphate, or sulfate.[57] Conversely, most cereal grains contain high levels of potassium salts that have the effect of producing alkaline urine.[50] The exception is corn gluten meal, which produces acidic urine because of its high concentration of sulfur amino acids.[62]

Diets that are moderate in caloric density and are highly digestible will be consumed in smaller amounts, thus lowering both DM and magnesium intake. The lower DM intake results in decreased fecal matter and fecal water and increased urine volume. Feeding a wet food with these characteristics may further contribute to increased urine volume and decreased urine specific gravity.[82] Although of less importance than urine pH and dilution, decreased magnesium intake results in lower concentrations of urine magnesium, which is necessary for struvite formation. The percentage of magnesium in the diet is not as important as the total amount of magnesium that a cat consumes. Although some researchers believe that magnesium concentration in the diet should be 0.1% or less on a DMB, others maintain that the risk of struvite formation is only increased when magnesium levels reach 0.25% or greater.[79,81,83] Because the cat's requirement for dietary magnesium is substantially lower than the amount usually found in cat food, a general rule of thumb is to select a food that contains 0.12% magnesium or less. There are several high-quality, nutritionally complete commercial cat foods that meet the criteria discussed. However, a cat food should not be selected only on the basis of its magnesium content. The food's caloric density, digestibility, and urine-acidifying properties should all be considered when selecting a maintenance cat food for the prevention of struvite urolithiasis (Box 30-3).

Risks Associated with Overacidification

Even though the maintenance of a urine pH of 6.6 or lower prevents the formation of struvite crystals, the production of urine that is too acidic can be detrimental to a cat's health. If more acid is consumed than an animal is capable of excreting, metabolic acidosis occurs. Several studies have shown that when cats are fed a severely acidifying diet for several months, they develop metabolic acidosis, decreased levels of serum potassium, and depletion of body potassium stores.[84,85] Other studies indicate that the long-term feeding of highly acidifying diets containing marginal levels of potassium causes hypokalemia and kidney disease in some cats.[86,87] For example, three out of nine cats fed an acidifying diet containing 40% protein and marginal levels of potassium developed chronic renal failure within 2 years.[86]

BOX 30-3 DIETARY MANAGEMENT FOR PREVENTION OF STRUVITE UROLITHIASIS

Perform surgical removal or medical dissolution of uroliths (initial treatment).

Treat and prevent recurrence of bacterial urinary tract infection (if present).

Select a food that produces acidified urine (pH 6.0 to 6.5).

Avoid overacidification of urine.

Select a food with a reduced magnesium content (<0.12% dry-matter basis for cats).

Select a food that is highly digestible and moderate in caloric density.

Feed either a canned food or add water to a dry food to increase water intake.

Feed free choice or provide many small meals throughout the day.

Do not feed other foods, supplements, or treats.

The consumption of an acidifying diet or urine-acidifying agents that cause acidosis results in increased urinary losses of potassium and calcium and may compromise electrolyte balance.[55] When acid intake is too high, the body will reestablish acid-base balance at a decreased blood bicarbonate concentration. Carbonate and phosphate are resorbed from bone to supply cations, and the calcium that is resorbed is excreted in the urine. Prolonged losses of calcium as a result of renal acidosis may eventually lead to bone demineralization and osteoporosis.[88,89] Urinary acidifying agents have been shown to have detrimental effects on bone mineralization in cats. When a diet containing 3% ammonium chloride was fed to growing kittens, urine pH was significantly decreased, but the kittens also exhibited impaired growth, decreased blood pH, increased urine calcium excretion, and bone demineralization of the caudal vertebrae. Similar changes were reported when adult cats were fed a diet containing 1.5% ammonium chloride.[90]

In contrast, a 2-year study found that adult cats that were fed two acidifying diets ad libitum maintained normal ranges for all hematological and serum biochemical profiles, as well as normal blood gas values.[91] Although cats fed the two acidifying diets had slightly lower serum phosphorus, bicarbonate, and base excess values, these values all remained within laboratory reference ranges. Measurement of bone mineral density after 2 years of feeding also showed no effect of diet. When fed ad libitum, the diet used in this study resulted in the production of urine with an average pH of 6.2. Another study using 1.7% phosphoric acid to induce moderate acidification of urine also reported a lack of detrimental effects after 1 year of feeding.[92] An important difference between these studies and those discussed previously is that the more recent studies used diets that included corn gluten meal, animal protein, and/or phosphoric acid as urine-acidifying components. Feeding a diet that contains ingredients that promote moderate urine acidification appears to present less risk for overacidification than does supplementing a cat's diet with a urine-acidifying agent such as ammonium chloride.

Another effect of acidified urine may be to promote the formation of another type of urolith. Although struvite is soluble in acidic urine, acid pH may increase the likelihood of calcium oxalate formation. The prolonged feeding of a highly acidified diet leads to a loss of calcium in the urine, making this mineral available for the formation of calcium-containing uroliths. Acidified urine also contains lower levels of citrate, which normally inhibits the formation of calcium oxalate by preferentially interacting with calcium and making it unavailable to bind with oxalate.[93] Similarly, feeding a low-magnesium diet can exacerbate this problem because urine magnesium also appears to inhibit calcium oxalate formation.[94] As discussed previously, the incidence of calcium oxalate urolithiasis in cats increased while struvite urolithiasis decreased over time until the last few years. It is theorized that the widespread feeding of acidifying diets that contain low levels of magnesium may have been an important contributing factor to this trend.

Even though the maintenance of urine pH of 6.6 or lower prevents the formation of struvite crystals, the production of urine that is too acidic can be detrimental to a cat's health. Problems associated with overacidification include metabolic acidosis, decreased levels of serum potassium, and depletion of body potassium stores. Long-term effects can cause hypokalemia, increased risk for developing calcium oxalate urolithiasis, and kidney disease.

STRUVITE UROLITHIASIS IN DOGS

Until late in the twentieth century, there was very limited information available regarding the incidence of urolithiasis and the prevalence of different types of uroliths in dogs. However, analysis of data collected at the Minnesota Urolith Center and the Urinary Stone Analysis Laboratory in California has provided valuable information regarding the age, breed, and sex of affected dogs and the mineral composition and location of calculi.[15,95] Struvite urolithiasis in both dogs and cats has proportionately decreased over the last 20 years compared to calcium oxalate urolithiasis.[96] But struvite uroliths are still the most commonly reported canine urolith.[14] Similar to its occurrence in cats, struvite urolithiasis is a disease of primarily adult dogs, although infection-induced struvite uroliths occur in some young dogs.[9,95] As stated previously, the mean age of diagnosis is between 4 and 6 years, and female dogs are disproportionately more likely to be affected than males (see p. 360).

Sterile versus Infection-Induced Struvite

Struvite urolithiasis in dogs is primarily a disease associated with infection, in contrast to struvite uroliths in cats.[96] Urease-producing bacteria such as *Staphylococcus, Escherichia coli, Streptococcus,* and *Proteus* are often found in dogs with struvite uroliths.[97] This association between urinary tract infection and struvite urolithiasis in dogs is well documented.[98-100] In contrast, urinary tract infections are often absent in dogs with calcium oxalate–, cystine-, urate-, or silica-containing calculi.[101] A study of more than 11,000 canine urinary calculi specimens found *Staphylococcus intermedius* in 30% of affected males and in 54% of affected females.[95,97] There is a significant correlation between the presence of struvite calculi and a positive culture for this organism in both sexes. It has been suggested that dogs producing urine with a high concentration of urea may be more susceptible to infection-induced struvite urolithiasis because bacterial urease converts the urea to ammonia. An increase in ammonia levels contributes one of the components of struvite and also to increased urinary pH.

Infection-induced struvite is the most common urolith in dogs less than 1 year of age.[9] Female dogs show a higher incidence of infection-induced struvite when compared with males.[97] One potential cause for this difference is anatomical. The shorter urethra of the female dog may facilitate the ability of opportunistic bacteria to move up the urethra and into the bladder to cause infection.[102] It has also been suggested that dogs confined indoors may have longer periods of urine retention, increasing the potential for bacterial growth within the urinary tract.

Struvite urolithiasis in dogs is primarily a disease associated with infection. Urease-producing bacteria are often found in dogs with struvite uroliths while urinary tract infections are often absent in dogs with calcium oxalate calculi. Possibly because of anatomical differences, female dogs show a higher incidence of infection-induced struvite when compared with male dogs.

Dietary Management

Surgical removal of uroliths is necessary in most cases of struvite urolithiasis in dogs, especially if the uroliths are obstructing the ureters or renal pelvis. An advantage to surgical intervention is that clinical signs are quickly relieved and treatment can then focus on eliminating urinary tract infections and preventing recurrence. Urethral uroliths are usually flushed into the bladder by retrograde hydropropulsion where they can be removed surgically or dissolved medically.[9]

Medical dissolution of struvite uroliths using an acidifying, restricted protein, calculolytic diet has also been used with dogs. The intent of restricting protein is to decrease urinary urea, an important substrate for urease-positive bacteria and the source of increased ammonia. However, proper antimicrobial treatment is more effective than protein restriction for controlling bacterial populations in the canine urinary tract.[103] In addition, restricted-protein diets have been associated with low palatability and acceptance by dogs. Because most struvite calculi found in dogs contain significant amounts of nonstruvite minerals, which may not dissolve in response to an acidifying diet, medical (dietary) dissolution is no longer recommended for most cases of canine struvite urolithiasis.[104] In all cases, appropriate antimicrobial therapy must be instituted if urinary tract infection is present. This should be continued for 3 to 4 weeks after the removal of uroliths.

The protocol for averting recurrence of struvite urolithiasis includes preventing urinary tract infection while feeding a diet that produces moderately acidic urine and reduces the concentration of struvite components.[104] A food that promotes the production of urine with a pH between 6.4 and 6.6 is recommended. Once an appropriate acidifying food has been selected, no other foods, supplements, or treats should be fed. The diet should also contain sufficient but not excessive amounts of high-quality protein. Keeping the dog's urinary tract free of bacterial infection is the most important factor for prevention of infection-induced struvite urolithiasis. Following a complete course of full-dose antimicrobial therapy, a reduced therapeutic dose of an antimicrobial agent is often administered for up to 6 months. Periodic urine cultures should be conducted every 2 to 3 months to monitor the effectiveness of the regimen, and these should be continued for up to 2 years following the completion of antibiotic treatment.

Surgical removal of uroliths is necessary in most cases of struvite urolithiasis in dogs, especially if the uroliths are obstructing the ureters or renal pelvis. Keeping the dog's urinary tract free of bacterial infection is the most important factor for prevention of infection-induced struvite urolithiasis in dogs. To decrease the likelihood of recurrence, a food that promotes the production of urine with a pH between 6.4 and 6.6 and contains sufficient but not excessive amounts of high-quality protein should be fed.

CALCIUM OXALATE UROLITHIASIS IN CATS

As discussed previously, during the past two decades, the prevalence of feline calcium oxalate uroliths has been increasing, and the prevalence of struvite uroliths has been substantially decreasing. A suggested cause of this trend is the increased use of urine-acidifying diets containing low levels of magnesium. The inappropriate feeding of diets formulated to prevent struvite formation in the subpopulation of cats that are actually at risk for calcium oxalate crystalluria may result in an increased incidence of clinical calcium oxalate urolithiasis.[105] Cats with this type of urolithiasis usually produce a concentrated urine (specific gravity of 1.040) that is slightly acidified (pH 6.3 to 6.7).[106] Mild acidemia is reported in some, but not all, cats with calcium oxalate urolithiasis.

In cats, calcium oxalate uroliths are found most often in the urinary bladder, but they also occur in various combinations in the urethra, kidneys, and ureters. The vast majority of feline ureteral calculi contain calcium oxalate.[21] The number of reported upper urinary tract uroliths is increasing, and these uroliths have been associated with chronic renal failure.[107] However, as an emerging clinical syndrome, acute ureteral obstruction remains poorly understood.[18] Clinical signs of ureteral calculi are nonspecific and include anorexia, lethargy, weight loss, polyuria, polydipsia, vomiting, and hematuria.[21] Metabolic changes may include azotemia, hyperphosphatemia, and, in a small number of cases, hypercalcemia. Interestingly, ultrasonography of the contralateral kidney of cats with unilateral ureteral calculi often revealed preexisting renal parenchymal disease.[21]

Risk Factors

Several dietary components are potential contributors to the development of calcium oxalate calculi in cats.[36,104,106] Factors that may be important include the food's urine-acidifying properties and levels of moisture, protein, potassium, phosphorous, magnesium, calcium, sodium, and vitamin B_6. As with struvite, the focus has been on factors that either increase or decrease the concentration of the calculi's components in the urine (in this case, calcium and oxalate) and those that affect the solubility of calcium oxalate crystals. Urine supersaturation with calcium and oxalate is one factor to consider regarding calcium oxalate urolith formation.[4] When sodium chloride is added to deionized water, the solution is considered saturated at the point where the addition of any more salt will result in crystals, unless some other change takes place, such as with temperature or pH. But urine is more complex than salt and water. Ions, proteins, and perhaps as yet unidentified substances form a complex solution in urine, one that apparently allows calcium and oxalate to remain in solution at high concentrations. Thus, when compared with water, normal feline urine may be supersaturated with calcium and oxalic acid.[32] In this state calcium oxalate crystals do not precipitate, but if crystals are already present they will be maintained or even grow. Because of the complex relationships between urine components, the exact initiating cause of calcium oxalate formation in feline urine is not completely understood.[108]

A study of urine samples from cats fed a variety of diets found that reduction of urine pH and magnesium concentration significantly increased struvite solubility but concurrently decreased calcium oxalate solubility.[109] In addition, in vitro studies have shown that increased amounts of urinary magnesium reduce the formation of calcium oxalate crystals. This observation has led to the use of magnesium supplementation in humans to prevent the formation of calcium oxalate calculi. However, because increased dietary magnesium is a risk factor for struvite urolithiasis in cats, increasing dietary magnesium with the intent of preventing calcium oxalate formation is contraindicated in this species. Similarly, providing a diet that has an alkalinizing effect upon urine pH may prevent calcium oxalate urolith formation but is an important risk factor for struvite formation.

Several factors may affect the concentrations of calcium and oxalate in urine. The consumption of high amounts of sodium leads to increased renal excretion of calcium.[106] Vitamin D and ascorbic acid levels in the diet may be important because vitamin D promotes intestinal absorption of calcium, and ascorbic acid is a precursor of oxalate. Vitamin B_6 has been identified as a potentially important nutrient because experimentally induced vitamin B_6 deficiency has been associated with hyperoxaluria and the formation of renal calcium oxalate calculi in kittens.[110] However, naturally occurring hyperoxaluria has not been reported in cats. Moreover, supplementation with vitamin B_6 for cats that are not deficient does not reduce urinary oxalate excretion.[106]

A final possible risk factor is the presence of hypercalcemia. As discussed previously, some cats with calcium oxalate urolithiasis have mild acidemia. A slight but persistent acidemia promotes the mobilization of carbonate and phosphorus from bone to buffer the excess hydrogen ions. The concomitant mobility of

calcium leads to increased serum calcium and hypercalciuria. It has been postulated that because hypercalcemia promotes urinary excretion of calcium, it may predispose the precipitation of calcium oxalate calculi. While serum concentration of minerals, including calcium, are normal in most cats with calcium oxalate urolithiasis, moderate hypercalcemias (11 and 13 milligrams [mg]/deciliter [dl]) have been reported.[106] This observation warrants routine evaluation of serum calcium concentrations in affected patients, because hypercalcemia promotes urinary calcium excretion and may promote the formation and precipitation of calcium oxalate crystals (Box 30-4).

Dietary Management

Unlike struvite uroliths, calcium oxalate uroliths in cats cannot be dissolved using a calculolytic diet. Therefore this type of urolith must be removed from the urinary tract using surgical intervention, lithotripsy, or urohydropropulsion.[111,112] In some cases, very small urocystoliths may be retrieved through catheterization. If hypercalcemia is present, appropriate treatment to correct the underlying cause must be instituted. Following removal of uroliths and recovery from surgery, emphasis is placed on preventing recurrence though the use of an appropriate diet.

Goals of dietary management include reducing urinary concentrations of calcium and oxalate and maintaining dilute urine with a pH between 6.3 and 6.9.[113] The food that is selected should contain ingredients that are highly digestible and include optimal levels of

---

BOX 30-4   DIETARY RISK FACTORS FOR CALCIUM OXALATE UROLITHIASIS IN CATS

Urine-acidifying properties (production of an acidified urine)

Excess vitamin D and ascorbic acid intake

Low water intake and balance

Reduced sodium content

Reduced potassium content

Any factor that may contribute to hypercalciuria or hypercalcemia

calcium and magnesium. Restriction of dietary calcium is not recommended unless absorptive hypercalcemia exists. In those cases, moderate restriction is advocated to prevent negative calcium balance. Although increased urine magnesium concentration reduces the formation of calcium oxalate crystals, this is also a risk factor for struvite urolith formation. Therefore magnesium levels in the diet should be adequate but not high. Because the consumption of excess levels of sodium may induce increased renal excretion of calcium, moderate restriction of dietary sodium has been recommended.[112] The production of a dilute urine can be achieved by feeding a diet that is high in digestibility and moisture. Feeding a canned ration or adding water to a high-quality, highly digestible dry food is the best way to achieve this. Potassium citrate is often included in diets that are formulated to prevent recurrence of calcium oxalate urolithiasis. Potassium citrate has an alkalinizing effect on urine pH, and when excreted in the urine, citrate forms a soluble salt with calcium, reducing its availability to form a complex with oxalate (Box 30-5).[36,106,113]

In recent years, the effect of reducing urine relative supersaturation (RSS) has been examined as an approach for preventing the formation of both calcium oxalate and struvite uroliths in cats.[114] Studies with experimental diets have shown that feeding foods that maintain RSS below a target RSS value (i.e., undersaturation) effectively reduces the crystallization potential for both types of urinary crystals. Urine pH, which is an important factor in struvite formation, has not been found to be a strong predictor of calcium oxalate formation.[114] Recent evidence also suggests that urine RSS is more strongly correlated with struvite precipitation potential than is urine pH.[115] Therefore a "single-diet" approach that effectively prevents both types of urolith formation has been suggested and is characterized by foods that produce a dilute (reduced RSS values) and moderately acidified urine. These changes are accomplished by increasing diet moisture (canned or pouched foods) and, in some cases, by moderately increasing sodium chloride to increase water consumption.[116-118]

CALCIUM OXALATE UROLITHIASIS IN DOGS

Like struvite uroliths, calcium oxalate uroliths can develop in dogs of any age, but it is primarily a disease of adult animals. More than half of the cases occur in dogs between the ages of 5 and 12 years.[119] In contrast to struvite urolithiasis, male dogs are more likely than females to be affected. The incidence of calcium oxalate urolithiasis in both sexes has increased dramatically in the past 25 years, possibly in response to the increased use and availability of dog foods that promote the production of acidified urine.

Risk Factors

Risk factors are similar to those for cats and include mild acidemia, decreased urine pH, hypercalciuria, production of concentrated urine, and possibly consumption of an acidifying diet or excessive amounts of vitamin C. Miniature Schnauzers are most commonly affected, accounting for about 25% of cases of calcium oxalate urolithiasis in dogs.[114] Other breeds that are more frequently affected include the Lhasa Apso, Yorkshire Terrier, Miniature Poodle, Shih Tzu, and Bichon Frise. Hypercalcemia is not common, but it is seen with primary hyperparathyroidism, pseudohyperparathyroidism, malignant lymphoma, and hyperthyroidism. Hypercalcemia is associated with increased urine

---

BOX 30-5	**DIETARY MANAGEMENT FOR PREVENTION OF CALCIUM OXALATE UROLITHIASIS**

Perform removal of uroliths through surgery, urohydropropulsion, or catheterization (initial treatment).

Treat hypercalcemia (if present).

Select a food that produces neutral or slightly acidified urine (pH 6.3 to 6.9).

Select a food with optimal calcium and magnesium levels.

Select a food that is highly digestible and moderate in caloric density.

Select a food with moderate sodium and supplemental potassium citrate.

Feed either a canned food or add water to a dry food to increase water intake.

Do not feed other foods, supplements, or treats.

calcium excretion, normal serum calcium values, and normal or low serum parathyroid hormone concentration.[120] There is also evidence that the presence of hyperadrenocorticism increases a dog's risk for developing calcium oxalate urolithiasis.[121] Hypercalciuria may also be associated with administration of glucocorticoids, urinary acidifiers, vitamin D, and diuretics that act on the ascending loop of Henle.[2]

Dietary Management

As in cats, the only effective treatment for dogs with clinically active calcium oxalate uroliths is removal via surgery, lithotripsy, or urohydropropulsion. If hypercalciuria is present, the underlying cause, if known, should be addressed. If an acidifying food or supplemental vitamin C is being fed, the dog should be switched to a food that promotes a neutral urine pH and contains ingredients that are high in quality and digestibility. All vitamin supplements should be discontinued. Increased water intake is recommended to promote the production of dilute urine and reduce supersaturation of urine with calcium oxalate.[112] This can usually be accomplished through either feeding a canned diet or adding water to a dry food immediately before feeding. As with cats, potassium citrate is often included in diets that are formulated to prevent recurrence of calcium oxalate urolithiasis in dogs because of its urine-alkalinizing effect and ability to sequester calcium and inhibit calcium oxalate formation (see Box 30-5).

OTHER DIET-RESPONSIVE URINARY CONDITIONS IN CATS

Other mineral types found in feline uroliths include ammonium urate, xanthine, cystine, silica, brushite, potassium magnesium pyrophosphate, dried solidified blood (DSB), and calcium phosphate.[6,122] Ammonium urate and xanthine uroliths make up a relatively small fraction of uroliths seen in cats and are most commonly located in the urinary bladder. Although the underlying cause is usually not known, the production of acidic, highly concentrated urine and the consumption of a food high in purine precursors (such as liver) may be risk factors for these types of urolith. Xanthuria in cats

is extremely uncommon. Recently a cat with xanthine urolithiasis was evaluated for hereditary xanthuria but was found not to be homozygous for a recessive mutant xanthine dehydrogenase allele.[123] This is in contrast to an autosomal recessive trait for xanthuria that has been described in humans and dogs. Treating feline xanthuria is limited to feeding a high-moisture food containing reduced purines and monitoring xanthine concentration in urine.

Calcium phosphate is found in 1% or less of naturally occurring feline uroliths.[124] A primary risk factor for this type of urolith in other species is the presence of primary hyperparathyroidism. However, this association has not been reported in cats.[125] Cats with cystine uroliths have increased urine concentration of the amino acids cystine, arginine, lysine, and ornithine.[29] Although medical protocols for the dissolution of this type of urolith have not been developed, cystine is soluble in alkaline urine and precipitates in acidified urine. Therefore urine-acidifying foods should not be fed to cats with this type of urolith.

Another type of FLUTD that is not urolith-related but may respond to dietary management is found in a subpopulation of cats affected by a disease that is similar to interstitial cystitis in humans. In cats, the disorder has been termed *idiopathic cystitis* to reflect its unknown etiology. A diagnosis is made based upon clinical signs of lower urinary tract disease, abnormalities of urinalysis, and urinary tract lesions identified by imaging studies. Clinically, a diagnosis of idiopathic cystitis is a diagnosis of exclusion in cats that present with signs of lower urinary tract disease for which no obvious cause can be found. Current evidence suggests that feline idiopathic cystitis represents a syndrome that has a number of different underlying causes, some of which may occur simultaneously and be interrelated.[126] Treatment and prevention strategies will therefore vary according to the underlying mechanisms involved. The currently recommended dietary management of idiopathic cystitis is to change the cat's diet to promote production of more dilute urine. This can be accomplished by adding water to a dry food or switching to a canned ration. Potential benefits of producing less-concentrated urine include the dilution of any noxious substances that may contribute to the disorder, more frequent urination patterns that decrease bladder contact time with urine, and removal of any excess crystals (if they exist).

OTHER TYPES OF UROLITHS FOUND IN DOGS

Other mineral types found in the urinary calculi of dogs include urate (usually in Dalmatians; see Chapter 27, pp. 305-306), calcium phosphate, silica, and cystine. Xanthine urolithiasis in dogs is most often iatrogenic, associated with allopurinol treatment, especially in cases in which dietary recommendations limiting purine are not followed. Although much less common, xanthine urolithiasis can be caused by a heritable defect in the enzyme xanthine oxidase. There have been case reports of this condition in Dachshunds, Cavalier King Charles Spaniels, Australian Shepherds, and Dalmatians.[127-129] Calcium phosphate is the third most common type of mineral found in canine uroliths; this type occurs more often in females than males. In most cases, calcium phosphate is found as a component of mixed-mineral uroliths with either struvite or calcium oxalate. Because calcium phosphate is typically considered to be a secondary component, dietary management is usually directed toward preventing the recurrence of the primary mineral.

Silica crystals are also often found in association with other types of minerals, but these are seen more often in males than females.[130] Certain breeds of dog appear to have an increased risk for silica urolithiasis. These include the German Shepherd Dog, Old English Sheepdog, Miniature Schnauzer, Shih Tzu, Lhasa Apso, Yorkshire Terrier, and Golden Retriever. Surgical removal is the conventional treatment. A measure used to prevent recurrence is increasing water consumption to produce more dilute urine.

Cystine urolithiasis is relatively rare in dogs, but when it occurs it is almost always in males. Certain breeds are at increased risk, and it is associated with reduced renal tubular reabsorption of several basic amino acids such as lysine, arginine, ornithine, and citrulline. The Newfoundland breed has been used as a model to study cystinuria.[131] Following surgical removal, preventive measures include feeding a urine-alkalinizing diet and increasing water consumption to promote the production of less-concentrated urine.

References

1. Senior D: Lower urinary tract disease—feline. In *WSAVA Proc*, 2006.

2. Bartges J: Canine lower urinary trace cases. In *ACVIM Proc*, 2003.

3. Zoran DL: Role of diet in feline and canine urolithiasis. Presented at *Western veterinary conference*, Las Vegas, 2006.

4. Bartges JW: Lower urinary tract disease in older cats: what's common, what's not, *Vet Clin Nutr* 3:57–62, 1996.

5. Ling GV, Franti CE, Ruby AL, and others: Urolithiasis in dogs. I: Mineral prevalence and interrelations of mineral composition, age, and sex, *Am J Vet Res* 59:624–629, 1998.

6. Cannon AB, Westropp JL, Ruby AL, and others: Evaluation of trends in urolith composition in cats: 5,230 cases (1985-2004), *J Am Vet Med Assoc* 231:570–576, 2007.

7. Lekcharoensuk C, Lulich JP, Osborne CA, and others: Patient and environmental factors associated with calcium oxalate urolithiasis in dogs, *J Am Vet Med Assoc* 217:515–519, 2000.

8. Picavet P, Detilleux J, Verschuren S, and others: Analysis of 4495 canine and feline uroliths in the Benelux. A retrospective study: 1994-2004, *J Anim Physiol Anim Nutr (Berl)* 91:247–251, 2007.

9. Seaman R, Bartges JW: Canine struvite urolithiasis, *Compend Contin Educ Pract Vet* 23:407–420, 2001.

10. Willeberg P: A case-control study of some fundamental determinants in the epidemiology of the feline urological syndrome, *Nord Vet Med* 27:1–14, 1975.

11. Lekcharoensuk C, Lulich JP, Osborne CA, and others: Association between patient-related factors and risk of calcium oxalate and magnesium ammonium phosphate urolithiasis in cats, *J Am Vet Med Assoc* 217:520–525, 2000.

12. Ling GV, Franti CE, Ruby AL, and others: Urolithiasis in dogs. II. Breed prevalence, and interrelations of breed, sex, age, and mineral composition, *Am J Vet Res* 59:630–642, 1998.

13. Willeberg P, Priester WA: Feline urological syndrome: associations with some time, space and individual patient factors, *Am J Vet Res* 37:975–978, 1976.

14. Houston DM, Moore AE, Favrin MG, and others: Canine urolithiasis: a look at over 16 000 urolith submissions to the Canadian Veterinary Urolith Centre from February 1998 to April 2003, *Can Vet J* 45:225–230, 2004.

15. Weichselbaum RC, Feeney DA, Jessen CR, and others: Evaluation of the morphologic characteristics and prevalence of canine urocystoliths from a regional urolith center, *Am J Vet Res* 59:379–387, 1998.

16. Lekcharoensuk C, Osborne CA, Lulich JP, and others: Trends in the frequency of calcium oxalate uroliths in the upper urinary tract of cats, *J Am Anim Hosp Assoc* 41:39–46, 2005.

17. Ross S, Osborne C, Polzin D, and others: Epidemiology of feline nephroliths and ureteroliths. Presented at *23rd annual forum of the American College of Veterinary Internal Medicine conference,* 2005.

18. Cowgill LD: Ureteral obstruction: a new dilemma in feline nephrology. Presented at *23rd annual forum of the American College of Veterinary Internal Medicine conference,* 2005.

19. Ling GV, Ruby Al, Johnson DK: Renal calculi in dogs and cats: prevalence, mineral type, breed, age and gender interrelationships (1981-1992), *J Vet Intern Med* 12:11–21, 1998.

20. Stoller ML, Meng MV, Abrahams HM, and others: The primary stone event: a new hypothesis involving a vascular etiology, *J Urol* 171:1920–1924, 2004.

21. Kyles AE, Hardie EM, Wooden BG, and others: Clinical, clinicopathologic, radiographic, and ultrasonographic abnormalities in cats with ureteral calculi: 163 cases (1984-2002), *J Am Vet Med Assoc* 226:932–936, 2005.

22. Langston C, Gisselman K, Palma D, and others: Diagnosis of urolithiasis, *Compend Contin Educ Vet* 30:447–455, 2008.

23. Chew DJ, Buffington T: Diagnosis and medical treatment of non-obstructive feline lower urinary tract disease. In *Proc WSAVA,* 2000, pp 15–20.

24. Gaskell C: Feline urological syndrome (FUS)—theory and practice, *J Small Anim Pract* 31:519–522, 1990.

25. Osborne CA, Johnston GR, Polzin DJ, and others: Feline urologic syndrome: a heterogenous phenomenon? *J Am Anim Hosp Assoc* 20:17–32, 1984.

26. Bovee KC, Reif JS, Maguire TG, and others: Recurrence of feline urethral obstruction, *J Am Vet Med Assoc* 174:93–96, 1979.

27. Jackson OF: The treatment and subsequent prevention of struvite urolithiasis in cats, *J Small Anim Pract* 12:555–568, 1971.

28. Bohonowych RO, Parks JL, Greene RW: Features of cystic calculi in cats in a hospital population, *J Am Vet Med Assoc* 173:301–303, 1978.

29. Osborne CA, Lulich JP, Thumchai R, and others: Feline urolithiasis. Etiology and pathophysiology, *Vet Clin North Am Small Anim Pract* 26:217–232, 1996.

30. Buffington CA, Rogers QR, Morris JG: Effect of diet on struvite activity product in feline urine, *Am J Vet Res* 51:2025–2030, 1990.

31. Buffington CA, Cook NE, Rogers QR, and others: The role of diet in feline struvite urolithiasis syndrome. In Burger IH, Rivers JPW, editors: *Nutrition of the dog and cat,* Cambridge, United Kingdom, 1989, Cambridge University Press.

32. Osborne CA, Lulich JP, Kruger JM, and others: Medical dissolution of feline struvite urocystoliths, *J Am Vet Med Assoc* 196:1053–1063, 1990.

33. Bartges JW: Rock 'n' roll cats: feline urolithiasis. Presented at *Atlantic Coast veterinary conference,* 2006.

34. Osborne CA, Kruger JM, Lulich JP, and others: Disorders of the feline lower urinary tract. In Osborne CA, Finco DR, editors: *Canine and feline nephrology and urology,* Baltimore, 1995, Williams & Wilkins.

35. Osborne CA, Polzin DJ, Abdullahi SU, and others: Struvite urolithiasis in animals and man: formation, detection, and dissolution, *Adv Vet Sci Comp Med* 29:1–101, 1985.

36. Lekcharoensuk C, Osborne CA, Lulich JP, and others: Association between dietary factors and calcium oxalate and magnesium ammonium phosphate urolithiasis in cats, *J Am Vet Med Assoc* 219:1228–1237, 2001.

37. Lewis LD, Morris ML Jr: Diet as a causative factor of feline urolithiasis, *Vet Clin North Am Small Anim Pract* 14:513–527, 1984.

38. Bushman DH, Emerick RJ, Embry LB: Experimentally induced ovine phosphatic urolithiasis: relationships involving dietary calcium, phosphorus and magnesium, *J Nutr* 87:499–504, 1965.

39. Chow FHC, Brase JL, Hamar DW, and others: Effect of dietary supplements and methylene blue on urinary calculi, *J Urol* 104:315–319, 1970.

40. Rich LJ, Dysart I, Chow FHC, and others: Urethral obstruction in male cats: experimental production by addition of magnesium and phosphate to diet, *Feline Pract* 4:44–47, 1974.

41. Lewis LD, Chow FH, Taton GF, and others: Effect of various dietary mineral concentrations on the occurrence of feline urolithiasis, *J Am Vet Med Assoc* 172:559–563, 1978.

42. Kallfelz FA, Bressett JD, Wallace RJ: Urethral obstruction in random source and SPF male cats induced by high levels of dietary magnesium or magnesium and phosphorus, *Feline Pract* 10:25–35, 1980.

43. National Research Council: *Nutrient requirements of dogs and cats*, Washington, DC, 2006, National Academy Press.

44. Association of American Feed Control Officials (AAFCO): Pet food regulations. *AAFCO official publication*, Atlanta, 2008, AAFCO.

45. Finco DR, Barsanti JA, Crowell WA: Characterization of magnesium-induced urinary disease in the cat and comparison with feline urologic syndrome, *Am J Vet Res* 46:391–400, 1985.

46. Ross LA: Feline urologic syndrome: understanding and diagnosing this enigmatic disease, *Vet Med* 85:1194–1203, 1990.

47. Osborne CA, Kruger JP, Lulich JP, and others: Feline matrix crystalline urethral plugs: a unifying hypothesis of causes, *J Small Anim Pract* 33:172–177, 1992.

48. Buffington CA, Rogers QR, Morris JG, and others: Feline struvite urolithiasis: magnesium effect depends upon urinary pH, *Feline Pract* 15:29–33, 1985.

49. Cook NE: The importance of urinary pH in the prevention of feline urologic syndrome, *Pet Food Ind* 27:24–31, 1985.

50. Tarttelin MF: Feline struvite urolithiasis: factors affecting urine pH may be more important than magnesium levels in food, *Vet Rec* 121:227–230, 1987.

51. Taton GF, Hamar DW, Lewis LD: Urinary acidification in the prevention and treatment of feline struvite urolithiasis, *J Am Vet Med Assoc* 184:437–443, 1984.

52. Taton GF, Hamar DW, Lewis LD: Evaluation of ammonium chloride as a urinary acidifier in the cat, *J Am Vet Med Assoc* 184:433–436, 1984.

53. Chan JCM: Nutrition and acid-base metabolism, *Fed Proc* 40:2423–2428, 1981.

54. Klahr SD: Disorders of acid-base metabolism. In Chan JCM, Gill JR, editors: *Disorders of mineral, water, and acid-base metabolism*, New York, 1982, Wiley and Sons.

55. Kane E, Douglass GM: The effects of feeding a dry commercial cat food on the urine and blood acid-base balance of the cat, *Feline Pract* 16:9–13, 1986.

56. Holzworth J: Nutrition and nutritional disorders. In Holzworth J, editor: *Diseases of the cat: medicine and surgery*, vol 1, Philadelphia, 1987, Saunders.

57. Harrington JT, Lemann J Jr: The metabolic production and disposal of acid and alkali, *Med Clin North Am* 54:1543–1554, 1970.

58. Funaba M, Uchiyama A, Takahashi K, and others: Evaluation of effects of dietary carbohydrate on formation of struvite crystals in urine and macromineral balance in clinically normal cats, *Am J Vet Res* 65:138–142, 2004.

59. Funaba M, Yamate T, Hashida Y, and others: Effects of a high-protein diet versus dietary supplementation with ammonium chloride on struvite crystal formation in urine of clinically normal cats, *Am J Vet Res* 64:1059–1064, 2003.

60. Funaba M, Yamate T, Narukawa Y, and others: Effect of supplementation of dry cat food with D, L-methionine and ammonium chloride on struvite activity product and sediment in urine, *J Vet Med Sci* 63:337–339, 2001.

61. Funaba M, Hashimoto M, Yamanaka C, and others: Effects of a high-protein diet on mineral metabolism and struvite activity product in clinically normal cats, *Am J Vet Res* 57:1726–1732, 1996.

62. Skoch ER, Chandler EA, Douglas GM, and others: Influence of diet or urine pH and the feline urological syndrome, *J Small Anim Pract* 32:413–419, 1991.

63. Funaba M, Matsumoto C, Matsuki K, and others: Comparison of corn gluten meal and meat meal as a protein source in dry foods formulated for cats, *Am J Vet Res* 63:1247–1251, 2002.

64. Funaba M, Tanak T, Kaneko M, and others: Fish meal vs. corn gluten meal as a protein source for dry cat food, *J Vet Med Sci* 63:1355–1357, 2001.

65. Funaba M, Oka Y, Kobayashi S, and others: Evaluation of meat meal, chicken meal, and corn gluten meal as dietary sources of protein in dry cat food, *Can J Vet Res* 69:299–304, 2005.

66. Anderson RS: Water balance in the dog and cat, *J Small Anim Pract* 23:588–598, 1982.

67. Gaskell CJ: Nutrition in diseases of the urinary tract in the dog and cat, *Vet Ann* 25:383–390, 1985.

68. Thrall BE, Miller LG: Water turnover in cats fed dry rations, *Feline Pract* 6:10–17, 1976.

69. Seefeldt SL, Chapman TE: Body water content and turnover in cats fed dry and canned rations, *Am J Vet Res* 40:183–185, 1979.

70. Sauer LS, Hamar D, Lewis LD: Effect of diet composition on water intake and excretion by the cat, *Feline Pract* 15:16–21, 1985.

71. Allen TA: Measurement of the influence of diet on feline urinary pH, *Vet Clin North Am Small Anim Pract* 26:363–368, 1996.

72. Kane E, Rogers QR, Morris JG, and others: Feeding behavior of the cat fed laboratory and commercial diets, *Nutr Res* 1:499–507, 1981.

73. Hart BL: Feline behavior, *Feline Pract* 9:10–12, 1979.

74. Finco DR, Adams DD, Crowell WA, and others: Food and water intake and urine composition in cats: influence of continuous versus periodic feeding, *Am J Vet Res* 47:1638–1642, 1986.

75. Finke MD, Litzenberger BA: Effect of food intake on urine pH in cats, *J Small Anim Pract* 33:261–265, 1992.

76. Osborne CA, Lulich JP, Thumchai R, and others: Diagnosis, medical treatment, and prognosis of feline urolithiasis, *Vet Clin North Am Small Anim Pract* 26:589–627, 1996.

77. Hamar DW, Chow FHC, Dysart MI, and others: Effect of sodium chloride in prevention of experimentally produced phosphate uroliths in male cats, *J Am Anim Hosp Assoc* 12:514–517, 1976.

78. Osborne CA, Polzin DJ: Prospective clinical evaluation of feline struvite urolith dissolution, *Proc Am Coll Vet Int Med* 1:4-11, 14-16, 1986.

79. Buffington CA: Acid questions: potential dangers associated with cat food acidification, *Pet Food Ind* 4–8, 1983.

80. Osborne CA, Polzin DJ, Lulich JP, and others: Relationship of nutritional factors to the cause, dissolution, and prevention of canine uroliths, *Vet Clin North Am Small Anim Pract* 19:583–619, 1989.

81. Osborne CA, Kruger JM, Polzin DJ, and others: Medical dissolution of feline struvite uroliths, *Minn Vet* 24:22–32, 1984.

82. Buffington CAT, Chew DJ: Lower urinary tract diseases in cats: the Ohio State experience. Presented at *Annual conference veterinary internal medicine forum*, 1997, pp 339–343.

83. Burger IH: Nutritional aspects of the feline urological syndrome (FUS), *J Small Anim Pract* 28:447–452, 1987.

84. Dow SW, Fettman MJ, LeCouteur RA, and others: Potassium depletion in cats: renal and dietary influences, *J Am Vet Med Assoc* 191:1569–1575, 1987.

85. Dow SW, Fettman MJ, Roger QR: Taurine depletion induced by experimental dietary potassium depletion and acidification of cats. Presented at *American College of Veterinary Internal Medicine*, San Diego, 1989, p 1040.

86. DiBartola SP, Buffington CA, Chew DJ, and others: Development of chronic renal disease in cats fed a commercial diet, *J Am Vet Med Assoc* 202:744–751, 1993.

87. Fettman MJ: Feline kaliopenic polymyopathy/nephropathy syndrome, *Vet Clin North Am Small Anim Pract* 19:415–432, 1989.

88. Buffington CA: Feline struvite urolithiasis: effect of diet. Presented at *European Society of Veterinary Nephrology and Urology annual symposium,* Barcelona, Spain, 1988, Intercongress.

89. Kurtz I, Maher T, Hulter HN, and others: Effect of diet on plasma acid-base composition in normal humans, *Kidney Int* 24: 670–680, 1983.

90. Ching SV, Fettman MJ, Hamar DW, and others: The effect of chronic dietary acidification using ammonium chloride on acid-base and mineral metabolism in the adult cat, *J Nutr* 119:902–915, 1989.

91. Jackson JR, Kealy RD, Lawler DF, and others: Long-term safety of urine acidifying diets for cats, *Vet Clin Nutr* 2:100–107, 1995.

92. Fettman MJ, Coble JM, Hamar DW, and others: Effect of dietary phosphoric acid supplementation on acid-base balance and mineral and bone metabolism in adult cats, *Am J Vet Res* 53:2125–2135, 1992.

93. Tetrick MA: The role of diet in managing feline lower urinary tract diseases. In *Proc WSAVA,* 2000, pp 20–24.

94. Schwille PO, Herrmann U: Environmental factors in the pathophysiology of recurrent idiopathic calcium urolithiasis (RCU), with emphasis on nutrition, *Urol Res* 20:72–83, 1992.

95. Ling GV, Franti CE, Johnson DL, and others: Urolithiasis in dogs. IV. Survey of interrelations among breed, mineral composition, and anatomic location of calculi, and presence of urinary tract infection, *Am J Vet Res* 59:650–660, 1998.

96. Kirk CA, Biourge VC: Managing struvite/oxalate urolithiasis: point/counterpoint. Presented at *North American veterinary conference,* Orlando, Fla, 2006, pp 749–752.

97. Ling GV, Franti CE, Johnson DL, and others: Urolithiasis in dogs. III. Prevalence of urinary tract infection and interrelations of infection, age, sex, and mineral composition, *Am J Vet Res* 59:643–649, 1998.

98. Osborne CA, Klausner JS, Polzin DJ, and others: Etiopathogenesis of canine struvite urolithiasis, *Vet Clin North Am Small Anim Pract* 16:67–86, 1986.

99. Weaver AD, Pillinger R: Relationship of bacterial infection in urine and calculi to canine urolithiasis, *Vet Rec* 97:48–50, 1975.

100. Clark WE: Staphylococcal infection of the urinary tract and its relations to urolithiasis in dogs, *Vet Rec* 97:204–206, 1974.

101. Osborne CA, Lulich JP, Bartges JW, and others: Canine and feline urolithiasis: relationship to etiopathogenesis to treatment and prevention. In Osborne CA, Finco DR, editors: *Canine and feline nephrology and urology,* Baltimore, 1995, Williams & Wilkins.

102. Escolar E, Bellanato J, Medina JA: Structure and composition of canine urinary calculi, *Res Vet Sci* 49:327–333, 1990.

103. Rinkardt NE, Houston DM: Dissolution of infection-induced struvite bladder stones by using a noncalculolytic diet and antibiotic therapy, *Can Vet J* 45:838–840, 2004.

104. Ling GV: Urinary stone disease. In Ling GV, editor: *Lower urinary tract disease of dogs and cats,* St Louis, 1995, Mosby.

105. Osborne C: Feline calcium oxalate urolithiasis: perspectives from the Minnesota Urolith Center. Presented at *Petfood forum,* Chicago, 1997, Watts Publishing.

106. Osborne C, Lulich J, Thumchai R, and others: Feline calcium oxalate uroliths: pathophysiology, clinical findings, diagnosis, treatment, and prevention, *Vet Clin Nutr* 1:105–114, 1994.

107. Lulich J: Feline urolithiasis—managing the consequences of an epidemiological shift in urolith type. Presented at *Hill's European symposium on advances in feline medicine,* Brussels, 2006.

108. Westropp JL: How to manage calcium oxalate urolithiasis in cats and dogs. Presented at *North American veterinary conference,* Orlando, Fla, 2007, pp 717–718.

109. Buffington CAT: *Nutritional diseases and nutritional therapy in the cat,* ed 2, London, 1995, Churchill Livingstone.

110. Bai SC, Sampson DA, Morris JG, and others: Vitamin B-6 requirement of growing kittens, *J Nutr* 119:1020–1027, 1989.

111. Lulich JP, Osborne CA, Carlson M, and others: Nonsurgical removal of urocystoliths in dogs and cats by voiding urohydropropulsion, *J Am Vet Med Assoc* 203:660–663, 1993.

112. Osborne CA, Lulich JP, Forrester D, Albasan H: Paradigm changes in the role of nutrition for the management of canine and feline urolithiasis, *Vet Clin North Am Small Anim Pract* 39:127–141, 2009.

113. Marone CC, Wong NL, Sutton RA, and others: Effects of metabolic alkalosis on calcium excretion in the conscious dog, *J Lab Clin Med* 101:264–273, 1983.

114. Biourge V: Urine dilution: a key factor in the prevention of struvite and calcium oxalate uroliths, *Vet Focus* 17:41–44, 2007.

115. Tournier C, Malandain E, Esperandieu M, and others: Relative supersaturation: a better predictor of struvite urolith dissolution kinetics than urinary pH. In *Proc ECVIM*, 2008, p 205.

116. Lulich JP, Osborne CA, Lekcharoensuk C: Effects of diet on urine composition of cats with calcium oxalate urolithiasis, *J Am Anim Hosp Assoc* 40:185–191, 2004.

117. Hawthorne AJ, Markwell PJ: Dietary sodium promotes increased water intake and urine volume in cats, *J Nutr* 134:2128S–2129S, 2004.

118. Lekcharoensuk C, Osborne CA, Lulich JP: Association between dietary factors and calcium oxalate and magnesium phosphate urolithiasis in cats, *J Am Vet Med Assoc* 219:1228–1237, 2001.

119. Lulich J, Osborne C, Thumchai R, and others: Epidemiology of canine calcium oxalate urolithiasis: case study. Presented at *Annual conference veterinary internal medicine forum*, 1995, pp 490–492.

120. Lulich JP, Osborne CA, Smith CL: Canine calcium oxalate urolithiasis: risk factor management. In Kirk RW, Bonagura JD, editors: *Current veterinary therapy XI*, Philadelphia, 1992, Saunders.

121. Hess RS, Kass PH, Ward CR: Association between hyperadrenocorticism and development of calcium-containing uroliths in dogs with urolithiasis, *J Am Vet Med Assoc* 212:1889–1891, 1998.

122. Houston DM, Moore AE, Favrin MG, and others: Feline urethral plugs and bladder uroliths: a review of 5484 submissions 1998-2003, *Can Vet J* 44:974–977, 2003.

123. Tsuchida S, Kagi A, Koyama H, and others: Xanthine urolithiasis in a cat: a case report and evaluation of a candidate gene for xanthine dehydrogenase, *J Feline Med Surg* 9:503–508, 2007.

124. Osborne CA, Thumchai R, Lulich JP, and others: Epidemiology of feline urolithiasis, *Proc Ann Conf Vet Intern Med Forum*, 1979.

125. Klausner JS, Osborne CA: Canine calcium phosphate uroliths, *Vet Clin North Am Small Anim Pract* 16:171–184, 1986.

126. Kruger JM, Osborne CA, Lulich JP: Changing paradigms of feline idiopathic cystitis, *Vet Clin North Am Small Anim Pract* 39:15–40, 2009.

127. Ling GV, Ruby AL, Harrold DR, and others: Xanthine-containing urinary calculi in dogs given allopurinol, *J Am Vet Med Assoc* 198:1935–1940, 1991.

128. van Zuilen CD, Nickel RF, van Dijk TH, and others: Xanthinuria in a family of Cavalier King Charles Spaniels, *Vet Q* 19:172–174, 1997.

129. Flegel T, Freistadt R, Haider W: Xanthine urolithiasis in a Dachshund, *Vet Rec* 143:420–423, 1998.

130. Aldrich J, Ling GV, Ruby AL, and others: Silica-containing urinary calculi in dogs (1981-1993), *J Vet Intern Med* 11:288–295, 1997.

131. Robinson MR, Norris RD, Sur RL, and others: Urolithiasis: not just a 2-legged animal disease, *J Urol* 179:46–52, 2008.

31

Nutritionally Responsive Dermatoses

The skin (integument) is the largest organ in the body; together skin, hair, and dermis make up 24% of the body weight (BW) of a newborn puppy and 12% of the BW of an adult dog.[1] The integument is metabolically active. It provides sensory input, acts as a barrier to protect the body from physical and infectious injury, is important for normal temperature control and immunoregulation, and serves as a reservoir for certain nutrients. The health of a pet's skin and hair coat can be affected by a variety of nutrients, most importantly protein, vitamin A, vitamin E, the essential fatty acids (EFAs), and zinc (Figure 31-1). Dogs and cats that are consuming high-quality, complete, balanced pet foods are unlikely to suffer from a serious deficiency or excess of any of these nutrients. However, feeding a poorly formulated or stored commercial food, or preparing a homemade diet that is not correctly balanced, can contribute to skin disorders. In addition, any metabolic or functional disease that affects a pet's ability to digest, absorb, or use nutrients can cause secondary nutrient imbalances that may manifest as dermatoses. A third way nutrition can affect the health of the skin relates to inflammatory skin disease. The development of an adverse reaction to one or more components in the diet can be the cause of inflammatory dermatoses in dogs and cats. In addition, diet can be an important component in the management of other forms of inflammatory skin disease in dogs and cats such as atopic dermatitis and feline miliary dermatitis.

PROTEIN AND SKIN HEALTH

The importance of protein for the maintenance and development of skin and coat health is well documented. Hair is more than 90% protein and contains high amounts of the sulfur amino acids, methionine and cystine. Normal turnover of skin cells and keratinization also impose a demand for protein. Together, skin and coat needs account for up to 30% of an animal's daily protein requirement.[2] Although uncommon,

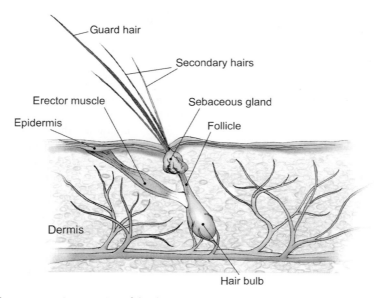

Figure 31-1   Cross-section of the skin and associated structures and the role of nutrients.

protein deficiency in dogs and cats can be seen in association with starvation, as a result of disease-induced anorexia, or in response to prolonged feeding of an inadequate diet. Changes to the skin and hair coat that develop during protein deficiency include abnormal keratinization, depigmentation of hair shafts, and changes in sebaceous and epidermal lipids. Coat hairs become brittle and break off easily, and coat growth slows or stops. The lipid layer of the epidermis becomes abnormal and loses its function as a protective barrier. The skin becomes scaly, greasy, and susceptible to secondary bacterial infections. When healthy pets are fed balanced, complete pet foods, signs of protein deficiency are highly unlikely.

Dietary protein may also affect skin health in terms of hypersensitivity response and effects upon subcutaneous lipid metabolism. The importance of dietary protein for pets with adverse food reactions is discussed later in this chapter (pp. 396-402). It has also been theorized that feeding different types of proteins may affect skin and serum lipid concentrations in dogs. For example, plant proteins have been reported to be hypocholesterolemic compared with animal proteins, when fed to monkeys and rabbits.[3,4] In a study with dogs, six different protein sources (chicken, pork, lamb, fish, beef, and soy) were sequentially fed to a group of 12 dogs.[5] No differences were observed between protein treatment groups in skin histology, signs of inflammation or pruritus, or skin fatty acid levels. Several of the dogs fed pork showed an increase in scale production and a decrease in hair regrowth following skin biopsies, suggesting that pork should be avoided as a protein source in dogs with seborrhea. However, additional research is needed to further investigate the role of pork in skin health in dogs and cats.

Another study compared the effects of feeding soy protein versus a meat-based protein source and soy oil versus poultry fat on serum cholesterol, serum lipids, and cutaneous fatty acid concentrations in dogs.[6] Dietary protein had no effect upon serum cholesterol concentration and only marginal effects upon serum and skin fatty acid concentrations. However, dogs fed soy oil–containing diets had higher linoleic acid (LA) and lower oleic acid concentrations in skin and serum when compared with dogs fed diets containing poultry fat. Dogs fed diets containing poultry fat also had higher concentrations of serum arachidonic acid (AA).

An important finding of this study is that while the type of fat significantly influenced serum and skin fatty acid and cholesterol concentrations in this study, the protein source did not affect lipid profiles.

The results of these two studies indicate that protein source does not significantly affect changes in fatty acid values or skin architecture in the dog. The effects of dietary protein on inflammatory skin disease in dogs are more related to allergenicity and frequency of exposure rather than to an influence upon fatty acid metabolism or homeostasis (see pp. 397-398). While it is possible that fat content in various protein sources may affect cutaneous and plasma fatty acid concentrations, such effects are associated with the protein's fatty acid composition and not with protein characteristics per se.

VITAMIN A–RESPONSIVE DERMATOSES

Vitamin A is necessary for normal epithelial cell differentiation and maintenance and for the process of keratinization (see Section 1, pp. 27-29). Both deficiencies and excesses of this vitamin cause skin lesions in dogs and cats. Signs include hair loss and poor coat condition, hyperkeratinization of the epidermis and hair follicles, scaling of the skin, and an increased susceptibility to secondary bacterial infections of the skin.[1] Vitamin A toxicity is most commonly caused by feeding an all-liver diet or by oversupplementation with cod liver oil. Nutritional deficiencies of vitamin A (retinol) are uncommon and are accompanied by visual and digestive problems.[2]

More common than deficiencies or excesses, however, are certain types of skin disorders that are responsive to treatment with supplemental vitamin A or retinoids (natural and synthetic vitamin A analogs). The administration of vitamin A and the retinoids appears to have both physiological and pharmacological effects. These compounds have been used successfully in humans and animals to treat cases of idiopathic seborrhea that are not caused by a vitamin A deficiency.[7,8] Seborrhea is a general term that describes the overproduction of oils and other protective secretions by the sebaceous glands in the skin. The skin usually becomes flaky, greasy, or both. Because the epidermal lipid layer is abnormal, the animal becomes prone to secondary bacterial skin infections that can cause pruritus and further damage to the skin. Treatment of seborrhea in companion animals is usually directed toward determining the underlying cause and correcting it. However, in a substantial number of cases, an underlying mechanism cannot be identified and treatment is directed primarily toward the relief of clinical signs.

Certain types of seborrhea in dogs and cats respond favorably to vitamin A. The most common form is idiopathic seborrhea in Cocker Spaniels, which can often be kept in complete remission with vitamin A therapy.[9-11] The disorder and response to vitamin A therapy has also been reported in Labrador Retrievers and Miniature Schnauzers.[10,12] Vitamin A–responsive seborrhea is characterized by dry and scaly skin that progresses to oily changes. Affected dogs eventually develop large, hyperkeratotic plaques (composed of sebum and keratin) and marked follicular plugging. Lesions are most prominent on the underside of the thorax and abdomen. Hair loss and skin changes are accompanied by secondary bacterial folliculitis. Pruritus and inflammation may or may not be present. Almost all reported cases also show moderate to severe otitis externa.

Cases of vitamin A–responsive seborrhea usually do not respond to the traditional treatments for seborrhea, which include medicated shampoos, antibiotic therapy, and glucocorticoid therapy. Although clinical signs can be used in support of a diagnosis, the diagnosis of vitamin A–responsive seborrhea can only be confirmed through favorable response to supplementation. A dose of 10,000 international units (IUs) per day is suggested, although levels as high as 50,000 IUs/day have been used.[9-12] A decrease in clinical signs is usually seen within 4 weeks, with complete remission within 2 to 6 months of starting treatment. Attempts to reduce the level of vitamin A, or to withdraw therapy, result in a relapse of clinical signs, indicating that lifelong therapy is necessary. The dosages used represent 6 to 10 times the dog's normal requirement for vitamin A. However, no signs of vitamin A toxicity have been observed in the reported cases, even after several years of therapy. Other studies have indicated that much higher levels of vitamin A are necessary to induce clinical signs of vitamin A toxicity in dogs.[13,14]

A second skin disorder that has been shown to be responsive to vitamin A supplementation is sebaceous adenitis. This chronic skin disease is characterized by the development of lymphocytic, granulomatous, or pyogranulomatous inflammation of the sebaceous glands, resulting in scaling, skin lesions, and hair loss. Over time, sebaceous glands are progressively destroyed, and inflammation diminishes. Sebaceous adenitis is genetically influenced. Standard Poodles, Akitas, Chow Chows, and Vizslas are more frequently affected with this disorder than the general population of dogs.[15,16] In Poodles, the disease is believed to be transmitted by an autosomal recessive gene.[17] Some of the treatments used to manage sebaceous adenitis include antiseborrheic shampoos, topical application of propylene glycol or EFAs, and systemic administration of cyclosporine or synthetic retinoids (vitamin A derivatives).

A study of 30 dogs examined the efficacy of using two synthetic retinoids, isotretinoin and etretinate, to treat the clinical signs of sebaceous adenitis.[18] Dogs that had been diagnosed with the disorder were treated for a minimum of 2 months with one of the two retinoids. Forty-seven percent of the dogs given isotretinoin and 53% of the dogs given etretinate were successfully treated and were maintained on retinoid therapy indefinitely. Although it was previously thought that Akitas respond poorly to synthetic retinoids, this study reported successful treatment in 10 of the 11 Akitas included in the study.[18,19] These results suggest that retinoids may be an effective treatment for some dogs with sebaceous adenitis. An initial dosage of 1 milligram (mg)/kilogram (kg) of BW per day of either isotretinoin or etretinate is recommended.

It is important to note that these skin conditions are not caused by a vitamin A deficiency. In all reported cases, the dogs were being fed a high-quality, complete and balanced, commercial dog food. Moreover, serum levels of vitamin A were normal, and no other signs of vitamin A deficiency were observed. One group of investigators also reported that the skin changes seen in cases of vitamin A–responsive dermatosis differed significantly from those seen with a true vitamin A deficiency.[9] It is likely that the effect of vitamin A is the result of a pharmacological action of the vitamin on epithelial cells, rather than a result of the vitamin's role as an essential nutrient.[7]

Some cutaneous disorders that respond to vitamin A therapy are not actually caused by a vitamin A deficiency. In these cases vitamin A therapy is required throughout the pet's life, but therapeutic dosages have not been found to be toxic. It is believed that there is a genetic basis for vitamin A–responsive seborrhea in Cocker Spaniels and for sebaceous adenitis in Standard Poodles, Akitas, Chow Chows, and Viszlas.

VITAMIN E–RESPONSIVE DERMATOSES

The term *vitamin E* refers to a group of compounds called the *tocopherols* that act as biological and food antioxidants. Alpha-tocopherol is the most biologically active form of vitamin E. Within the body, vitamin E functions as a free-radical scavenger, protecting cell membranes and tissues from oxidative stress. An animal's dietary requirement for vitamin E is dependent upon dietary intake of polyunsaturated fatty acids (PUFAs), with an increase in requirement occurring when high levels of PUFAs are fed (see Section 1, p. 31 and Section 2, p. 110). Vitamin E deficiency is uncommon in dogs, but has been reported in cats fed high-fat diets and results in a pathological condition called *pansteatitis* (see Chapter 26, p. 279 for a complete discussion). Although a poor hair coat may be seen in cats with pansteatitis, the primary manifestations of vitamin E deficiency are related to the necrosis and inflammatory changes in subcutaneous and intraabdominal fat.

Conversely, supraphysiological doses of vitamin E have some efficacy in the management of a skin condition called *primary acanthosis nigricans* in Dachshunds. This disorder is characterized by hair loss and extreme hyperpigmentation (blackening) and thickening of the skin. As the disease progresses, varying degrees of greasiness, crusting, rancid odor, and secondary bacterial infections develop. Pruritus is usually absent or mild during the early stages of the disorder, but it may become more pronounced as secondary infections occur. In one study, a group of eight Dachshunds with acanthosis nigricans were given 200 IUs of alpha-tocopherol daily.[20] All eight dogs showed improvement within 60 days. Skin inflammation, crusting, and pruritus completely subsided, although hyperpigmentation did not improve. Clinical signs did not reappear in any of the dogs within follow-up periods of 7 months to 3 years. All of the dogs were maintained on the vitamin E supplementation throughout this time. None of the owners attempted to decrease the dose or withdraw the supplementation, so it is not known if long-term vitamin E supplementation is necessary in all cases.

A medium-sized (20-kg) adult dog has a minimum daily requirement for vitamin E of about 10 IUs. Most commercial pet foods will supply a 20-kg dog with between 20 and 50 IUs/day. The levels that were fed in this study represent 4 to 10 times the dog's normal daily intake of vitamin E, but no toxicity signs were observed in any of the eight dogs. The authors concluded that vitamin E may offer a therapeutic alternative for some cases of primary canine acanthosis nigricans. In all cases, the disorder is chronic and persistent, and therapy is directed toward control rather than cure. Many dogs with acanthosis nigricans respond favorably to systemic treatment with corticosteroids. However, concern over the immediate and long-term side effects of corticosteroid therapy dictates the need to find alternative or adjunctive treatments, one of which may be supplemental vitamin E.

Vitamin E therapy has also been used with varying levels of success in dogs with discoid lupus erythematosus and dermatomyositis.[21,22] However, not all dogs with these disorders respond to vitamin E therapy, and additional research needs to be conducted to determine an effective dose range of vitamin E. Conversely, vitamin E supplementation has been shown to be ineffective as an antiinflammatory and antipruritic agent for the treatment of atopic dermatitis (allergic dermatitis) in dogs (Table 31-1).

ZINC-RESPONSIVE DERMATOSES

The essential mineral zinc has several functions that affect skin health and coat quality. As an integral component of several metalloenzymes and a cofactor for both ribonucleic acid (RNA) and deoxyribonucleic acid (DNA) polymerases, zinc plays an important role

TABLE 31-1   VITAMIN E–RESPONSIVE DERMATOSES

DISORDER	BREEDS	SUCCESS OF VITAMIN E SUPPLEMENTATION
Demodicosis	All	Variable
Primary acanthosis nigricans	Dachshunds	Yes
Discoid lupus erythematosus	All	Variable
Dermatomyositis	Collies, Shetland Sheepdogs	Variable

in regulating cellular metabolism and cell division. Zinc is also needed for the synthesis of fatty acids and is essential for immune system health and normal inflammatory responses. In adult animals, a deficiency of zinc manifests principally as changes to skin and coat health. In young animals, skin changes are accompanied by impaired growth, inappetance, and other health problems.

Dermatoses that respond to zinc supplementation occur in companion animals for a number of reasons. Genetic disorders are responsible for impaired zinc absorption and metabolism in several breeds of dogs.[23] A defect in the mucosal transfer system for zinc in the small intestine occurs in Alaskan Malamutes, Siberian Huskies, and American Eskimos. Bull Terriers with lethal acrodermatitis also have an inability to absorb dietary zinc (see Chapter 27, pp. 299-300 for a complete discussion). Zinc deficiency can also result from inadequate levels of the mineral in the diet and from the presence of other nutrients or components that interfere with zinc absorption.[24,25] Specifically, increased levels of calcium and phytate will interfere with the bioavailability of dietary zinc and can lead to zinc deficiency.[26] Naturally occurring cases of zinc-responsive dermatoses are rare in dogs and have not been reported in cats. The reported cases in dogs have all been associated with feeding foods that contain either marginal levels of zinc, cereal-based foods containing high levels of phytate, poor-quality foods containing high amounts of calcium, or a combination of these factors. Growing dogs are most susceptible to zinc deficiency, and

excessive supplementation with calcium during growth also has the potential to result in dermatoses associated with zinc deficiency.[25,27]

> *In dogs, cases of diet-induced zinc deficiency are associated with feeding foods that contain either marginal levels of zinc, cereal-based foods that contain high levels of phytate, poor quality foods that contain high amounts of calcium, or a combination of these factors. Growing dogs are most susceptible to zinc deficiency, and excessive supplementation with calcium during growth also has the potential to result in dermatoses associated with zinc deficiency.*

The skin lesions of zinc-responsive dermatosis are seen on the face, over pressure points, and on the foot pads (Figure 31-2).[28,29] In extreme cases, the lesions eventually spread over the entire body. Affected areas are characterized by hair loss, redness, inflammation, crusting, and pruritus. Secondary skin infections are also seen. Diagnosis is usually made by diet history, breed, physical examination, and skin biopsy. Positive response to oral zinc supplementation without changing the diet can be used to confirm a diagnosis.[28] However, because dogs vary considerably in response and because a wide range of effective dosages has been reported, it is difficult to make recommendations for appropriate dosages of zinc to use. In addition, zinc requirements and response to supplementation are influenced by the animal's physiological state, the presence of inhibitory components in the diet, and the form of zinc that is used.[30] A dose of 10 mg of zinc sulfate/kg per day or 1.7 mg of zinc methionine/kg per day is recommended by some authors.[22,28] The smaller dose of zinc methionine was suggested because of presumed increased bioavailability of the organic form. However, increased bioavailability of zinc methionine appears to be significant only when there is high metabolic demand such as during growth or when there are inhibitory components in the food.[31,32] Other authors suggest an initial dosage that provides 2 to 3 mg/kg BW of elemental zinc/day.[23] The initial dose should be administered for at least a 30-day period to determine the response to treatment. A response should be seen within 6 weeks of initiation of supplementation and,

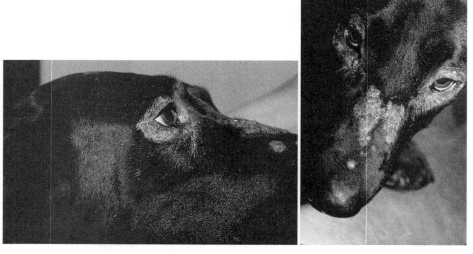

Figure 31-2　Zinc deficiency in an adult male Labrador Retriever, caused by a diet of generic dog food. (Courtesy Candace Sousa, DVM, Animal Dermatology Clinic, Sacramento, Calif.)

in most cases, skin lesions show a rapid response, with complete healing within 2 weeks.

Zinc supplementation confirms a diagnosis of zinc-responsive dermatosis and aids in rapid recovery. In cases that occurred as a result of an inadequate diet (i.e., presence of inhibitory substances) or excessive supplementation, feeding a high quality complete and balanced food that supplies adequate levels of zinc is recommended. Additionally, there is some evidence that increasing EFAs may have a synergistic effect with zinc in some animals.[23,33] In other species, supplementation with EFAs has been shown to ameliorate the clinical effects of zinc deficiency.[34] This may occur because clinical signs of EFA and zinc deficiencies are similar. The presence a deficiency in both nutrients negatively affects sebum production and skin health. It is possible that a subclinical EFA deficiency occurred in dogs that reportedly showed an additive response to zinc and EFA (LA). This would be expected if the underlying cause of zinc deficiency was a poor diet. Alternatively, fat absorption may be reduced in dogs with zinc-responsive dermatoses, which could lead to a subclinical deficiency state.[35] Continued supplementation with zinc after correction of the diet is necessary when an inherited problem with zinc metabolism exists.

ESSENTIAL FATTY ACIDS AND SKIN DISEASE

As components of cell-membrane phospholipids and precursors for a variety of regulatory compounds, the EFAs maintain the health and integrity of epithelial tissue in the body. The omega-6 fatty acids that are considered to be essential nutrients include LA in dogs and LA and AA in cats (see Section 2, pp. 81-83). Although the essential nature of omega-3 fatty acids has been controversial, alpha-linolenic acid (ALA) is considered by most nutritionists to be conditionally essential for dogs and cats.[36] LA is specifically responsible for maintaining the cutaneous water permeability barrier, while AA, as a prostaglandin precursor, is needed for normal epidermal proliferation. Other nutrients that may be important to support a healthy epidermal barrier in dogs include pantothenate, choline, nicotinamide, histidine, and inositol.[37] The long-chain omega-3 fatty acids, eicosapentaenoic acid (EPA) and docosahexaenoic acid (DHA), support normal cell membrane fluidity and also have antiinflammatory and immunostimulatory properties. Because of these functions and the skin's rapid cell turnover rate, the skin is especially susceptible to EFA deficiencies.[38]

In dogs and cats, signs of EFA deficiency become apparent within 2 to 3 months of consuming a deficient diet. Initial signs include a reduction in surface lipid production, which results in a dry, dull coat; hair loss; and the eventual development of skin lesions. Over time, the skin becomes greasy, pruritic, and susceptible to infection. A change in the surface lipids in the skin compromises the permeability layer, alters the normal bacterial flora, and predisposes the animal to secondary bacterial infections.[2] Epidermal peeling, interdigital exudation, and otitis externa have also been reported in EFA-deficient dogs. When EFA deficiency is uncomplicated by other nutrient imbalances, skin lesions show a response to dietary correction within 1 to 2 months.[2]

Naturally occurring skin disease as a result of EFA deficiency is rare in dogs and cats today. Healthy companion animals that are fed high-quality foods are not at risk of developing an EFA deficiency. When a deficiency does occur, it is usually the result of feeding a food that is either poorly formulated or has been stored improperly. If the food has been stored at high temperatures or beyond the stated expiration date, there is a risk of EFA loss as a result of oxidative damage to the food. When an EFA deficiency is suspected, it is better to change the diet to a food that is well formulated and has been stored properly, rather than to attempt to correct a deficiency by adding supplemental fatty acids.

Therapeutic Role of Omega-6 and Omega-3 Fatty Acids

EFA supplementation and dietary manipulation of EFA metabolism appear to have some efficacy in the treatment of certain skin disorders that are not the result of a dietary EFA deficiency. The PUFAs are divided into several series based on the position of the first double bond in the carbon chain. Of greatest interest are the omega-3 and omega-6 series of fatty acids. The omega-3 (or n-3) fatty acids have the first double bond located at the third carbon atom from the terminal methyl group. The omega-6 fatty acids have the first double bond at the sixth carbon atom (see Section 1, p. 19). The effects of both types of fatty acids upon cell membrane fluidity and permeability, and their availability for synthesis of new compounds, are affected by the molecule's chain length, the degree of saturation, and the position of the first double bond.

TABLE 31-2 SOURCES OF OMEGA-3 AND OMEGA-6 FATTY ACIDS IN PET FOODS

OMEGA-6 FATTY ACID SOURCES	OMEGA-3 FATTY ACID SOURCES
Corn oil (70% linoleic acid)	Coldwater fish oils (12%-15% EPA)
Safflower oil (78% linoleic acid)	Flaxseed (57% alpha-linolenic acid)
Sunflower oil (69% linoleic acid)	Canola oil (8% alpha-linolenic acid)
Cottonseed oil (54% linoleic acid)	Soybean oil (7% alpha-linolenic acid)
Soybean oil (54% linoleic acid)	

Note: The following fats and oils are poor sources of omega-6 and omega-3 fatty acids: lard, mutton fat, coconut oil, and olive oil.
EPA, Eicosapentaenoic acid (20:5n-3).

Algae synthesize large amounts of omega-3 fatty acids. As a result, most marine animal tissues contain high concentrations of the omega-3 PUFAs. Sources of omega-3 fatty acids in pet foods include cold-water fish oils as well as whole-fat flax (flax oil is an enriched source of ALA). Land animals, in contrast, have higher concentrations of the omega-6 fatty acids in their tissues because most plants consumed by these animals contain greater amounts of omega-6 than omega-3 fatty acids.[39] Enriched sources of omega-6 fatty acids in pet foods include corn, safflower, sunflower, and cottonseed oils. Soy and canola oils contain high levels of omega-6 fatty acids, as well as some ALA. Another omega-6 fatty acid, gamma-linolenic acid (18:3n-6) (GLA), is found in borage, black currant, and evening primrose oil.[40] Oils containing a large proportion of monounsaturated fatty acids, such as olive oil, and saturated animal fats are not considered enriched in either omega-3 or omega-6 fatty acids (Table 31-2).

Fatty Acids as Eicosanoid Precursors

In addition to providing structural integrity and fluidity to cell membranes, membrane fatty acids also have specific roles in the regulation of cell functions. The PUFAs AA, GLA, EPA, and DHA are all precursors for the synthesis of eicosanoids. Eicosanoids are immunoregulatory molecules that have local and short-lived

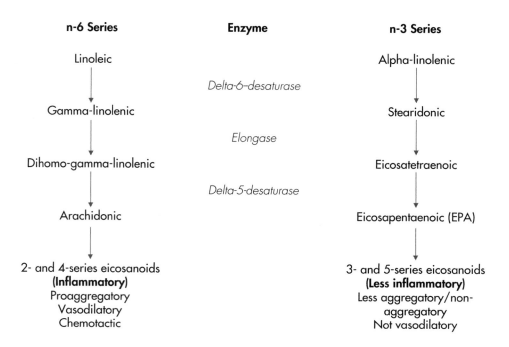

n-6 Series	**Enzyme**	**n-3 Series**

Linoleic

Delta-6–desaturase

Alpha-linolenic

Gamma-linolenic

Stearidonic

Elongase

Dihomo-gamma-linolenic

Eicosatetraenoic

Delta-5-desaturase

Arachidonic

Eicosapentaenoic (EPA)

2- and 4-series eicosanoids
(Inflammatory)
Proaggregatory
Vasodilatory
Chemotactic

3- and 5-series eicosanoids
(Less inflammatory)
Less aggregatory/non-
aggregatory
Not vasodilatory

Figure 31-3   Metabolism of omega-3 and omega-6 series fatty acids.

hormonelike effects. The four primary types of eicosanoids are prostaglandins, leukotrienes, prostacyclins, and thromboxanes. Eicosanoids are involved in inflammatory reactions, immunoregulation, and epidermal cell proliferation. When cellular injury occurs, membranes release their component fatty acids, which are then metabolized to eicosanoids. The amount and type of eicosanoid synthesized is determined by the availability and type of fatty acid precursor from the cell membrane and by the activities of the two metabolic enzyme systems, cyclooxygenase and lipoxygenase. The omega-3 and omega-6 fatty acids produce different families of eicosanoids and also compete for these two metabolic pathways.[41]

During an inflammatory response, the release and metabolism of omega-6 fatty acids produces the 2-series prostaglandins, the 4-series leukotrienes, hydroxyeicosatetraenoic acid, and thromboxane A_2 (Figure 31-3). These agents are immunosuppressive at high levels, are proinflammatory, promote platelet aggregation, and act as potent mediators of inflammation in type-I hypersensitivity reactions.[42,43] In contrast, the release and metabolism of omega-3 fatty acids (specifically, EPA) produces

mediators with much less inflammatory activity. Those compounds are antiaggregatory, not immunosuppressive at levels normally found in the body, and vasodilatory. They include the 3-series prostaglandins, the 5-series leukotrienes, hydroxyeicosapentaenoic acid, and thromboxane A_3. For example leukotriene B_5 (LTB_5), produced from EPA, is approximately 10-fold less potent as a neutrophil chemoattractant than leukotriene B_4 (LTB_4), which is produced from AA.[44] In addition to being less biologically active than LTB_4, there is evidence that LTB_5 may inhibit the action of LTB_4, possibly via competition for cell membrane receptors.[45,46] These data suggest that the ratio of leukotrienes produced from AA to leukotrienes produced from EPA may be more important than absolute amounts of these compounds.

Influence of Dietary Omega-6 and Omega-3 Fatty Acids on Eicosanoid Production

Research studies with humans, laboratory animals, and companion animals have shown that levels of omega-6 and omega-3 fatty acids present in tissue cell membranes can be manipulated by diet, and that these manipulations influence the inflammatory response. Increasing the amount of omega-3 fatty acids in skin and other tissues leads to decreased production and activity of the proinflammatory eicosanoids and increased synthesis of the less-inflammatory metabolites.[47] Several factors are responsible for this effect. First, as discussed previously, omega-6 and omega-3 fatty acids compete directly for the same enzyme systems. Therefore increasing the amount of available omega-3 fatty acids competitively inhibits the metabolism of omega-6 fatty acids when fatty acids are released from membranes during an inflammatory reaction. Second, the compounds produced from the metabolism of omega-3 fatty acids are less inflammatory than those produced from AA.[48] Finally, two of the end products of EPA metabolism are LTB$_5$ and 15-hydroxyeicosapentaenoic acid. There is evidence that these compounds inhibit the potent proinflammatory action of omega-6–derived leukotrienes.

The amount and type of omega-3 and omega-6 fatty acids and the ratio of these two classes of fatty acids in the diet must be considered when determining effects on plasma and tissue levels and consequent eicosanoid synthesis.[49-51] For example, an early study with healthy dogs showed that feeding a diet containing an omega-6 to omega-3 ratio between 5:1 and 10:1 resulted in the production of significantly lower levels of LTB$_4$ and significantly higher levels of the less inflammatory metabolite LTB$_5$ in the skin, when compared with levels that were produced when the dogs were fed a diet with ratios of 28:1 or higher.[52] Similarly, the neutrophils of dogs fed diets containing the lowest omega-6 to omega-3 ratios (5:1 and 10:1) had decreased LTB$_4$ and increased LTB$_5$ concentrations (Figure 31-4). Cells from lipopolysaccharide-stimulated (LPS) skin biopsy samples synthesized 48% to 62% less LTB$_4$ and 48% to 79% more LTB$_5$ when compared with samples obtained prior to feeding the experimental diets. Similar changes were observed in neutrophils. These responses were considered to be clinically significant because decreases in tissue LTB$_4$ concentrations of 50% or more are typically large enough to attenuate an inflammatory response.

Additional research corroborated these results and further refined understanding of the specific types and amounts of omega-3 fatty acids that can modulate the inflammatory response. Healthy elderly Beagles fed diets that were supplemented with fish oil to achieve

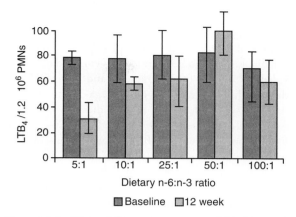

Figure 31-4 Effect of dietary omega-6 to omega-3 fatty acid ratio on leukotriene B$_4$ (*LTB$_4$*) synthesis. *PMNs,* Polymorphonuclear leukocytes.

(From Reinhart GA, Davenport GM: Omega-3 fatty acids and inflammation management. In *Proceedings of fourth world congress of veterinary dermatology,* 2000, p 32.)

an omega-6 to omega-3 fatty acid ratio of 1.4:1 had altered plasma fatty acids (increased DHA and EPA and decreased AA) and had reduced prostaglandin E$_2$ (PGE$_2$) production by peripheral blood mononuclear cells.[53] Fish oil–supplemented dogs also showed a reduction in response to a delayed-type hypersensitivity (DTH) skin test and a blunted response to immunization with a novel protein.[54] A follow-up study was conducted to examine the relationship between plasma fatty acid concentrations and leukotriene production by peripheral blood neutrophils in dogs fed these diets for 36 weeks.[55] Plasma concentrations of EPA and AA reflected dietary intake, and a strong and significant correlation was found between the plasma ratio of EPA:AA and the ratio of LTB$_5$ to LTB$_4$ produced by stimulated neutrophils. Specifically, plasma EPA increased, plasma AA decreased, and LTB$_5$ produced by stimulated neutrophils increased in dogs fed fish oil–supplemented diets. The same researchers demonstrated an interaction between dietary vitamin E intake and intake of omega-3 fatty acids, suggesting that the benefits of vitamin E on DTH response are reduced when the intake of omega-3 fatty acids is very high.[56] Together, these studies suggest that there is an optimal level of omega-3 fatty acid intake and an omega-6 to omega-3 ratio that can modify the production of proinflammatory compounds but that is not high enough to negatively impact other immune system functions or vitamin E status.

In a study, a group of 15 healthy adult dogs were fed a base diet supplemented with either sunflower oil (source of LA), fish oil (source of EPA and DHA), or fish oil plus vitamin E.[57] The fish oil–enriched diets provided 1.75 grams (g) EPA/kg diet and 2.2-g DHA/kg diet, resulting in an omega-6 to omega-3 ratio of 3.4:1. After 12 weeks of feeding the test diets, in vivo measurement of the serum of dogs fed fish oil–enriched foods showed a blunted inflammatory response to LPS when compared with the response observed in dogs fed the sunflower oil–enriched diet. These results are especially significant because this was the first report that used an in vivo assay to examine LPS-stimulated cytokine response after feeding omega-3 fatty acid enriched diets. Additional studies of the same dogs showed that increasing omega-3 fatty acids in the diet did not significantly increase plasma concentrations of lipid peroxides or cause a reduction in serum vitamin E concentrations.[58] These results indicate that the dogs did not experience increased oxidative stress in response to the altered fatty acid ratios and increased intake of EPA and DHA.

Although changing the ratio of omega-6 to omega-3 fatty acids is an effective approach to modifying the production of proinflammatory and less inflammatory compounds, there is also evidence that when an equal ratio is fed and kept constant, increasing the omega-3 dose alone influences the plasma fatty acid profile.[59] Healthy dogs were fed diets containing an omega-6 to omega-3 ratio of 1:1, with varying concentrations of each class of fatty acid, supplied by corn oil and fish oil, respectively. Plasma concentrations of omega-3 fatty acids increased with increasing total intake of omega-3 fatty acids, up to a certain level of intake, regardless of the fact that omega-6 fatty acids were also increasing. These results suggest a dose-dependent response to omega-3 intake that was independent of the ratio of the two classes of fatty acids. However, it is important to note that the diets that were fed in this study already contained an "adjusted" fatty acid ratio (1:1). It is unknown (and questionable) whether a similar response would have occurred if the ratio was more similar to that seen in many commercial foods (i.e., 15:1 or greater). Second, the omega-3 fatty acids in this study were supplied as EPA and DHA (fish oil), while the omega-6 fatty acid was supplied as primarily LA (corn oil). Therefore the dose response may reflect

a selective favoring of highly unsaturated fatty acids for esterification into phospholipids when compared with their precursors. It is not known if these effects would have been observed if increased omega-6 fatty acids had been supplied as AA instead of as LA. Regardless, these results suggest that when a favorable ratio is included in the diet, increasing the source of EPA and DHA while maintaining a constant omega-6 to omega-3 ratio positively affects plasma fatty acid profiles and, presumably (although not yet reported), the production of less inflammatory eicosanoids.

Research studies show that levels of omega-6 and omega-3 fatty acids in pets' diets influence tissue levels of these fatty acids and these modifications influence the inflammatory response. Increasing the amount of omega-3 fatty acids in skin and other tissues leads to decreased production and activity of the proinflammatory eicosanoids and increased synthesis of the less inflammatory metabolites.

Dietary Fatty Acids and Atopic Dermatitis

Dogs and cats are susceptible to a wide range of inflammatory skin diseases. In dogs, these include allergic disorders, parasitic infestations, bacterial infections, and adverse reactions to food. Cats show the same disorders with the addition of miliary dermatitis and eosinophilic granuloma complex. Inflammatory skin disorders that are associated with immunoglobulin E (IgE)-mediated type-1 hypersensitivity (allergic) responses are most likely to respond favorably to modifications of dietary fatty acid concentrations. In dogs, these include atopic dermatitis (atopy), flea-bite hypersensitivity, and food hypersensitivity (discussed below). In cats, allergic skin disease also manifests as miliary dermatitis.[60] Because flea-bite hypersensitivity is best treated via stringent flea-control programs, current research studies have focused on the use of fatty acid therapy to control atopic disease in dogs and cats.

In dogs, atopic dermatitis is considered to be the most frequently diagnosed form of allergic skin disease.[61] Many animals with atopy are sensitized to multiple environmental allergens, which may include house dust mites or dust, molds, weeds, grasses, and trees. In addition, a substantial proportion of dogs with atopic dermatitis are simultaneously affected by an adverse food reaction.[62] Recent studies suggest that dogs with atopic disease have almost four times greater risk of developing concurrent food allergy than dogs without atopy. For these reasons, differential diagnosis of allergic skin disorders must always include consideration of the presence of both atopy and adverse food reaction and the role that multiple allergens and the pruritic threshold plays in the development of clinical signs.

Atopy is characterized by pruritus, self-trauma to the skin, and secondary bacterial or yeast infection.[63,64] Chronic otitis externa is also a common finding. Diagnosis of atopic dermatitis in dogs typically uses the criteria of Willemse, which includes case history information and clinical signs.[65] Observations of breed and family predilections, along with results of limited breeding trials, indicate that some dogs are genetically predisposed to develop atopy.[66] Breeds identified as being at increased risk include Chinese Shar-Peis, Dalmatians, Irish Setters, Golden Retrievers, Boxers, Labrador Retrievers, Belgian Tervurens, and several Terrier and toy breeds. Cats with atopic disease often develop miliary dermatitis, which is characterized by small papules and crusts found most frequently on the head and neck.

Clinical signs develop when the animal is exposed to the offending antigen(s) and IgE-sensitized mast cells in the skin degranulate and release a host of inflammatory mediators. These compounds include histamine, heparin, proteolytic enzymes, chemotactic factors, and various types of eicosanoids. As discussed previously, the type and proportions of fatty acids present in the cell membranes and activity of the cyclooxygenase and lipoxygenase enzyme systems determine the specific type of eicosanoids that will be produced during an inflammatory response. In pets with atopy, the immediate-type hypersensitivity response (IgE-mediated) is followed by a late-phase response that develops 6 to 12 hours following mast cell activation.[67] In addition, some of the released cytokines function to recruit inflammatory cells to the local area, which can persist for several days and are responsible for the chronic inflammatory skin changes seen in atopic animals.

Although IgE-mediated immediate-type and delayed (late-phase) hypersensitivities are responsible for the cascade of inflammatory agents after exposure to offending allergens in most patients, it appears that other factors are also involved.[68] The most important of these is epidermal barrier function. Human subjects with atopic dermatitis have irregularities in the lipid and ceramide components of their stratus corneum (the uppermost protecting layer of the epidermis).[69] A defect in this layer can affect the skin's function as a protective barrier, leading to increased transepidermal water loss and increased risk of penetration by allergens and infectious agents. Although these changes have not been definitely demonstrated in dogs, there is evidence that the stratum corneum of atopic dogs has structural differences when compared with normal canine skin and that these differences may involve the lipid-containing ceramides.[70] It is theorized that a stratum corneum with an impaired lipid barrier predisposes an animal to the development of hypersensitive response to contact allergens because foreign agents are able to penetrate further into the skin. Another potentially influencing factor is the presence of a defect in fatty acid metabolism. There is evidence that dogs with atopy may have compromised ability to metabolize omega-6 fatty acids due to reduced activity of delta-5 and/or delta-6 desaturase enzymes.[71,72]

Increased understanding of the role of an optimally functioning skin barrier has implications for both the prevention and treatment of atopic disease. While it was previously believed that inhalant allergens were the most common cause of atopy, new evidence suggests that contact allergens are most important. Avoidance of known allergens and frequent bathing to reduce time of exposure and penetration into the skin are now routinely recommended for pets with atopic disease.[73] Because secondary staphylococcal infections may be responsible for many of the clinical signs of atopy, antimicrobial treatment is also an important component of management. Glucocorticoid or cyclosporine therapies are typically prescribed to control inflammation. Fatty acid therapy that helps to restore defects in the intercellular ceramides of the stratum corneum may also be helpful and may allow reduction or discontinuation of the use of these antiinflammatory medications. In recent years, fatty acid therapy for atopic disease has focused both on modulating the inflammatory response by altering the types of eicosanoids produced by the mast cells and other skin cells involved in the inflammatory response (keratinocytes and cutaneous antigen-presenting cells), and providing nutrients that support a healthier skin barrier.[74]

Fatty Acid Supplementation

Supplements that are enriched with omega-3 fatty acids are frequently recommended in the management of inflammatory skin disease in dogs and cats. Omega-3 fatty acids included in these supplements are the PUFAs, EPA (20:5n-3), and DHA (22:6n-3), which are found in certain types of fish oil. ALA (18:3n-3), found in flax, has also been used. However, the limited ability of adult animals to convert ALA to long-chain PUFAs for incorporation into cell membranes suggests that this omega-3 fatty acid has less value as a supplement for affecting the production of inflammatory mediators. In addition to omega-3 fatty acids, the omega-6 fatty acid LA is needed for normal epidermal lipid barrier function. Therefore supplementation with LA may result in reduced transepidermal water loss.[33]

A second, less common omega-6 fatty acid that has been studied for its antiinflammatory effects is GLA. Once consumed, GLA is readily converted to dihomo-gamma-linolenic acid in the liver, where it is then further metabolized to either the monoenoic prostaglandins and thromboxanes or to AA (Figure 31-5). The more active pathway is toward the production of the monoenoic prostaglandins (PGE_1) because the rate-limiting delta-5-desaturase step for AA production is quite slow in animals.[41] Like the eicosanoids that are produced from EPA, PGE_1 is less inflammatory than the dienoic prostaglandins that are produced from AA. Therefore it is expected that providing supplemental GLA will promote the formation of dihomo-gamma-linolenic acid and the monoenoic prostaglandins, rather than the formation of AA and its more inflammatory metabolites.

When dogs' diets are supplemented with GLA, plasma levels of dihomo-gamma-linolenic acid increase.[75] Similarly, when dogs with atopy that had been controlled by feeding a supplement containing omega-3 fatty acids and GLA were switched to a supplement containing only olive oil (a poor source of both omega-3 and omega-6 fatty acids), plasma levels of dihomo-gamma-linolenic acid subsequently decreased.[76] A return of clinical signs in these dogs paralleled the reduction in dihomo-gamma-linolenic acid. As stated previously, it has been theorized that one factor that may contribute to atopic disease in some dogs is low activity of the enzyme delta-6-desaturase, the rate-limiting step for conversion of LA to GLA.[77] Providing GLA to this subpopulation of dogs would be expected to bypass this step of fatty acid metabolism and provide substrate for the production of the monoenoic prostaglandins. However, not all studies have shown a benefit of providing GLA to pruritic dogs. A study comparing pruritic and healthy dogs found that the unmedicated dogs with signs of atopy naturally had higher concentrations of dihomo-gamma-linolenic acid in subcutaneous fat when compared with levels in the dogs with healthy skin.[78] These results suggest that some dogs with atopy may have an abnormality in dihomo-gamma-linolenic metabolism caused by a deficiency in delta-5-desaturase. Together these studies suggest that there may be several underlying causes and influencing factors that contribute to atopy in dogs. While some atopic animals show abnormal fat absorption and clearance, others may have deficiencies of delta-6- and/or delta-5-desaturase activities, and/or, as examined more recently, impairments that affect the epidermal barrier.

Using supplementation of pets' regular diets with omega-3 and omega-6 fatty acids to manage the pruritus and inflammatory responses associated with atopy has met with variable success. A review of five separate clinical tests of a commercial supplement (DVM Derm Caps) shows that fatty acid supplementation was effective in controlling pruritus in 11% to 27% of dogs with inflammatory skin disease.[79-83] This supplement contains EPA, DHA, LA, and GLA. In one study, 93 dogs with a diagnosis of atopic dermatitis were supplemented at a dose that provided 15 mg EPA per 9 kg

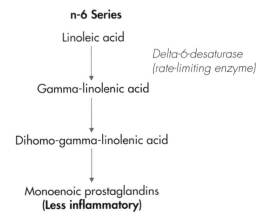

n-6 Series

Linoleic acid

Delta-6-desaturase (rate-limiting enzyme)

Gamma-linolenic acid

Dihomo-gamma-linolenic acid

Monoenoic prostaglandins
(Less inflammatory)

Figure 31-5   Production of gamma-linolenic acid metabolites.

(20 pounds [lb]) of BW.[79] One third of the dogs showed a good or excellent response to the supplement, and 17 dogs (18%) required no additional therapy. A second study using the same supplement reported that 11% of dogs with atopy, food allergy, or flea-bite allergy were adequately controlled by the supplement alone with no other treatment necessary.[80] Because these studies did not control dogs' regular diets, variability of the background fatty acid intake among dogs fed different commercial foods may have significantly influenced response rate. A more recent study fed 22 atopic dogs the same balanced homemade food and administered a daily supplement containing 17 mg/kg BW EPA, 5 mg/kg BW DHA, and 35 mg/kg BW GLA.[84] Supplementation resulted in an overall omega-6 to omega-3 ratio of 5.5:1. The dogs in this study were also divided into two groups: early stage (preimmunotherapy) and late-stage (nonresponsive to immunotherapy). More than half (53%) of the early-stage dogs responded positively to fatty acid supplementation, compared with only one dog from the group of seven dogs that had chronic and refractory atopy. Interestingly, plasma fatty acid profiles also differed between the two categories of atopic dogs, even though they were fed the same diets and supplements. This difference supports the theory that subpopulations of atopic dogs exist, whose disease is influenced by different factors, which in turn could affect clinical response to supplementation.

There is also evidence that supplementation with a combination of evening primrose oil (a source of GLA) and fish oil (a source of EPA and DHA) is effective in the control of inflammatory skin disease in some cats.[85] When the diets of 14 cats that had a diagnosis of miliary dermatosis were supplemented with various combinations of evening primrose oil and fish oil, improvements in clinical signs were observed in 11 of 14 cats fed a combination of 80% evening primrose oil and 20% fish oil.[86] Supplementation with fish oil alone was not effective. A second study with cats found that 40% of cats with nonlesional pruritus and 67% of cats with eosinophilic granuloma complex responded favorably to dietary supplementation with a product that contained EPA, GLA, DHA, safflower oil, natural glycerin, and vitamin E.[87] It has been speculated that cats may differ from dogs in their response to omega-3 fatty acids because cats have been shown to lack omega-3 fatty acid activity in the skin and because they have a lower

activity of the enzyme delta-6-desaturase (see Section 2, pp. 81-83).

While a small number of allergic pets have been shown to require no additional therapy when provided with a dietary fatty acid supplement, most that respond still require concurrent treatment with antihistamines, corticosteroids, or cyclosporine to control pruritus.[88,89] However, there is some evidence that fatty acid supplementation can have an additive or synergistic effect when used in combination with systemic antiinflammatory medications, particularly corticosteroids.[90] A well-controlled double-blind study of 60 dogs with atopy found that that after 2 months of supplementation, dogs fed a fatty acid product containing borage seed oil and fish oil required lower dosages of prednisolone to control signs of pruritus when compared with dogs supplemented with a placebo.[91] After the initial lag period, this benefit continued and became more pronounced until the end of the study period at 84 days.

Finally, a substantial proportion of dogs and cats with atopic disease show no response at all to fatty acid supplementation. There are several possible reasons for the variable responses that have been observed. First, there are a number of different agents that mediate inflammation and pruritus in dogs and cats with allergic dermatitis. Recent studies support the theory that atopy is not a single disease, but rather a syndrome that may have multiple contributing factors and causes, leading to several population subsets of atopic animals. Therefore the manipulation of fatty acids would not be expected to work in all individuals. A second factor may involve the manner in which fatty acid therapy is administered and the length of time of the test period. As mentioned previously, supplementing a companion animal's diet with a fatty acid–containing capsule does not account for the levels or proportions of fatty acids present in the regular diet. The exact quantities and ratio of fatty acids in the regular diet are often unknown. If the regular diet contains very high levels of omega-6 fatty acids, providing an omega-3 fatty acid supplement may not effectively change the proportion of these types of fatty acids present in the tissues. There also appears to be a time lag for response that may be as long as 8 to 12 weeks in some animals.[91] A final factor, and one that may be true for diet modification as well, is that other skin factors such as bacterial or yeast infections, the degree of erythema and presence of skin lesions, and presence of otitis externa may all be important contributors to clinical signs; their presence or absence may significantly influence an individual animal's degree of response to fatty acid supplementation.[92]

Dietary supplements that are enriched with omega-3 fatty acids and certain omega-6 fatty acids (gamma-linolenic acid and possibly linoleic acid) may be helpful in controlling pruritus and other signs of atopy in some dogs and cats. Although a complete amelioration of signs is not usually seen, fatty acid supplementation may complement other therapies and allow reduced dosages of antiinflammatory medications. Still, because the effects of supplementation depend upon the fatty acid levels in the pet's normal diet and because many factors appear to affect the development of atopy, not all animals respond to fatty acid supplementation.

Diet Modification

When modifying dietary fatty acid levels to manage inflammatory disease, the goal is to supply optimal amounts of LA to meet a dog's essential dietary requirement and at the same time produce a potentially less inflammatory fatty acid metabolic profile. Using a dietary approach in which the quantity and the ratio of omega-6 and omega-3 fatty acids are controlled may be an effective means of altering tissue eicosanoid profiles and reducing pruritus in some allergic pets. For example, results of an experiment with healthy adult dogs showed that feeding a food that contained an omega-6 to omega-3 ratio between 5:1 and 10:1 led to changes in skin leukotriene concentrations that are considered to be clinically significant.[52] Omega-3 fatty acid–enriched diets have also been shown to modify the biochemical components of the inflammatory stage of wound healing in the skin of dogs.[93] Specifically the concentration of antiinflammatory fatty acids and eicosanoids in 4-day-old skin wounds increased, and the concentration of proinflammatory fatty acids and eicosanoids decreased as the proportion of omega-3 fatty acids in the diet increased. The omega-3 fatty acid concentrations that were fed in these studies did not negatively impact platelet reactivity, coagulation assays, fibrinogen concentration, or antithrombin III activity.[94]

Clinical studies have examined the effectiveness of varying the dietary omega-6 to omega-3 fatty acid ratio in managing inflammatory skin disease. In one study, 31 pruritic dogs were fed a veterinary-exclusive commercial food containing an adjusted fatty acid ratio of 5:1 for a period of 8 weeks.[95] All of the dogs had been diagnosed with atopy, adverse reactions to food, or a combination of these two conditions. Twenty-eight dogs completed the trial, and 14 dogs (45%) showed a good-to-excellent response to the therapeutic food. Another feeding trial was conducted with 18 non–food-allergic, atopic dogs fed a lamb-and-rice diet containing an omega-6 to omega-3 fatty acid ratio of 5.3:1.[96] The dogs' clinical responses were evaluated by both a veterinarian and the owner. In this study, 44% of the dogs (8 of 18) had a good or excellent response to the test diet within 7 to 21 days of feeding. Upon refeeding the original diet, all showed a return of clinical signs. Pruritus was again alleviated by reintroduction of the test diet in all eight dogs. An important result of this study was the positive response in dogs that had previously been unresponsive to a dietary fatty acid supplement containing omega-3 and omega-6 fatty acids. Of 11 dogs that had been previously treated unsuccessfully with the supplement, 7 (65%) had a good or excellent response to the test diet.

A double-blind study compared three commercial dog foods that were formulated specifically to control signs of inflammatory skin disease in dogs.[97] A group of 50 dogs with atopic dermatitis were randomly assigned one of the three therapeutic foods or to the control diet, a commercial adult maintenance food. Dogs were fed their assigned food for 12 weeks. After 8 weeks of feeding, dogs fed two of the three therapeutic foods showed a significant reduction in pruritus. Dogs fed the control food also showed some improvement in overall severity of atopy. One of the therapeutic foods also significantly improved coat luster. This food contained the highest levels of LA and ALA, which corroborates other evidence that LA contributes positively to coat shine and luster.[33] All three of the therapeutic foods used in this study had omega-6 to omega-3 fatty acid ratios of between 3:1 and 5:1, while the control food had a ratio of 14:1. Although other dietary factors also changed from the dogs' regular diets (i.e., protein source, digestibility), these data support the use of modified fatty acid profiles to manage atopy in dogs. The authors of this study also noted that the production of less inflammatory leukotrienes may not have been the only (or most crucial) mechanism of action of the omega-3 fatty acids included in these foods. There is recent evidence that increasing a diet's PUFAs may also exert an effect by improving the skin's epidermal barrier, and may positively affect the immune system by regulating signal transduction or transcription.[98,99] Therefore some of the response that was seen may have been due to increasing the total amount of PUFA in the food, as opposed to an effect of omega-3 fatty acids alone.

Recommended Doses and Ratios

Several studies have shown that allergic pruritus is not effectively controlled in most dogs using the recommended doses of omega-3 fatty acid supplements.[100] Other studies have reported that 2 to 10 times the recommended dose may be necessary to achieve clinical results in pruritic dogs.[76,77] High doses of supplements increase the risk of causing an imbalanced fatty acid ratio in the diet and can become cost-prohibitive for some clients. Fatty acid supplements have also been associated with undesirable side effects such as lethargy, vomiting, diarrhea, and urticaria in some dogs and cats.[87,100] An added risk with use of omega-3 fatty acids is oversupplementation, which may lead to decreased platelet aggregation and increased blood clotting time.[101]

Documentation of appropriate doses of supplements and ratios of fatty acids to include in pet foods is lacking and an exact effective dose range has not been identified. Experimental data show that changes in skin concentrations of fatty acids are maximized after 3 to 12 weeks of supplementation or feeding a new diet and reflect dietary concentrations.[6] However, great variability is seen with the type and ratio of fatty acids that are used. One problem is that there are currently no canine or feline recommended daily allowances for omega-3 fatty acids. The Association of American Feed Control Officials' (AAFCO's) LA minimum requirement is 1% dry matter (DM) for dogs and 0.5% for cats. In many commercial pet foods, omega-6 fatty acids contribute more than 4% of the food's energy. It is therefore possible that excessive levels of omega-6 fatty acids may obfuscate an effective

dose of omega-3 fatty acids, even when high levels are supplemented.

A review of several therapeutic foods commonly recommended for pets with skin or gastrointestinal inflammation found that the omega-3 fatty acid concentration typically provided between 0.6% and 2% of the daily energy intake, with one food containing as high as 4%.[40] It was suggested that a daily dietary omega-3 intake of between 2% and 4% of energy effectively increases membrane and plasma omega-3 concentrations. Likewise, a reasonable starting dose for a fatty acid supplement is one that supplies 175 mg of total omega-3 fatty acids per kg of BW per day (EPA +DHA). This recommended dose is substantially higher than those recommended on the labels of most commercial fatty acid supplements.

As discussed previously, the ratio of dietary omega-6 to omega-3 fatty acids may be as important as the total amount of omega-3 fatty acids. The easiest and most effective way to modulate this ratio is by incorporating it directly into the pet's normal diet. Based on current studies, a ratio between 5:1 and 10:1 seems to be the most effective in altering tissue lipid and eicosanoid concentrations and modifying the inflammatory response. However, evidence suggests that reducing the ratio to as low as 3:1 may be even more effective.[97] The omega-6 fatty acid content should meet the EFA requirements of dogs and cats, but it should not exceed 4% of the metabolizable energy (ME) calories. Several additional benefits of a total dietary approach include improved client compliance, achievement of a specifically targeted omega-6 to omega-3 ratio, and safety (no danger of oversupplementation).

Another approach to managing atopic disease in dogs and cats is a dietary approach in which both the quantity and the ratio of omega-6 and omega-3 fatty acids are controlled. Studies show that increasing polyunsaturated fatty acids (PUFAs) and providing omega-6 to omega-3 fatty acid ratios between 3:1 and 10:1 are most effective. Increasing omega-3 fatty acids and overall long-chain PUFAs in the food may effectively decrease the production of proinflammatory agents, improve epidermal barrier function, and positively influence the immune response.

TABLE 31-3　CAUSES OF ADVERSE FOOD REACTIONS IN DOGS AND CATS

CLASSIFICATION	MECHANISM
Food hypersensitivity	Immune-mediated adverse reaction to a food component
Food intolerance	Nonimmunological adverse rea ction of a metabolic, idiosyncratic, toxic, or pharmacological nature to a food component
Metabolic adverse reaction	Abnormal metabolic response to a food component, usually due to an inborn error of metabolism
Food idiosyncrasy	Abnormal response to a food substance; resembles a hypersensitivity response but does not have an immunological basis
Food toxicity (poisoning)	Adverse reaction to a contaminating organism or toxin present in a food
Pharmacological reaction	Due to pharmacological or druglike effect of a food component (e.g., histamine in poorly preserved fish)

CUTANEOUS ADVERSE FOOD REACTIONS

Dogs and cats can have adverse reactions to dietary ingredients for a number of reasons (Table 31-3). Those that manifest as inflammatory dermatologic disease are collectively termed *cutaneous adverse food reactions*.[102] These include both immune-mediated and non–immune-mediated reactions. Dietary (or food) hypersensitivity is an immune-mediated response to one or more components in the diet. The majority of food hypersensitivities are an IgE-mediated type-1 hypersensitivity, involving mast cell degranulation (see p. 397). A *food intolerance* refers to an abnormal physiologic response to a food ingredient that is not immune-mediated. Food intolerances include problems such as a lack of the intestinal enzyme lactase, food toxicities, and pharmacological reactions to dietary ingredients. Because a clinical distinction is rarely made between adverse food reactions that are immune mediated and those that are not, and because the exact proportion of each type of dermatological reaction in the pet population is not known, the more inclusive term of "adverse food reaction" is currently recommended instead of the traditional terms *food allergy* or *food hypersensitivity*.[103]

Description and Incidence

It is estimated that adverse food reactions account for between 1% and 5% of all dermatoses, and between 10% and 15% of inflammatory dermatoses that are diagnosed in dogs and cats.[104,105] A recent study using data from a referral veterinary practice reported that adverse food reactions were responsible for 20% to 35% of nonseasonal dermatitis cases in dogs.[106] There is evidence that dogs with adverse food reactions have an increased likelihood of developing atopic dermatitis.[103] The coexistence of these two disorders may explain some of the positive responses to dietary intervention with atopic dogs (see pp. 390-391).

Adverse reactions to food can develop at any age. Unlike atopic disease and flea-bite dermatitis, which often take several years to develop, signs of an adverse food reaction often first occur in pets that are less than 1 year old. In two reports, 19% and 33% of dogs developed initial clinical signs when they were less than 1 year old.[107,108] Another study of 25 dogs diagnosed with food allergy found that more than 50% were less than 1 year old at the onset of clinical signs.[109] These data suggest that adverse reactions to food should always be considered when an immature pet exhibits a nonseasonal and persistent dermatitis.

The onset of adverse food reactions can be seen at any time of the year and are not typically associated with a recent dietary change. In one study, 68% of the dogs had been fed the offending pet food for 2 years or more before clinical signs developed.[110] No significant sex or age predilections have been observed. Although the presence of a genetic component has not been proven, one study did find that among purebred dogs, German Shepherd Dogs and Golden Retrievers appeared to be overrepresented when compared with a general veterinary hospital population.[109] This difference was not significant but suggests the possibility of a genetic predilection in these breeds. Other breeds that may be at increased risk include the Soft-Coated Wheaton Terrier, Dalmatian, West Highland White Terrier, Collie, Chinese Shar-Pei, Lhasa Apso, Cocker Spaniel, English Springer Spaniel, Miniature Schnauzer, and Labrador Retriever.[111]

Dogs and cats can have adverse reactions to dietary ingredients that include both immune-mediated and non–immune-mediated reactions. Adverse food reactions are nonseasonal, show no sex or age predilection, and do not have a clear genetic cause (although certain dog breeds may have increased susceptibility). A pet may also develop an adverse food reaction to a food that has been fed regularly for months or years. In most cases, adverse food reactions manifest as dermatological problems, with the most common sign an intense pruritus.

Etiology

In cases of immune-mediated adverse food reaction, the underlying immunological mechanisms are only partly understood. The disorder is currently considered to be the result of type-I and/or type-III immediate hypersensitivity responses. A type-I response is responsible for the severe pruritus that is seen after ingesting the offending dietary antigen. A type-III response, on the other hand, is thought to be responsible for the acute intestinal signs (diarrhea) that are seen in a small number of animals.[112] Delayed (type-IV) hypersensitivities, which occur several hours to days after ingesting the offending antigen, may also be involved.

Food antigens are generally proteins, glycoproteins, or lipoproteins. Although all food proteins are potentially antigenic (i.e., foreign to the body), the capacity of a given protein to induce an allergic reaction is influenced by the permeability of the intestinal mucosa to the protein and the protein's capacity to stimulate IgE production and eventually histamine release from mast cells.[113] Mast cell degranulation requires cross-linking between the allergen and two or more IgE molecules that are bound to IgE receptors present on sensitized mast cell membranes. This condition places a minimum size limit on molecules that are capable of causing an IgE-mediated reaction. The majority of allergens that have been identified in dogs and cats are proteins of large molecular weight, between 40 and 70 kilodaltons (kD).[114] However, it is possible that smaller protein molecules may act as haptens, allowing a much smaller protein molecule to be allergenic. Protein molecules that are larger than 70 kD are less likely to be absorbed

intact across the intestinal mucosa and so are unlikely to become food allergens. In dogs and cats, beef, soy, and dairy products are the most common food allergens.[115] Other dietary ingredients to which dogs and cats develop adverse reactions include wheat, pork, chicken, corn, horse meat, egg, and fish. It appears that these ingredients are common allergens because they are often used in pet foods, thus increasing the likelihood of exposure, as opposed to any characteristics that confer unique antigenicity.[116]

There is some evidence that the processing procedures used to produce commercial pet foods may influence the antigenicity of certain dietary components.[117] This provides one explanation for the observation that some allergic pets tolerate homemade diets but develop an allergic response to commercial foods that contain the same ingredients.[108] Heat treatment causes a change in the 3-dimensional structure of proteins, which can destroy some epitopes (antigenic determinants) or simultaneously expose others.[118] In addition, heat-processing can cause Maillard reactions. Some of the byproducts of the Maillard reaction (melanoidins) may be more allergenic than the uncooked version of the contributing protein.[119] In a study, healthy adult cats were fed two protein sources (soy and casein) that were either unprocessed and in an aqueous suspension or heat-processed into a canned ration.[120] After 21 days of feeding, both forms of dietary protein stimulated an increase in serum IgG but the degree of response was affected by protein source. Cooked soy protein produced a lower IgG response than did unprocessed soy, suggesting that, in the case of soy protein, cooking caused a reduction in the protein's antigenicity. Conversely, the serum IgG response to casein was not affected by processing. However, cooked casein (but not soy) caused a significant increase in salivary IgG levels. The authors interpreted this to suggest that cooking increased the immunogenicity of this protein source, although no adverse reactions were observed in any of the cats during the study.

Animals may react to a single or multiple ingredients or nutrients in food, although there are conflicting reports regarding the frequency at which multiple sensitivities are observed in dogs and cats. While some researchers have reported finding many instances of multiple hypersensitivities, others report that these are rare.[110,121] A study of 25 dogs with signs consistent with food hypersensitivity reported that the mean number of allergens per dog was 2.4, and 64% of the dogs reacted adversely to two or more dietary ingredients when challenged.[15] In addition, a study found that dogs with diagnosed adverse food reactions had circulating IgE antibodies against bovine IgG, a protein found in cow's milk. These IgE molecules cross-reacted to beef and lamb proteins, suggesting that cross-reactivity may be the mechanism underlying some multiple hypersensitivities.[114] Regardless of the underlying cause, these results indicate that multiple hypersensitivities should always be considered when diagnosing and treating adverse food reactions in dogs and cats.

It has been proposed that early weaning of puppies or kittens may predispose some pets to the development of food allergies later in life.[112] In healthy animals, the small intestine possesses a protective barrier that limits the absorption of macromolecules. In young puppies and kittens, this protective barrier is not completely functional. When foreign food proteins are introduced to the immature gut, some may pass across the intestinal barrier, penetrate the lymphoid tissue, and trigger an immunological response and loss of oral tolerance.[122] Disease states that disrupt the small intestine's immunological barrier may have a similar effect. This theory may explain the early onset of food allergies in some pets. Further research is needed to determine the exact role that early weaning or the disruption of the intestine's protective barrier may play in the development of adverse food reactions.

Clinical Signs

The most common dermatological sign of adverse food reaction in dogs and cats is an intense pruritus.[123] Initially, this usually occurs between 4 and 24 hours after ingesting the offending antigen. Over time, chronic cases show constant pruritus with no evident association between eating and an exacerbation of signs. The onset of pruritus is not accompanied by other skin changes. However, the dog's intense scratching, biting, and self-trauma quickly lead to secondary lesions. In dogs, areas of the body most often affected are the feet, axillae, and inguinal area.[108,109,123] Cats are affected most intensely around the head, neck, and ears. In severe cases in both species, generalized pruritus over the entire body is seen. Excessive scratching and licking leads to hair loss and reddening of the skin. Papular eruptions occur in

approximately 40% of reported cases, and secondary bacterial infections are seen in about 20% of cases.[124] Other secondary changes may include chronic inflammation, crusting, seborrhea, and hyperpigmentation.

Persistent otitis externa, with or without infection, is often seen in both dogs and cats, and in some cases it is the only presenting sign. A small number of cases have also been reported that showed only a recurrent pyoderma that is not associated with pruritus. The pyoderma subsided with antibacterial therapy but continued to recur until the diet was changed. Skin disease caused by an adverse food reaction is usually nonseasonal. However, if multiple sensitivities are present (e.g., adverse food reaction plus atopy or flea-bite allergy), the adverse food reaction may not manifest clinically until another sensitivity is also triggered and the dog or cat reaches its pruritic threshold. This situation can cause the signs to appear to be seasonal in nature (Table 31-4).[117,124]

Although not common, gastrointestinal signs may accompany the dermatological signs of adverse food reaction. Reportedly, German Shepherd Dogs, Chinese Shar-Peis, and Irish Setters with adverse food reaction have an increased likelihood of showing gastrointestinal symptoms.[122] Diarrhea and, less frequently, vomiting are the most common forms of gastrointestinal signs. Some dogs show pruritus and skin changes and increased frequency of defecations per day (four or more).[121] Diarrhea that is associated with adverse food reactions is often chronic and intermittent.

TABLE 31-4 SIGNS OF ADVERSE FOOD REACTIONS IN DOGS AND CATS

Dogs	Cats
Intense pruritus (on the feet, axillae, and inguinal area)	Intense pruritus (on the head and neck)
Self-induced skin trauma	Self-induced trauma
Chronic inflammation of skin	Ulcerative dermatitis
Papular eruptions	Miliary dermatitis
Hair loss	Hair loss
Hyperpigmentation/scaling	Cutaneous hyperesthesia
Otitis externa	Seborrhea
Secondary bacterial infections (e.g., recurrent pyoderma)	Vomiting/diarrhea
Vomiting/diarrhea	

Diagnosis and Treatment

Diagnosis of adverse food reaction involves first ruling out other potential causes of the allergic dermatosis. These causes include atopy, flea-bite dermatitis, and drug hypersensitivities. Obtaining a full diet history is essential and is needed for all phases of the diagnostic and management program. When adverse food reaction is suspected, the standard method of diagnosis includes three phases: (1) a food trial that involves feeding a food that contains novel ingredients (called an *elimination diet*) and demonstrating an amelioration of clinical signs, (2) rechallenging the pet with the original diet and observing a return of clinical signs, and (3) a provocation test—feeding selected ingredients to identify the specific offending dietary antigens (Box 31-1). Generally, intradermal skin testing and serological testing have been shown to be unreliable in diagnosing food hypersensitivities in dogs and cats.[115,125,126]

An elimination diet contains a single protein source and a single carbohydrate source to which the pet has not previously been exposed. In most cases, this means selecting a food that contains ingredients not typically included in commercial pet foods. The most commonly used ingredients in commercial dog and cat foods include chicken, beef, lamb, fish, egg, soy, milk, corn, rice, and wheat. Other protein-containing ingredients that are less common but included in some products include turkey, venison, rabbit, oat, kelp, barley, flax, alfalfa, and potatoes. The wide range of ingredients found in commercial pet foods today makes it increasingly difficult to compose a suitable elimination diet for many pets and emphasizes the importance of including a complete diet history during the initial diagnostic workup. Today, three types of elimination diet can be used; a homemade diet, a commercial limited-ingredient food, or a commercial hydrolyzed-protein food.

HOMEMADE DIET A homemade pet food is often recommended for the elimination phase of diagnosis because some pets with adverse food reaction will still react to commercial diets and because few nonprescription commercial pet foods contain only one carbohydrate and one protein source. For example, 20% of dogs that were asymptomatic when fed a homemade diet of lamb and rice became pruritic again when fed a commercial preparation containing the same ingredients.[108] Another controlled study showed that 16% of dogs with diagnosed food hypersensitivity developed allergic reactions to a commercial food that was manufactured as an elimination diet for the diagnosis of dietary hypersensitivity.[104] These differences suggest that the processing of some commercial pet foods may enhance the antigenicity of certain food components. It is thought that the inclusion of poor-quality ingredients that are partially resistant to heat treatment or digestion may also increase the antigenicity of proteins in some economic brands of food. If a homemade elimination diet is used, common protein sources are lamb (if the pet has not been previously exposed), rabbit, venison, or tofu. Potential carbohydrates include rice (if not previously exposed) or potatoes. For dogs, a ratio of 1:2 to 1:4 parts protein source to carbohydrate source can be used. In cats, baby food composed of a single (or limited) protein and carbohydrate source is often used successfully.

An advantage of using a homemade elimination diet is that the food can be easily formulated in response to the patient's diet history and, if needed, modified to meet individual needs. Many pet owners also appreciate having some control over the diagnostic and treatment

---

BOX 31-1 THREE PHASES OF FOOD HYPERSENSITIVITY DIAGNOSIS

1. **Feeding the elimination diet.** The food should consist of a single protein and a single carbohydrate source to which the animal has not been previously exposed. The diet should be introduced gradually over a 4-day period. Improvement in clinical signs is usually observed within 3 weeks but may take up to 10 weeks.
2. **Feeding a challenge diet to confirm.** The pet's original food or a food that is known to cause an allergic reaction in the animal should be fed. If pruritus occurs within 4 hours to 14 days, a diagnosis of food hypersensitivity is confirmed.
3. **Identifying the offending dietary ingredients.** One suspected offending ingredient should be added to the elimination diet. The animal should be monitored for signs of allergic response. This process should be repeated for all suspected ingredients. Common pet food ingredients are most likely to be the cause of food hypersensitivity (e.g., beef, soy, chicken, egg, dairy, wheat, corn).

process and enjoy being able to contribute to their pet's recovery.[122] However, preparing a homemade diet is time consuming and can be expensive, depending on the type of ingredients that are used and the size of the dog. Owner compliance may also be low when a homemade diet is required by the practicing veterinarian for diagnosis. For example, a research study that mandated owners to use a homemade food for initial diagnosis of food allergy reported a drop-out rate of almost 40% due to owner noncompliance.[127] Last, with few exceptions, homemade foods used as elimination diets are not nutritionally balanced, and so cannot be fed for more than the period of time required for diagnosis. For example, a survey study that examined the homemade diet recipes prescribed by veterinarians as elimination diets reported that the vast majority (>90%) were nutritionally inadequate.[128] Therefore, once a diagnosis is made, another diet change is needed, which increases the risk of relapse if all possible allergens were not properly identified through provocation (see pp. 401-402).

COMMERCIAL LIMITED-INGREDIENT FOOD

A variety of commercial limited-ingredient (also called *limited-antigen*) foods are available for dogs and cats. Most of these contain a single protein and single carbohydrate source. These foods are formulated to be nutritionally complete and balanced and are advertised as appropriate for both the diagnostic phase and for long-term feeding for dogs and cats with adverse food reactions. However, owners and veterinarians should be aware that not all of these products have been thoroughly tested as elimination diets and so may not be suitable for use in diagnosis. In addition, a variety of protein sources are used in different products, which warrants careful selection using the pet's diet history as a guide. For example, 50% of dogs diagnosed with adverse food reactions relapsed when fed a limited-ingredient food that contained fish and potatoes.[127] Limited-ingredient products are most often used in the diagnostic phase when owners are not able or willing to prepare a homemade elimination diet, when the dog is so large as to make a homemade food cost prohibitive, or when an animal does not tolerate or accept a homemade food.

COMMERCIAL HYDROLYZED PROTEIN DIET

These foods are based upon the theory that reducing protein size via enzymatic hydrolysis effectively reduces the size (molecular weight) of the protein, thereby reducing or completely eliminating its antigenicity.[129] Products vary in the source of protein and the degree of hydrolysis and reduction in protein size that results.[130] Soy, chicken, casein, and liver protein are most commonly used as source proteins in these products.[131] Although not all hydrolyzed proteins have been tested, one study showed that 11 out of 14 dogs with confirmed adverse reactions to soy protein and corn showed no signs of adverse reaction to a food containing soy hydrolysate and cornstarch.[132] Other researchers have reported that the efficacy of hydrolyzed protein foods did not significantly differ from that of a homemade food when used as elimination diets to diagnosis adverse food reaction.[106,133,134] Owner compliance when using the commercial products was very good and the authors reported completion rates that were as good as or greater than completion rates reported in studies that used a homemade elimination diet. However, because some hydrolyzed proteins may still be allergenic, a product that includes a protein source that the patient is known or suspected to be sensitized to should be avoided if possible. Similar to limited-ingredient foods, these hydrolyzed protein products are formulated to be nutritionally complete and so are suitable for long-term feeding of dogs and cats with confirmed adverse food reactions.

Limitations of hydrolyzed protein diets include the potential for retained immunogenicity (i.e., the pet has an adverse reaction to the food), acceptability to the pet, and expense.[135] The small peptides and amino acids produced from protein hydrolysis have a variety of flavors, ranging from sweet to extreme bitterness. These can subsequently affect the palatability of the formulated food. Bitter flavors are caused in part by the hydrophobicity (water-insoluble) components of the protein and the degree to which these are exposed during hydrolysis. Conversely, some protein hydrolysates contain peptides and amino acids that are highly palatable to dogs and cats and which, in fact, have been used for many years as diet palatability enhancers. Although studies have reported acceptability problems in up 10% of dogs fed protein hydrolysate diets, some authors maintain that these percentages are no higher than those reported for conventional pet foods.[133,134] Finally, the required extra processing and use of purified carbohydrate sources (for example, corn starch) in these foods incur significantly higher costs to the manufacturer, which are then passed along to the consumer. In general, hydrolyzed protein diets cost substantially more than limited-ingredient products, which may make the expense of using them for diagnosis cost prohibitive for some pet owners.

FEEDING THE ELIMINATION DIET   The pet's diet should be gradually changed to the selected food over a period of 3 to 4 days. The elimination diet should then be fed exclusively, with no additional treats or table scraps. In addition, all chew toys that are made of animal products must be removed, and chewable vitamins or heartworm medication must be replaced with pure forms of medication. Some dogs and cats will show improvement within a few weeks after eating the elimination diet, while others may not begin to show signs for 6 to 10 weeks. A study of 51 dogs with a food allergy reported that only 25% responded to an elimination diet after 3 weeks of feeding, but more than 90% responded by 10 weeks.[111] In general, a 50% or greater reduction of pruritus and skin disease is accepted as diagnostic for dietary hypersensitivity.[63] Some pets may have a dietary hypersensitivity occurring concomitantly with other pruritic dermatoses, such as flea-bite allergy or atopy. When this occurs, feeding an elimination diet often causes a decrease in pruritus and skin disease but does not result in the complete resolution of signs. If pruritus is not diminished during the elimination phase, then either food allergy is not the diagnosis or the elimination diet being used still contains an ingredient to which the pet is allergic.

An elimination diet contains a single protein source and a single carbohydrate source to which the pet has not previously been exposed. For most pets, this means selecting a food that contains ingredients not typically included in commercial pet foods. Three types of elimination diet can be used; a homemade diet, a commercial limited-ingredient food, or a commercial hydrolyzed protein food. The pet's food should be gradually changed to the selected food over a period of 3 to 4 days and the elimination diet should then be fed exclusively for 6 to 10 weeks, while the pet is monitored for a change in clinical signs.

RECHALLENGE WITH ORIGINAL DIET
A conclusive diagnosis can only be made if the pet's former diet is reintroduced as a challenge diet and the previous clinical signs again develop. Pets with an adverse food reaction will usually show pruritus within 4 hours to 3 days of refeeding their original food. When the dog or cat has been fed the elimination food for 4 weeks or more, the response may be delayed for up to a week.[109,112] Some pet owners may be reluctant to conduct this portion of the diagnostic program, especially if they have seen a dramatic improvement. However, the challenge test is important to rule out a placebo effect of the elimination diet and to confirm (or negate) an adverse food reaction as the underlying cause of the pet's symptoms.

PROVOCATION TEST   The final phase of diagnosis, identification of specific antigens, is accomplished by adding single food items to the elimination diet and assessing for a return of clinical signs. Because beef, soy, and dairy products account for many of the adverse food reactions in dogs and cats, these ingredients should be tested first. It is generally accepted that only a very small amount of allergen is necessary to evoke a hypersensitivity response.[136] Adding powdered milk at a level of ½ to 2 tablespoons (tbsp) per meal provides exposure to the antigens found in dairy products.[137] If no return of signs is seen after 10 to 14 days, the next ingredient can be tested. Food items that are readily available to pet owners can be easily tested. Cooked beef, wheat flour, and soy meal can each be tested by adding 1½ to 2 tbsp per meal. Only one new substance should be added and tested at a time, and if a food causes an allergic reaction, the elimination diet should be fed until all signs are resolved before proceeding to another item. If no clinical signs are observed within 14 days of adding a test ingredient, the pet is probably not allergic to that food. Because a substantial number of animals are allergic to more than one food component, testing should include as many common pet food proteins as possible.

The identification phase of diagnosis can be very tedious and time-consuming for many pet owners. In addition, some owners are reluctant to risk the recurrence of clinical signs in their pet. After completing the elimination and challenge phases and arriving at a diagnosis of food allergy, some pet owners choose to simply find a balanced and complete food that their pet tolerates without attempting to identify the specific ingredients to which the pet reacts. Simply changing to a new, commercial pet food is rarely effective because most commercial foods contain similar ingredients. A food that contains a single protein and carbohydrate source to which the pet has not been exposed and that is not expected to cause a reaction should be selected. Feeding the elimination diet as a long-term maintenance diet is acceptable if this diet has been determined to be complete and balanced.

A conclusive diagnosis of adverse food reaction can only be made if the pet's former diet is reintroduced as a challenge diet and clinical signs (pruritus) again develop. The final phase of diagnosis, identification of specific antigens, is accomplished by adding single food items to the elimination diet and assessing for a return of clinical signs. However, because many pet owners are reluctant to risk the recurrence of signs in their pet, some opt to not complete a provocation test. Feeding the elimination diet as a long-term maintenance diet is acceptable if this diet has been determined to be complete and balanced.

Long-Term Management

The lifetime nutritional management of pets with adverse food reactions requires feeding a food that is palatable, complete, and balanced, and that does not contain the offending antigen or antigens. The protein included in the diet should be of high quality and highly digestible. Poorly digested proteins are more likely to retain their inherent antigenicity during heat processing of the product. In addition, incomplete digestion within the gastrointestinal tract may result in increased antigenicity in some poor-quality proteins. The inclusion of a reduced omega-6 to omega-3 fatty acid ratio may also help manage inflammation and pruritus.

Although homemade diets may be used safely for the elimination phase of diagnosis, these are not recommended for long-term maintenance because they are expensive and inconvenient and may not be complete and balanced. Commercial products offer economy and convenience, and unlike most homemade diets, they are guaranteed to be nutritionally complete and balanced.

Some pets with diagnosed adverse food reactions eventually develop additional sensitivities to ingredients in the new diet.[124] In these cases, the identification phase must be repeated, and another suitable diet must be found. Similarly, it is possible for the original sensitivity to become diminished and allow the pet to once again consume a diet containing that ingredient. Because adverse food reactions do not always respond to corticosteroid therapy and because of the long-term side effects of corticosteroids, emphasis is placed on strict adherence to dietary management rather than on drug therapy. Any small dietary indiscretion on the part of the owner or the pet does not cause direct harm but may lead to damage from pruritus and self-induced trauma. In some cases, repeated failures to adhere to the new diet decrease the chance of obtaining relief when fed an elimination diet. It is therefore very important that pet owners are aware of the need for strict compliance in order to control clinical signs.

Long-term nutritional management of pets with adverse food reactions requires feeding a food that is palatable, complete, and balanced, and that does not contain any offending food antigens. No other foods can be fed. The protein included in the diet should be of very high quality and highly digestible, and including a reduced omega-6 to omega-3 fatty acid ratio may help manage inflammation and pruritus. Because any small dietary indiscretion on the part of the owner or the pet can lead to relapse, pet owners must understand the need for strict compliance in order to control clinical signs.

References

1. Kirk RW: Nutrition and the integument, *J Small Anim Pract* 32:283–288, 1991.

2. Scott DW, Miller WH Jr, Griffin CE: Allergic skin disease in dogs and cats. In Scott DW, Miller WT Jr, Griffin CE, editors: *Muller and Kirk's small animal dermatology*, ed 6, Philadelphia, 2001, Saunders.

3. Terpstra AHM, West CE, Fennis JTCM: Hypocholesterolemic effect of dietary soy protein versus casein in rhesus monkeys, *Am J Clin Nutr* 39:1–7, 1984.

4. Bauer JE, Covert SJ: The influence of protein and carbohydrate type on serum and liver lipids and lipoprotein cholesterol in rabbits, *Lipids* 19:844–850, 1984.

5. White SD, Rosychuk RAW, Scott KV, and others: Effects of various proteins in the diet on fatty acid concentrations in the skin, cutaneous histology, clinicopathology and thyroid function in dogs. In Carey DP, Norton SA, Bolser SM, editors: *Recent advances in canine and feline nutritional research, Proceedings of the Iams international nutrition symposium*, Wilmington, Ohio, 1996, Orange Frazer Press.

6. Campbell KL, Czarnecki-Maulden GL, Schaeffer DJ: Effects of animal and soy fats and proteins in the diet on fatty acid concentrations in the serum and skin of dogs, *Am J Vet Res* 56:1465–1469, 1995.

7. Fadok VA: Treatment of canine idiopathic seborrhea with isotretionin, *Am J Vet Res* 47:1730–1733, 1986.

8. Strauss JS, Stranieri AM: Changes in long-term sebum production from isotretionin therapy, *J Am Acad Dermatol* 6:751–755, 1982.

9. Scott DW: Vitamin A-responsive dermatosis in the Cocker Spaniel, *J Am Anim Hosp Assoc* 22:125–129, 1986.

10. Ihrke PJ, Goldschmidt MH: Vitamin A-responsive dermatosis in the dog, *J Am Vet Med Assoc* 182:687–690, 1983.

11. Power HT, Ihrke PJ, Stannard AA, and others: Use of etretinate for treatment of primary keratinization disorders (idiopathic seborrhea) in Cocker Spaniels, West Highland White Terriers, and Basset Hounds, *J Am Vet Med Assoc* 201:419–429, 1992.

12. Parker W, Yager-Johnson JA, Hardy MH: Vitamin A responsive seborrheic dermatosis in the dog: a case report, *J Am Anim Hosp Assoc* 19:548–554, 1983.

13. Cho DY, Frey RA, Guffy MM, and others: Hypervitaminosis A in the dog, *Am J Vet Res* 36:1597–1603, 1975.

14. Cline JL, Czarnecki-Maulden GL, Losonsky JM, and others: Effect of increasing dietary vitamin A on bone density in adult dogs, *J Anim Sci* 75:2980–2985, 1997.

15. Stewart LJ, White SD, Carpenter JL: Isotretinoin in the treatment of sebaceous adenitis in two Vizslas, *J Am Anim Hosp Assoc* 27:65–71, 1991.

16. Rosser EJ Jr: Sebaceous adenitis. In Kirk RW, Bonagura JD, editors: *Current veterinary therapy XI*, Philadelphia, 1992, Saunders.

17. Rosser EJ Jr, Dunston RW, Breen PT, and others: Sebaceous adenitis with hyperkeratosis in the Standard Poodle: a discussion of 10 cases, *J Am Anim Hosp Assoc* 23:341–345, 1986.

18. White SD, Rosychuk AS, Scott KV, and others: Sebaceous adenitis in dogs and results of treatment with isotretinoin and etretinate: 30 cases (1990-1994), *J Am Vet Med Assoc* 207:197–200, 1995.

19. Power HT, Ihrke PJ: Synthetic retinoids in veterinary dermatology, *Vet Clin North Am Small Anim Pract* 20:1525–1539, 1990.

20. Scott DW, Walton DK: Clinical evaluation of oral vitamin E for the treatment of primary canine acanthosis nigricans, *J Am Anim Hosp Assoc* 21:345–356, 1985.

21. Ayres S, Mihan R: Is vitamin E involved in the autoimmune mechanism? *Cutis* 21:321–325, 1978.

22. Watson TDG: Diet and skin disease in dogs and cats, *J Nutr* 128:2783S–2789S, 1998.

23. White SD, Bourdeau R, Rosychuk RAW, and others: Zinc-responsive dermatosis in dogs: 41 cases and literature review, *Vet Dermatol* 12:101–109, 2001.

24. Van den Broek AHM, Thoday KL: Skin disease in dogs associated with zinc deficiency: a report of five cases, *J Small Anim Pract* 27:313–323, 1986.

25. Sousa CA, Stannard AA, Ihrke PJ: Dermatosis associated with feeding generic dog food: 13 cases (1981-1982), *J Am Vet Med Assoc* 192:676–680, 1988.

26. Thoday KL: Diet-related zinc-responsive skin disease in dogs. A dying dermatoses? *J Small Anim Pract* 30:213–215, 1989.

27. Codner EC, Thatcher CD: Nutritional management of skin diseases, *Compend Contin Educ Pract Vet* 15:411–424, 1993.

28. Kunkle GA: Zinc-responsive dermatoses in dogs. In Kirk RW, editor: *Current veterinary therapy VII*, Philadelphia, 1980, Saunders.

29. Colombini S, Dunstan RW: Zinc-responsive dermatosis in northern-breed dogs: 17 cases (1990-1996), *J Am Vet Med Assoc* 211:451–453, 1997.

30. Wedekind KJ, Lowry SR: Effects of zinc source, calcium level and fiber on zinc bioavailability in puppies, *J Nutr* 128:2593S–2595S, 1998.

31. Wedekind KJ, Clookings G, Hancock J: The bioavailability of zinc methionine relative to zinc sulfate is affected by calcium level, *Poultry Sci* 73:114, 1994.

32. Wedekind KJ, Hortin AE, Baker DH: Methodology for assessing zinc bioavailability: efficacy estimates for zinc methionine, zinc sulfate and zinc oxide, *J Anim Sci* 70:178–187, 1992.

33. Marsh KA, Ruedisueli FL, Coe SL, Watson TDG: Effects of zinc and linoleic acid supplementation on the skin and coat quality of dogs receiving a complete and balanced diet, *Vet Dermatol* 11:277–284, 2000.

34. Cunnane SC, Sella GE, Horrobin DF: Essential fatty acid supplementation inhibits the effect of dietary zinc deficiency, *Adv Prostaglandin Thromboxane Res* 8:1797–1798, 1980.

35. Van den Broek AHM, Simpson JW: Fat absorption in dogs with demodicosis or zinc-responsive dermatosis, *Res Vet Sci* 52:117–119, 1992.

36. National Research Council: *Nutrient requirements of dogs and cats*, Washington, DC, 2006, National Academy Press.

37. Watson AL, Fray TR, Bailey J, and others: Dietary constituents are able to play a beneficial role in canine epidermal barrier function, *Exp Dermatol* 15:74–81, 2006.

38. Lloyd DH: Essential fatty acids and skin disease, *J Small Anim Pract* 30:207–212, 1989.

39. Logas D, Beale KM, Bauer JE: Potential clinical benefits of dietary supplementation with marine-life oil, *J Am Vet Med Assoc* 199:1631–1636, 1991.

40. Remillard RL: Omega 3 fatty acids in canine and feline diets: a clinical success or failure? *Vet Clin Nutr* 5:6–11, 1998.

41. Schoenherr WD, Jewell DE: Nutritional modification of inflammatory diseases, *Semin Vet Med Surg (Small Anim)* 12:212–222, 1997.

42. Bibus DM: Dietary control of eicosanoids. In *Proceedings of the petfood forum*, Chicago, 1997, Watts Publishing.

43. Yammamoto S, Hayashi Y, Takahashi Y: Reactions of mammalian lipoxygenases and cycloxygenases with various polyunsaturated fatty acids. In Sinclair A, Gibson R, editors: *Essential fatty acids and eicosanoids*, Urbana, Ill, 1992, AOCS Press.

44. Calder PC: Dietary fatty acids and the immune system, *Nutr Rev* 56:S70–S83, 1998.

45. James MJ, Givson RA, Cleland LG: Dietary polyunsaturated fatty acids and inflammatory mediator production, *Am J Clin Nutr* 71:343S–348S, 2000.

46. Kragballe K, Voorhees JJ, Goetzl EJ: Inhibition by leukotrienes B5 of leukotriene B4-induced activation of human keratinocytes and neutrophils, *J Invest Dermatol* 88:555–558, 1987.

47. Lands WEM: Control of eicosanoid response intensity. In Vanderhoek J, editor: *Frontiers in bioactive lipids*, New York, 1996, Plenum Press.

48. Lands WEM, LeTellier RP, Rome LH, and others: Inhibition of prostaglandin biosynthesis, *Adv Biosci* 9:15–27, 1973.

49. Boudreau MD, Chanmugam PS, Hart SB, and others: Lack of dose response by dietary n-3 fatty acids at a constant ratio of n-3 to n-6 fatty acids in suppressing eicosanoid biosynthesis from arachidonic acid, *Am J Clin Nutr* 54:111–117, 1991.

50. Waldron MK, Bauer JE, Hannah SS: Dietary PUFAs effects on neutrophil functions. In *Proc Ann Conf Vet Intern Med Forum*, 1996, p 753.

51. Bauer JE, McAlister K, Harte J: Differential metabolism of dietary omega-3 fatty acids by LCAT in polyunsaturated fat-supplemented dogs, *J Vet Intern Med* 9:213, 1995.

52. Vaughn DM, Reinhart GA, Swaim SF, and others: Evaluation of dietary n-6 to n-3 fatty acid rations on leukotriene B synthesis in dog skin and neutrophils, *Vet Dermatol* 5:163–173, 1994.

53. Wander RC, Hall JA, Gradin JL, and others: The ratio of dietary (n-6) to (n-3) fatty acids influences immune system function, eicosanoid metabolism, lipid peroxidation and vitamin E status in aged dogs, *J Nutr* 127:1198–1205, 1997.

54. Hall JA, Wander RC, Gradin JL, and others: Effect of dietary n-6 to n-3 fatty acid ratio on complete blood and total white blood cell counts and T-cell subpopulations in aged dogs, *Am J Vet Res* 60:319–327, 1999.

55. Hall JA, Henry LR, Jha S, and others: Dietary (n-3) fatty acids alter plasma fatty acids and leukotrienes B synthesis by stimulated neutrophils from healthy geriatric Beagles, *Prostaglandins Leukot Essent Fatty Acids* 73:335–341, 2005.

56. Hall JA, Tooley KA, Gradin JL, and others: Effects of dietary n-6 and n-3 fatty acids and vitamin E on the immune response of healthy geriatric dogs, *Am J Vet Res* 64:762–772, 2003.

57. LeBlanc CJ, Horohov DW, Bauer JE, and others: Effects of dietary supplementation with fish oil on in vivo production of inflammatory mediators in clinically normal dogs, *Am J Vet Res* 69:486–492, 2008.

58. LeBlanc CJ, Dietrich MA, Horohov DW: Effects of dietary fish oil and vitamin E supplementation on canine lymphocyte proliferation evaluated using a flow cytometric technique, *Vet Immunol Immunopathol* 119:180–188, 2007.

59. Hall JA, Picton RA, Skinner MM, and others: The (n-3) fatty acid dose, independent of the (n-6) to (n-3) fatty acid ratio, affects the plasma fatty acid profile of normal dogs, *J Nutr* 136:2338–2344, 2006.

60. Rees CA: Canine and feline atopic dermatitis: a review of the diagnostic options, *Clin Tech Small Anim Pract* 16:230–232, 2001.

61. Scott DW, Paradis M: A survey of canine and feline skin disorders seen in a university practice (1987-1988), *Can Vet J* 31:830–835, 1990.

62. Ellis CJ: Food allergy, atopic dermatitis, or could it be both? *Vet Forum* 25:15–19, 2008.

63. Scott DW, Miller WH Jr, Griffin CE: Allergic skin disease in dogs and cats. In Scott DW, Miller WH Jr, Griffin CE, editors: *Muller and Kirk's small animal dermatology*, ed 5, Philadelphia, 1995, Saunders.

64. Chalmers S, Medleau L: Feline allergic dermatoses: diagnosis and treatment, *Vet Med* 84:399–403, 1989.

65. Willemse T: Atopic skin disease: a review and reconsideration of diagnostic criteria, *J Small Anim Pract* 27:771–778, 1986.

66. Schwartzman RM: Immunologic studies of progeny of atopic dogs, *Am J Vet Res* 45:375–379, 1984.

67. Olivry T, Dunston SM, Murphy KM, Moore PF: Characterization of the inflammatory infiltrate during IgE-mediated late phase reactions in the skin of normal and atopic dogs, *Vet Dermatol* 12:49–58, 2001.

68. DeBoer D: Canine atopic dermatitis: new targets, new therapies, *J Nutr* 134:2056S–2061S, 2004.

69. Fartasch M: Epidermal barrier disorders of the skin, *Microsc Res Tech* 38:361–372, 1997.

70. Inman AO, Olivry T, Dunston SM, and others: Electron microscopic observations of stratum corneum intercellular lipids in normal and atopic dogs, *Vet Pathol* 38:720–723, 2001.

71. Saevik BK, Thoresen SI, Taugbol O: Fatty acid composition of serum lipids in atopic and healthy dogs, *Res Vet Sci* 73:153–158, 2002.

72. Fuhrmann H, Zimmermann A, Guck T, Oechtering G: Erythrocyte and plasma fatty acid patterns in dogs with atopic dermatitis and healthy dogs in the same household, *Can J Vet Res* 70:191–196, 2006.

73. Nesbitt GH: Bathing is key to managing pruritus in dogs and cats, *Proc 2005 Central Vet Conf*, 2005.

74. Watson AL, Fray TR, Bailey J, and others: Dietary constituents are able to play a beneficial role in canine epidermal barrier function, *Exp Dermatol* 15:74–81, 2006.

75. Lloyd DH, Thomsett LR: Essential fatty acid supplementation in the treatment of canine atopy, *Vet Dermatol* 1:41–44, 1989.

76. Bond R, Lloyd DH: A double-blind comparison of olive oil and a combination of evening primrose oil and fish oil in the management of canine atopy, *Vet Rec* 131:558–560, 1992.

77. Campbell KL: Fatty acid supplementation and skin disease, *Vet Clin North Am Small Anim Pract* 20:1475–1486, 1990.

78. Taugbol O, Baddaky-Taugbol G, Saarem K: The fatty acid profile of subcutaneous fat and blood plasma in pruritic dogs and dogs without skin problems, *Can J Vet Res* 62:275–278, 1998.

79. Miller WH, Griffin GE, Scott DW, and others: Clinical trial of DVM derm caps in the treatment of allergic disease in dog: a nonblinded study, *J Am Anim Hosp Assoc* 25:163–168, 1989.

80. Scott DW, Buerger RG: Nonsteroidal anti-inflammatory agents in the management of canine pruritus, *J Am Anim Hosp Assoc* 24:425–428, 1988.

81. Miller WH, Scott DW, Wellington JR: Investigation on the anti-pruritic effects of ascorbic acid given alone and in combination with a fatty acid supplement to dogs with allergic skin disease, *Can Pract* 17:11–13, 1992.

82. Scott DW, Miller WH, Decker GA, and others: Comparison of the clinical efficacy of two commercial fatty acid supplements (EfaVet and DVM Derm Caps), evening primrose oil, and cold water marine fish oil in the management of allergic pruritus in dogs: a double-blinded study, *Cornell Vet* 82:319–329, 1992.

83. Paradis M, Lemay S, Scott DW: The efficacy of clemastine (Tavist), a fatty acid-containing product (DVM Derm Caps) and the combination of both products in the management of canine pruritus, *Vet Dermatol* 2:17–20, 1991.

84. Abba C, Mussa PP, Vercelli A, Raviri G: Essential fatty acids supplementation in different-stage atopic dogs fed on a controlled diet, *J Anim Physiol Anim Nutr* 89:203–207, 2005.

85. Harvey RG: Effect of varying proportions of evening primrose oil and fish oil on cats with crusting dermatosis (miliary dermatitis), *Vet Rec* 133:208–211, 1993.

86. Harvey RG: Management of feline miliary dermatitis by supplementing the diet with essential fatty acids, *Vet Rec* 128:326–329, 1991.

87. Miller WH Jr, Scott DW, Wellington JR: Efficacy of DVM Derm Caps Liquid in the management of allergic and inflammatory dermatoses of the cat, *J Am Anim Hosp Assoc* 29:37–40, 1993.

88. Scott DW, Miller WH: Nonsteroidal management of canine pruritus: chlorpheniramine and a fatty acid supplement (DVM Derm Caps) in combination, and the fatty acid supplement at twice the manufacturers' recommended dosage, *Cornell Vet* 80:381–387, 1991.

89. Bond R, Lloyd DH: Combined treatment with concentrated essential fatty acids and prednisolone in the management of canine atopy, *Vet Rec* 134:30–32, 1994.

90. Paradis M, Lemay S, Scott DW: The efficacy of clemastine (Tavist), a fatty acid-containing product (Derm Caps), and the combination of both products in the management of canine pruritus, *Vet Dermatol* 2:17–20, 1992.

91. Saevik B, Bergvall K, Holm BR, and others: A randomized, controlled study to evaluate the steroid sparing effect of essential fatty acid supplementation in the treatment of canine atopic dermatitis, *Vet Dermatol* 15:137–145, 2004.

92. Nesbitt GH, Freeman LM, Hannah SS: Correlations of fatty acid supplementation, aeroallergens, shampoo, and ear cleanser with multiple parameters in pruritic dogs, *J Am Anim Hosp Assoc* 40:270–284, 2004.

93. Mooney MA, Vaughn DM, Reinhart GA, and others: Evaluation of the effects of omega-3 fatty acid-containing diets on the inflammatory stage of wound healing in dogs, *Am J Vet Res* 59:859–863, 1998.

94. Boureaux MK, Reinhart GA, Vaughn D, and others: The effects of varying dietary n-6 to n-3 fatty acid ratios on platelet reactivity, coagulation screening assays, and antithrombin III activity in dogs, *J Am Anim Hosp Assoc* 33:235–243, 1997.

95. Schick MP, Schick RP, Reinhart GA: The role of polyunsaturated fatty acids in the canine epidermis: normal structural and functional components, inflammatory disease state components, and as therapeutic dietary components. In *Recent advances in canine and feline nutritional research, Proceedings of the Iams international nutrition symposium*, Wilmington, Ohio, 1996, Orange Frazer Press.

96. Scott DW, Miller JR, Reinhart GA, and others: Effect of an omega-3/omega-6 fatty acid-containing commercial lamb and rice diet on pruritus in atopic dogs: results of a single-blinded study, *Can J Vet Res* 61:145–153, 1997.

97. Glos K, Kinek M, Loewenstein C, and others: The efficacy of commercially available veterinary diets recommended for dogs with atopic dermatitis. *Vet Dermatol* 19:280–287, 2008.

98. Hwang D: Fatty acids and immune responses—a new perspective in searching for clues for mechanism, *Ann Rev Nutr* 20: 431–456, 2000.

99. Stehle ME, Goebel T, Hancaruk M, Mueller RS: The influence of polyunsaturated fatty acids on the T cell response in dogs with atopic dermatitis, *Vet Dermatol* 18:194, 2007.

100. Scott DW, Buerger RG: Nonsteroidal anti-inflammatory agents in the management of canine pruritus, *J Am Anim Hosp Assoc* 24:425–428, 1988.

101. Vaughn DM, Reinhart GA: Dietary fatty acid ratios and eicosanoid production, *Proc Ann Conf Vet Intern Med Forum*, 1995.

102. Anderson JA: The establishment of common language concerning adverse reactions to foods and food additives, *J Allergy Clin Immunol* 78:140–144, 1986.

103. Hillier A, Griffin CE: The ACVD task force on canine atopic dermatitis (X): is there a relationship between canine atopic dermatitis and cutaneous adverse food reactions? *Vet Immunol Immunopathol* 81:227–231, 2001.

104. Carlotti DN, Remy I, Prots C: Food allergy in dogs and cats: a review and report of 43 cases, *Vet Dermatol* 1:55–62, 1990.

105. Ackerman L: Food hypersensitivity: a rare, but manageable disorder, *Vet Med* 83:1142–1148, 1988.

106. Chesney CJ: Food sensitivity in the dog: a quantitative study, *J Small Anim Pract* 43:203–207, 2002.

107. Rosser EJ: Food allergy in the dog: a retrospective study of 51 dogs. In *Proceedings of the annual meeting of the American College of Veterinary Dermatology*, San Francisco, 1990, p 47.

108. White SD: Food hypersensitivity in 30 dogs, *J Am Vet Med Assoc* 188:695–698, 1986.

109. Harvey RG: Food allergy and dietary intolerance in dogs: a report of 25 cases, *J Small Anim Pract* 34:175–179, 1993.

110. Walton GS: Skin responses in the dog and cat due to ingested allergens: observations on one hundred confirmed cases, *Vet Rec* 81:709–713, 1967.

111. Rosser EJ: Diagnosis of food allergy in dogs, *J Am Vet Med Assoc* 203:259–262, 1993.

112. August JR: Dietary hypersensitivity in dogs: cutaneous manifestations, diagnosis and management, *Compend Contin Educ Pract Vet* 7:469–477, 1985.

113. Taylor SL, Lemanske RJ, Bush RK, Busse WW: Food allergens: structure and immunologic properties, *Ann Allergy* 59:93–99, 1987.

114. Martin A, Sierra MP, Gonzalez JL, Arevalo MA: Identification of allergens responsible for canine cutaneous adverse food reactions to lamb, beef and cow's milk, *Vet Dermatol* 15:349–356, 2004.

115. Jeffers JG, Shanley KJ, Meyer EK: Diagnostic testing of dogs for food hypersensitivity, *J Am Vet Med Assoc* 198:245–250, 1991.

116. Jeffers JG, Meyer EK, Sosis EJ: Responses of dogs with food allergies to single-ingredient dietary provocation, *J Am Vet Med Assoc* 209:608–611, 1996.

117. Hodgkins E: Food allergy in cats: considerations, diagnosis and management, *Pet Vet*, pp 24–28, Nov/Dec 1991.

118. Oobatake M, Ooi T: Hydration and heat stability effects on protein unfolding, *Prog Biohys Mol Biol* 39:237–284, 1993.

119. Otani H, Morita SI, Tokita F: Studies on the antigenicity of the browning product between beta-lactoglobulin and lactose, *Jpn J Zootech Sci* 56:1–74, 1983.

120. Cave NJ, Marks SL: Evaluation of the immunogenicity of dietary proteins in cats and the influence of the canning process, *Am J Vet Res* 65:1427–1433, 2004.

121. Paterson S: Food hypersensitivity in 20 dogs with skin and gastrointestinal signs, *J Small Anim Pract* 36:529–534, 1995.

122. Verlinden A, Hesta M, Millet S, Janssens GPJ: Food allergy in dogs and cats: a review, *Crit Rev Food Sci Nutr* 46:259–273, 2006.

123. Wills J, Harvey R: Diagnosis and management of food allergy and intolerance in dogs and cats, *Aust Vet J* 71:322–326, 1994.

124. Halliwell REW: Management of dietary hypersensitivity in the dog, *J Small Anim Nutr* 33:156–160, 1992.

125. Kunkle G, Horner S: Validity of skin testing for diagnosis of food allergy in dogs, *J Am Vet Med Assoc* 200:677–680, 1992.

126. Mueller R, Tsohalis J: Evaluation of serum allergen-specific IgE for the diagnosis of food adverse reactions in the dog, *Vet Dermatol* 9:167–171, 1998.

127. Tapp T, Griffin C, Rosenkrantz W, and others: Comparison of a commercial limited-antigen diet versus home-prepared diets in the diagnosis of canine adverse food reaction, *Vet Ther* 3:244–251, 2002.

128. Roudebush P, Cowell CS: Results of a hypoallergenic diet survey of veterinarians in North America with a nutritional evaluation of homemade diet prescriptions, *Vet Dermatol* 3:23–28, 1992.

129. Cordle CT: Control of food allergies using protein hydrolysates, *Food Technol* 48:72–76, 1994.

130. Olson ME, Hardin JA, Buret AG: Hypersensitivity reactions to dietary antigens in atopic dogs. In *Recent advances in canine and feline nutritional research, Proceedings of the Iams international nutrition symposium*, Wilmington, Ohio, 2000, Orange Frazer Press, pp 69–77.

131. Loeffler A, Soares-Magalhaes R, Bond R, Lloyd DH: A retrospective analysis of case series using home-prepared and chicken hydrolysate diets in the diagnosis of adverse food reactions in 181 pruritic dogs, *Vet Dermatol* 17:272–279, 2006.

132. Jackson HA, Jackson MW, Coblentz L: Evaluation of the clinical and allergen specific serum immunoglobulin E responses to oral challenge with cornstarch, corn, soy and a soy hydrolysate diet in dogs with spontaneous food allergy, *Vet Dermatol* 14:151–157, 2003.

133. Biourge VC, Fontaine J, Vroom MW: Diagnosis of adverse reactions to food in dogs: efficacy of a soy-isolate hydrolysate-based diet, *J Nutr* 134:2062S–2064S.

134. Loeffler A, Lloyd DH, Bond R, and others: Dietary trials with a commercial chicken hydrolysate diet in 63 pruritic dogs, *Vet Rec* 154:519–522, 2004.

135. Cave NJ: Hydrolyzed protein diets for dogs and cats, *Vet Clin Small Anim Pract* 36:1251–1268, 2006.

136. Walton GS: Skin diseases of domestic animals: skin manifestations of allergic response in domestic animals, *Vet Rec* 82:204–207, 1968.

137. Johnson LW: Food allergy in a dog: diagnosis by dietary management, *Mod Vet Pract* 68:236–239, 1987.

32

Chronic Renal Failure

DESCRIPTION AND CLINICAL SIGNS

Chronic renal failure in dogs and cats is characterized by an irreversible and progressive loss of kidney function and the development of clinical signs that reflect the kidneys' decreasing ability to perform normal regulatory and excretory functions. There are many potential causes for the initial kidney damage that leads to chronic disease. These causes include, but are not limited to, trauma, infection, immunological disease, neoplasms, renal ischemia (decreased blood flow to the kidneys), genetic anomalies, and exposure to toxins. Although renal disease can develop at any age, chronic renal disease is most frequently diagnosed in older pets.[1] In most cases the initial underlying cause of renal damage is no longer present when the pet develops chronic renal failure. This is due to the ability of the kidney to compensate for large proportions of functional tissue loss. However, over time these compensatory mechanisms may break down, leading to progressive loss of kidney function and signs of chronic disease.

Nephrons are the functional units of the kidneys. Each nephron consists of a glomerulus and a system of tubules within which reabsorption and excretion occur. The glomerulus is a tuft of capillaries where water, waste products, and electrolytes from the blood are filtered. The tubules originate at the base of the glomerulus and selectively reabsorb many of the blood components present in the filtrate. When the filtrate reaches the final portion of the tubule, it contains only those compounds that are going to be excreted as waste in the urine. The healthy kidney contains thousands of nephrons and has a substantial functional reserve.

Blood flow through the kidneys is very high, with approximately one fourth of cardiac output filtered through the kidneys each minute. The waste products of protein catabolism, such as urea, creatinine, uric acid, and ammonia are removed and excreted in the urine. In addition, electrolytes and trace minerals are filtered, reabsorbed, and selectively excreted. The kidneys are also important in the normal regulation of fluid balance, pH, and blood pressure and for the production of the hormone erythropoietin and the active form of vitamin D. All of these functions can be affected in pets with chronic renal disease.

The compensatory mechanisms of the healthy nephrons that remain after initial renal injury allow the kidneys to function normally even after the loss of a large proportion of tissue. A loss of at least 70% to 85% of functional capacity usually occurs before a pet begins to show clinical signs of renal failure.[1,2] One of the first signs that most pet owners notice is increased water consumption and increased urination. This effect is caused by a reduced capacity to concentrate urine, resulting in an increased volume of urine and increased frequency of urination. Some dogs may appear to regress in their house-training and begin to house-soil or involuntarily empty their bladder while sleeping. Polydipsia accompanies increased urination because the dog compensates with increased water consumption to maintain fluid balance. Polyuria and polydipsia are less commonly observed in cats because cats usually become uremic before they lose the ability to concentrate urine.[3] In addition, owners of indoor cats that use litter boxes are less likely to notice increased urination when it does occur.

The kidneys have an enormous reserve capacity; at least 70% to 85% of functional loss occurs before a pet begins to show clinical signs of renal failure. Common initial signs include increased water consumption and increased urination. Some dogs may appear to regress in their house-training and begin to house-soil or involuntarily empty their bladder while sleeping. Indoor cats begin to use the litter box more often, but this change may not be noticed by owners.

Many of the clinical signs seen in dogs and cats with advanced renal failure are associated with the degree of azotemia or uremia that is present. This is commonly referred to as *uremic syndrome*.[4] *Azotemia* refers to the accumulation of nitrogenous waste products in the blood, waste products composed primarily of urea nitrogen and/or creatinine. The term *uremia* technically means elevated concentrations of urea in the blood, but it commonly refers to the collection of clinical signs associated with renal failure. Although urea is singularly only a minor uremic toxin, serum urea levels are associated with the adverse clinical signs that reduce quality of life and contribute to morbidity in patients with chronic renal failure.[5] These signs include decreased appetite or anorexia, vomiting, depression, electrolyte and pH disturbances, mucosal ulcers, and weight loss. Some pets also develop chronic diarrhea and neurological signs. Aberrations in phosphorus and calcium metabolism lead to secondary renal hyperparathyroidism, which causes renal osteodystrophy (bone demineralization) and deposition of calcium phosphate in soft tissues. In many cases of chronic renal failure, the inability of the kidneys to produce erythropoietin and a reduced lifespan of red blood cells lead to the development of a normocytic, normochromic anemia (Box 32-1).[6]

Diagnosis of chronic renal disease in dogs and cats is based on medical history, clinical signs, serum chemistry, and urinalysis. Pets with chronic renal failure develop elevated blood urea nitrogen (BUN) and plasma creatinine levels as a result of reduced glomerular function. Although BUN and creatinine measurements

have been used for many years as the primary indicator of renal health in dogs and cats, they are relatively insensitive tests and do not accurately reflect the magnitude of renal functional loss.[7,8] This occurs because the relationship between glomerular filtration rate (GFR) and serum urea and creatinine concentrations is not linear, and up to 75% of renal function must be lost before BUN and creatinine values increase above the normal range.[7] After this point, values rise rapidly in response to small additional losses of renal function. Of the two measures, plasma creatinine is a more sensitive indicator of renal dysfunction and is not affected by dietary protein intake. In contrast, BUN is strongly affected by the consumption of a protein-containing meal. A fasting BUN of greater than 35 milligrams (mg)/deciliter (dl) may be an indication of some level of kidney dysfunction.

In 2006 the International Renal Interest Society (IRIS) established a set of diagnostic guidelines for dogs and cats with suspected chronic renal disease.[9] IRIS algorithms use fasting plasma creatinine level, presence of proteinuria, and systemic blood pressure to diagnose and stage kidney disease in dogs and cats. Separate algorithms are used for each species. Results allow practitioners to classify patients into stages and substages of renal disease, each of which is associated with a set of recommended treatment protocols. For example, plasma creatinine levels of between 2.1 and 5.0 mg/dl in dogs or between 2.9 and 5.0 in cats are indicative of moderate renal azotemia. Levels higher than 5.0, in either species, indicate severe renal azotemia that is typically associated with multiple extrarenal signs of disease. Tests for proteinuria and multiple blood pressure measurements are used to further classify animals into substages. A loss of concentrating ability and elevated serum phosphorus (greater than 5 mg/dl) also provides supportive evidence for a diagnosis of chronic renal failure. Laboratory test results may also show a normocytic, normochromic anemia; lymphopenia; hypercholesterolemia; or metabolic acidosis. Both lipase and amylase may be increased in the absence of pancreatitis due to decreased renal filtration.

With chronic renal disease, the gradual decline in GFR is responsible for the inability of the kidneys to filter and excrete waste products efficiently. However, early detection of kidney dysfunction is difficult in dogs and cats because clinical signs of uremia only develop

---

BOX 32-1   CLINICAL SIGNS OF CHRONIC RENAL FAILURE

Polyuria

Increased frequency of urination

Polydipsia

Depression

Diarrhea

Vomiting

Anorexia

Renal osteodystrophy

Anemia

Neurological impairment

after a large proportion of renal function has been lost. The most accurate and sensitive method for detecting early changes in renal function and for monitoring disease progression is to measure GFR. This test requires 24-hour urine collection by a veterinarian and measures the rates at which blood is filtered through the kidneys and waste products are removed and excreted. An estimate of GFR can also be obtained by measuring the renal clearance of exogenous creatine.[10,11] Unfortunately, these tests usually require expensive equipment and are time consuming and tedious to perform, so they are not available in most clinical settings. Efforts to produce a simpler and less expensive method for measuring GFR have reported success with using iohexol, an iodine-based radiographic contrast compound or gadolinium diethylenetriamine pentaacetic acid (Gd-DTPA).[12-14] These tests may be especially important because early detection of a decreasing GFR can be the signal for nutritional interventions that can actually slow the progression of renal failure. Waiting for the appearance of azotemia or a loss of concentrating ability delays the use of these measures.

> BUN and serum creatinine provide veterinary practitioners with a rapid screening test for assessing glomerular function in clinically affected patients. A fasting BUN of greater than 35 mg/dl is an indication of some level of kidney dysfunction. Plasma creatinine levels higher than 5.0 mg/dl indicate advanced failure or end-stage disease. IRIS guidelines also use blood pressure and presence of proteinuria to stage renal disease. The most accurate and sensitive method for detecting early changes in renal function is to measure GFR. Early detection of a decreasing GFR is important because it may allow early nutritional interventions that can slow the progression of renal failure.

PROGRESSIVE NATURE

The occurrence of chronic renal failure is preceded by some type of renal insult or injury that causes a loss of nephrons. Following this initial episode, the kidneys undergo structural and functional compensatory adaptations. Specifically, these changes include increased glomerular capillary hypertension, increased single nephron glomerular filtration rate (SNGFR), and renal hypertrophy (growth of remnant nephrons).[15,16] The increase in GFR in the surviving nephrons causes the kidneys' total GFR to be higher than the level that would be predicted following the reduction in renal mass. These changes enable a damaged kidney to compensate and function for variable and extended periods of time at normal or near-normal capacity. During this compensatory phase, clinical signs of renal disease are not evident.

Depending on the extent of the damage to the kidneys and on other factors that can influence the progression of disease, renal function may eventually begin to decline. When this occurs, the progressive and irreversible loss of functioning nephrons causes a gradual reduction in total GFR and in the kidneys' ability to excrete waste products from the body. The inability to excrete waste products and the compromised regulatory functioning of the kidneys lead to clinical signs of renal failure. Renal failure can progress to end-stage disease even after the initial cause of injury has been resolved and in the absence of active renal disease. It appears that the loss of a certain critical mass of nephrons can result in self-perpetuating, progressive renal disease. Studies in dogs have indicated that between ¾ and ¹⁵⁄₁₆ of renal mass must be destroyed before progression occurs.[17] However, great variability is seen among individuals. Some dogs and cats never develop progressive disease, even when an extremely high proportion of renal mass has been destroyed.

Many factors may contribute to the progression of renal disease in dogs and cats. Evidence from early studies with rats suggested that the alterations that compensate for the initial loss of active tissue may eventually contribute to progressive deterioration of the remaining tissue.[18] These studies led to the hypothesis that hyperfiltration and hypertension of surviving nephrons ultimately would cause cellular injury, resulting in progressive glomerulosclerosis and a loss of nephron function. This hypothesis has been termed the *hyperfiltration theory* and appears to explain the progressive nature of renal disease in several strains of laboratory rat.[19,20] However, while glomerular hypertrophy and hypertension occur in dogs and cats with decreased renal function, the role of these changes in disease progression is unclear.[21,22] Studies with dogs indicate that the adaptive changes that occur following a loss of renal tissue do not lead to the progressive glomerulosclerosis that has been reported in rats.[23,24] In contrast, therapies that reduce glomerular hypertension have been shown to protect the kidneys from further damage in dogs with experimentally induced diabetic nephropathy.[25,26] These results suggest that a reduction in glomerular hypertension may be beneficial to dogs with chronic renal disease.

Role of Diet in Progression

Other factors that may contribute to spontaneous progression of renal disease in dogs and cats include systemic hypertension, hyperparathyroidism, intrarenal inflammation, hyperlipidemia, renal mineralization, and renal ammoniagenesis. Each of these factors is influenced to some degree by the animal's diet and nutritional status. Chronically elevated serum phosphate levels can contribute to hyperparathyroidism and renal mineralization; dietary fatty acids affect serum lipid levels, intrarenal blood pressure, and inflammation; dietary sodium may influence the development of systemic hypertension; and metabolic acidosis affects ammonia production in the kidneys.

The goals of dietary management of chronic renal failure are to ameliorate clinical signs of uremia (see p. 417) and, if possible, slow or stop the progression of the disease. Historically, dietary protein was the major nutrient identified as important in slowing disease progression. However, studies have shown that protein is not an important factor in disease progression in dogs and cats, while other nutrients play a more significant role. Dietary components that can influence the rate of progression of chronic renal failure in dogs and cats include phosphorus, the type of fatty acids included in the diet, and nutritional factors that affect the body's acid-base status.

PROTEIN   Feeding a high-protein diet results in increased renal blood flow and increased postprandial GFR in all species that have been studied, including the dog.[19,27] This effect is seen in both healthy animals and animals with compromised kidney function. A series of early studies reported that dietary protein restriction reduced these effects and slowed the progression of chronic renal disease in a susceptible strain of male rats

with experimentally reduced renal mass.[19] Restricting dietary protein also slowed the development of progressive disease in healthy Fischer 344 rats that were genetically predisposed to develop chronic renal disease as they aged.[28,29]

These effects have not been observed in dogs. In contrast to rats, feeding elevated protein levels has not been shown to cause a progression of renal disease in dogs with either experimentally induced or naturally occurring renal disease.[23,24,30-32] In an early long-term study, diets containing either 19%, 27%, or 56% protein were fed to dogs with experimentally induced ¾ reduction in renal mass for a period of 4 years.[30] The dogs that were fed the high-protein diet (56% protein) had higher GFR and renal plasma flow rates than the dogs that were fed the low-protein diet (19% protein). However, significant morphological or functional deterioration in the remaining nephrons of the kidneys was not observed in any dogs. The investigators were unable to establish a cause and effect relationship between protein feeding and the progression of renal disease in the dogs that were studied. Feeding the high-protein (56%) and the low-protein (19%) diets was associated with slight proteinuria, but the 27%-protein diet did not cause this effect. In contrast to the rats that were studied, none of the dogs in this study developed elevated BUN levels or clinical signs of chronic renal disease in response to consuming moderate- or high-protein diets.

In another study, three groups of dogs with induced renal failure were fed three diets varying in protein, fat, carbohydrate, and mineral content.[32] Over a 40-week period, dogs that were fed the high-protein, high-phosphorus diet (44.4% protein, 2.05% phosphorus) showed the highest mortality rate. However, mortality was associated with uremia caused by the increased protein, rather than uremia caused by the development of progressive nephron destruction. There was no evidence of a decline in GFR (an indication of progressive renal disease) in the dogs fed the high-protein diet. These results indicate that the increased mortality was caused by the extrarenal, clinical effects of feeding high amounts of protein to dogs with renal failure and not to an enhanced progression of renal disease caused by the diet.

The previous studies do not support the hypothesis that protein affects the progression of chronic renal failure in dogs. Additional evidence comes from studies that fail to demonstrate that restricting dietary protein inhibits the initial development or progression of renal disease. Early studies with rats reported that feeding low-protein diets prolonged life and delayed the development of chronic renal disease.[19,33,34] However, follow-up studies found that benefits that had been attributed to low protein were actually a result of low energy intake throughout life.[29,35] Reduced energy consumption significantly slowed growth (which continues throughout life in rats) and retarded the progression of chronic renal disease. Unfortunately, the belief that feeding a low-protein diet prevents the development and the progression of renal disease had already been applied to several other species, including companion animals. This theory is without supportive scientific evidence in either dogs or cats.

In dogs, moderate restriction of dietary protein is not effective in modifying glomerular hypertrophy after a loss of kidney function. When dogs with a $15/16$ loss of kidney function were fed a moderately restricted diet containing 16% protein, the adaptive changes of hyperfiltration, capillary hypertension, and glomerular hypertrophy still occurred.[15] A second study of dogs with a $7/8$ loss of functional kidney tissue reported that renal lesions were indistinguishable between dogs that were fed a diet containing 15% protein and those that were fed a diet containing 31% protein over a 14-month period.[36]

Studies with cats have reported similar results. When cats with experimentally induced renal failure were fed either a high-protein diet (51.7%) or a low-protein diet (27.6%), cats consuming the low-protein diet showed fewer and less severe glomerular lesions in the remnant kidney.[37] However, the low-protein diet was less palatable, and cats consuming this diet had significantly lower caloric intakes than those consuming the high-protein diet, leading to weight loss and signs of protein deficiency. Because of this confounding effect, the authors of the study concluded that restriction of calories and protein led to less glomerular injury in cats with induced renal failure when compared with cats fed a diet replete in calories and protein.

A subsequent study was undertaken to elucidate the separate effects of protein and calorie intake on the progression of renal disease in cats.[38] A group of 28 adult female cats with experimentally induced renal failure was divided into four groups according to initial GFR.

Each group received one of four diets for a 12-month period: low protein/low calorie, low protein/high calorie, high protein/low calorie, or high protein/high calorie. GFR did not decrease in any of the groups during the 12-month study period. Mild to moderate renal glomerular lesions were observed in all groups, but their development was not affected by either protein level or caloric intake. On the other hand, nonglomerular lesions in the kidneys were reported in cats fed the high-calorie diets but not in those fed the high-protein diets. The cat appears to be similar to the dog in that feeding a diet containing adequate protein does not exacerbate chronic renal disease.

Because of the early research studies with rats and because it has been hypothesized that elderly pets experience some loss of renal function as a normal process of aging, it became popular during the 1980s to advocate feeding low-protein diets to older animals, with the intent of slowing the rate of renal deterioration. However, no research has shown that there is an obligatory loss of kidney function with aging in either dogs or cats.[39-41] Elderly pets require adequate levels of high-quality protein to help to minimize losses of protein reserves and satisfy their maintenance needs (see Section 4, pp. 268-270). Long-term restriction of dietary protein in both dogs and cats is associated with several inherent dangers. Protein deficiency results in impaired immunological response and resistance to infection, reduced hemoglobin production and anemia, decreased plasma protein levels, and muscle wasting.[42,43] Restricting protein in older pets when it is not necessary can lead to further loss of protein reserves, malnutrition, and clinical signs associated with protein or amino acid deficiency. Finally, foods with severely reduced protein are low in palatability, which can lead to reduced intake that can further exacerbate protein deficiency. For example, when a diet containing 27.6% protein was fed to cats with $5/6$ renal ablation, the cats consumed significantly less food when compared with cats fed 51.7% protein.[37] The cats fed the low-protein diet lost weight and developed hypoalbuminemia, a clinical sign of protein malnutrition. In contrast, cats fed the high-protein diet gained weight and did not develop protein deficiency. Consideration of the detrimental effects of protein restriction is particularly important in cats because this species does not readily adapt to reduced-protein diets (see Section 2, pp. 92-95).

Current evidence suggests that mechanisms that can alter the progression of renal disease in the rat do not have the same effect in the dog and cat. Dogs appear to be resistant to the glomerulosclerosis and loss of renal function associated with aging and adaptive changes in nephrons and protein-feeding in the rat.[39] Although high-protein feeding can exacerbate clinical signs by leading to azotemia in dogs with advanced renal failure, these effects occur because the loss of renal function leads to an accumulation in the blood of nitrogenous and nonnitrogenous end products of protein metabolism, not due to direct damage to the kidneys.[44] There is no evidence that dietary protein causes a progressive destruction of nephron functioning in the remaining normal tissue. It is hypothesized that the absence of systemic hypertension in dogs with renal disease and the fact that dogs do not normally develop the same type of renal disease as rats explain the differences between dogs and rats. In addition, unlike the rat, the dog does not continue to grow throughout its life and typically consumes only one to two meals per day, compared with the nibbling regimen of the rat. In dogs, hyperfiltration following the consumption of a meal that contains protein lasts for a short time, as opposed to continuously throughout a 24-hour period in the rat. The cat appears to be similar to the dog; routine restriction of protein in cats with chronic renal disease with the intent of slowing disease progression is not supported.

Dietary protein is not a contributor to either the initiation or progression of chronic renal disease in dogs and cats. Although high-protein feeding can exacerbate clinical signs by leading to azotemia in animals with advanced renal failure, these effects occur because the loss of renal function leads to an accumulation in the blood of nitrogenous and nonnitrogenous end products of protein metabolism, not due to increased damage to the kidneys.

PHOSPHORUS   A dietary factor that is involved in the progression of renal disease in companion animals is the level of phosphorus in the diet. As chronic renal failure progresses, GFR declines and leads to a decreased ability to excrete phosphorus. Declining kidney function also leads to an inability to produce calcitriol (active vitamin D) and to degrade parathyroid hormone (PTH). Collectively, these changes result in aberrations in phosphorus and calcium metabolism and can ultimately result in hyperphosphatemia, bone demineralization (osteodystrophy), and the deposition of calcium phosphate crystals in soft tissues. The deposition of calcium and phosphorus in renal tissue causes inflammation, scarring, and subsequent loss of nephrons.[45] Therefore the restriction of dietary phosphorus may help to control renal secondary hyperparathyroidism, resulting in decreased mineralization and less damage to the remaining functioning nephrons, ultimately slowing the progression of renal disease.

Studies with rats have shown that phosphorus restriction is effective in minimizing or preventing proteinuria and in slowing the structural and functional changes that occur in the remaining healthy nephrons.[46] Similar studies with dogs have found that the dietary restriction of phosphorus can slow the progression of clinical disease and prolong survival in azotemic dogs with induced chronic renal failure.[47] In addition, when diets containing 32% protein and varying levels of phosphorus were fed to dogs with induced renal failure, the dogs that were fed the low-phosphorus diets had significantly higher GFR values when compared with dogs fed the high-phosphorus diets.[48] However, over time, renal lesions developed that were not influenced by the level of phosphorus in the diet, indicating that other factors were involved in the progression of the disease. Beneficial effects of phosphorus restriction that are independent of the level of protein in the diet were found in a study comparing the effects of high and low dietary protein and phosphorus in dogs with a 15/16 reduction in renal mass.[49] Survival time and GFR stability were enhanced in dogs fed reduced phosphorus (0.4%) but were not affected by the level of protein fed. There is also evidence that normal phosphorus intake in cats with induced renal disease causes increased mineralization of renal tissue, and that dietary restriction can prevent these changes.[50] Current evidence suggests that high dietary phosphorus contributes to the progression of renal disease in dogs and cats and that phosphorus restriction can reduce damage to renal tissue and disease progression (see p. 420). However, because other factors are involved, progression of disease can still occur even with restricted dietary phosphorus.

A dietary factor that is involved in the progression of renal disease in companion animals is the level of phosphorus in the diet. Declining kidney function leads to an inability to excrete phosphorus, produce calcitriol, and degrade parathyroid hormone. Restriction of dietary phosphorus helps to control renal secondary hyperparathyroidism, resulting in decreased mineralization and less damage to the remaining functioning nephrons, ultimately slowing the progression of renal disease.

DIETARY LIPIDS The amount and type of fat in a pet's diet may affect the progression of renal disease. Hyperlipidemia has been identified as a causal factor in uremic renal failure in some species.[51,52] Like rats and humans, dogs and cats with renal dysfunction often exhibit elevated serum cholesterol and triglycerides. In addition, the degree of hyperlipidemia has been shown to be directly related to further losses of renal function in dogs with experimentally induced renal disease. When dogs with induced renal failure were fed a diet enriched in polyunsaturated fatty acids (PUFAs) (safflower oil or menhaden fish oil), they had lower blood lipid levels, compared with dogs fed a diet containing saturated fat.[53] These results indicate that replacing a proportion of saturated fat with polyunsaturated fat may be helpful in ameliorating the hyperlipidemia seen in pets with chronic renal disease.

A second factor affecting the progression of renal disease is the presence of increased vascular pressure in the kidneys, specifically within the glomerular capillaries. In rats, manipulations that increase glomerular pressure contribute to the progression of chronic renal failure, and factors that reduce glomerular hypertension are renoprotective.[19,54] Modification of the level of omega-3 fatty acids in the diet affects glomerular pressure and the progression of renal disease in rats. However, while some researchers report benefits of feeding omega-3 fatty acids, others found that feeding this class of fatty acid was associated with a worsening of disease in rats.[55-57] Similarly, while some human patients with immune-mediated forms of renal disease have benefited

from supplementation with omega-3 fatty acids, others have shown no change in condition.[58,59]

Like rats and humans, dogs and cats with chronic renal disease develop glomerular hypertension.[16,21] A study of diabetic dogs demonstrated that therapies aimed at reducing glomerular hypertension significantly slowed the progression of kidney disease.[25,26] It is speculated that lowering glomerular pressure may also be of benefit to dogs and cats with other forms of chronic renal failure.[55] Dietary lipids influence intrarenal pressure through the effects of renal eicosanoid metabolism. Eicosanoids, produced from fatty acids, are one of several mediators of inflammation in many different tissues of the body (see pp. 387-390). During an inflammatory response, the release and metabolism of omega-6 fatty acids produces the 2-series prostaglandins, the 4-series leukotrienes, hydroxyeicosatetraenoic acid, and thromboxane A_2 (TXA_2). Two omega-6–derived eicosanoids, prostaglandin E_2 (PGE_2) and prostacyclin, are vasodilatory and proinflammatory and function in the kidney to increase renal blood flow and GFR. In contrast, TXA_2 causes vasoconstriction and has variable effects on GFR. Omega-3 fatty acid–derived eicosanoids are less potent inflammatory agents, and omega-3–derived thromboxanes have less vasoconstrictive and platelet-aggregating effects. Because omega-6 and omega-3 fatty acids compete for the same enzyme systems, increasing tissue concentrations of omega-3 fatty acids causes a diminution of the 2-series eicosanoids derived from the omega-6 fatty acid arachidonic acid, thus down-regulating intrarenal inflammatory responses.

A link between production of the 2-series of prostaglandins and thromboxanes and progressive renal disease has been proposed.[60] This theory is based on studies that suggest glomerular hypertension is affected by renal eicosanoids, and that supplementation with omega-3 fatty acids (marine fish oil) can reduce renal hypertension and may slow the progression of chronic renal disease.[61] One study measured the effects of three different types of fat on GFR in dogs with induced renal failure.[62] Dogs were fed a low-fat diet supplemented with either menhaden fish oil (a source of omega-3 fatty acids), safflower oil (a source of unsaturated omega-6 fatty acids) or beef tallow (a source of saturated omega-6 fatty acids) for a period of 20 months. Dogs fed the menhaden fish oil–supplemented diet had reduced proteinuria and lower serum creatinine, cholesterol, and triglyceride values when compared with dogs fed either safflower oil or beef tallow. While six out of seven dogs fed the diet enriched with omega-6 fatty acids showed progressive loss of renal function over the 20-week period, dogs fed the diet supplemented with omega-3 fatty acids did not exhibit signs of progression and actually had GFR test values indicating a slight increase in renal function at the end of the trial (Figure 32-1). These results suggested that omega-3 fatty acids may be renoprotective, while supplementation with omega-6 fatty acids may contribute to disease progression.

A second study examined the effects of fatty acid supplementation in dogs with naturally occurring chronic renal failure.[63] Dogs were fed fatty acid supplements containing either safflower oil or menhaden fish oil for a 6-week period. Dogs fed the omega-3 supplement maintained GFR for the entire 6-week period and exhibited decreased levels of urinary PGE_2. The dogs supplemented with safflower oil had increased GFR and increased urinary PGE_2 concentrations. Although dogs fed safflower oil had higher GFR values, it is theorized that this was a short-lived effect caused by increased

renal blood flow. The rise in PGE_2 is indicative of increased intrarenal pressure, which over time may contribute to the progression of disease.

OTHER CONTRIBUTING NUTRIENTS A high level of dietary sodium has been identified as a potentially exacerbating factor in progression of chronic renal failure through enhancement of systemic hypertension. There is evidence in rats that sodium restriction can slow the progression of chronic renal disease.[64] For this reason, moderate sodium restriction has been recommended for dogs and cats with chronic renal failure. However, sodium restriction is not universally accepted because systemic hypertension is not a consistent finding in dogs and cats with renal failure. In addition, studies of risk factors and of the effects of reduced sodium intake in dogs and cats with compromised renal function have not shown a clear benefit of sodium restriction.[65-67] The unnecessary restriction of dietary sodium may exacerbate compromised renal concentrating ability due to reduced intrarenal sodium content, and may cause increased production of angiotensin in

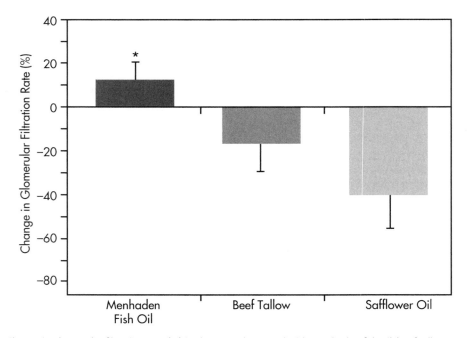

Figure 32-1   Change in glomerular filtration rate (%) in dogs supplemented with menhaden fish oil, beef tallow, or safflower oil. *, $P < .05$.

(From *New concepts in management of renal failure*, Dayton, Ohio, 1998, The Iams Company.)

response to lowered systemic levels of sodium. Because the ideal dietary sodium intake for pets with chronic renal failure is not well defined and because of the risks of severe restriction, current recommendations are to provide a food that contains normal or moderately restricted amounts of sodium to pets with chronic renal disease (see p. 423).[68]

Metabolic acidosis occurs commonly in pets with chronic renal failure and is caused by the reduced ability of the kidneys to excrete acids. For example, a retrospective study of cats with naturally occurring renal failure reported that approximately 80% of cats had metabolic acidosis at the time of diagnosis.[69] The development of acidosis in cats may be exacerbated by the acidifying nature of many commercial maintenance diets. Acidosis contributes to renal injury and uremia and leads to increased renal tubular generation of ammonia. These changes may all contribute to a progressive loss of renal function. In addition, there is an apparent association between metabolic acidosis and negative potassium balance in cats, which may further contribute to disease progression.[70]

DIETARY MANAGEMENT

When chronic renal disease has been diagnosed in a dog or cat, medical management is directed toward normalizing blood pressure, preventing or reducing proteinuria, normalizing plasma phosphate (if dietary restriction is not sufficient), and preventing or correcting metabolic acidosis.[9] Dietary management is implemented with the goals of minimizing the clinical, biochemical, and physiological consequences of the loss of kidney function. Alterations in the kidneys' ability to excrete waste products and to regulate metabolism of certain nutrients and hormones are the cause of the clinical signs that the animal experiences. Although dietary therapy does not cure chronic renal disease, it can minimize clinical signs and contribute to a pet's health, well-being, and longevity. In addition, the modification of certain essential nutrients in the diet may slow the progression of disease. A major goal of dietary management is to minimize the accumulation of protein catabolites in the blood while still providing adequate protein for the pet's maintenance needs. To this end, adequate calories from nonprotein sources must be provided to minimize the use of either body tissues or dietary protein for energy.

Other nutrients of concern include dietary fat, fiber, phosphorus, sodium, potassium, and water-soluble vitamins (Box 32-2). In all cases, medical and dietary management should be customized to address the needs of the individual patient and modified as a patient's stage of disease changes.[9]

Protein

A distinction must be made between restricting protein with the proposed purpose of slowing or stopping the progression of renal disease and restricting protein with the purpose of managing clinical signs. Although early studies with rats indicated that protein restriction was beneficial in slowing the progression of chronic renal disease, research does not support this effect in dogs and cats (see pp. 412-414).[38,41] In contrast, when chronic renal disease has been definitively diagnosed in a dog or cat through the appearance of clinical signs, diminished GFR, and changes in blood chemistry data, modification of dietary protein may be beneficial and is recommended for the management of clinical signs.

The accumulation of the nitrogenous end products of protein and amino acid metabolism causes many of the clinical and metabolic signs of chronic renal failure. Urea is the most abundant of these metabolites and can be readily measured in the blood. Although urea is only a mild uremic toxin, its concentration parallels the levels of other, more potent nitrogenous toxins and can be used as an index to monitor the extent of disease and clinical signs.[71] Together these components produce nausea, vomiting, osmotic diuresis, and a decreased

---

BOX 32-2   **GOALS OF DIETARY MANAGEMENT OF CHRONIC RENAL DISEASE**

Maintain nitrogen balance by providing optimal protein nutrition.

Provide adequate nonprotein calories.

Minimize azotemia and associated clinical signs.

Normalize serum phosphorus.

Normalize blood pH.

Normalize electrolyte balance and good hydration.

lifespan of red blood cells. Normalizing the levels of urea and other nitrogenous waste products in the blood through moderate restriction of dietary protein contributes to a return of appetite, weight gain, and a lessening of other clinical signs.

The generation of urea is directly proportional to the daily turnover of dietary and body protein. Protein that is ingested in excess of the animal's requirement is metabolized for energy, producing urea and other end products that must then be excreted by the kidneys. Similarly, when inadequate calories are ingested or when an animal is in a catabolic state, body protein is used for energy, also resulting in the synthesis of urea. A reduction in the excretory capacity of the kidneys results in an elevation of urea and other components in the blood, because they are retained by the body. A primary goal of dietary therapy is to provide an optimal amount of protein and adequate nonprotein calories to prevent the breakdown of body tissue for energy. These changes minimize the amount of urea and other nitrogenous end products that are produced. In most cases, this necessitates a moderate restriction of dietary protein and a change in the type of protein included in the diet.

Minimum protein and amino acid requirements for pets with chronic renal failure have not been established. Therefore the decision to control protein intake is determined by the patient's clinical signs and degree of impairment of renal function. Protein restriction is suggested only when a pet's BUN is greater than 65 to 80 mg/dl and when serum creatinine is greater than 2.5 mg/dl.[72,73] Although the normal range for fasting BUN is between 10 and 24 mg/dl, most dogs do not show clinical signs of renal disease until BUN exceeds 60 to 80 mg/dl. Pets that have only slightly elevated BUN values (30 to 60 mg/dl) and are not showing clinical signs do not benefit from protein restriction.[74]

The goal of dietary protein restriction is to maintain the animal's BUN below a level of 60 mg/dl. In dogs and cats, as in other animals, a direct relationship exists between the BUN to serum creatinine ratio and dietary protein. The current National Research Council's minimum protein requirement for adult dogs is 80 grams (g) of crude protein per kilogram (kg) diet (8.0% by weight), when high-quality proteins are fed.[75] Early recommendations were to feed very low levels of protein to uremic dogs.[76,77] However, a study of dogs with induced renal disease found that feeding a

diet containing 1.6 g/kg of protein or less caused signs of protein deficiency.[78] This is equivalent to feeding a diet containing just 8.2% protein on a dry-matter basis (DMB). Increasing the protein level to 2 g/kg still aided in the control of BUN levels and clinical signs of renal disease but did not cause protein malnutrition.[79] The potential to induce protein deficiency necessitates conservative restriction of dietary protein in dogs with renal disease. Because uremic animals tend to be in a catabolic state, their minimum protein requirement may be even slightly higher than that of a healthy animal. In addition, dogs with proteinuria may require more dietary protein than dogs without proteinuria. In all cases, the highest level of protein that results in an amelioration of clinical signs and controls BUN levels without compromising protein and amino acid nutrition should be fed.

In dogs with mild to moderate renal disease, a diet containing between 12% and 28% protein on a DMB is recommended, with the exact level dependent on the animal's clinical and biochemical response. In cases of severe renal disease, when GFR has deteriorated to only 10% to 20% of normal, protein must be progressively restricted to approach a level that is close to the pet's minimum daily requirement. Depending on the degree of clinical signs and the energy level of the diet, a pet food containing between 10% and 15% protein may be needed, provided that the protein is of high biological value.[79] At this level of renal dysfunction, a balancing act occurs between providing a diet that will ameliorate clinical signs yet will still provide adequate amounts of nutrients. Once a modified diet has been selected and found to be acceptable to the pet, progressive improvement of clinical signs such as a reduction in vomiting, improved appetite, weight gain, and improved physical activity is generally seen within 2 to 4 weeks. Weekly monitoring of BUN and serum creatinine and evaluation of clinical response should be used to determine the need for either increasing or decreasing dietary protein level.

Modification of dietary protein for cats with chronic renal failure must account for the cat's naturally higher protein requirement and its inability to adapt to low-protein diets (see Section 2, pp. 92-95). Although the efficacy of feline renal diets containing several nutrient modifications has been studied in recent years (see pp. 424-425), the effectiveness of restricted protein intake alone in managing clinical signs of chronic renal disease in cats has not been studied extensively. In one study, when cats with naturally occurring renal failure were fed a diet containing either normal or reduced levels of protein and phosphorus, the group fed lower protein and phosphorus exhibited decreasing BUN and serum phosphorus levels over the 6-week study period.[80] However, the health of cats fed both high and low protein and phosphorus deteriorated during the study. Subjective changes in health were assessed as being less severe in the cats fed the restricted diet, but long-term survival and the rate of disease progression were not reported. Moreover, the design of this study (and of subsequent studies) does not allow separation of the effects of low protein from those of reduced phosphorus. A general recommendation is that, similar to dogs, cats with chronic renal failure should be fed the maximum level of protein that will control uremia/azotemia and its associated clinical signs. It is especially important to monitor cats that are consuming reduced protein diets for signs of protein malnutrition.[81] Signs of protein deficiency include hypoalbuminemia, anemia, weight loss, and loss of lean body mass. If these signs occur, dietary protein should be increased to a level that corrects these abnormalities.

In both dogs and cats, the type of protein included in the restricted protein diet is very important. Only protein sources that are highly digestible and of high biological value should be fed. These sources include eggs, dairy products, soy protein isolates, and some lean muscle meats. Poor-quality proteins and ingredients that are not highly digestible should be avoided. The therapeutic diet can be either a commercially prepared renal diet or a homemade diet. Advantages of using a commercially prepared diet include convenience, the assurance of consistency in the formulation, and adequate testing (see pp. 424-425). However, preparing a homemade diet may allow greater flexibility in the level of protein and other nutrients that are included, thus providing a diet that is specifically formulated to meet a pet's individual needs. Homemade diets may also be more palatable for some pets than some commercially prepared products. Because of their tendency to develop anorexia, cats with renal disease should be fed diets that are highly palatable and acceptable. Commercial feline maintenance diets should be avoided because many are formulated to be acidifying and so may contribute to an exacerbation of metabolic acidosis in cats with renal disease. Decisions regarding the type of diet to use can be made based on the veterinarian's recommendation, the pet's response to treatment, and the capabilities and preferences of the owner.

The decision to control protein intake in dogs and cats with chronic renal failure is determined by the patient's clinical signs and degree of impairment of renal function. The highest level of protein that results in an amelioration of clinical signs and controls blood urea nitrogen levels, without compromising protein and amino acid nutrition, should be fed. In cats, modification of dietary protein must also account for the cat's naturally higher protein requirement and its inability to adapt to low-protein diets. Only protein sources that are highly digestible and of high biological value should be fed to pets with renal disease; examples include eggs, dairy products, soy protein isolates, and some lean muscle meats.

Fat

It is important that diets formulated for pets with chronic renal disease contain enough nonprotein calories to spare protein from being used as an energy source. Fat is an excellent energy source for dogs and cats and also promotes diet palatability. The type of fat included in the diet is also very important. Hyperlipidemia has been shown to be causally linked to the progression of chronic renal disease in dogs and other species.[47,51,82] Additionally, hyperlipidemia in dogs with induced renal failure can be ameliorated by feeding a food that is enriched in PUFAs, supplied as either safflower oil or fish oil from cold-water fish species.[83,84] Unsaturated fatty acids in the omega-3 family (e.g., certain marine fish oils, flax oil) may be the preferred source because of the beneficial effects that this class of fatty acids have on intrarenal hemodynamics and inflammation. Diets rich in omega-3 fatty acids may help to slow the progression of this disease in dogs and cats (see pp. 415-416).

It is currently recommended that fatty acid supplements containing omega-6 fatty acids not be administered to pets with chronic renal failure. Conversely, increasing omega-3 fatty acids in the diet may be beneficial. While one method of increasing omega-3 fatty acids is to add a supplement to the diet, another approach is to adjust the ratio of omega-6 to omega-3 fatty acids in the food. Although an ideal ratio for pets with renal disease has not been identified, current evidence suggests that feeding a diet containing a ratio of 5:1 is beneficial.[83]

Phosphorus

The decrease in GFR that occurs during renal failure results in a decreased ability to excrete phosphorus. This decreased ability leads to phosphorus retention, hyperphosphatemia, and renal secondary hyperparathyroidism. These factors are believed to promote the formation of calcium phosphate crystals and the deposition of these crystals in the kidneys and other soft tissues, which may lead to further loss of nephrons and progression of disease (see pp. 414-415).[45,46,85] Additionally, the chronic elevation of PTH that is caused by retention of phosphorus results in excessive demineralization of bone and pathological changes that are associated with bone loss.

A goal of dietary therapy is to normalize serum phosphorus concentration and prevent bone demineralization and deposition of calcium phosphate crystals in soft tissues. In moderate cases of renal disease, when serum phosphorus is slightly elevated, a decrease in the level of phosphorus in the diet may be sufficient to achieve normalization of serum phosphorus. Because dietary protein is a principal source of phosphorus, restriction of protein and the use of reduced phosphorus protein sources contribute to this dietary modification. However, as the disease progresses, dietary restriction does not always control blood phosphorus levels and may not be sufficient to control the long-term effects of secondary hyperparathyroidism and bone disease. Intestinal phosphate-binding agents must then be used in conjunction with reduced dietary phosphorus to normalize the serum phosphorus concentration.[50,74,85] These agents are administered with a meal and limit the gastrointestinal absorption of phosphorus. The compounds most commonly used are aluminum hydroxide and aluminum carbonate.

Blood phosphorus concentration should be monitored regularly, and the pet's food (and when applicable, binding agents) should be adjusted until normalization of serum phosphorus is achieved. Calcium supplementation and vitamin D supplementation should be avoided until serum phosphorus levels are under control. Providing additional calcium in the presence of hyperphosphatemia may further contribute to soft tissue mineralization. Once serum phosphorus concentration has been normalized, calcium and/or vitamin D (calcitriol) can be supplemented to aid in the control of renal hyperparathyroidism and bone disease. Calcium carbonate at a dosage of 100 mg/kg of body weight is recommended.

Although some studies with dogs showed that restriction of dietary phosphorus prevented or reversed renal secondary hyperparathyroidism, most research indicates that dietary restriction alone does not consistently reduce serum PTH levels.[74,86] Moreover, serum phosphorus does not appear to be a sensitive predictor of renal secondary hyperparathyroidism.[74] It has been hypothesized that chronically elevated PTH may be more affected by decreased levels of active vitamin D (calcitriol) than by elevated phosphorus. As kidney function declines, the ability to produce calcitriol is compromised. Subsequently, low calcitriol levels stimulate the release of PTH. It therefore appears that restriction of dietary phosphorus alone may not be sufficient to prevent hyperparathyroidism in some pets with chronic renal failure. Phosphate-binding agents, calcium supplementation, and administration of calcitriol may be necessary to treat the hyperparathyroidism of renal disease in these animals.[87]

A goal of dietary therapy in pets with chronic renal disease is to normalize serum phosphorus concentration and control or reverse secondary hyperparathyroidism. In moderate cases of renal disease, when serum phosphorus is slightly elevated, a decrease in the level of phosphorus in the diet may be sufficient to achieve normalization of serum phosphorus. However, as the disease progresses, intestinal phosphate-binding agents are often needed. Compounds most commonly used are aluminum hydroxide and aluminum carbonate. Once hyperphosphatemia is controlled, calcium supplementation and administration of calcitriol may be initiated.

Dietary Fiber

The reduced ability of the kidneys to excrete nitrogenous end products of protein catabolism is a major cause of the uremic signs and laboratory abnormalities seen in animals with chronic renal failure. As discussed previously, providing moderately reduced dietary protein that is of very high quality can decrease the body's need to oxidize dietary amino acids and excrete the nitrogenous end products. An additional approach to managing nitrogen excretion is to alter the route of excretion. There is evidence showing that the amount and type of fiber included in the diet influences nitrogen excretion and urea concentrations in the blood. Specifically, feeding fermentable fiber alters the flux of urea and ammonia in the large intestine and cecum, resulting in a shift of urea excretion from the kidneys via urine to the large intestine via feces. Because an alternative route of urea excretion is available, BUN values decrease. Feeding fermentable fibers has been shown to cause a repartitioning of nitrogen into the feces of several species, including humans, rats, dogs, and cats.[88-92]

The underlying mechanism involves the effects of dietary fiber on bacterial growth in the gastrointestinal tract. Feeding fermentable fiber results in increases in bacterial growth and activity in the large intestine. This is accompanied by increased colonic blood flow, tissue weights, surface area, and nitrogen excretion.[91,93-95] The increased fecal nitrogen is primarily due to excretion of a greater proportion of bacterial mass. The intestinal bacteria that proliferate synthesize the enzyme urease, which converts urea to ammonia and carbon dioxide. The ammonia is subsequently used by bacteria as a source of nitrogen for protein synthesis. This process functions to remove urea nitrogen from circulation and incorporate it into bacterial protein, which is ultimately excreted via the feces (Figure 32-2).

The effect of fermentable fiber on patterns of nitrogen excretion has been studied in dogs. When healthy adult dogs were fed a diet containing a blend of fermentable fibers (beet pulp, fructooligosaccharides [FOS], and gum arabic), apparent digestibility of dry matter (DM) and organic matter decreased slightly due to excretion of nonfermentable fiber components and increased bacterial mass.[43] This was accompanied by a

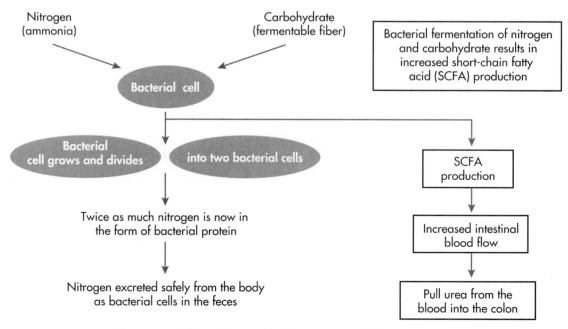

Figure 32-2   Effect of fermentable fiber on patterns of nitrogen excretion.
(From *New concepts in management of renal failure*, Dayton, Ohio, 1998, The Iams Company.)

slight decrease in apparent protein digestibility (91.3% versus 88.2%). Dogs fed the fiber-containing diet had excellent stool scores, with no adverse effects such as diarrhea or formation of soft stools. Changes in protein digestibility due to feeding fermentable fibers to dogs have been shown to be caused by the increased excretion of bacterial nitrogen as opposed to a decreased digestibility of dietary protein within the small intestine.[91,96] These results support the theory that fermentable fiber can be used to repartition nitrogen excretion through intestinal bacterial protein in dogs.

The efficacy of repartitioning nitrogen excretion using fermentable fiber in the diet for dogs with chronic renal disease has also been examined. Because fermentable fiber is capable of repartitioning nitrogen excretory patterns away from the kidneys and toward the large intestine, it is possible that more dietary protein can be fed without negatively impacting azotemia and its associated signs. When dogs with experimentally induced renal insufficiency were fed either a control food or a food supplemented with a fermentable fiber blend, GFR was unchanged, while BUN values and urinary excretion of urea nitrogen decreased (Figures 32-3 and 32-4).[97] Because there was no change in renal function, this indicates that the reduced concentration of urea in the blood was a result of enhanced fecal nitrogen excretion.

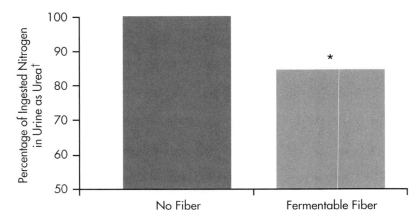

Figure 32-3   Effect of feeding fermentable fiber on percent nitrogen in urine. *, P <.05; †, expressed as a percent of no-fiber value. (From World Small Animal Veterinary Association: *Clinical nutrition symposium proceedings*, Dayton, Ohio, 1998, The Iams Company.)

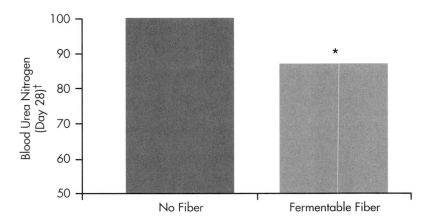

Figure 32-4   Effect of feeding fermentable fiber on blood urea nitrogen. *, P <.05; †, expressed as a percent of no-fiber value. (From World Small Animal Veterinary Association: *Clinical nutrition symposium proceedings*, Dayton, Ohio, 1998, The Iams Company.)

In another study, the clinical response to feeding a low- or moderate-protein diet containing a fermentable fiber blend to dogs in various stages of chronic renal failure was examined.[98] All of the dogs in the study had previously been fed a conventional renal diet that was severely restricted in protein (14% DM). At the start of the study, the dogs were switched to either a moderate-protein (21.1%) or low-protein (17.5%) renal diet, based upon initial BUN and creatinine values. In addition to fiber content and higher protein level, the two experimental diets also had an adjusted omega-6 to omega-3 fatty acid ratio of approximately 5:1, compared with a ratio of 22:1 in the conventional renal diet. All of the foods also contained reduced levels of phosphorus. Blood chemistries, hematocrit and hemoglobin counts, and overall health were monitored for a 10-week period and compared with values collected at the start of the study.

Results indicated that the inclusion of dietary fiber in the two experimental renal diets successfully partitioned nitrogen excretion away from the kidneys. For example, none of the dogs fed the moderate protein had increased BUN values, and two showed reduced blood ammonia values, even though the diet contained approximately 50% more protein than the conventional renal diet that had previously been fed. It appears that adequate protein to meet the nutritional recommendation for adult maintenance was provided to these dogs without the side effect of exacerbating azotemia. The dogs also showed a trend toward lower serum triglyceride values presumed to be a result of the lower percentage of calories provided by fat and the adjusted omega-6 to omega-3 fatty acid ratio. Owners reported an overall improvement in the quality of their dog's coat in all of the reported cases, again reflecting better protein nutrition in these dogs. The dogs with more advanced renal disease were fed the second experimental renal diet, which contained approximately 25% more protein than the conventional renal diet. Similar to the first group of dogs, these dogs either maintained or lowered BUN and creatinine values over the 10-week period.

These results suggest that including a blend of fermentable fiber sources in the diet of dogs with chronic renal failure is efficacious because it can allow higher levels of protein to be fed to uremic dogs, thus providing optimal protein nutrition and preventing the development of protein deficiency. Dogs tolerate a blend of fermentable fibers with no adverse effects on gastrointestinal function or fecal score. Although less research has been conducted with cats, there is evidence that including moderate levels fermentable fibers in cats' diets results in increased fecal nitrogen and decreased urinary nitrogen excretion, suggesting a repartitioning of nitrogen that would be beneficial for cats with renal disease.[99]

Other Nutrients

Additional nutrients that are of concern in the diets of dogs and cats with renal disease include sodium, potassium, the water-soluble vitamins, and, possibly, bicarbonate. The major route of sodium excretion in dogs is through the urine.[100] Hypertension is commonly diagnosed in dogs and cats with renal disease and has been associated with disease progression.[101,102] The risk of experiencing a uremic crisis also increases in hypertensive dogs with renal disease. However, restriction of dietary sodium as an approach to controlling hypertension associated with kidney disease has not been shown to be singularly effective in dogs and cats.[103,104] Moreover, pets with renal disease demonstrate limited renal responsiveness and have a decreased tolerance to sudden changes of sodium content in the diet.[68] Therefore, while renal diets for dogs and cats often contain normal or moderately reduced sodium concentrations, the recommended treatment for high blood pressure is usually medical, rather than dietary.[9]

Potassium deficiency (hypokalemia) is seen in cats with chronic renal failure as a result of increased urinary loss and reduced intake, but is rare in dogs with renal disease.[70,105] However, because not all cats with chronic renal failure are hypokalemic, potassium status should be monitored closely and dietary potassium intake adjusted on an individual basis. Potassium can be added as a dietary supplement as potassium gluconate or potassium citrate, or can be added to subcutaneous fluids when necessary.[106] In both dogs and cats, when polyuria is present, supplementation with water-soluble vitamins is advisable because of excessive losses of these vitamins in the urine.

Antioxidant vitamins may also be beneficial. The tissues of cats with spontaneous renal disease that were fed a renal diet that included increased concentrations of vitamin E, vitamin C, and beta-carotene had significantly reduced oxidative deoxyribonucleic acid (DNA) damage.[107] It is known that human subjects with chronic renal disease have increased free radical production and reduced antioxidant status, changes that may contribute to disease progression.[108] Supplementation with antioxidant vitamins reduces measures of oxidative stress in humans with kidney disease.[109] Although it has not been demonstrated in dogs and cats, there is evidence from studies with rats that supplementation with vitamin E slows renal disease progression.[110]

Reduced renal mass is associated with an increase in the production of ammonia by the renal tubules. This results in a rise in renal tissue ammonia concentration, which can cause local toxic and inflammatory effects and further contribute to renal damage.[76] In severe cases, systemic metabolic acidosis may occur as a result of compromised capacity to regulate acid-base balance. Supplementation with sodium bicarbonate or potassium citrate may ameliorate some of the damage as a result of increased ammonia production in the kidneys and will aid in the treatment of metabolic acidosis. A dosage of 5 to 10 grains of sodium bicarbonate, given orally every 10 to 12 hours, is recommended (Box 32-3).

Additional nutrients that are of concern for dogs and cats with renal disease include sodium, potassium, the water-soluble and antioxidant vitamins, and, possibly, bicarbonate. Renal diets for dogs and cats contain normal or moderately reduced sodium concentrations to help to control high blood pressure (although the principal treatment is medical). Dietary potassium intake is adjusted on an individual basis and is supplemented as needed. When polyuria is present, supplementation with water-soluble vitamins is advisable. Antioxidant vitamins (vitamin E, vitamin C, and beta-carotene) may also be beneficial. Finally, supplementation with sodium bicarbonate or potassium citrate aids in the control of metabolic acidosis.

Efficacy of Dietary Management (Clinical Studies)

Commercial prescription diets for the management of chronic renal disease in dogs and cats are typically formulated to include moderately reduced protein

---

BOX 32-3 PRACTICAL FEEDING TIPS: DIETARY MANAGEMENT OF CHRONIC KIDNEY DISEASE

Provide the highest dietary protein that will maintain a blood urea nitrogen of less than 60.

Provide a highly digestible, high–biological value protein source.

Provide an adequate amount of nonprotein calories.

Restrict dietary phosphorus and regularly monitor serum phosphorus level.

Feed a diet that has an adjusted omega-6 to omega-3 fatty acid ratio of 5:1.

Feed a diet containing a moderate level of fermentable fiber to aid in the control of azotemia.

Provide intestinal phosphate binding agents, if necessary.

When necessary, provide supplemental calcium and active vitamin D (calcitriol) once serum phosphorus is normalized.

Monitor intake of sodium bicarbonate, potassium, and water-soluble vitamins closely.

Adjust diet as necessary.

---

that is of high biological value, restricted phosphorus, increased omega-3 fatty acids (and in some, an adjusted omega-6 to omega-3 fatty acid ratio), and normal or moderately reduced sodium. In recent years, controlled clinical studies have been conducted to examine the efficacy of these foods when fed to pets with naturally occurring renal disease.

In a double-blind, controlled study of 38 dogs with naturally occurring renal disease, half of the dogs were fed a commercial maintenance diet and half of the dogs a prescription renal diet, all for 24 months.[111] Dogs fed the renal diet had significantly fewer uremic episodes, reduced risk of death from renal disease, and an increased median interval of time before experiencing their first uremic emergency when compared with dogs fed the maintenance food. Median survival time in dogs fed the renal diet was three times longer than the survival time of dogs that were fed the maintenance food.

Similar positive results have been reported in cats. When a group of 50 cats with stable, naturally occurring renal disease were fed either a prescription renal food (reduced protein, low phosphate) with or without an intestinal phosphate binding agent, or their normal, non-prescription maintenance diet, the 29 cats fed the renal diet had a significantly longer median survival time than cats fed their normal food (633 days versus 264 days).[112] In another study, cats with stage 2 or stage 3 kidney disease were fed either an adult maintenance diet or a renal diet. Similar to the study with dogs, feeding a renal diet significantly reduced the number of uremic crises and significantly extended lifespan and reduced mortality in cats with spontaneous renal disease.[113] Finally, a retrospective study of survival times in cats fed seven different prescription renal diets, or the pets' conventional maintenance diet, reported that all of the renal diets resulted in longer survival times and owner-reported improvement in quality of life in cats with renal disease when compared with cats with renal disease that were fed maintenance diets.[114] An interesting correlation found in this study was that the food that was associated with the longest survival time (~23 months) also contained the highest level of the omega-3 fatty acid, eicosapentaenoic acid.

Collectively, these studies show that dietary management is an indispensable component of the treatment protocol for pets with chronic renal disease. The primary dietary modifications include changes in protein, phosphorus, fats, and essential vitamin levels. Once an appropriate food has been selected, regular and consistent monitoring of the patient's response is essential for continued well-being and long-term management. It is generally recommended that dogs and cats with chronic renal disease be reevaluated within 2 weeks of initial diagnosis and beginning dietary treatment. Biweekly visits should continue until the pet has stabilized and has accepted the dietary change. Once the pet has stabilized, veterinary assessments can be conducted every 3 months, and continue to be crucial for successful management for the remainder of the pet's life.

References

1. Polzin DJ, Osborne CA, Bartges JW, and others: Chronic renal failure. In Ettinger SJ, Feldman EC, editors: *Textbook of veterinary internal medicine*, ed 4, Philadelphia, 1995, Saunders.

2. Squires RA: Uraemia. In Bainbridge J, Elliott J, editors: *BSAVA manual of canine and feline nephrology and urology*, Ames, Iowa, 1996, Iowa State University Press.

3. Ross LA, Finco DR: Relationship of selected clinical renal function tests to glomerular filtration rate and renal blood flow in cats, *Am J Vet Res* 42:1023–1026, 1981.

4. Langston CE, May SN: Managing chronic renal failure, *Compend Contin Educ Pract Vet* 28:853–861, 2006.

5. Reinhart GA, Sunvold GD: New methods for managing canine chronic renal failure. In *Proc Cong World Small Anim Vet Assoc*, 1998, pp 46–51.

6. Bovee KC: The uremic syndrome: patient evaluation and treatment, *Compend Contin Educ Pract Vet* 1:279–283, 1979.

7. Krawiec DR: Quantitative renal function tests in cats, *Compend Contin Educ Pract Vet* 16:1279–1284, 1994.

8. Carey DP: Clinical assessment of chronic renal failure. In Reinhart GA, Carey DP, editors: *Recent advances in canine and feline nutrition, Iams nutrition symposium proceedings*, vol 2, Wilmington, Ohio, 1998, Orange Frazer Press.

9. International Renal Interest Society: *Staging of CKD and treatment recommendations* (website). http://www.iris-kidney.com. Accessed 2006.

10. Finco DR, Coulter DB, Barsanti JA: Simple, accurate method for clinical estimation of glomerular filtration rate in the dog, *Am J Vet Res* 42:1874–1877, 1981.

11. Finco DR, Brown SC, Crowell WA, and others: Exogenous creatinine clearance as a measure of glomerular filtration rate in dogs with reduced renal mass, *Am J Vet Res* 52:1029–1032, 1991.

12. Watson ADJ, Lefebre HP, Laroute V, and others: Comparison of clearance tests to assess glomerular filtration rate in dogs. In *Proc Ann Conf Vet Intern Med Forum*, 1998, p 711.

13. Brown SA, Finco DR, Boudinot FD: Evaluation of a single injection method, using inoxol, for estimating glomerular filtration rate in cats and dogs, *Am J Vet Res* 57:105–110, 1996.

14. Nolan BG, Ross LA, Vaccaro DE, and others: Estimation of glomerular filtration rate in dogs by plasma clearance of gadolinium diethylenetriamine pentaacetic acid as measured by use of an ELISA, *Am J Vet Res* 70:547–552, 2009.

15. Brown SA, Finco DR, Crowell WA, and others: Dietary protein intake and the glomerular adaptations to partial nephrectomy in dogs, *J Nutr* 121:S125–S127, 1991.

16. Brown SA, Finco D, Crowell WA: Single-nephron adaptations to partial renal ablation in the dog, *Am J Physiol* 258:F495–F503, 1990.

17. Churchill J, Polzin D, Osborne C, and others: The influence of dietary protein intake on progression of chronic renal failure in dogs, *Semin Vet Med Surg Small Anim* 7:244–250, 1992.

18. Anderson S, Brenner BM: The role of intraglomerular pressure in the initiation and progression of renal disease, *J Hypertens* 4(Suppl 5):S236–S238, 1986.

19. Brenner BM, Meyer TW, Hostetter TH: Dietary protein intake and the progressive nature of renal disease: the role of hemodynamically mediated glomerular injury in the pathogenesis of progressive glomerular sclerosis in aging, renal ablation and intrinsic renal disease, *N Engl J Med* 307:652–659, 1982.

20. Shimamura T, Morrison AB: A progressive glomerulosclerosis occurring in partial five-sixths nephrectomized rats, *Am J Pathol* 79:95–106, 1975.

21. Brown SA, Brown CA: Single-nephron adaptations to partial renal ablation in cats, *Am J Physiol* 269:R1002–R1008, 1995.

22. Gonin-Jmaa D, Senior DF: The hyperfiltration theory: progression of chronic renal failure and the effects of diet in dogs, *J Am Vet Med Assoc* 207:1411–1415, 1995.

23. Finco DR, Crowell WA, Barsanti JA: Effects of three diets on dogs with induced chronic renal failure, *Am J Vet Res* 46:646–653, 1985.

24. Polzin DJ, Leininger JR, Osborne CA, and others: Development of renal lesions in dogs after 11/12 reduction in renal mass, *Lab Invest* 58:172–183, 1988.

25. Brown SA, Walton C, Crawford P, and others: Long-term effects of anti-hypertensive regimens on renal hemodynamics and proteinuria in diabetic dogs, *Kidney Int* 43:1210–1218, 1993.

26. Gaber L, Walton C, Brown S, and others: Effects of antihypertensive agents on the morphologic progression of diabetic nephropathy in dogs, *Kidney Int* 46:161–169, 1994.

27. Bourgoignie JJ, Gavellas G, Martinex E, and others: Glomerular function and morphology after renal mass reduction in dogs, *Lab Clin Med* 109:380–388, 1987.

28. Maeda H, Gleiser CA, Masoro EJ, and others: Nutritional influences on aging of Fischer 344 rats. II. Pathology, *J Gerontol* 40:671–688, 1985.

29. Masoro EJ, Iwasaki K, Gleiser CA, and others: Dietary modulation of the progression of nephropathy in aging rats: an evaluation of the importance of protein, *Am J Clin Nutr* 49:1217–1227, 1989.

30. Bovee KC, Kronfeld DS, Ramberg CF, and others: Long term measurement of renal function in partially nephrectomized dogs fed 56, 27 or 19% protein, *Invest Nephrol* 16:378–385, 1979.

31. Robertson JL, Goldschmidt M, Kronfeld DS, and others: Long term renal responses to high dietary protein in dogs with 75% nephrectomy, *Kidney Int* 29:511–519, 1986.

32. Polzin DJ, Osborne CA, Hayden DW: Influence of reduced protein diets on morbidity, mortality, and renal function in dogs with induced chronic renal failure, *Am J Vet Res* 45:506–517, 1984.

33. Tucker SM, Mason RL, Beauchene RE: Influence of diet and feed restriction on kidney function of aging male rats, *J Gerontol* 31:264–270, 1976.

34. Berg BN, Simms HS: Nutrition and longevity in the rat. II. Longevity and onset of disease with different levels of food intake, *J Nutr* 71:255–263, 1960.

35. Tapp DC, Kobayoshu S, Fernandes S: Protein restriction or calorie restriction? A critical assessment of the influence of selective calorie restriction on the progression of experimental renal disease, *Semin Nephrol* 9:343–353, 1989.

36. White JV, Finco DR, Brown SA, and others: Effect of dietary protein on kidney function, morphology, and histopathology during compensatory renal growth in dogs, *Am J Vet Res* 52:1357–1365, 1990.

37. Adams LG, Polzin DJ, Osborne CA, and others: Effects of dietary protein and calorie restriction in clinically normal cats and in cats with surgically induced chronic renal failure, *Am J Vet Res* 54:1653–1662, 1993.

38. Finco DR, Brown SC, Brown CA, and others: Protein and calorie effects on progression of induced chronic renal failure in cats, *Am J Vet Res* 59:575–582, 1998.

39. Finco DR: Renal function in geriatric dogs—are there dietary protein effects? *Vet Clin Nutr* 1:66–68, 1994.

40. Sheffy BE, Williams AJ, Zimmer JF, and others: Nutrition and metabolism of the geriatric dog, *Cornell Vet* 75:324–347, 1985.

41. Finco DR, Brown SA, Crowell WA, and others: Effects of aging and dietary protein intake on uninephrectomized geriatric dogs, *Am J Vet Res* 55:1282–1290, 1994.

42. Osborne CA, Polzin DJ, Abdullahi S, and others: Role of diet in management of feline chronic polyuric renal failure: current status, *J Am Anim Hosp Assoc* 18:11–20, 1982.

43. Reinhart GA, Sunvold GD: New methods for managing chronic renal failure. In *Proc North Am Vet Conf*, Orlando, Fla, 1998, pp 17–20.

44. Laflamme DP: Pet food safety: dietary protein, *Top Companion Anim Med* 23:154–157, 2008.

45. Polzin DJ, Osborne CA, Lulich JP: Effects of dietary protein/phosphate restriction in normal dogs and dogs with chronic renal failure, *J Small Anim Pract* 32:289–295, 1991.

46. Lau K: Phosphate excess and progressive renal failure: the precipitation-calcification hypothesis, *Kidney Int* 36:918–937, 1989.

47. Brown SA, Crowell WA, Barsanti JA: Beneficial effects of dietary mineral restriction in dogs with marked reduction of functional renal mass, *J Am Soc Nephrol* 1:1169–1179, 1991.

48. Finco DR, Brown SA, Crowell WA, and others: Effect of phosphorus/calcium-restricted and phosphorus/calcium-replete 32% protein diets in dogs with chronic renal failure, *Am J Vet Res* 53:157–163, 1992.

49. Finco DR, Brown SC, Crowell WA, and others: Effects of dietary phosphorus and protein in dogs with chronic renal failure, *Am J Vet Res* 153:2264–2271, 1992.

50. Ross LA, Finco DR, Crowell WA: Effect of dietary phosphorus restriction on the kidneys of cats with reduced renal mass, *Am J Vet Res* 43:1023–1026, 1982.

51. French SW, Yamanaka W, Ostwald R: Dietary induced glomerulosclerosis in the guinea pig, *Arch Pathol* 83:204–210, 1967.

52. Heifets M, Morrissey JJ, Parkerson ML, and others: Effect of dietary lipids on renal function in rats with subtotal nephrectomy, *Kidney Int* 32:335–341, 1987.

53. Brown SA: Managing chronic renal failure: the role of dietary polyunsaturated fatty acids. In *Proc NAVC*, Orlando, Fla, 1998, pp 5–8.

54. Fries JWU, Sandstrom DJ, Meyer TW, and others: Glomerular hypertrophy and epithelial cell injury modulate progressive glomerulosclerosis in the rat, *Lab Invest* 60:205–218, 1989.

55. Barcelli U, Miyata J, Ito Y, and others: Beneficial effects of polyunsaturated fatty acids in partially nephrectomized rats, *Prostaglandins* 32:211–219, 1986.

56. Clark WF, Parbani A, Philbrick DJ, and others: Chronic effects of omega-3 fatty acids (fish oil) in a rat 5/6 renal ablation model, *J Am Soc Nephrol* 1:1343–1353, 1991.

57. Logan JL, Michael UF, Benson B: Dietary fish oil interferes with renal arachidonic acid metabolism in rats: correlation with renal physiology, *Metabolism* 41:382–389, 1992.

58. Donadio JV, Bergstralh EJ, Offord KP, and others: A controlled trial of fish oil in IgA nephropathy, *N Engl J Med* 331:1194–1199, 1994.

59. Clark WF, Parabtani A, Maylor CD, and others: Fish oil in lupus nephritis: clinical findings and methodological implications, *Kidney Int* 44:75–86, 1993.

60. Brown SA: Influence of dietary fatty acids on intrarenal hypertension. In Reinhart GA, Carey DP, editors: *Recent advances in canine and feline nutrition, Iams nutrition symposium proceedings,* vol 2, Wilmington, Ohio, 1998, Orange Frazer Press.

61. Bauer JE, Markwell PJ, Rawlings JM: Effects of dietary fat and polyunsaturated fatty acids in dogs with naturally developing chronic renal failure, *J Am Vet Med Assoc* 215:1588–1591, 1999.

62. Brown SA, Brown CA, Crowell WA, and others: Beneficial effects of chronic administration of dietary omega-3 polyunsaturated fatty acids in dogs with renal insufficiency, *J Lab Clin Med* 131:447–455, 1998.

63. Bauer J, Crocker R, Markwell P, and others: Dietary n-6 fatty acid supplementation improves ultrafiltration in spontaneous canine chronic renal failure (abstract), *J Vet Intern Med* 11:2, 1997.

64. Dworkin L, Benstein J, Tolbert E, and others: Salt restriction inhibits renal growth and stabilizes injury in rats with established renal disease, *J Am Soc Nephrol* 7:437–442, 1996.

65. Greco DS, Les GE, Dzendzel G: Effect of dietary sodium intake on glomerular filtration rate in partially nephrectomized dogs, *Am J Vet Res* 55:152–159, 1994.

66. Burankarl C, Amathur S, Cartier L: Effects of dietary sodium chloride (NaCl) supplementation on renal function and blood pressure in normal cats and in cats with induced renal insufficiency. In *Proc 28th World Cong WSAVA,* October 24, 2003.

67. Hughes KL, Slater MR, Geller S: Diet and lifestyle variables as risk factors for chronic renal failure in pet cats, *Prev Vet Med* 55:1–15, 2002.

68. Elliott DA: Nutritional management of chronic renal disease in dogs and cats, *Vet Clin North Am Small Anim Pract* 36:1377–1384, 2006.

69. Lulich J, Osborne C, O'Brien T, and others: Feline renal failure: questions, answers, questions, *Compend Contin Educ Pract Vet* 14:127–152, 1992.

70. Dow SW, Fettman MJ, Smith KR, and others: Effects of dietary acidification and potassium depletion on acid-base balance, mineral metabolism, and renal function in adult cats, *J Nutr* 120:569–578, 1990.

71. Langston CE: Managing chronic renal failure, *Compend Contin Educ Pract Vet* 28:123–128, 2006.

72. Finco DR: Chronic renal failure: dietary protein and phosphorus. In *Proc NAVC,* Orlando, Fla, 1998, pp 9–10.

73. Carey DP: Clinical assessment of chronic renal failure. In Reinhart GA, Carey DP, editors: *Recent advances in canine and feline nutrition, Iams nutrition symposium proceedings,* vol 2, Wilmington, Ohio, 1998, Orange Frazer Press.

74. Hansen B, DiBartola SP, Chew DJ, and others: Clinical and metabolic findings in dogs with chronic renal failure fed two diets, *Am J Vet Res* 53:326–334, 1992.

75. National Research Council: *Nutrient requirements of dogs and cats,* Washington, DC, 2006, National Academy Press.

76. Polzin DJ, Osborne CA: Current progress in slowing progression of canine and feline chronic renal failure, *Comp Anim Pract* 3:52–62, 1988.

77. Bovee KC: Diet and kidney failure. In *Kal Kan symposium for the treatment of dog and cat diseases,* Vernon, Calif, 1977.

78. Polzin DJ, Osborne CA, Stevens JB, and others: Influence of modified protein diets on the nutritional status of dogs with induced chronic renal failure, *Am J Vet Res* 44:1694–1702, 1983.

79. Devaux C, Polzin DJ, Osborne CA: What role does dietary protein play in the management of chronic renal failure in dogs? *Vet Clin North Am Small Anim Pract* 26:1247–1267, 1996.

80. Harte J, Markwell P, Moraillion R, and others: Dietary management of naturally occurring chronic renal failure in cats, *J Nutr* 124:2660S–2662S, 1994.

81. Polzin DJ, Osborne CA, Lulich JP: Diet therapy guidelines for cats with chronic renal failure, *Vet Clin North Am Small Anim Pract* 26:1269–1275, 1996.

82. Keane WF, Kasiske BL, O'Donnell MP: Hyperlipidemia and the progression of renal disease, *Am J Clin Nutr* 47:157–160, 1987.

83. Brown SC, Brown CA, Crowell WA, and others: Does modifying dietary lipids influence the progression of renal failure? *Vet Clin North Am Small Anim Pract* 26:1277–1285, 1996.

84. Brown SC, Brown CA, Crowell WA, and others: Effects of dietary polyunsaturated fatty acid supplementation in early renal insufficiency in dogs, *J Lab Clin Med* 135:275–286, 2000.

85. Barber PJ, Rawlings JM, Markwell PJ: Effect of dietary phosphate restriction on renal secondary hyperparathyroidism in the cat, *J Small Anim Pract* 40:62–70, 1999.

86. Kaplan MA, Canterbury JM, Bourgoignie JJ: Reversal of hyperparathyroidism in response to dietary phosphorus restriction in the uremic dog, *Kidney Int* 15:43–48, 1979.

87. Nagode LA, Chew DJ, Podell M: Benefits of calcitriol therapy and serum phosphorus control in dogs and cats with chronic renal failure, *Vet Clin North Am Small Anim Pract* 26:1293–1331, 1996.

88. Titens I, Livesey G, Eggum BO: Effects of the type and level of dietary fibre supplements on nitrogen retention and excretion patterns, *Br J Nutr* 75:461–469, 1996.

89. Younes H, Remesey C, Behr S, and others: Fermentable carbohydrate exerts a urea-lowering effect in normal and nephrectomized rats, *Am J Physiol* 272:G515–G525, 1997.

90. Bliss DZ, Stein TP, Schleifer CR, and others: Supplementation with gum arabic fiber increases fecal nitrogen excretion and lowers serum urea nitrogen concentration in chronic renal failure patients consuming a low-protein diet, *Am J Clin Nutr* 63:392–398, 1996.

91. Howard MD, Sunvold GD, Reinhart GA, and others: Effect of fermentable fiber consumption by the dog on nitrogen balance and fecal microbial nitrogen excretion, *FASEB J* 10:A257, 1996.

92. Vickers RJ, Sunvold GA, Reinhart GA: Effect of selected fiber blends on repartitioning of nitrogen disposal in the cat. In *Proc 9th Ann ESVIM Forum*, 1999, pp 178–179.

93. Sunvold GD, Fahey GC Jr, Merchen NR, and others: Dietary fiber for dogs. IV. In vitro fermentation of selected fiber sources by dog fecal inoculum and in vivo digestion and metabolism of fiber-supplemented diets, *J Anim Sci* 73:1099–1109, 1995.

94. Hallman JE, Moxley RA, Reinhart GA, and others: Cellulose, beet pulp and pectin/gum arabic effects on canine colonic microstructure and histopathology, *J Vet Clin Nutr* 2:137–142, 1995.

95. Howard MD, Kerley MS, Mann FA, and others: Dietary fiber sources alter colonic blood flow and epithelial cell proliferation of dogs, *J Anim Sci* 75:170, 1997.

96. Muir HE, Murray SM, Fahey GC Jr, and others: Nutrient digestion by ileal cannulated dogs as affected by dietary fibers with various fermentation characteristics, *J Anim Sci* 74:1641–1648, 1996.

97. Brown SA, Reinhart GA, Haag M, and others: Influence of dietary fermentable fiber on nitrogen excretion in dogs with chronic renal insufficiency. In Reinhart GA, Carey DP, editors: *Recent advances in canine and feline nutrition, Iams nutrition symposium proceedings,* vol 2, Wilmington, Ohio, 1998, Orange Frazer Press.

98. Tetrick MA, Sunvold GD, Reinhart GA: Clinical experience with canine renal patients fed a diet containing a fermentable fiber blend. In Reinhart GA, Carey DP, editors: *Recent advances in canine and feline nutrition, Iams nutrition symposium proceedings,* vol 2, Wilmington, Ohio, 1998, Orange Frazer Press.

99. Sunvold GD, Vickers RJ, Reinhart GA: Effect of fermentable fiber blends on nitrogen repartitioning in the feline. In *Proc NAVC*, 2000, pp 20–24.

100. Smith RC, Haschem T, Hamlin RL, and others: Water and electrolyte intake and output and quantity of feces in the healthy dog, *Vet Med Small Anim Clin* 59:743–748, 1964.

101. Syme HM, Barber PJ, Markwell PJ: Prevalence of systolic hypertension in cats with chronic renal failure at initial evaluation, *J Am Vet Med Assoc* 220:1799–1804, 2002.

102. Jacob F, Polzin DJ, Osborne CA: Association between initial systolic blood pressure and risk of developing an uremic crisis or of dying in dogs with chronic renal failure, *J Am Vet Med Assoc* 222:322–329, 2003.

103. Greco DS, Lees GE, Dzendzel G: Effects of dietary sodium intake on blood pressure measurements in partially nephrectomized dogs, *Am J Vet Res* 55:160–165, 1994.

104. Burankarl C, Mathur S, Cartier L: Effects of dietary sodium chloride (NaCl) supplementation on renal function and blood pressure in normal cats and cats with induced renal insufficiency. In *Proc WSAVA*, October 2003.

105. Polzin DJ, Osborne CA, Ross S: Dietary management of feline chronic renal failure: where are we now? In what direction are we headed? *J Feline Med Surg* 3:75–82, 2000.

106. Polzin DJ, Osborne CA, Ross S: Chronic kidney disease. In Ettinger SJ, Feldman EC, editors: *Textbook of veterinary internal medicine*, ed 6, St Louis, 2005, Saunders.

107. Yu S, Paetau-Robinson I: Dietary supplements of vitamins E and C and betacarotene reduce oxidative stress in cats with renal insufficiency, *Vet Res Commun* 30:403–413, 2006.

108. Hasselwander O, Young IS: Oxidative stress in chronic renal failure, *Free Radical Res* 29:1–11, 1998.

109. Peuchant E, Delmas-Beauvieux MC, Dubourg L: Antioxidant effects of a supplemented very low protein diet in chronic renal failure, *Free Radical Biol Med* 22:313–320, 1997.

110. Hahn S, Krieg RJ Jr, Hisano S: Vitamin E suppresses oxidative stress and glomerulosclerosis in rat remnant kidney, *Pediatr Nephrol* 13:195–198, 1999.

111. Jacob F, Polzin DJ, Osborne CA, and others: Clinical evaluation of dietary modification for treatment of spontaneous chronic renal failure in dogs, *J Am Vet Med Assoc* 220:1163–1170, 2002.

112. Elliott J, Rawlings JM, Markwell PJ: Survival of cats with naturally occurring chronic renal failure: effect of dietary management, *J Small Anim Pract* 41:235–242, 2000.

113. Ross SJ, Osborne CA, Kirk CA, and others: Clinical evaluation of dietary modification for treatment of spontaneous chronic kidney disease in cats, *J Am Vet Med Assoc* 229:949–957, 2006.

114. Plantinga EA, Everts H, Kastelein AMC, Beynen AC: Retrospective study of the survival of cats with acquired chronic renal insufficiency offered different commercial diets, *Vet Rec* 157:185–187, 2005.

33

Feline Hepatic Lipidosis

Feline hepatic lipidosis (FHL) is an acquired disorder caused by the excessive accumulation of triglycerides in the cells of the liver, which ultimately interferes with the liver's ability to function.[1] It is one of the most common hepatobiliary disorders of cats and was historically associated with a very high mortality rate.[2,3] However, the long-term prognosis of cats with hepatic lipidosis has dramatically improved, due in large part to the use of early and aggressive tube feeding, which successfully reverses the condition in many cats.[4,5] Still, the underlying cause of hepatic lipidosis is not completely understood. Its onset is almost universally preceded by a period of anorexia and most, but not all, cats that develop FHL are overweight or obese.[6] Less commonly, hepatic lipidosis occurs secondarily to other pathological conditions such as inflammatory bowel disease, renal disease, or diabetes mellitus.

INCIDENCE AND CAUSE

In healthy animals, a dynamic relationship exists among the fatty acids that are located in adipose tissue, traveling in the blood, and stored in the liver. Circulating fatty acids are taken up by the liver, where they are either metabolized for energy or converted to triglycerides and secreted back into the circulation. If the supply of fatty acids to the liver exceeds the liver's capacity to oxidize or secrete them, lipidosis develops.[7] Several studies support the theory that the origin of excess hepatic triglycerides in cats with FHL is from fatty acids mobilized from adipose tissue.[8-10] Metabolic changes that may contribute to hepatic lipidosis include impaired mitochondrial or peroxisomal oxidation of fatty acids in hepatocytes and reduced liver secretion of the very–low-density lipoproteins (VLDLs) that carry triglycerides in the bloodstream. Support for reduced fatty acid oxidation is provided from a study of induced FHL in adult female cats.[11] Cats began to accumulate hepatic lipids during the weight gain phase of the study, and this increase was associated with a reduction in mitochondrial numbers in liver cells. Liver lipid accumulation continued during the weight loss stage of the study, presumably as a result of impaired fatty acid oxidation. Another study reported that overweight cats experiencing rapid weight loss did not demonstrate reduced VLDL transport from the liver, nor was there a pronounced increase in triglyceride synthesis.[12] Most researchers agree that the pathogenesis of FHL is probably multifactorial, involving factors that affect fatty-acid mobilization to the liver as well as the oxidation of fatty acids or synthesis and, possibly, secretion of VLDLs.[3,4]

FHL is relatively common and is usually seen in middle-aged cats with a history of obesity. Females are reported to be twice as likely to be affected as males, but this may reflect a higher incidence of obesity in the females that were studied, rather than a true gender difference.[6] There is also evidence that spayed females tend to consume more food, which may predispose them to overweight conditions.[13] In the majority of cases, a cat will have experienced a period of stress followed by partial or complete anorexia. Although obesity in cats is not consistently associated with hepatic accumulation of lipids, the metabolic changes caused by prolonged fasting can lead to rapid and severe hepatic fat accumulation and the clinical signs associated with liver disease. For example, when five healthy but obese cats were fasted for a period of 4 to 6 weeks, three of the cats remained healthy and two developed overt clinical and laboratory signs of FHL.[14] Subsequent studies by the same group reported that voluntary fasting could be induced by changing the diets of obese cats from a highly palatable commercial diet to a less palatable purified diet.[15] In this study, all of the cats refused to eat the new diet and developed histological signs of hepatic lipidosis over a period of 4 to 7 weeks.

Feline idiopathic hepatic lipidosis is fairly common among middle-aged, obese cats. It most often occurs after a period of partial or complete anorexia, usually brought on by stress.

Although prolonged fasting appears to be a consistent finding in cats that develop FHL, the exact metabolic changes responsible for the rapid accumulation of lipid in the liver have not been completely elucidated. Cats diagnosed with FHL typically show signs of protein malnutrition such as muscle wasting, anemia, and hypoalbuminemia. It has been hypothesized that deficiencies of arginine and methionine, secondary to anorexia and protein malnutrition, are involved in the onset of FHL. The cat requires a dietary source of the amino acid arginine for the production of urea in the liver. When the cat stops eating, prolonged anorexia leads to a deficiency of arginine. Urea cycle activity is depressed, and ammonia begins to accumulate in the blood. Byproducts of this disruption in the urea cycle can interfere with lipoprotein synthesis in the liver.[16] Moreover, a deficiency of one or more essential amino acids may limit the synthesis of the proteins needed for production of lipoproteins by the liver, leading to an accumulation of triglycerides.[17] For example, methionine contributes to the development of hepatic lipidosis in rats.[18] In addition, taurine supplementation, which is synthesized from methionine by most species, has been shown to reduce liver lipid concentrations in obese children.[19] Because taurine is an essential nutrient for cats, it has been speculated that low levels of dietary taurine may contribute to FHL and providing supplemental taurine to the diet may help to prevent its development.[11] Supportive research for the role of protein and essential amino acids has shown that the administration of small amounts of protein to obese cats during fasting helps to prevent the accumulation of hepatic lipids.[20]

Carnitine is a compound that is synthesized from methionine and lysine, primarily in the liver. It is necessary for the transport of long-chain fatty acids into cellular mitochondria for oxidation. Human subjects with carnitine deficiency show severe fat accumulation in the liver and other organs and develop signs of liver disease.[21] Carnitine concentrations have been shown to be increased in the muscle and liver of obese women and also during periods of starvation in humans and rats.[22-24] Because of this association in other species and because of evidence of reduced fatty acid oxidation in the liver of obese cats, it had been theorized that a deficiency of carnitine may be a contributing factor to

FHL. However, carnitine concentrations in the plasma, liver, and skeletal muscle of cats with hepatic lipidosis have been reported to be normal.[25,26] Another study reported increased plasma concentrations of carnitine during a period of weight gain in cats fed a diet containing normal carnitine levels, but liver carnitine did not increase.[27] The change in plasma concentration was attributed to increased food consumption during weight gain. Conversely, liver carnitine levels were not higher in obese cats when compared with lean cats. It is possible that increased liver carnitine is necessary during the overweight condition to support normal fatty acid oxidation in the liver and that insufficient levels may contribute to the onset of FHL during periods of anorexia and rapid weight loss (see p. 433).

CLINICAL SIGNS AND DIAGNOSIS

Clinical signs of FHL include complete or partial anorexia with a duration of 7 days or longer, depression, jaundice, weight loss, and muscle wasting.[28-30] Vomiting and/or diarrhea are occasionally reported. Owners usually report that the cat suddenly stopped eating following a period of lifestyle change or stress. Commonly reported stresses include a move to a new house, the arrival of new pets into the household, or a sudden change in diet. Laboratory findings show increased serum activities of liver-associated enzymes, increased serum bilirubin and bile acid concentrations, and, in some cases, increased blood urea nitrogen (BUN) and plasma ammonia concentration.[28] A nonregenerative anemia characterized by irregularly shaped erythrocytes is typically seen.[4] The initial diagnosis of FHL is made using medical history, clinical signs, and the results of laboratory tests. The diagnosis is confirmed by a liver biopsy or fine-needle aspirate showing excessive lipid accumulation in the sampled hepatocytes.

TREATMENT

Regardless of the metabolic cause of FHL, it is essential for the cat's recovery that an early diagnosis is made and that supportive fluid and nutritional therapy is started as soon as possible. Aggressive tube feeding is the treatment of choice because afflicted cats will not eat voluntarily. Force-feeding is not recommended because it can further stress the cat and does not provide an accurate measure of the pet's caloric intake. For these reasons, tube feeding with a nasogastric tube or PEG (percutaneous endoscopic gastrostomy) tube is preferred by most veterinarians.[31,32] The use of a gastrostomy tube involves direct surgical entry into the cat's stomach. This procedure allows accurate and consistent delivery of nutrients and does not interfere with the cat's ability to swallow.[29,31] Although surgical complications are a risk, most cats tolerate gastrostomy and esophagostomy tubes better than nasogastric tubes.

The composition of an ideal therapeutic diet for cats recovering from FHL has not been determined. A variety of diets have been recommended, including blenderized high-protein cat diets, human enteral products, and veterinary enteral products.[32,33] Because it is generally accepted that the provision of optimal levels of dietary protein is essential, a high-protein, high-fat product is needed. Veterinary foods that are formulated for recovery are often appropriate because they contain high levels of protein and are energy dense. Cats that show clinical signs of hepatoencephalopathy initially need to be fed a reduced-protein diet. Protein content can be gradually increased as neurological signs resolve.

In addition to providing adequate protein, there is evidence that supplementation with L-carnitine may improve fatty acid oxidation in overweight cats that are predisposed to FHL.[11,27] Cats that were supplemented with L-carnitine (1000 milligram/kilogram [mg/kg] diet) during a weight gain and fasting protocol designed to induce FHL had significantly increased plasma, muscle, and liver carnitine concentrations compared with unsupplemented cats during the weight gain phase of the study.[27] When cats were fasted, supplementation with carnitine ameliorated fasting ketosis in cats that did not develop FHL, but did not have this affect in cats that developed FHL. Conversely, unsupplemented cats showed dramatic increases in plasma free fatty acids and became ketotic during fasting, whether or not FHL developed. Another study showed that providing increased dietary L-carnitine to obese cats that were fed for weight loss enhanced weight loss and improved fatty acid oxidation, but did not affect hepatic lipidosis.[11] These studies suggest that L-carnitine may help to protect overweight cats from fasting-induced FHL, but may be less effective therapeutically, once FHL has developed and aggressive treatment is needed.

The initial tube feeding should provide ¼ to ½ of the cat's calculated metabolizable energy (ME) requirement. This is gradually increased over a 1-week period to the cat's ME requirement. A minimum of four feedings should be provided per day. Signs of hepatic dysfunction begin to resolve as soon as the cat is receiving adequate protein and energy intake. However, most cats require 3 to 6 weeks of intense dietary therapy before laboratory values normalize, clinical improvement occurs, and the cat's appetite returns. Because it appears that acquired food aversion is a component of the anorexia seen in many cats with FHL, oral feeding should not be introduced until tube feeding is well established and the cat voluntarily shows a strong interest in food when it is presented.

The cat's owner must be willing to assist with the nursing care of the pet because cats with hepatic lipidosis may not eat well for several months. As the cat's appetite returns, the frequency of tube feedings should be slowly decreased until the cat is consuming adequate calories voluntarily. When vomiting can be controlled and long-term adequate protein and calorie intake is ensured, treatment is usually successful. However, because many cats refuse to eat voluntarily for a period of weeks to several months, management can be difficult for pet owners, and prognosis will be guarded until the cat begins to eat voluntarily. Supportive treatment involves minimizing any stress that the animal may experience and, in some cases, administering appetite stimulants. Although some investigators advocate supplying supplemental carnitine during tube feeding, recent evidence indicates that this is probably less important than providing adequate carnitine to cats that may be at high risk, such as overweight cats and spayed females.[11,13,27]

Throughout the treatment period, frequent monitoring of liver-associated enzymes in serum can be used as an indicator of hepatic recovery. Because most cats with FHL have a history of obesity, it is prudent to prevent weight regain following recovery. If the cat is still overweight, a weight loss protocol that allows a slow rate of weight loss and includes a diet containing optimal levels of protein should be followed (see Chapter 28, pp. 328-335). Veterinary supervision is warranted to ensure a slow rate of weight loss and prevent the recurrence of FHL. Most importantly, the cat's lifestyle and living conditions should be managed to minimize or prevent stressful events that may lead to subsequent episodes of anorexia.

Early diagnosis is essential for successful treatment of feline hepatic lipidosis (FHL). Tube feeding is the treatment of choice, using either a nasogastric tube or gastrostomy. The dietary solution should include high levels of protein and energy. Most cats require 3 to 6 weeks of intense dietary therapy before improvement is seen and the cat's appetite returns. Owner commitment and compliance is important during treatment of FHL because affected cats may not eat well for several months.

References

1. Hubbard BS, Vulgamott JC: Feline hepatic lipidosis, *Compend Contin Educ Pract Vet* 14:459–464, 1992.

2. Zawie D, Garvey M: Feline hepatic disease, *Vet Clin North Am Small Anim Pract* 14:1201–1230, 1984.

3. Dimski DS, Taboada J: Feline idiopathic hepatic lipidosis, *Vet Clin North Am Small Anim Pract* 25:357–373, 1995.

4. Center SA, Crawford MA, Guida L, and others: A retrospective study of 77 cats with severe hepatic lipidosis, *Am J Vet Res* 5:724–731, 1993.

5. Biourge V, Pion P, Lewis J, and others: Spontaneous occurrence of hepatic lipidosis in a group of laboratory cats, *J Vet Intern Med* 7:194–197, 1993.

6. Center SA: Feline hepatic lipidosis, *Vet Ann* 33:244–254, 1993.

7. Thornburg LP, Simpson S, Digilo K: Fatty liver syndrome in cats, *J Am Anim Hosp Assoc* 18:397–400, 1982.

8. Hall JA, Barstad LA, Voller BE, and others: Lipid composition of liver and adipose tissues from normal cats and cats with hepatic lipidosis (abstract), *J Vet Intern Med* 6:127, 1992.

9. Hall JA, Barstad LA, Connor WE: Lipid composition of hepatic and adipose tissues from normal cats and cats with idiopathic hepatic lipidosis, *J Vet Intern Med* 11:238–242, 1997.

10. Pazak HE, Bartges JW, Cornelius LC, and others: Characterization of serum lipoprotein profiles of healthy, adult cats and idiopathic feline hepatic lipidosis patients, *J Nutr* 128:2747S–2750S, 1998.

11. Ibrahim WH, Bailey NB, Sunvold GD, Bruckner GG: Effects of carnitine and taurine on fatty acid metabolism and lipid accumulation in the liver of cats during weight gain and weight loss, *Am J Vet Res* 64:1265–1277, 2003.

12. Ibrahim WH, Szabo J, Sunvold GD: Effect of dietary protein quality and fatty acid composition on plasma lipoprotein concentrations and hepatic triglyceride fatty acid synthesis in obese cats undergoing rapid weight loss, *Am J Vet Res* 61:566–572, 2000.

13. Flynn MF, Hardie EM, Armstrong PJ: Effect of ovariohysterectomy on maintenance energy requirement in cats, *J Am Vet Med Assoc* 209:1572–1581, 1996.

14. Biourge V: Sequential findings in cats with hepatic lipidosis, *Feline Pract* 21:25–28, 1993.

15. Biourge V, Groff JM, Munn R, and others: Experimental induction of feline hepatic lipidosis, *Am J Vet Res* 55:1291–1302, 1994.

16. Hardy PM: Diseases of the liver and their treatment. In Ettinger SJ, editor: *Textbook of veterinary internal medicine*, ed 3, Philadelphia, 1989, Saunders.

17. Alpers DH, Sabesin SM: Fatty liver: biochemical and clinical aspects. In Schiff L, Schiff ER, editors: *Diseases of the liver*, ed 6, Philadelphia, 1987, Lippincott.

18. Aoyama Y, Yasui H, Ashida K: Effect of dietary protein and amino acids in a choline-deficient diet on lipid accumulation in rat liver, *J Nutr* 101:739–745, 1971.

19. Obinata K, Maruyama T, Hayashi M: Effect of taurine on the fatty liver of children with simple obesity, *Adv Exp Med Biol* 403:607–613, 1996.

20. Biourge VC, Massat B, Groff JM, and others: Effects of protein, lipid, or carbohydrate supplementation on hepatic lipid accumulation during rapid weight loss in obese cats, *Am J Vet Res* 55:1405–1415, 1994.

21. Chapoy PR, Angelini C, Brown WJ: Systemic carnitine deficiency—a treatable inherited lipid storage disease presenting as Reye's syndrome, *N Engl J Med* 303:1389–1394, 1980.

22. Harper P, Wadstrom C, Beckman L, Cederblad G: Increased liver carnitine content in obese women, *Am J Clin Nutr* 61:81–25, 1995.

23. Sandor A, Cseko J, Kispal G, Alkonyi I: Surplus acylcarnitines in the plasma and liver of starved rats derive from the liver, *J Biol Chem* 265:22313–22316, 1990.

24. Hoppel CL, Genuth SM: Carnitine metabolism in normal-weight and obese human subjects during fasting, *Am J Physiol* 238:E409–E415, 1980.

25. Jacobs G, Cornelius L, Keene B, and others: Comparison of plasma, liver, and skeletal muscle carnitine concentrations in cats with idiopathic hepatic lipidosis and in healthy cats, *Am J Vet Res* 51:1349–1351, 1991.

26. Jacobs G, Cornelius L, Allen S, and others: Treatment of idiopathic hepatic lipidosis in cats: 11 cases (1986-1987), *J Am Vet Med Assoc* 195:635–638, 1989.

27. Blanchard G, Pargon BM, Milliat F, Lutton C: Dietary L-carnitine supplementation in obese cats alters carnitine metabolism and decreases ketosis during fasting and induced hepatic lipidosis, *J Nutr* 132:204–210, 2002.

28. Cornelius LM, Rogers K: Idiopathic hepatic lipidosis in cats, *Mod Vet Pract* 66:377–380, 1985.

29. Evans KL, Cornelius LM: Dietary management of feline idiopathic hepatic lipidosis, *Feline Pract* 18:5–10, 1990.

30. Biourge V: Feline hepatic lipidosis. In *Proceedings of the petfood forum*, Chicago, 1996, Watts Publishing.

31. Armstrong P, Hand M, Frederick G: Enteral nutrition by tube, *Vet Clin North Am Small Anim Pract* 20:237–275, 1990.

32. Biourge B, MacDonald M, King L: Feline hepatic lipidosis: pathogenesis and nutritional management, *Compend Contin Educ Pract Vet* 12:1244–1258, 1990.

33. Center S: Feline liver disorders and their management, *Compend Contin Educ Pract Vet* 8:889–902, 1986.

34

Dental Health and Diet

Periodontal disease and inflammation of the gingivae are common disorders in dogs and cats.[1] Gingivitis is caused by the formation and persistence of dental plaque on the surface of the teeth. If untreated, this can progress to periodontal disease, which affects the gingivae, periodontal ligament, cementum, and alveolar bone. Periodontal disease is associated with oral pain, malodorous breath, ulceration, and the loss of alveolar bone and teeth. The bacteremia that often accompanies periodontitis may also lead to damage to other organs in the body. Although a direct causal relationship has not been proven, periodontal disease has been implicated as contributing to systemic diseases involving the kidneys, cardiovascular system, lungs, and immune system.[2,3] Because periodontal disease is a common and serious disorder in dogs and cat, studies have focused on nutrition and diet as risk factors for its development and as potential means for reducing gingivitis and calculus formation, preventing its progression to periodontal disease and supporting long-term dental health.

INCIDENCE AND DESCRIPTION

The types of dental health problems that occur in dogs and cats differ somewhat from those typically seen in humans. Because of the sharp inclined planes of their dentition, dogs and cats are not susceptible to the formation of tooth caries (i.e., cavities). In dogs, demineralization of teeth is not common because of the alkaline nature of their saliva. Cats, in comparison, can produce saliva with a more acidic pH, making tooth demineralization possible in this species. Overall, the three primary dental problems that are seen in dogs and cats are oral malodor, gingivitis, and periodontitis. The term *periodontal disease* typically refers to gingivitis and periodonitis together. Odontoclastic resorptive lesions in cats also are associated with gingival inflammation and periodontal disease (Figures 34-1 and 34-2).[4,5]

Periodontal disease is one of the most common diseases observed by small-animal practitioners, and it is the most prevalent type of oral disorder. It has been reported in domestic pets for at least 80 years and is considered a worldwide problem. For example, gingival inflammation and heavy calculus deposits were found in 95% of research colony dogs, 2 years old or older, in a study conducted more than 40 years ago.[6] Another early study reported moderate to severe periodontal disease in 75% of necropsied pet dogs that were between 4 and 8 years of age.[7] Recent survey studies of dogs and cats living in several different areas of the world consistently report prevalence rates of periodontal disease of 60% to 80%.[1,8-10]

Periodontal disease is strongly associated with increasing age in both dogs and cats. In dogs, increasing age is positively correlated with several measures of periodontal disease severity, including the intensity of gingival inflammation, the quantity of calculus that is deposited, and the degree of bone resorption and tooth mobility.[11] Similarly, a study with cats found evidence of periodontal disease in 60% of cats older than 3 years, and another found that 40% of cats older than 7 years of age had advanced periodontitis.[12,13] Feline odontoclastic resorptive lesions (FORLs) are also a commonly diagnosed dental disorder of cats as they age. A study of 145 adult cats found evidence of FORLs in 48% of the animals studied.[14] Other groups have found FORL incidence values between 23% and 67%.[15] The progressive nature of periodontal disease and the likelihood that supragingival changes may go unnoticed by owners until there is significant damage to the periodontium may explain the increased incidence in older animals.

Mouth size is a significant risk factor for periodontal disease in dogs. Although all dogs can be affected, the small and toy breeds are more likely to develop periodontitis at an early age and tend to show more severe disease when compared with large breed dogs.[3,11] The reduced jaw size and resultant crowding of teeth of small dogs may be predisposing factors to this prevalence. In addition, toy-breed dogs are more likely to have malocclusion problems, which may facilitate the deposition of subgingival plaque that is more difficult to remove either via chewing or through homecare by

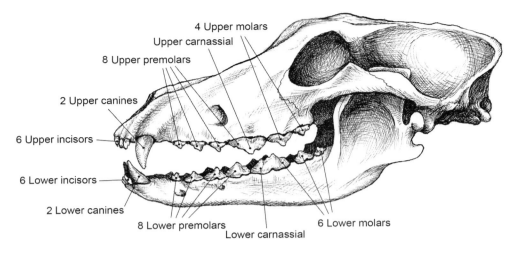

Figure 34-1 Dentition of the dog.

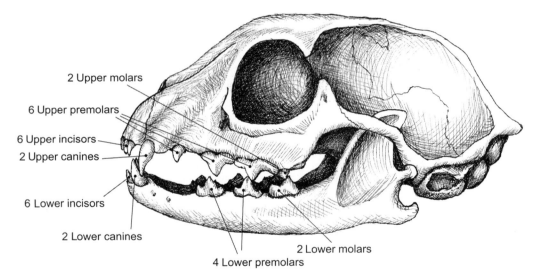

Figure 34-2 Dentition of the cat.

the owner. As periodontal disease progresses, there is destruction and loss of alveolar bone along the roots of teeth. Because small dogs have a lower ratio of the size of the mandible (lower jaw) to the volume of teeth when compared with large-breed dogs, the loss of bone from the jaw has a greater impact.[16] Alveolar bone loss in small dogs can destabilize the jaw, leading to weakness and eventually to increased risk of fracture.[17]

Periodontal disease is the most prevalent type of oral disorder seen by veterinarians. Survey studies of dogs and cats consistently report prevalence rates of periodontal disease of 60% to 80%. Risk increases as pets age, and small and toy breeds of dogs tend to be more severely affected than larger breeds. In cats, feline odontoclastic resorptive lesions are also a commonly diagnosed dental disorder.

Oral Malodor

Oral malodor (halitosis) is commonly reported in dogs and cats and is perceived by many owners to be a significant problem.[18] Moreover, malodor is considered to be a precursor or manifestation of more serious dental disease and is often the first clinical sign that owners report to their veterinarians. As in humans, halitosis in dogs and cats can be caused by oral or nonoral factors. Nonoral etiologies include gastrointestinal, lung, and systemic disease. In the majority of cases in dogs and cats, the predominant source of halitosis is within the oral cavity. Microbial metabolism of protein-containing substances such as food debris, exfoliated epithelium, saliva, and blood result in the production of volatile sulfur compounds (VSCs).[19,20] These compounds, particularly methyl mercaptan, dimethyl sulfide, and hydrogen sulfide, produce breath malodor when exhaled.[20] They may also have detrimental effects on the structural integrity of epithelial tissue in the mouth, further contributing to the pathogenesis and progression of periodontal disease.[21]

In addition to the microbial flora in the mouth, two other factors that influence the production of malodor in human subjects are the pH and glucose concentration of the saliva. Specifically, saliva with a low pH and a relatively high glucose concentration suppresses odor formation, while the production of saliva with an alkaline pH and low glucose concentration is associated with increased production of odor.[22] Although not reported in dogs and cats, it is presumed that these factors influence breath odor in these species in a similar manner.

Breath malodor is consistently associated with gingivitis and periodontitis. Two independent studies with dogs demonstrated significant correlations between the production of VSCs in the mouth and the amount of plaque and calculus accumulation on the tooth surface.[20,23] While the earlier study reported that degree of halitosis was a consistent predictor of the severity of gingivitis, the more recent study did not find a linear relationship with inflammation severity. Another study found that dogs with a high degree of oral malodor were more likely to have moderate to severe periodontal disease when compared with dogs having less malodor.[24] This association is further demonstrated by evidence that veterinary periodontal therapy causes a significant

reduction in previously established halitosis in dogs.[25] One explanation for this is that chronic inflammation and tissue damage provides increased protein substrate for microorganisms in the mouth, enhancing the production of VSCs. The heavier plaque that occurs with dental disease may also provide a favorable anaerobic environment and additional substrate for the formation of VSCs.[26]

> *Oral malodor (halitosis) is commonly reported in dogs and cats and is perceived by many owners to be a significant problem. Bad breath is also a sign of more serious dental disease and is often the first problem that owners report to their veterinarians.*

Gingivitis and Periodontal Disease

Gingivitis is a nonspecific term referring to inflammation of the gingivae (gums). It is considered to be the reversible stage of periodontal disease and can be prevented by regular plaque removal and control. When a clean tooth surface is exposed to saliva and gingival fluids, a pellicle, composed of a thin layer of proteins and glycoproteins, forms within minutes. Oral debris and plaque-forming bacteria, which are part of the normal oral flora, rapidly adhere to the pellicle and begin to proliferate. Within 24 hours, a smooth layer of plaque covers the entire tooth surface. Newly formed plaque is a soft, gelatinous material composed of bacteria and their metabolic byproducts, oral debris, and salivary components. It is generally thickest along the gingival margin because frictional cleaning associated with normal mastication is much less in this area when compared with the apex of the tooth.

Left undisturbed, aerobic and facultative anaerobic bacteria proliferate as the plaque thickens and matures. As bacterial populations increase, the pellicle becomes more firmly attached to the surface of the tooth and bacterial colonies begin to stratify within the plaque layers. The outer surface of the plaque will contain primarily aerobic, gram-positive species, while the interior surface supports anaerobic populations of bacteria.[27] Species of bacteria that tend to proliferate in dental plaque are classified as "periodontopathogens" because their proliferation and metabolic products contribute to progression of periodontal disease. In dogs, the most commonly isolated periodontopathogens are three species of the black-pigmented anaerobic genus *Porphyromonas: P. gluae, P. salivosa,* and *P. denticans.* [28]

Over time, salivary minerals, in particular calcium carbonate and calcium phosphate, are deposited within the plaque, producing calculus. Calculus is a hard deposit that provides a rough and porous surface, promoting accumulation of more plaque and also contributing to tissue irritation as it extends into the gingival sulcus.

Gingivitis develops when contact between the plaque bacteria and gingival tissues leads to tissue damage and an inflammatory response. Initially, only supragingival plaque, which is found on the visible portion of the teeth along the gingival margin, is present. As dental plaque matures, it begins to spread under the gingivae. This form of plaque, called *subgingival plaque,* forms within the gingival sulcus. Left untreated, the gingival sulcus enlarges into a periodontal pocket and the area provides an oxygen-depleted environment that allows proliferation of gram-negative, anaerobic bacteria. Periodontal disease becomes established when the periodontal ligament is exposed to plaque, bacteria, and bacterial byproducts.

Periodontal disease is a plaque-induced, progressive inflammatory disease affecting the gingiva, periodontal ligaments (connective tissue between the tooth root and socket), and alveolar bone. The presence and proliferation of certain species of anaerobic bacteria and the inflammatory responses of the host contribute to the progressive destruction of the periodontium.[1] As the supporting connective tissues and adjacent bone are weakened, teeth become loose and may be lost. Periodontal disease itself causes discomfort and pain and, if left untreated, can lead to bacteremia. For example, a study of 39 dogs with periodontal disease found that 15% of the dogs had bacteremia upon presentation.[29] This increased to 67% after veterinary dental manipulation. The transient increase in bacteremia following dental cleaning was a result of the release of bacteria from disturbed periodontal pockets. There is also evidence that dogs with severe periodontal disease have increased blood bacteria levels immediately following mastication of a meal.[30] Cats with periodontitis are similarly susceptible to bacteremia.[31] As stated previously, the bacteremia associated with periodontal

disease is a risk factor for kidney disease, bacterial endocarditis, and pulmonary disease, especially in older animals.

Mature plaque is not removed by normal actions of the tongue or by rinsing of the mouth. Rather, removal requires mechanical abrasion from chewing, regular tooth brushing, and if necessary, veterinary dental cleaning. Therefore pets who do not receive regular home care or veterinary prophylaxis will eventually develop gingivitis. In some animals, gingivitis persists without progressing into periodontitis. However, in most, untreated gingivitis eventually progresses to periodontal disease. Clinical signs of gingivitis and periodontal disease include oral malodor, gingival sensitivity and bleeding, tooth loss, and difficulty eating.

Gingivitis (inflammation of the gums) is considered to be the reversible stage of periodontal disease and can be prevented by regular plaque removal and control. Periodontal disease is a plaque-induced, progressive inflammatory disease affecting the gingiva, periodontal ligaments, and alveolar bone. Untreated gingivitis will eventually progress to periodontal disease in most dogs and cats. Clinical signs of gingivitis and periodontal disease include oral malodor, gingival sensitivity and bleeding, tooth loss, and difficulty eating.

Feline Odontoclastic Resorptive Lesions

Although rare in dogs, odontoclastic resorptive lesions (feline tooth resorption) are one of the most common dental problems reported in the domestic cat.[32,33] These lesions are also called *neck lesions* or *cervical line lesions,* because the dental defect is often found at the neck area of the tooth. They are characterized by odontoclastic resorption of the tooth's enamel, dentin, or cementum.[34]

Mandibular premolars and molars are the most frequently affected teeth, although canine teeth and incisors may also develop these lesions. As with periodontal disease, the incidence of FORLs is strongly associated with increasing age.[35] Although the underlying etiology of odontoclastic lesions in cats is not completely understood, it is clear that these lesions are not dental caries. Several theories have been advanced to explain FORLs. One study suggested that cats infected with feline immunodeficiency virus were more likely to develop FORLs, which supported virus-induced immunosuppression as an underlying cause.[36] However, other more extensive studies have failed to find corroborating evidence for this theory.[37,38] Another theory postulates that FORLs develop in response to localized inflammatory responses associated with gingivitis and periodontal disease.[39] For this reason these lesions are often classified as a form of periodontal disease in the cat. Dietary influences such as the food's acidifying effects, diet texture (dry versus wet), feeding noncommercial foods, and vitamin D content may also play a role in FORLs (see p. 447).

Because resorptive lesions are very painful to the cat, difficulties in eating and refusal to eat are often the first signs reported by owners. Other signs include oral malodor, gingivitis, and excessive salivation. Gingival inflammation and proliferation are commonly observed in cats with dental lesions, but it is not known if this is a result of the resorptive lesion or an underlying cause. The inflammation associated with FORLs may provide a favorable environment for plaque formation and bacterial proliferation, which lead to gingivitis and possible periodontitis. Alternatively, resorptive lesions may develop in response to the localized and chronic inflammation of gingivae that is associated with periodontal disease. It is known that activity of odontoclasts, the cells responsible for tooth demineralization, is stimulated by chronic inflammation and also by an acidic environment.[34,40] In addition to dietary influences in oral pH, bacterial populations associated with chronic inflammatory disease in the cat's mouth may contribute to an acidic microenvironment necessary for the tooth decalcification that occurs with resorptive lesions.

Initial physical evaluation of a cat's mouth may not reveal damage to the tooth because of the progressive nature of the disorder. Over time, there is eventual loss of the tooth crown and root. Diagnosis usually requires dental examination and radiographs.[41] FORLs are typically categorized into four stages, with treatment and management procedures dependent upon the stage of the disease at the time of diagnosis.[42,43] Although dental prophylaxis and application of a fluoride cavity varnish may stop or slow progression of the early stages,

extraction of the tooth is usually necessary in more advanced stages of the disease.

> *Feline odontoclastic resorptive lesions (FORLs) are one of the most common dental problems reported in the domestic cat. Although the underlying cause is not completely understood, risk of developing a FORL increases in older cats. These lesions are painful and lead to difficulty or refusal to eat in affected cats. Other signs include oral malodor, gingivitis, and excessive salivation. Over time, there is eventual loss of the tooth crown and root; extraction of the tooth is usually necessary in more advanced stages of the disease.*

ROLE OF DIET IN THE DEVELOPMENT OF DENTAL DISEASE

The most important factor that influences the development of gingivitis and periodontal disease in dogs and cats is the presence and persistence of undisturbed plaque on tooth surfaces. Therefore management and feeding practices that minimize plaque and calculus formation or aid in their removal are important in the prevention of periodontal disease. Factors that are important include the frequency of tooth brushing, the type of diet that is fed, whether or not table scraps or noncommercial foods are fed, and the frequency of access to chew toys, dental chews, and biscuits.

Once plaque has been deposited on the surface of the tooth, it is most efficiently removed mechanically through the abrasion provided by diet, tooth brushing, or chewing on supplemental chew toys or foods. Chemical agents such as rinses, pastes, and sprays can also be helpful but will not replace the necessary abrasion. For example, the antimicrobial agent chlorhexidine digluconate is effective for the reduction of breath malodor, plaque accumulation, and gingivitis in dogs.[44,45] However, the effectiveness of chlorhexidine and other antimicrobial agents is greatly enhanced when they are used in conjunction with brushing. The use of a chemical mouthwash or gel alone is not effective in removing the hardened calculus that forms when plaque is allowed to accumulate. For this reason, an approach that provides frequent and consistent mechanical removal of plaque and calculus is always recommended (see pp. 447-449).

Type of Food: Dry versus Wet

Historically, the form of food that is fed has been implicated as a potential risk factor for the development of dental disease in dogs and cats. Early studies reported that dogs fed a soft (wet) diet developed clinical and histological signs of periodontal disease earlier in life than those fed dry foods.[46,47] The severity of disease in dogs fed a soft diet was also greater than that observed in dogs fed a dry biscuit diet. In another early study, dogs fed a food that required mastication did not develop gingivitis during the 1-month trial period.[48] In contrast, dogs fed the same diet in a minced, soft form developed gingivitis and had signs associated with developing periodontal disease.

Survey studies have also been used to identify dietary risk factors associated with periodontal disease in dogs. Data from a group of 63 pet dogs in the United States showed that gingivitis and calculus were less common in dogs fed dry dog food as the major portion of their diet, compared with those fed canned food.[49] However, indicators of tooth mobility, tooth loss, and periodontal disease did not differ significantly with the type of diet fed. Another study conducted by the Japanese Small Animal Veterinary Association collected data from more than 2600 dogs.[50] Analysis showed that dental calculus was found in 34% of dogs fed primarily dry food and 42% of dogs fed primarily canned or home-cooked food. Most recently, a study conducted in Poland provided oral examinations to client-owned dogs recruited by a group of private veterinary practices.[51] Data were collected for almost 30,000 dogs. Following an adjustment for a possible confounding age effect, the data showed that dogs fed only wet food were significantly more likely to have dental calculus and periodontal disease than dogs fed only dry food or a mixture of dry and wet food. Results from these studies indicate that feeding canned foods only may increase risk or severity of periodontal disease. However, the form of the food alone does not completely protect against dental disease; dogs can still accumulate plaque and develop gingivitis and periodontal disease when fed a dry diet.

A similar relationship between wet and dry diet and the development of dental disease was reported in an early study with cats.[52] In this study, the gingivae of growing kittens fed a dry cat food remained healthy, showing little inflammation or accumulation of calculus. In contrast, kittens fed a canned food for the same period developed oral malodor, gingivitis, and calculus. Another group reported that cats had greater plaque accumulation when fed a canned diet, compared with plaque accumulation in cats fed a dry commercial food for a period of only 2 weeks.[53] The Polish survey discussed previously also included 9074 cats.[51] Cats fed wet food only were less likely to be free of dental deposits or periodontal disease than were cats fed dry foods or a mixture of dry and wet food. However, similar to dogs, cats fed dry foods were still at risk of developing dental disease. Current indications are that soft foods such as canned commercial diets or home-prepared foods are less effective than hard, dry foods in providing the abrasion needed to remove plaque that normally forms on teeth. However, the mechanical abrasion provided by feeding a normal dry pet food does not effectively prevent the development of gingivitis and periodontal disease, since in most studies a substantial proportion of animals fed dry diets still developed signs associated with progressive dental disease.

The exclusive feeding of a wet (canned) food or a soft home-prepared diet is less effective at providing the needed mechanical abrasion of chewing to help remove dental plaque than feeding a dry food. However, by itself, the mechanical abrasion from consuming a normal dry pet food cannot effectively prevent the development of gingivitis and periodontal disease in dogs and cats.

Opportunities for Chewing

The dental health benefits afforded by feeding dry pet foods are related to having frequent opportunities for chewing and its associated mechanical cleaning action on the surface of teeth. A study of 1350 dogs in North America examined the relationship between the occurrence and severity of calculus and periodontal disease and the type of diet and chew toys that dogs received.[54] There was a significant linear relationship between decreasing calculus score and increasing number of chewing materials. Although less significant, this trend was also observed for gingivitis. When the type of food alone was considered, there was no significant association between feeding a diet made up exclusively of dry pet food and the degree of calculus, gingivitis, or tooth attachment loss. However, in dogs that were fed dry food, access to rawhide chews and other types of chewing materials was significantly associated with a reduced accumulation of calculus and less gingival inflammation and attachment loss. Rawhide chew materials were the most effective in preventing dental disease, followed by various types of hard bones. In this study, feeding regular (nondental) hard biscuits as a supplement to the dry diet did not provide any additional dental benefit. In contrast, dogs that were not exclusively fed dry food obtained little or no dental benefit from additional chew materials. The authors concluded that there was a consistent (if not always significant) trend toward a widespread protective effect of access to supplemental chewing materials in dogs that were fed dry pet food, compared with dogs fed primarily soft food or a mixture of food types.

A smaller study of 67 dogs showed similar results.[55] Providing dogs with rawhide chews as a supplement to their normal dry diet led to significant removal of preexisting supragingival calculus over a period of 3 weeks. Providing cereal biscuits instead of rawhide was somewhat helpful, but less so than providing rawhide chews. Two other studies examined the dental effects of feeding a rawhide chew that was specifically formulated to promote dental hygiene.[56,57] In the first study, dogs were fed a dry maintenance dog food and provided with tooth brushing every other day.[56] Half of the dogs also received one rawhide chew per day. Dental health was assessed over a period of 3 weeks. While plaque accumulation and gingivitis occurred in all of the dogs, significantly less gingivitis developed when the rawhide chew was added to the regimen. After the study period, deposits of calculus and stain were greater with tooth brushing only, compared with the degree of calculus and stain when the teeth were brushed and the chew was provided. In the second study, the effects of the chew on dental health were measured in the absence of regular tooth brushing.[57] Similar results were reported. While gingivitis developed in both groups of dogs, the daily provision of chewing materials significantly decreased the severity. A follow-up study by the same group found that the dental hygiene chew maintained a benefit to oral malodor and the degree of plaque and calculus throughout a 21-month period of offering one chew per day.[58] These results indicate that chewing materials are helpful in reducing the degree of gingivitis through direct mechanical cleaning of the tooth surfaces. However, because dogs given the dental chews still showed some level of plaque accumulation and gingivitis, it appears unlikely that this level of reduction can completely prevent the development of calculus, gingivitis, and periodontitis, even when given to dogs that are exclusively fed a dry diet.

In recent years, dental chew toys that provide mechanical abrasion, and which also include agents to reduce the formation of calculus or inhibit the growth of oral bacteria, have been developed. For example, rawhide treats coated with polyphosphate salts may help to reduce the formation of dental calculus by sequestering salivary calcium.[59] Polyphosphates are also used as coatings on dental diets and have shown some efficacy in reducing calculus formation (see pp. 445-446). Another approach is to add an antibacterial agent, such as chlorhexidine, to a dental chew. The intended effect is to reduce bacterial populations present in plaque and reduce their contribution to gingivitis and disease progression. Although one study reported a reduction in plaque accumulation in dogs given this type of chew device, another reported no added efficacy when a toy with an added antimicrobial agent was compared to the same toy without the agent.[60,61] It is important that both the efficacy and the safety of supplemented dental chew toys be critically evaluated prior to making any recommendations for their use.

The variable results associated with specific types of chewing toys and different effects on mandibular and maxillary teeth suggest that owners should provide a variety of different types of chewing materials to their dogs. It appears that a cumulative effect is afforded by feeding a dry food and providing additional and varied chew toys. Ideally, dogs fed a dry pet food should have at least one and, if possible, two or more opportunities for extended chewing each day. The additive effect of consuming a dry food plus having frequent access to chew toys may surpass a relative "chewing threshold" that affords some level of protective effect not reached when a canned or soft food is fed and little opportunity to chew is provided. It is also possible that dogs fed dry pet foods may by nature or through learning be more frequent or vigorous "chewers." This theory is supported by data showing that dogs given rawhide chews varied significantly in their level of interest and in the speed with which they chewed and consumed the rawhide.[62] Videotaping chewing episodes allowed the authors to divide dogs into categories of slow and fast chewers. Dogs classified as slow chewers had less dental calculus accumulation at the end of the 12-month test period when compared with fast chewers, indicating that the amount of time a dog spends chewing each day is an important factor.

While providing chewing toys is beneficial for dental health in dogs, this is generally not an approach that can be used for cats. Although individual cats that enjoy chewing on hard bones or rawhide may exist, most pet cats do not engage in frequent or prolonged bouts of chewing. An examination of the cats' evolutionary history provides a possible explanation for this difference. Unlike dogs, which evolved from a species that hunted large ungulates and spent a great deal of time chewing bones and tough connective tissue, the cat evolved from the small African wild cat (*Felis libyca*), which hunts primarily small rodents, such as mice. The wild cat's prey is rapidly consumed, with minimal chewing, and numerous mice are caught and eaten each day. As a result, our domestic cat (*Felis catus*) has neither the dentition nor (it appears) the desire to spend large amounts of time chewing on bones or other types of chew toys.

Dogs can be offered regular opportunities for chewing by feeding a dry food and providing daily chew bones and dental chews. For best results, a variety of forms and types of dental chews should be selected. However, while these activities can help to reduce plaque, calculus, and gingivitis, they will not completely prevent plaque formation in most dogs. Because cats do not typically engage in prolonged or regular chewing, this is generally not an approach that can be used for cats.

Dental Diets and Biscuits

It is generally accepted that the development of plaque and gingivitis can be somewhat reduced (but not completely prevented) by feeding dry foods and providing frequent chewing opportunities. Historically, the primary mechanism of action has been the mechanical friction and scraping on the surface of the teeth as the animal consumes the kibble or chews on the toy. In recent years, specific "dental diets" have been formulated to expand these effects by modifying the texture, shape and size of the kibble pieces. However, while mechanical abrasion can be effective for reducing plaque on the chewing surfaces, it may have limited or no value for nonchewing tooth surfaces in the mouth. Therefore an additional approach is to include agents in the food that provide dental benefits by chemically influencing the formation of dental plaque or calculus throughout the oral cavity. A group of compounds that have been shown to be effective via this approach are the polyphosphates, which affect the formation of dental calculus.

FOOD TEXTURE AND KIBBLE SIZE/ SHAPE Food texture and kibble characteristics can affect the oral environment by controlling dental plaque and presumably reducing the risk of developing periodontal disease. Factors that are believed to be important include the size, shape, and density of the food's pieces; the food's moisture level; and the modification of certain nutrients, such as dietary fiber.[63] Theoretically, a dry food has the potential to mechanically remove plaque if the shape and size of the pieces are designed for both the species (dog or cat) and for the size of the animal's mouth. To allow maximal mechanical cleansing, the texture of the food must also allow the tooth to penetrate deeply into the kibble before it breaks or crumbles, and the size of the kibbles must promote chewing prior to swallowing. Although exact formulations are often not reported, several studies have examined the efficacy of dental diets formulated to enhance mechanical tooth cleansing in dogs and in cats.

In one study, an adult maintenance food that was formulated to reduce plaque, stain, and calculus formation was compared with a conventional dry adult maintenance food.[63] Dogs were fed each diet for a period of 3 weeks. At the end of the test period, dogs fed the specially formulated dental diet had 19% less plaque, 44% less stain, and 32% less calculus accumulation when compared with dogs fed the maintenance food. However, signs of gingivitis and periodontitis were not reported. A previous study by the same group found that dogs fed the oral care diet developed less oral malodor after a 1-week feeding period.[64] A follow-up study examining long-term effects of the same food reported statistically significant reductions in dental plaque (39%) and gingival inflammation (36%) over a 6-month feeding period.[65] The authors concluded that the type of processing and ingredients used in the test food helped to reduce the accumulation of plaque, stain, and calculus but did not completely prevent their occurrence. However, the clinical significance of these results is not known, because the effect of this level of reduction on the development of gingivitis or periodontal disease has not been studied.

Because of the documented importance of providing chewing materials for promoting dental health, a second study was conducted to compare the aforementioned oral care diet with feeding a conventional dry dog food plus an oral hygiene rawhide chew.[66] During the 3-week test period, dental plaque, calculus, and gingivitis increased similarly in all of the dogs, regardless of feeding regimen. Because a control group of dogs was not included in this study, no comparison could be made between dental changes in dogs fed these two regimens and dogs fed a conventional maintenance dog food. An additional finding was that dogs fed the oral care diet lost significant amounts of body weight during the treatment period. This effect was associated with poor acceptance of the food and a failure to eat the entire ration each day. As in the previous study, these data showed that neither regimen effectively maintained clinically healthy gingivae over a 3-week period, again suggesting that dietary approaches to oral hygiene, while helpful, cannot replace other methods of dental care such as tooth brushing and veterinary dental prophylaxis.

A variety of food bars and consumable bones have also been developed as dental health supplements in recent years. These products are typically marketed to be used as a snack or treat, and have the added benefit of promoting dental health. Unlike biscuits, many of these products are formulated to have an elastic and resistant texture that facilitates mechanical abrasion of the entire tooth surface and promotes extended periods of chewing. Some companies have produced dental chews specifically for small and toy breeds of dogs, recognizing that these are the dogs that are most seriously affected by periodontal disease. For example, a study

of the effectiveness of a dental chew designed for small dogs reported a reduction in plaque and calculus when dogs were fed one chew per day throughout a 4-month period.[67] These types of chews may also be preferable to providing harder chew bones, which some veterinarians believe are more likely to splinter or cause slab fractures to the carnassial teeth.[68]

Specially formulated dental or oral care pet foods are formulated to have kibble texture, shape, and size characteristics that promote chewing and provide the mechanical abrasion needed to remove plaque from the surface of teeth. Other dental care products include supplemental food bars, biscuits, and bones with a chewy or resistant texture that encourages prolonged bouts of chewing. Some companies have produced dental chews specifically for small and toy breeds of dogs, recognizing that these are the dogs that are most seriously affected by periodontal disease.

POLYPHOSPHATES   The polyphosphates are a group of compounds that act to sequester salivary calcium, making it unavailable for the formation of calculus within the plaque pellicle of the teeth. One of the most commonly studied forms, sodium hexametaphosphate (HMP), has been incorporated into the outer coating of kibble or snack biscuits.[69,70] It is theorized that when small amounts of HMP are included in food, chewing allows the HMP to adhere to plaque, form soluble complexes with calcium, and then be washed away. Because the inorganic portion of tooth calculus in dogs contains predominantly calcium carbonate and small amounts of calcium phosphate, inclusion of HMP helps to prevent or decrease calculus formation.[71]

A series of studies compared the dental effects of daily supplementation with HMP-coated biscuits to dogs fed either dry dog food or dry dog food moistened with water.[69,70] After pretreatment with dental prophylaxis (scaling and polishing), dogs were supplemented daily with either conventional biscuits, experimental biscuits coated with HMP, or no biscuits. In both types of feeding regimens (dry and moistened diet), the daily ingestion of HMP-coated biscuits reduced but did not completely prevent the formation of calculus. A more pronounced reduction of calculus occurred in dogs fed the moistened diet than in those fed a dry maintenance diet. Overall, reductions in calculus formation varied between 30% and 63%. The degree of gingivitis was not measured in this study, nor was it possible to predict the clinical significance of the reported reductions in calculus.

Several studies have examined the efficacy of incorporating microcrystalline polyphosphate coatings onto the outer coating of the kibbles in a complete and balanced dog or cat food.[72,73] In a set of studies with adult dogs and cats, diets were formulated to contain the polyphosphate coating and were compared with the same food formulated without the coating.[72] There was no difference in kibble shape, size, or texture between the control and the test diets, to ensure that any observed dental effects would be due to a chemical effect of the polyphosphate as opposed to a mechanical effect from chewing. Following initial dental prophylaxis, animals were fed either the test diet or the control diet for a 4-week period, using a crossover experimental design. Following the first 4-week period, a second dental prophylaxis was performed and dietary treatments were switched. Including a polyphosphate coating on the dry food's kibbles was well accepted by both dogs and cats. In both of these studies, dogs and cats had significantly lower mean tooth calculus scores after consuming food with added polyphosphates, when compared with calculus scores derived after feeding the normal maintenance diet. A follow-up study was conducted to examine the effectiveness of incorporating the same type of polyphosphate microcrystals into a complete and balanced food designed for senior dogs.[73] Similar to the earlier studies, adding an outer coating of polyphosphate to the food significantly reduced calculus accumulation when measured during a 5-week feeding period.

Because the mechanism of action of polyphosphates is to sequester salivary calcium, including these compounds in pet foods, biscuits, or chews is not expected to influence either plaque accumulation or the oral microflora populations that are responsible for many of the pathological effects of dental disease. Therefore, while polyphosphates have shown some efficacy in controlling calculus formation, complete dental care must also include methods that control plaque and the pathogenic bacterial populations to maintain long-term oral health.

> *The inclusion of polyphosphates such as hexametaphosphate in dental diets or biscuits can promote dental health by reducing calculus formation. These compounds work by sequestering salivary calcium, making it unavailable for precipitation as dental calculus.*

OTHER INGREDIENTS   In recent years, a number of unconventional supplemental ingredients have been identified as having potential dental health benefits for dogs and cats. The polyphenols are a large group of compounds, several of which are found in green tea. One in particular, epigallocatechin gallate (catechin), has been shown to have bacteriostatic action against canine dental plaque bacteria.[74,75] Incorporating green tea into dog food may be helpful in reducing the growth of *Porphyromonas* bacteria in the oral cavity.[76] Most recently, a pilot study with 29 cats found that feeding cats a cat food that included catechin caused a reduction in gingival inflammation, oral malodor, and decreased *Porphyromonas* numbers when compared with these measures in cats fed a control diet.[77] Soluble zinc salts such as zinc ascorbate and zinc gluconate have been shown to control plaque when included in cleansing gels and rinses for cats, although no studies of their use in pet foods or treats have been reported.[78] Finally, there is some evidence that certain types of oils, such as eucalyptus, lavender, and rosemary oil, have an inhibitory effect on oral malodor and gingivitis. The effect on breath malodor is attributed to both a masking effect and to a reduction of VSCs. There is also evidence that eucalyptus oil may inhibit the growth of periodontopathogens.[79] Although of interest, each of these ingredients and compounds requires additional controlled studies to elucidate both their potential for dental health benefits and for long-term safety when fed to dogs and cats before recommendations can be made.

VOHC SEAL OF ACCEPTANCE   The nutrient composition and processing methods of oral health foods and chews that have been studied are rarely described in published studies. These limitations should be taken into consideration when evaluating the efficacy of specially formulated diets or making recommendations regarding diet components that might affect the dental health of pets. One helpful guide that veterinarians and pet owners can use when selecting a dental diet is the Seal of Acceptance awarded by the Veterinary Oral Health Commission (VOHC). The VOHC was established in 1997 with the objective of providing independent overviews of pet products that are marketed for the mechanical control of plaque or the mechanical and/or chemical control of calculus. The VOHC provides a set of efficacy protocols for companies to use; data are then submitted to the VOHC for review. Products that are approved by the VOHC carry the "VOHC Seal of Acceptance" on their label and may make a claim for plaque, tartar (calculus), or plaque and tartar control when fed. The VOHC website also maintains a current list of accepted products. In 2009 there were 22 products on the VOHC list; these include complete and balanced foods, dental chews and treats, and a water additive.

DIET AND FELINE TOOTH RESORPTION (FORL)

There is some evidence that an association exists between dental resorptive lesions and certain aspects of a cat's diet. A study that examined risk factors for the development of odontoclastic lesions in 145 adult cats reported that the two most important factors associated with resorptive lesions were increasing age and feeding a cat food that contained low levels of magnesium.[14] In addition, cats that had their teeth cleaned at least twice a week and were fed diets containing higher levels of magnesium, calcium, phosphorus, and potassium were less likely to develop oral lesions. Neither the type of diet fed (soft versus hard) nor the number of feedings provided per day was associated with the development of dental lesions. Although limited data are available, a positive association has also been reported between resorptive lesions and feeding noncommercial (homemade) diets, cat treats, table foods, and diets containing low amounts of calcium or high amounts of vitamin D.[80-82]

The increased use of acid sprays as a coating on dry cat foods and of urine-acidifying diets for the prevention of struvite urolithiasis in cats led to speculation that some commercial cat foods may reduce the oral pH and promote an environment that is favorable for tooth demineralization. To examine this theory, a study was conducted to determine whether the pH of a cat food and that of a cat's tooth surfaces after eating are correlated.[83] Cats with resorptive lesions were found to have lower tooth surface pH values than cats without lesions (7.93 versus 8.65). However, no relationship was found between the pH of the food that was fed and the incidence or severity of FORLs. Although the surface pH values for the commercial diets studied were all acidic (pH range between 4.9 and 6.3), ingestion caused only a very slight and transient decrease in tooth surface pH. The authors speculated that cats' saliva quickly neutralized the acidic coating of the kibble pieces, and thus resulted in only very slight alterations in tooth surface pH. Moreover, even the transient change in tooth surface pH that was observed cannot be considered clinically significant because physiological decalcification of bone and teeth occur only at a pH between 4 and 5.[84,85]

Systemic acidosis that may lead to a persistently acidic environment in the mouth has also been suggested as a potential contributor to FORLs. Recent in vitro studies have reported that cultured feline osteoclasts become highly proliferative and cause in vitro bone resorption when exposed to an acidic environment.[86] However, research demonstrating a direct relationship between a cat's diet, metabolic acid-base balance, and the development of FORLs is lacking. More studies of a possible connection between the urine acidifying characteristics of a cat food, oral pH, and risk of FORLs are needed to further explore this potential factor. Similarly, while one study reported that cats with FORL had significantly higher levels of circulating vitamin D (25-hydroxy-cholecalciferol) when compared with cats that did not have FORL, a subsequent study using the same design found no association between FORL and vitamin D status.[82,87] Studies that are designed to examine the potential relationship between dietary levels of vitamin D and the development of FORL are needed.

PREVENTION OF DENTAL DISEASE AND HOME MAINTENANCE CARE

Current evidence supports a significant role of diet in the maintenance of dental health and prevention of plaque and calculus formation. However, simply feeding a dry pet food or a food formulated as an oral care diet cannot replace regular and consistent prophylactic dental care. The primary approach for preventing the development of gingivitis and periodontal disease includes a program of regular home care, periodic veterinary dental prophylaxis, and provision of carefully chosen and varied types of chewing materials (for dogs). Feeding a dry diet or an oral care diet is considered to be adjunctive to these procedures.

Veterinary dental prophylaxis is conducted under general anesthesia and includes supragingival and subgingival scaling and polishing.[88,89] The scaling removes calculus and plaque that has formed above and below the gingival interface, and polishing removes micropitting on the tooth that provides a favorable surface for plaque deposition. The frequency of treatment depends upon the pet's rate of plaque accumulation, the degree of established gingivitis or periodontal disease, and the pet's age. Because moderate to severe dental disease is most commonly seen in older dogs and cats, the risk of frequent anesthesia administration must always be considered.[90] Generally, veterinary dental cleaning every 12 to 18 months is recommended for pets with healthy gingiva. Pets with chronic gingivitis or periodontitis will benefit from more frequent cleaning, usually every 6 to 12 months.[89] It is important for pet owners to be informed that when established dental disease is present, frequent veterinary cleaning is still necessary even in the face of optimal home care. Although daily tooth brushing can effectively remove plaque, it cannot affect the degree of subgingival disease and may even mask the progression of disease below the gingival surface.[91] Therefore regular and continued professional therapy is essential for dogs and cats diagnosed with periodontal disease.

The most effective method of home dental care is regular tooth brushing. Brushing prevents plaque accumulation and the development of gingivitis.[88,92] Current evidence shows that the frequency of brushing necessary to maintain clinically healthy gingivae depends on the initial condition of the tissue. For example, in studies of dogs with established gingivitis, brushing daily was effective in returning the gums to health, but brushing three times per week was not sufficient.[92-94] Conversely, brushing three times per week can successfully maintain dental health in dogs with no signs of gingivitis or periodontal disease.[92,95] As

discussed previously, providing various types of chew materials such as rawhides, dental devices, and, possibly, some types of hard biscuits, can augment but not replace the effectiveness of brushing.

Dental care products that contain oral disinfectants such as chlorhexidine gluconate or chlorhexidine acetate have been shown to effectively reduce breath malodor and plaque formation in dogs.[96-98] In addition, long-term use of chlorhexidine can effectively reduce gingivitis and slow the progression of periodontal disease.[96] There is also recent evidence that the antimicrobial agent cetylpyridinium chloride may effectively control oral malodor, and reduce plaque and calculus accumulation in dogs when applied to teeth as a dental solution or gel.[99] However, long-term studies of this agent are needed before recommendations for its use can be made. The effectiveness of chlorhexidine is maximized when it is applied as a tooth-brushing solution, as this allows the mechanical removal of plaque. However, studies with dogs have also shown that applying a chlorhexidine-containing spray or gel prevents plaque accumulation, improves breath, and helps prevent gingivitis and periodontal disease, even when not accompanied by brushing.[100] This is a distinct advantage for owners whose dog or cat will not tolerate frequent sessions of tooth brushing. The only reported side effects of chlorhexidine-containing dental products are an unpleasant taste and brown staining of the teeth in some animals. The staining occurs after long-term use and, though it may be aesthetically displeasing to some owners, is not harmful or pathogenic.

Regardless of the type of dental agent used, all pet owners should receive instructions on home dental care and should be encouraged to maintain a consistent preventive program throughout their pet's life. Although meticulous home care does not necessarily preclude the need for regular professional prophylaxis, it can reduce the accumulation of plaque, the deposition of calculus, and the development of gingivitis. This may effectively prevent periodontitis and allows a reduced frequency of veterinary dental prophylaxis. Additional care involves providing a variety of chew toys and products for dogs and feeding a dry food. Diets consisting primarily of wet food with no opportunities for chewing hard kibble or biscuits should be avoided unless another health condition requires their use or the pet will not accept a dry pet food. If a soft or canned food provides the primary basis of a pet's diet, frequent tooth brushing, the provision of chew toys, and veterinary prophylaxis are doubly important (Box 34-1).

Lifelong dental care for dogs and cats should include regular veterinary examinations and cleaning (scaling and polishing), consistent home dental care (brushing, ideally daily), and the provision of a variety of chew toys and hard biscuits to pets who enjoy them. Although it cannot replace regular dental care, feeding an oral care pet food contributes to healthy gums and teeth.

References

1. Logan EL: Dietary influences on periodontal health in dogs and cats, *Vet Clin North Am Small Anim Pract* 36:1385–1401, 2006.

2. DeBowes LJ, Mosier D, Logan E, and others: Association of periodontal disease and histologic lesions in multiple organs from 45 dogs, *J Vet Dent* 13:57–60, 1996.

3. Watson ADJ: Diet and periodontal disease in dogs and cats: part 2, *Vet Clin Nutr* 5:11–13, 1998.

4. Okuda A, Harvey CE: Etiopathogenesis of feline dental resorptive lesions, *Vet Clin North Am Small Anim Pract* 22:1385–1404, 1992.

5. Lyon KF: Subgingival odontoclastic resorptive lesions: classification, treatment, and results in 58 cats, *Vet Clin North Am Small Anim Pract* 22:1417–1432, 1992.

6. Rosenberg HM, Rehfeld CE, Emmering TE: A method for the epidemiologic assessment of periodontal health-disease state in a Beagle hound colony, *J Periodontol* 37:208–213, 1966.

7. Lindhe J, Hamp SE, Löe H: Plaque induced periodontal disease in Beagle dogs: a 4-year clinical, roentgenographical and histometrical study, *J Periodontal Res* 10:243–255, 1975.

8. Hoffman TH, Gaengler P: Epidemiology of periodontal disease in poodles, *J Small Anim Pract* 37:309–316, 1996.

9. Kyllar M, Witter K: Prevalence of periodontal disease in pet dogs, *Vet Med (Czech)* 50:496–505, 2005.

10. Verhaert L, Wetter CV: Survey of oral diseases in cats in Flanders, *Vlaams Diergeneeskundig Tijdschrift* 73:331–341, 2004.

11. Harvey CE, Shofer FS, Laster L: Association of age and body weight with periodontal disease in North American dogs, *J Vet Dent* 11:94–105, 1994.

12. Crossley DA: Survey of feline dental problems encountered in a small animal practice in NW England, *Br Vet Dent Assoc J* 2:2–6, 1991.

13. Gengler W, Dubielzig R, Ramer J: Physical examination and radiographic analysis to detect dental and mandibular bone resorption in cats: a study of 81 cases from necropsy, *J Vet Dent* 12:97–100, 1995.

14. Lund EM, Bohacek LK, Dahlke JL: Prevalence and risk factors for odontoclastic resorptive lesions in cats, *J Am Vet Med Assoc* 212:392–395, 1998.

15. Van Wessum R, Harvey CE, Hennet P: Feline dental resorptive lesions: prevalence patterns, *Vet Clin North Am Small Anim Pract* 22:1405–1417, 1992.

16. Gioso MA, Shofer F, Barros PS: Mandible and mandibular first molar tooth measurements in dogs: relationship of radiographic height to body weight, *J Vet Dent* 18:65–68, 2001.

17. Shim Km, Kim SE, Yoo KH, and others: Case studies of repair of pathological mandibular fracture due to periodontal disease in dogs, *J Vet Clinics* 24:653–657, 2007.

18. Perez G: Results from a home audit survey of pets and their care, *Watham Centre Pet Nutr Data*, 1996.

19. Spouge JD: Halitosis: a review of its cause and treatment, *Dent Pract Dent Rec* 15:307–317, 1964.

20. Kim SE, Shim KM, Yoo KH, and others: Association between halitosis and periodontal disease related parameters in dogs, *J Vet Clinics* 24:192–196, 2007.

21. Ng W, Tonzetich J: Effect of hydrogen sulfide and methyl mercaptan on the permeability of oral mucosa, *J Dent Res* 63:994–997, 1984.

22. DeBoever EH, Deuzeda M, Losche WJ: Relationship between volatile sulfur compounds, BANA-hydrolyzing bacteria and gingival health in patients with and without complaints of oral malodor, *J Clin Dent* 4:114–119, 1994.

23. Culham N, Rawlings JM: Oral malodor and its relevance to periodontal disease in the dog, *J Vet Dent* 15:165–168, 1998.

24. Hennet PR, Delille B, Davor JL: Oral malodor measurements on a tooth surface of dogs with gingivitis, *Am J Vet Res* 59:255–257, 1998.

25. Culham N, Rawlings JM: Studies of oral malodor in the dog, *J Vet Dent* 15:169–173, 1998.

26. Kleinberg I, Westbay G: Oral malodor, *Crit Rev Oral Bio Med* 1:247–260, 1990.

27. Watson ADJ: Diet and periodontal disease in dogs and cats: part 1, *Vet Clin Nutr* 4:135–137, 1997.

28. Hardham J: Pigmented-anaerobic bacteria associated with canine periodontitis, *Vet Microbiol* 106:119–128, 2005.

29. Nieves MA, Hartwig P, Kinyon JM, Riedesel DH: Bacterial isolates from plaque and from blood during and after routine dental procedures in dogs, *Vet Surg* 26:26–32, 1997.

30. Geerts S, Nys M, DeMoi P: Systemic release of endotoxins induced by gentle mastication: associations with periodontitis severity, *J Periodontol* 73:73–78, 2002.

31. Colmery B, Frost P: Periodontal disease: etiology and pathogenesis, *Vet Clin North Am Small Anim Pract* 16:817–834, 1986.

32. Reiter AM, Mendoza K: Feline odontoclastic resorptive lesions—an unsolved enigma in veterinary dentistry, *Vet Clin North Am Small Anim Pract* 32:791–837, 2002.

33. American Veterinary Dental College: *Position statement: feline tooth resorption* (website). http://www.avdc.org/position-statements.html. Accessed April 2007.

34. Okuda A, Harvey CE: Etiopathogenesis of feline dental resorptive lesions, *Vet Clin North Am Small Anim Pract* 22:1385–1401, 1992.

35. Ingham KE, Gorrel C, Blackburn J: Prevalence of odontoclastic resorptive lesions in a population of clinically healthy cats, *J Small Anim Pract* 42:430–443, 2001.

36. Hofmann-Lehmannn R, Berger M, Sigrist B: Feline immunodeficiency virus (FIV) infection leads to increased incidence of feline odontoclastic resorptive lesions (FORL), *Vet Immunol Immunpathol* 65:299–309, 1998.

37. Malik R, Kendall K, Cridland J, and others: Prevalence of feline leukaemia virus and feline immunodeficiency virus infections in cats in Sydney, *Aust Vet J* 75:323–327, 1997.

38. Scarlett JM, Saidla J, Hess J: Risk factors for odontoclastic resorptive lesions in cats, *J Am Anim Hosp Assoc* 35:188–192, 1999.

39. Reichart PA, Durr UM, Triadan H, and others: Periodontal disease in the domestic cat: a histopathologic study, *J Periodontal Res* 19:67–75, 1984.

40. Muzylak M, Arnett TR, Price JS, Horton MA: The in vitro effect of pH on osteoclasts and bone resorption in the cat: implications for the pathogenesis of FORL, *J Cell Physiol* 213:144–150, 2007.

41. Holstrom SE: External osteoclastic resorptive lesions, *Feline Pract* 20:7–11, 1992.

42. Okuda A, Asari M, Harvey CE: Challenges in treatment of external odontoclastic resorptive lesions in cats, *Compend Conin Educ Pract Vet* 17:1461–1469, 1995.

43. Lyon KF: Subgingival odontoclastic resorptive lesions: classification, treatment and results in 58 cats, *Vet Clin North Am Small Anim Pract* 22:1417–1432, 1992.

44. Hamp SF, Löe H: Long-term effect of chlorhexidine on developing gingivitis in the Beagle dog, *J Periodontal Res* 8:63–70, 1973.

45. Robinson JGA: Chlorhexidine gluconate—the solution for dental problems, *J Vet Dent* 12:29–31, 1995.

46. Burwasser P, Hill TJ: The effect of hard and soft diets on the gingival tissues of dogs, *J Dent Res* 18:389–393, 1939.

47. Engelberg J: Local effect of diet on early plaque formation and development of gingivitis in dogs, *Odont Rev* 16:31–50, 1965.

48. Krasse B, Brill N: Effect of consistency of diet on bacteria in gingival pockets in dogs, *Odont Rev* 11:152–156, 1960.

49. Golden AL, Stoller N, Harvey CE: A survey of oral and dental diseases in dogs anaesthetized at a veterinary hospital, *J Am Anim Hosp Assoc* 18:891–899, 1982.

50. Japanese Small Animal Veterinary Association: *Survey on the health of pet animals*, 1985.

51. Gawor JP, Reiter AM, Jodkowska K, and others: Influence of diet on oral health in cats and dogs, *J Nutr* 136:2021S–2023S, 2006.

52. Studer E, Stapley RB: The role of dry foods in maintaining healthy teeth and gums in the cat, *Vet Med Small Anim Clin* 68:1124–1126, 1973.

53. Boyce EN: Feline experimental models for control of periodontal disease, *Vet Clin North Am Small Anim Pract* 22:1309–1321, 1982.

54. Harvey CE, Shofer FS, Laster L: Correlation of diet, other chewing activities and periodontal disease in North American client-owned dogs, *J Vet Dent* 13:101–105, 1996.

55. Lage A, Lausen N, Tracy R, and others: Effect of chewing rawhide and cereal biscuit on removal of dental calculus in dogs, *J Am Vet Med Assoc* 197:213–219, 1990.

56. Gorrel C, Rawlings JM: The role of tooth-brushing and diet in the maintenance of periodontal health in dogs, *J Vet Dent* 13:139–143, 1996.

57. Gorrel C, Rawlings JM: The role of a "dental hygiene chew" in maintaining periodontal health in dogs, *J Vet Dent* 13:31–34, 1996.

58. Gorrel C, Bierer TL: Long-term effects of a dental hygiene chew on the periodontal health of dogs, *J Vet Dent* 16:109–113, 1999.

59. Warrick JM, Stookey GK, Inskeep GA: Reducing calculus accumulation in dogs using an innovative rawhide treat system coated with hexametaphosphate. In *Proc 15th Ann Vet Dent Forum*, 2001, pp 379–382.

60. Rawlings JM, Gorrel C, Markwell PJ: Effect of canine oral health of adding chlorhexidine to a dental hygiene chew, *J Vet Dent* 15:129–134, 1998.

61. Brown WY, McGenity P: Effective periodontal disease control using dental hygiene chews, *J Vet Dent* 22:16–19, 2005.

62. Goldstein GS: The effect of rawhide strips on the removal and prevention of plaque and calculus. In *Proc Vet Dent*, Auburn, Ala, 1993.

63. Jensen L, Logan E, Finney O, and others: Reduction in accumulation of plaque, stain, and calculus in dogs by dietary means, *J Vet Dent* 12:161–163, 1995.

64. Simone A, Jensen L, Setser C, and others: Assessment of oral malodor in dogs, *J Vet Dent* 11:71–74, 1994.

65. Logan EI, Finney O, Herrerrenn JJ: Effects of a dental food on plaque accumulation and gingival health in dogs, *J Vet Dent* 19:15–18, 2002.

66. Rawlings JM, Gorrel C, Markwell PJ: Effect of two dietary regimens on gingivitis in the dog, *J Small Anim Pract* 38:147–151, 1997.

67. Hennet P, Servet E, Venet C: Effects of feeding a daily oral hygiene chew on dental deposits in small breed dogs: a 4-month trial. In *Proc 13th Europ Cong Vet Dent*, 2004, pp 47–48.

68. Carmichael DT: Periodontal disease—strategies for preventing the most common disease in dogs. In *Proc NAVC*, January 13-27, 2007, pp 357–359.

69. Stookey GK, Warrick JM, Miller LL, and others: Hexametaphosphate-coated biscuits significantly reduce calculus formation in dogs, *J Vet Dent* 13:27–30, 1996.

70. Stookey GK, Warrick JM, Miller LL: Sodium hexametaphosphate reduces calculus formation in dogs, *Am J Vet Res* 56:913–918, 1995.

71. Legeros RZ, Shannon IL: The crystalline components of dental calculi: human vs. dog, *J Dent Res* 58:2371–2377, 1979.

72. Johnson RB, Cox ER, Lepine AJ: Dietary technology for inhibition of calculus formation in companion animals. In *Proc World Vet Dent Cong*, 2003.

73. Lepine AJ, Murray SM, Cox ER: Clinical investigation of dental diet efficacy in the senior dog. In *Proc World Vet Dent Cong*, 2003.

74. Hirasawa M, Kakada K, Makimura M: Improvement of periodontal status by green tea catechin using a local delivery system: clinical pilot study, *J Periodontal Res* 37:433–438, 2002.

75. Sakanaka S, Okada Y: Inhibitory effects of green tea polyphenols on the production of a virulence factor of the periodontal-disease-causing anaerobic bacterium *Porphyromonal gingivalis*, *J Agric Food Chem* 52:1688–1692, 2004.

76. Isogai E, Isogai H, Kimura K: Effect of Japanese green tea extract on canine periodontal diseases, *Microbiol Ecol Heath Dis* 8:57–61, 1995.

77. Isogai H, Isogai E, Takahashi K, Kurebayashi Y: Effect of catechin diet on gingivitis in cats, *Intern J Appl Res Vet Med* 6:82–86, 2008.

78. Clarke DE: Clinical and microbiological effects of oral zinc ascorbate gel in cats, *J Vet Dent* 18:177–183, 2001.

79. Takarada K, Kimizuka R, Takahashi N: A comparison of the antibacterial efficacies of essential oils against oral pathogens, *Oral Microbiol Immunol* 19:61–64, 2004.

80. Donoghue S, Scarlett JM, Williams CA, and others: Diet as a risk factor for feline external odontoclastic resorption (abstract), *J Nutr* 124:2693S–2694S, 1994.

81. Zetner K, Steurer I: Role of commercial dry cat food in the pathogenesis of feline neck lesions, *Prakt Tierarzt* 73:289–297, 1992.

82. Reiter AM, Lyon KF, Nachreiner RF, Shofer FS: Evaluation of calcitropic hormones in cats with odontoclastic resorptive lesions, *Am J Vet Res* 66:1446–1452, 2005.

83. Zetner K, Steurer I: The influence of dry food on the development of feline neck lesions, *J Vet Dent* 9:4–6, 1992.

84. Hall TJ, Chambers TJ: Optimal bone resorption by isolated rat osteoclasts requires chloride/bicarbonate exchange, *Calcif Tissue Int* 45:378–380, 1989.

85. Dellmann HD, Brown EM: *Textbook of veterinary histology*, Philadelphia, 1987, Verlag Lea & Febiger.

86. Muzylak M, Arnett TR, Price JS, Horton MA: The in vitro effect of pH on osteoclasts and bone resorption in the cat: implications for the pathogenesis of FORL, *J Cell Physiol* 213:144–150, 2007.

87. Zhang P, Cupp C, Kerr W: Vitamin D status in cats with and without feline odontoclastic resorptive lesions, *Compend Contin Educ Pract Vet* 28:77, 2006.

88. Carmichael DT: Periodontal disease—strategies for preventing the most common disease in dogs. In *Proc NAVC*, 2007.

89. Aller S: Dental home care and preventive strategies, *Semin Vet Med Surg Small Anim* 8:204–212, 1993.

90. Hefferren JJ, Boyce E, Bresnahan ME: Aging and oral health, *Vet Clin Nutr* 3:97–100, 1996.

91. Korman KS: The role of supra gingival plaque in the prevention and treatment of periodontal disease, *J Periodontal Res* 16(Suppl):5–22, 1986.

92. Tromp JA, van Rijn LJ, Jansen J: Experimental gingivitis and frequency of tooth brushing in the Beagle dog model: clinical findings, *J Clin Periodontol* 13:190–194, 1986.

93. Corba NHC, Jansen J, Pilot T: Artificial periodontal defects and frequency of tooth-brushing in Beagle dogs. I. Clinical findings after creation of the defects, *J Clin Periodontol* 13:158–163, 1986.

94. Corba NHC, Jansen J, Pilot T: Artificial periodontal defects and frequency of tooth-brushing in Beagle dogs. II. Clinical findings after a period of healing, *J Clin Peridontol* 13:186–189, 1986.

95. Sanges G: A pilot study on the effect of tooth-brushing on the gingiva of a Beagle dog, *Scand J Dent Res* 84:106–108, 1976.

96. Briner W: Effect of chlorhexidine on plaque, gingivitis, and alveolar bone loss in Beagle dogs after seven years of treatment, *J Periodontal Res* 15:390–394, 1980.

97. Tepe JH, Loenard G, Singer R, and others: The long-term effect of chlorhexidine on plaque, gingivitis, sulcus depth, gingival recession and loss of attachment in Beagle dogs, *J Periodontal Res* 18:452–458, 1983.

98. Reed JH: A review of the experimental use of antimicrobial agents in the treatment of periodontitis and gingivitis in the dog, *Can Vet J* 29:705–708, 1988.

99. Kim SE, Shim KM, Yoo KH, and others: The effect of cetylpyridinium chloride on halitosis and periodontal disease-related parameters in dogs, *Biotech Bioproc Engineer* 13:252–255, 2008.

100. Cummins D, Creeth JE: Delivery of anti-plaque agents from dentifrices, gels and mouthwashes, *J Dent Res* 71:1439–1449, 1992.

Nutritional Management of Gastrointestinal Disease

Gastrointestinal disease in dogs and cats is composed of a group of disorders with varying and often unrelated underlying causes. Regardless of the cause, most gastrointestinal disorders manifest as acute or chronic diarrhea and, in some cases, vomiting or anorexia. Nutritional support is an important component of treatment because of the gastrointestinal tract's essential role in nutrient digestion and absorption. A primary goal of dietary therapy is to maintain delivery of nutrients and prevent nutrient deficiencies and malnutrition. In addition, long-term dietary management can help to repair the damaged intestinal lining, restore normal populations of intestinal microflora, promote normal gastrointestinal motility and function, support immune function, and reduce gastrointestinal inflammation.[1,2] While dietary management will not always cure the underlying disease, it can have a profound influence on the ability of the intestine to recover and is an important component of veterinary treatment for the control of many types of intestinal disease.

NUTRITIONALLY RESPONSIVE GASTROINTESTINAL DISEASES

Intestinal disorders in companion animals that have been shown to be responsive to dietary management include small intestinal bacterial overgrowth (SIBO)/ antibiotic-responsive diarrhea (ARD), pathogen overgrowth, exocrine pancreatic disease, several types of inflammatory disorders, and nonspecific acute diarrhea.

SIBO and ARD

SIBO occurs when there are quantitative and qualitative changes to bacterial populations in the lumen of the proximal (upper) part of the small intestine.[3,4] Some researchers have recently argued that SIBO should be renamed antibiotic-responsive diarrhea (ARD) because of the difficulty in SIBO diagnosis via bacterial population numbers, and because not all dogs that are treated successfully for SIBO show reduced intestinal bacterial counts following treatment.[4] The designation of ARD reflects the leading theory that antibiotic therapy and dietary treatments for SIBO support a change in the population dynamics of the intestinal flora, as opposed to simply a reduction in total number of microbes that are present. The goal is to shift the balance of the microbiota away from pathogens and toward the less pathogenic and beneficial species that are present in a healthy intestine. To reflect this change (and the lack of total consensus), the inclusive term *SIBO/ARD* will be used in this review.

Although some dogs with SIBO/ARD do not have persistent clinical signs, most develop chronic episodes of intermittent diarrhea that may be accompanied by vomiting or anorexia. SIBO/ARD may develop secondarily to a number of other intestinal disorders or be idiopathic. Factors that can lead to secondary SIBO include impaired gut motility, the prolonged or excessive use of oral antibiotics, and achlorhydria (decreased acid production in the stomach). In a healthy animal, bacterial populations increase in number proximally to distally in the gastrointestinal tract. Normal peristalsis helps to limit bacterial populations in the upper small intestine by regularly flushing bacteria distally through the gastrointestinal tract. Reduced motility allows increased substrate to be available to gut bacteria, which can lead to increased microbial populations and changes in the balance of normal flora. Numerous health problems can contribute to a reduction in gut motility and increase risk of developing secondary SIBO. These include intestinal obstruction, neuropathy, abdominal surgery, peritonitis, pancreatitis, uremia, hypokalemia, and endotoxemia. SIBO/ARD may also develop as a sequela to other forms of intestinal disease such as lymphocytic-plasmacytic enteritis and exocrine pancreatic insufficiency (EPI).[5,6] Animals with idiopathic SIBO/ARD will have a decrease in signs following the appropriate antibiotic regimen. Finally, SIBO may have a genetic component.

German Shepherd Dogs have been reported to have an unusually high incidence of SIBO, and this has been associated with a breed-specific deficiency of secretory immunoglobulin A.[7,8]

Historically, the gold standard for diagnosis of SIBO has been via microbiological culture of duodenal fluid obtained endoscopically or during a laparotomy. A culture showing more than 10^5 total or 10^4 anaerobic colony-forming units of bacteria per milliliter (CFU/ml) is considered to be consistent with SIBO.[9] However, the clinical relevance of these numbers has been questioned because some healthy dogs consistently have counts that are this high and because a proportion of dogs with ARD/SIBO that respond to antibiotic treatment do not show a reduction in total bacterial counts.[9-11] For this reason, a total bacterial count in excess of 10^7 to 10^8 CFU/ml has been suggested by some researchers as the standard for diagnosis of SIBO in dogs and cats.[10]

In addition, elevated serum folate, reduced serum cobalamin, and elevated deconjugated bile acids provide indirect supportive evidence for bacterial overgrowth in the proximal small intestine.[12-14] Although serum folate and cobalamin are individually not very sensitive indicators of SIBO, when these values are concurrently altered, these changes are considered specific for SIBO/ARD. Serum folate increases as bacteria numbers in the upper small intestine increase due to increased bacterial production of folate. Serum cobalamin concentration decreases because bacteria interfere with cobalamin binding to intrinsic factor and subsequently inhibit absorption of the vitamin into circulation. Intestinal bacteria also cause the deconjugation of bile salts, which are then reabsorbed, making them unavailable to participate in fat absorption. Deconjugated bile acids that remain in the intestinal lumen are also a significant contributor to the osmotic and secretory diarrhea seen in dogs with SIBO/ARD.

Qualitative changes in the bacterial flora of the small intestine of pets with SIBO/ARD are as significant as increased numbers, and these changes should always be assessed. Species of bacteria that typically increase in dogs with SIBO/ARD include coliforms, staphylococci, and enterococci, with *Clostridium* and *Bacteroides* species predominating. Although clinical SIBO is less common in cats, subclinical cases have been reported based upon earlier diagnostic criteria.[15] The most common species of bacteria found in cats with SIBO were *Bacteroides* species, eubacteria, fusobacteria, and *Pasteurella* species. In addition, the cat appears to be unique in the relatively high number of clostridia found in the intestine, as compared with other carnivorous species. Even when the challenges of defining and diagnosing SIBO/ARD are considered, it is still generally accepted that SIBO/ARD is an important cause of chronic diarrhea in dogs (and less commonly in cats), as well as a concomitant finding in several other forms of chronic intestinal disease.[16]

SIBO/ARD occurs when there are quantitative and qualitative changes to bacterial populations in the lumen of the proximal (upper) part of the small intestine. Clinical signs include chronic episodes of intermittent diarrhea that may be accompanied by vomiting or anorexia. SIBO/ARD may be a primary disease or can develop secondarily to a number of other intestinal disorders.

Pathogen Overgrowth

In healthy animals, the many genera and species of intestinal microbes exist in a commensal balance that promotes normal digestive and immune functioning.[17-19] When present in optimal numbers, bacterial species that are classified as beneficial inhibit the proliferation of harmful bacterial species, stimulate immune function, aid in the digestion or absorption of food, and synthesize essential vitamins.[20] These effects are achieved through competition for oxygen, luminal substrates, and living space within intestinal niches. In addition, some indigenous flora produce substances that directly inhibit the growth of other bacterial species. For example, saccharolytic species of intestinal microbes produce short-chain fatty acids (SCFAs) during the metabolism of carbohydrate. In turn, these SCFAs inhibit the growth of some pathogenic species of bacteria.[21]

An animal's intestinal microbial population is not static. Microbial populations are susceptible to change and can be affected by stress, infection, antibiotic administration, nutritional factors, motility problems, and immunosuppression. When a change in the normal population of microbes allows the proliferation of one or more pathogenic species of bacteria, clinical illness can result. Pathogen overgrowth may manifest as a single problem or can occur secondarily as a component of SIBO/ARD or another form of intestinal disease. The proliferation of pathogenic species of bacteria causes harm to the host animal by producing toxins, carcinogens, or putrefactive compounds. These compounds may directly affect the intestinal mucosa, cause systemic disease, and inhibit the growth of beneficial bacteria. One of the most common intestinal pathogens in companion animals is *Clostridium perfringens*.[19,22] Signs of an imbalanced intestinal microbe population or pathogen overgrowth include vomiting, diarrhea, weight loss, and, in some cases, systemic illness caused by the production of toxins.

Pancreatitis and Exocrine Pancreatic Insufficiency

Pancreatitis and EPI are well-defined gastrointestinal disorders in dogs and cats that can occur in acute and chronic forms.[23,24] Acute pancreatitis is a short-term, usually reversible illness in which there is no evidence of tissue fibrosis or acinar atrophy.[25] It may have an extremely rapid onset, and in severe cases may lead to rapid tissue necrosis and a potentially lethal outcome. Chronic pancreatitis is a continuous, usually progressive inflammatory disorder that is characterized by permanent damage to pancreatic structure and exocrine (and sometimes endocrine) function. Acute pancreatitis is the most common form that is diagnosed in dogs, while chronic pancreatitis is the primary manifestation seen in cats.[26] However, dogs treated for acute pancreatitis may subsequently develop chronic or subclinical pancreatitis. There is also recent evidence suggesting that many cases of chronic pancreatitis in dogs are undiagnosed.[27] Similarly, because feline pancreatitis may be subclinical or mild, cases of chronic feline pancreatitis may be easily missed.[28]

The underlying cause of many cases of pancreatitis is not determined, so many cases are classified as idiopathic. Identified risk factors for developing pancreatitis include being overweight or obese, hyperlipidemia, consuming a high-fat meal or experiencing one or more bouts of dietary indiscretion (dogs), and the presence of other forms of gastrointestinal disease such as inflammatory bowel disease or liver disease (cats), neoplastic

disease, and exposure to certain drugs or infectious agents.[25,29-31] Cats are susceptible to a generalized inflammatory syndrome called "triaditis," in which chronic pancreatitis occurs concurrently with inflammatory diseases of the liver and intestine.[31] In dogs, Miniature Schnauzers and Yorkshire Terriers may be at increased risk for developing pancreatitis, and a possible mode of inheritance has been identified in Miniature Schnauzers.[29,32]

EPI occurs when the exocrine pancreas produces inadequate amounts of digestive enzymes resulting in a maldigestion/malabsorption syndrome. In dogs, the most common underlying cause of EPI is selective atrophy of the pancreatic acinar cells, which are responsible for the production and storage of the digestive enzymes.[33] Canine EPI has a genetic basis; the majority of cases are diagnosed in German Shepherd Dogs and Rough Collies.[34] The mode of inheritance in these two breeds appears to be autosomal recessive. A recent report also found that Cavalier King Charles Spaniels and Chow Chows are also at increased risk for EPI when compared with the entire population of dogs, and there appears to be a juvenile-onset form of EPI in Greyhounds.[35,36] EPI is less common in cats, but can occur as a sequela to chronic pancreatitis. A genetic basis for EPI has not been reported in cats.

Although acute pancreatitis can be a medical emergency, most cases of chronic pancreatitis are classified as mild, with the pet showing transient but recurrent signs. The most common clinical signs of pancreatitis are complete or partial anorexia, depression and lethargy, vomiting, and weight loss.[24] Pets often present with abdominal pain, dehydration, icterus, and dyspnea. The clinical signs of EPI all relate to the reduced ability to digest and absorb dietary nutrients. Fat digestion and absorption is severely impaired, which can contribute to both acute and chronic intestinal symptoms.[37] Other changes in intestinal function include a decrease in protein synthesis within enterocytes, malabsorption of some vitamins, and secondary development of SIBO/ARD or pathogen overgrowth. Studies indicate that SIBO/ARD is found in more than 70% of dogs with a diagnosis of EPI.[38] Animals with EPI produce voluminous stools that are often loose and foul smelling. Frequent bouts of diarrhea and steatorrhea are common. Excessive weight loss and an emaciated appearance are classic signs of EPI, even while the pet demonstrates a voracious appetite and polyphagia. The diarrhea caused by EPI is typically osmotic due to the passage of malabsorbed diet components along the intestinal tract. However, secretory diarrhea of the lower small intestine and colon may also be present, as a result of bacterial deconjugation of bile acids and the metabolism of unabsorbed fat to hydroxy fatty acids.

While clinical signs and history are helpful in diagnosing pancreatitis and EPI, definitive diagnosis is made using results of the pancreatic lipase immunoreactivity assay (pancreatitis) or the serum trypsin–like immunoreactivity assay (EPI).[39-42] Immediate treatment of acute pancreatitis requires fluid therapy and correction of hypokalemia or other electrolyte or acid-base imbalances, if present.[25] Pain management is also important for pets with pancreatitis and is typically achieved via opioid administration or transdermal fentanyl patches. There is evidence that pancreatic enzyme supplementation is helpful at reducing pain in human patients with chronic pancreatitis. Although it has not been studied, this may be helpful in dogs and cats as well. Early nutritional intervention via enteral feeding also may be beneficial in acute cases of pancreatitis. An important component to the long-term management of both pancreatitis and EPI is diet modification. For pets with pancreatitis, reduction of overweight conditions (if present) is important, and possibly the control of dietary fat (see pp. 463-464). Long-term management of EPI includes providing supplemental enzyme extracts with meals and dietary modification to promote efficient digestion and reduce malabsorption. In addition, antibiotic therapy or dietary approaches to control SIBO are necessary for some animals.

Exocrine pancreatic insufficiency (EPI) is a specific type of pancreatic disease that occurs when the exocrine pancreas produces inadequate amounts of digestive enzymes. Clinical signs all relate to the reduced ability to digest and absorb dietary nutrients. Animals with EPI produce voluminous stools that are often loose and foul smelling, and diarrhea and steatorrhea are common. Excessive weight loss and an emaciated appearance are seen, even while the pet demonstrates a voracious appetite. Diagnosis of EPI is made using results of the serum trypsin–like immunoreactivity assay.

Inflammatory Bowel Disorders

Inflammatory diseases of the intestine are a diverse group of disorders that are generally categorized according to the type of inflammatory cell that predominates in the intestinal mucosa, the area of the intestine affected, or the underlying cause, if known. Colitis is a general term for a condition that describes irritation or inflammation of the large intestine, and it is considered the most frequently diagnosed disorder of the large intestine in dogs and cats.[43] Colitis is further classified into several forms, which include lymphocytic-plasmacytic, eosinophilic, histocytic, and granulomatous colitis. Lymphocytic-plasmacytic enterocolitis is the most common form of inflammatory bowel disorder (IBD) in dogs.[44] In recent years, a new classification has identified a subgroup of dogs with chronic idiopathic large bowel diarrhea (CILBD).[45] Although limited data are available, CILBD is presumed to be a stress-related disorder that may be concomitantly influenced by other factors such as inflammatory disease, dietary indiscretions, pathogen overgrowth, parasitic infection, and neoplasia. Clinical signs of colitis and CILBD are the result of dysfunction of the large intestine and include increased defecation frequency, tenesmus, and production of bloody or mucoid diarrhea. When IBD affects the small intestine, signs include production of large quantities of soft, bulky stools or diarrhea, with occasional steatorrhea. Contrary to large intestinal disease, weight loss and vomiting are common with small intestinal IBD.

IBD is considered to be a multifactorial disorder. Predisposing factors include genetics, exposure to luminal antigens and loss of immune tolerance, compromised colonocyte health, increased mucosal permeability, and impairment or insufficiency of the intestine's normal protective mechanisms.[46] A genetic basis may be involved in some forms of IBD; Boxers and German Shepherd Dogs are at increased risk of developing lymphocytic-plasmacytic enterocolitis while Basenjis are susceptible to a form called *immunoproliferative enteropathy*.[47-49] Several forms of IBD occur in the domestic cat, including lymphocytic-plasmacytic enteritis and eosinophilic enteritis, but no breed-specific predilections have been reported.[50,51] Additionally, distinguishing between IBD and gastrointestinal lymphoma can be diagnostically challenging in cats. Infection with an intestinal parasite or bacterial pathogen, bacterial overgrowth, or presence of a food antigen may all trigger an initial inflammatory response, which can persist even after the initial cause has been resolved. Once an immune response has been initiated in the small or large intestine, production of inflammatory eicosanoids and tissue ischemia may sustain the inflammatory response, resulting in a cycle of chronic illness.

Treatment of IBD and CILBD is directed toward eliminating the underlying cause (if one can be found), reducing inflammation, and achieving long-term remission. Medical therapy of IBD includes the use of antiinflammatory and immunosuppressive drugs such as corticosteroids (prednisone or prednisolone), sulfasalazine, and, in some cases, oral cyclosporine or metronidazole (cats).[52] However, these drugs are associated with undesirable and deleterious health effects when used for long periods. In recent years, new regimens have been developed that focus on dietary management (see pp. 461-472 for complete discussion).[52,53] While drug therapy is still often used in the initial treatment phase to reduce inflammation and allow healing of the intestinal tract, dietary management can often maintain remission and prevent relapse. Drug therapy is then only reinstated if clinical signs return.

Nonspecific Acute Diarrhea

Nonspecific acute diarrhea refers to short episodes of diarrhea for which a cause cannot be found. In most cases, the pet remains active, there is no evidence of systemic disease, and the clinical signs are self-limiting. In dogs, this condition is commonly caused by dietary indiscretions such as consuming garbage, animal feces, or carrion. Overeating or a sudden change in the type or brand of food that is fed can cause acute diarrhea in both dogs and cats. Feeding a poorly formulated or inadequately prepared homemade diet or excessive amounts of table scraps can also lead to small or large intestinal diarrhea. In these cases, the diarrhea can be treated symptomatically until the animal recovers or an underlying cause can be found and treated.

Gastric Dilatation-Volvulus

Gastric dilatation-volvulus (GDV), commonly referred to as *bloat,* is a life-threatening disorder characterized by rapid and abnormal distention of the stomach (dilatation). This disorder is often, but not always, accompanied by rotation of the stomach along its long axis (volvulus). Dilatation occurs when gas, fluid, and secretions accumulate within the stomach and are not expelled because of the occlusion of both the cardiac and pyloric sphincters. The condition rapidly worsens as the distended and rotated stomach places pressure on the major abdominal blood vessels, the portal vein, and caudal vena cava. This pressure causes a loss of blood flow to the stomach and other vital organs, decreased cardiac output, and the development of shock. At this point the dog's condition rapidly deteriorates, and if the GDV is not corrected quickly, shock and tissue damage become severe and death ensues. In addition, cardiac arrhythmias are observed in up to 40% of dogs with GDV and can cause death within weeks or months following apparent recovery from GDV.[54] Diagnosis is usually based on clinical signs, with radiographs used to distinguish between GDV and gastric dilatation without gastric torsion. Although the course of GDV can be quite variable among dogs, this disorder should always be treated as a medical emergency.

Bloat most often affects large, deep-chested dogs. The breeds that have been identified as being most susceptible include the Great Dane, Saint Bernard, Weimaraner, Irish Setter, Gordon Setter, Standard Poodle, and Basset Hound.[55] Although rare, the disorder can also occur in small breeds of dogs and cats.[56] Risk of GDV also increases as dogs age. A dog that is developing GDV will exhibit acute abdominal pain and distention, and it will often whine, pace, salivate, and appear anxious. The dog may attempt to vomit but will be unable to regurgitate any stomach contents. As the problem progresses, hypovolemic shock occurs, characterized by pale mucous membranes, a rapid and weak pulse, increased heart rate, and weakness. In all cases, veterinary care must be provided immediately.

Initial treatment of GDV involves decompression of the stomach and treatment for shock. Surgical intervention is usually also necessary and involves derotation and repositioning of the stomach, followed by prophylactic measures that help to prevent recurrence. Surgery also allows assessment of the damage to the stomach and other organs. Even with treatment, prognosis is often guarded. In a retrospective study of almost 2000 cases, the case fatality rate was 33.6% in dogs treated for GDV at veterinary teaching hospitals.[55] The strongest prognostic indicator appears to be the extent of gastric necrosis that has occurred. Death occurs either during surgery because of irreversible shock or within several days of surgery as a result of cardiac complications or gastric necrosis.[57] While nonsurgical treatment is associated with a high rate of recurrence, the use of gastropexy to surgically stabilize the stomach significantly reduces recurrence and postoperative mortality.[58]

GDV is considered to have a multifactorial etiology. Potential influencing factors that have been studied include genetic predisposition, dietary management practices, diet type and composition, and intrinsic abnormalities such as elevated serum gastrin or altered gastric motility. Genetics plays an important role in GDV to the degree that body type and structure are inherited characteristics. A study reported that the two most important risk factors affecting a breed's predisposition for development of GDV are a relatively high chest depth-to-width ratio and a large adult size.[59] Together, chest conformation and body size account for 76% of the variability in breed risk for GDV. Subsequent studies with Irish Setters have shown that there is a positive and significant correlation between increasing chest depth-to-width ratio and an individual dog's risk for developing GDV.[60] Because chest depth-to-width ratios are significantly influenced by genetics, it may be possible to reduce the incidence of GDV through selective breeding.[61] Studies of the genetics involved in GDV are complicated by the fact that it is often difficult or impossible to separate these effects from environmental influences such as husbandry practices, medical care, and feeding management. However, dogs that inherit a large, deep-chested body type have an increased susceptibility to this disease, and this conformation appears to have a high heritability in some breeds of dogs.

Other studies have identified additional risk factors for GDV.[62,63] While some of these, such as breed and conformation, are characteristics that are inherent to a particular dog, others are environmental factors over which owners have at least some measure of control. In one study, a group of 101 dogs that had acute episodes of GDV were individually matched with dogs of the same age, breed, and size.[63] Comparisons of the two groups showed that physical characteristics that significantly increased an individual dog's risk of GDV included gender, body weight, and temperament. Specifically, male dogs that were underweight and were

determined to have a nervous or fearful temperament were at higher risk for eventually developing GDV. In contrast, a study of 74 Irish Setters with GDV and a group of matched controls found that the risk of GDV was not associated with gender or temperament in that breed. The differences between these two studies may reflect differences between the general population of dogs and the subpopulation of a specific breed (Irish Setters). In both studies, however, the most significant precipitating factor identified was an episode of environmental change or a stress-inducing event within several hours preceding the onset of clinical signs. In the Irish Setters that were studied, two precipitating risks that were identified were recent kenneling and a recent car journey.

Several nutritional factors have been found to influence a dog's risk for GDV.[62,64] These include consuming only one meal per day, having a fast rate of eating, and experiencing aerophagia while eating. On the other hand, feeding table foods, having snacks available between meals, and adding canned food to a dog's diet all decreased the risk of GDV. This second group of practices all contribute to a more frequent meal schedule and are assumed to result in a decreased volume of food being fed during a single meal. These findings are in agreement with earlier reports that the majority of cases of GDV occur when the dog has recently consumed a large meal or quantity of water.[64] Finally, contrary to popular belief, using an elevated food bowl to feed dogs who are increased risk of GDV does not help to prevent bloat and may even increase risk.[65]

The mechanism through which meal frequency affects gastric health may have to do with the volume of food that is fed. A study with Irish Setters reported that dogs fed one large meal per day throughout growth developed larger, heavier stomachs than did dogs fed three meals per day during the same period.[64] Dogs that were fed once daily also had greater gastric distention than did dogs fed multiple meals, but no differences in gastric motility were seen between the two groups. The investigators concluded that feeding one time per day, rather than feeding multiple small meals per day, may contribute to changes associated with GDV in susceptible dogs. It has also been postulated that strenuous exercise, stress, or excitement may be contributing factors, especially before or after a meal or a large volume of water is consumed.

Composition of the diet or type of diet that is fed has received attention as a possible cause of GDV, but there are little actual data to support this theory. Dry dog foods were initially implicated because of the belief that they absorb water and expand while in the stomach, causing an abnormal amount of gastric distention. Another theory proposed that cereal-based, dry diets delay gastric emptying when consumed and contribute to the accumulation of gas in the stomach. The presence of soybean products in pet foods has also been proposed as a causative factor. It has been theorized that soy provides a fermentative substrate for *Clostridium* spp. bacteria within the stomach, which produces the gas responsible for GDV. However, a study with large breeds of dogs compared the effects of feeding a dry cereal-based diet, canned meat or canned, cereal-based diet on gastric motility and the rate of gastric emptying. Results showed no significant effect of diet on gastric function in any of the dogs that were studied.[66] Another clinical study involving 240 dogs that had been treated for GDV did not find any correlation between the type of food that was fed and the occurrence of GDV.[67] Lastly, although there is some disagreement, the fermentation theory has been largely refuted by the observation that the gas found in the stomachs of dogs with GDV is made up primarily of atmospheric gas, indicating that swallowed air is usually the source of the gas, not fermented stomach contents.[68,69] Production of fermentative gas in the stomach of dogs with GDV can occur after death and may lead to the erroneous conclusion that this gas was the initial cause of the disorder. For example, studies of postmortem tissue decomposition have been unable to demonstrate that the presence of *Clostridium* bacteria in the stomach is primary to the disease, rather than secondary. Currently, the studies that are available support the conclusion that GDV is not a dietary disorder per se, and that its development is not related to any component in pet foods nor to the type of food that is fed.

Although the type of diet and components within the diet are not causal factors in GDV, several feeding management practices can be used to help prevent GDV in dogs that are susceptible or have a history of GDV. In other words, although what the dog eats does not appear to affect the occurrence of GDV, how the dog is fed and the feeding environment can be managed to minimize the chances of GDV. Portion-controlled

---

BOX 35-1 PRACTICAL TIPS: PREVENTION OF GASTRIC DILATATION-VOLVULUS (GDV) IN SUSCEPTIBLE DOGS

Use portion-controlled meal feeding as the feeding regimen.

Feed several small meals per day to prevent overfilling of the stomach.

Do not allow the consumption of a large volume of water immediately before or after eating or exercise.

Feed susceptible dogs separately from other animals. If possible, supervise mealtimes.

Do not provide exercise for 1 hour before and 3 hours after meals.

Minimize stress and environmental changes.

If signs of GDV are observed, seek veterinary assistance immediately.

---

meal feeding should be used. Several small meals should be fed per day, as opposed to one large meal, to prevent overfilling of the stomach.[65] Similarly, although fresh water should be available at all times, dogs should not be allowed to drink a large volume of water before or after eating, or after exercise. Because dogs often increase their rate of eating or the amount that they eat when in the presence of other dogs, all susceptible dogs should be fed separately, and any stress that may be associated with the feeding environment should be minimized. If possible, feeding times should be scheduled so that the dog is supervised and can be observed for 1 to 2 hours after meals. Lastly, although exercise as a predisposing factor has not been confirmed, it is prudent to withhold exercise for 1 hour before and at least 3 hours after feeding. All dogs that have a susceptible body type or a history of GDV should be carefully monitored for signs of GDV. If signs are seen, veterinary care should be sought immediately (Box 35-1).

DIETARY MANAGEMENT OF INTESTINAL DISEASE

A diet used to manage gastrointestinal disease should be selected in accordance with the specific disease being treated, the area of the gastrointestinal tract affected, and the ability of the diet to promote healing and maintain remission. Specific diet characteristics that should be considered include protein and carbohydrate sources, level and type of fat, level and type of dietary fiber, potential benefits of prebiotics or probiotics, and diet digestibility.

Managing Acute Disease

The immediate nutritional management of acute gastrointestinal disease usually involves short-term fasting or severely reduced food intake with the intent of providing "gut rest." This approach is based upon the theory that slowing gastrointestinal tract function by withholding food allows normal gastric and peristaltic contractions to subside and promotes healing of the intestinal lining.[1] Traditionally, after a fasting period of 12 to 48 hours, a bland diet consisting of highly digestible ingredients has been recommended. However, while "resting the gut" may have benefits, especially when the animal is vomiting or diarrhea is severe, the use of "bland diet" has been questioned due to a lack of evidence for its efficacy.[2] Moreover, while use of the term "bland" to describe the refeeding diet enjoys ubiquitous usage, the definition of this term and the specific diet characteristics are vague and poorly defined. While a short-term fasting period to allow gut rest is helpful in the initial treatment stage of some intestinal disorders and may help to prevent hypersensitivities when altered mucosal permeability is present, studies of intestinal disease in dogs and cats show that the type of diet is very important and that diet characteristics other than "blandness" must be considered (see pp. 462-472). In the face of new information supporting the use of specifically formulated diets for the treatment and management of gastrointestinal disorders, it is advised that the term "blandness" be discontinued altogether when attempting to describe a therapeutic diet.

Long-Term Management—Diet Composition

PROTEIN SOURCE Diseases that affect the small intestine, such as EPI, SIBO/ARD, and some forms of inflammatory bowel disease, can impair protein digestion and absorption. Prolonged malabsorption of dietary protein can lead to protein malnutrition, which further exacerbates existing intestinal disease through reduced mucosal cell protein synthesis and impaired local immune function.[70] Most seriously, a syndrome called *protein-losing enteropathy* (PLE) occurs when there is rapid and severe loss of protein from the small intestine.[71] Although PLE is most commonly associated with idiopathic lymphangiectasia, it may also represent the end stage of several chronic intestinal disorders. Therefore the diet should provide a high-quality protein source that is easily digested and assimilated and contains all of the essential amino acids in their correct proportions to minimize the risk of protein malnutrition.

Any dietary protein that is not completely digested and assimilated in the small intestine travels to the large intestine, where it can be metabolized by gut microbes, causing changes in the intestinal microflora.[72] A healthy and balanced intestinal microflora is comprised predominantly of saccharolytic (carbohydrate fermenting) bacterial species, most of which are considered to be beneficial gut microbes.[73] Conversely, other species, such as *Bacteroides* spp. and *Clostridia* spp. are capable of fermenting polypeptides and amino acids. These organisms are normally present in low numbers; however, when partially digested protein is delivered to the large intestine it provides increased substrate for these pathogenic species, leading to their proliferation and to the production of ammonia, phenols, indoles, and gas. This can lead to large intestinal diarrhea, further exacerbating intestinal disease.

Dietary protein is also important because of its effect on immune-mediated responses in the gastrointestinal tract. In at least some animals, the development of colitis appears to be an immune-mediated response to food antigens that gain access to the colonic lamina propria and submucosa.[72] Once an immune response is triggered, the continuous exposure of the local immune system of the large intestine to an offending antigen results in persistent inflammation and disruption of intestinal function. Some dogs and cats with chronic gastrointestinal disease are also found to have an adverse food reaction or dietary sensitivity and respond positively to a pet food that contains a single and novel protein source (for a complete discussion of adverse food reactions see Chapter 31, pp. 396-402).[74]

For all of these reasons, the proteins that are included in diets for dogs and cats with intestinal disease must be highly digestible. When adverse food reaction is suspected, a single-source protein should be fed, preferably one to which the dog or cat has not previously been exposed. Highly digestible protein sources have reduced antigenicity because less intact dietary protein is absorbed into the mucosa of the small intestine and less arrives intact or partially digested in the large intestine. Providing a single protein source also minimizes the chance of feeding a protein to which the pet has been previously sensitized. Because of a possible connection between food antigens and colitis, some authors recommend feeding an elimination diet to treat colitis and other forms of inflammatory intestinal disease. Types of elimination diets and their use in the diagnosis and management of dietary hypersensitivity are described in detail in Chapter 31 (see pp. 399-402).

Several studies of dogs and cats with colitis have shown positive results when the animals are fed an elimination diet containing a single, novel protein source.[75,76] Although response rates vary among studies, between 30% and 85% of dogs with idiopathic colitis respond favorably to this type of regimen. Differences in response rates may reflect variations in the diets used with respect to protein source and digestibility. Animals that did not respond with complete remission to a novel protein source often showed some degree of improvement and required lower levels of antiinflammatory medications to achieve and maintain remission.[75] A number of suitable commercially prepared veterinary diets are available. Most are formulated to provide complete and balanced nutrition and include single-source, highly digestible protein (limited-antigen foods).

It has been suggested that animals with IBD are at increased risk of immunological sensitization to food proteins during the initial phase of treatment.[72] Chronic inflammation of the intestinal mucosa can lead to impaired protein digestion and damage to the intestinal lining. As a result, intact food proteins may have a greater chance of gaining access to the lamina propria and stimulating an immune response during periods of active disease.[43] Therefore the novel protein that is fed during the initial phase of therapy may have only short-term benefit. This theory has led to the concept of using an initial "sacrificial protein source" for the first 4 to 6 weeks of diet therapy. The protein source is then changed again to a second novel and highly available source to use as the pet's maintenance diet. The intent of this procedure is to introduce the second

protein only after mucosal inflammation and permeability has decreased, thus minimizing the risk of the second protein resulting in hypersensitivity. Although this approach has theoretical merit, there is currently no clinical or experimental evidence of its efficacy. Because using a sacrifice diet and protein source requires identifying two novel protein sources and changing the pet's food twice during treatment, most veterinarians and nutritionists are not currently recommending this treatment approach.[77]

Proteins that are included in diets for dogs and cats with intestinal disease must be of high quality and highly digestible. When adverse food reaction is suspected, a single-source protein should be fed, preferably one to which the dog or cat has not previously been exposed. Because of a possible connection between food antigens and colitis, it may be helpful to feed an elimination diet to treat colitis and other forms of inflammatory intestinal disease.

CARBOHYDRATE   Similar to protein, a single carbohydrate source that can be easily digested and assimilated should be included in foods formulated for pets with gastrointestinal disease. Because gluten-induced enteropathy is the cause of intestinal disease in some dogs, particularly Irish Setters, it has been suggested to include only gluten-free carbohydrates in diets formulated for intestinal disease.[78,79] Cooked and blended white rice is highly digestible and is gluten free.[80] Other gluten-free carbohydrate sources include potato, tapioca, and corn. Potato and tapioca starches are less digestible than rice, while corn may be contraindicated in dogs that have a hypersensitivity to this ingredient.[81] In contrast, wheat, oats, and barley all contain gluten.

LEVEL AND TYPE OF FAT   A reduced fat diet is often beneficial for dogs and cats with gastrointestinal disease. High-fat intake is specifically contraindicated in animals with EPI, postacute pancreatitis, and lymphangiectasia because these diseases all involve severe impairment of fat digestion and assimilation. A low-fat diet is also indicated whenever there is SIBO or reduced surface area in the small intestine. Malabsorption of dietary fat allows bacterial metabolism of unabsorbed

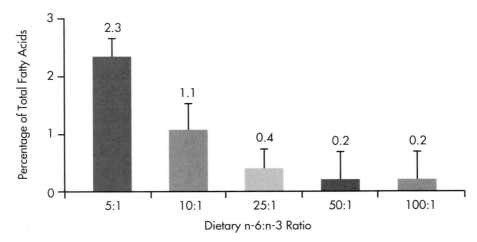

Figure 35-1   Effect of dietary omega-6:omega-3 fatty acid ratio on 12-week eicosapentaenoic acid concentrations in canine intestinal mucosa.

(From World Small Animal Veterinary Association: *Gastrointestinal health symposium*, Dayton, Ohio, 1997, The Iams Company.)

dietary fat to hydroxy fatty acids, while bacterial overgrowth contributes to deconjugation of bile salts, both of which stimulate secretory diarrhea in the distal small intestine and colon.[13] A general recommendation is to select a food that contains approximately 11% or 15% or less total fat (on a dry-matter basis [DMB]) for dogs and cats, respectively, with gastrointestinal disease.[82]

The well documented antiinflammatory benefits of omega-3 fatty acids suggest that there may be a role for this class of fatty acids in the management of inflammatory intestinal disease. In addition to demonstrated benefits for pets with inflammatory skin disease (see Chapter 31, pp. 386-394), there is also evidence that altering the omega-6 to omega-3 fatty acid ratio to favor production of omega-3 metabolites alters eicosanoid profiles in the intestinal mucosa (Figures 35-1 and 35-2).[82] When dogs were fed diets containing omega fatty acid ratios of 10:1 and 5:1, intestinal and colonic mucosa eicosapentaenoic acid (EPA) (20:5n-3) and docosapentaenoic acid (22:6n-3) concentrations increased and arachidonic acid levels decreased over an 8-week period. Regional differences were seen, with small-intestinal mucosa having a greater concentration of stearic acid (18:0) and linoleic acid (18:2n-6) than colonic mucosa, and colonic mucosa having greater concentrations of eicosatrienoic (20:3n-3) and arachidonic (20:4n-6) acids.

Additional studies with humans and laboratory animals have indicated that increasing dietary omega-3

fatty acids in the diet significantly affects clinical disease.[83,84] When the diets of human patients with ulcerative colitis were supplemented with fish oil, they showed a 56% reduction in colitis symptoms and a 30% reduction in colonic leukotriene B_4 (LTB_4) production.[85] Another study revealed that inclusion of fish oil in the diet of patients with IBD resulted in increased concentrations of EPA and docosahexaenoic acid (DHA) and decreased arachidonic acid in intestinal mucosa lipid membranes.[86] Similarly, when human subjects consumed a fish oil supplement containing 3.2 grams (g) of EPA and 2.1 g of docosapentaenoic acid per day, significant changes occurred in intestinal eicosanoids, and improvements in histological findings and body weight were reported.[87] Of particular interest in this study was the finding that the degree of reduction of intestinal LTB_4 was similar in magnitude to that observed in patients treated with prednisolone. This effect allowed a reduction in drug dosages in patients who were receiving the fish oil supplement.

While canine colonic lipid and eicosanoid production are demonstrably altered by increasing the proportion of dietary omega-3 fatty acids, the efficacy of this class of fatty acids in the treatment of intestinal disease has not been well studied in dogs or cats. However, positive results in humans and rats, as well as the responses of canine intestinal mucosa to dietary omega-3 fatty acids, support the use of diets containing optimized omega-6

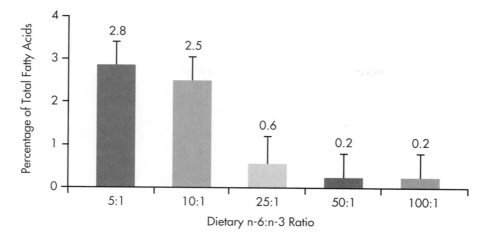

Figure 35-2   Effect of dietary omega-6:omega-3 fatty acid ratio on 12-week eicosapentaenoic acid concentrations in canine colonic mucosa.

(From World Small Animal Veterinary Association: *Gastrointestinal health symposium,* Dayton, Ohio, 1997, The Iams Company.)

to omega-3 fatty acid ratios as an aid in managing the inflammation associated with intestinal disease. Clinical studies of dogs and cats with naturally occurring intestinal disease are necessary to further define the role of omega-3 fatty acids in the management of these disorders.

DIETARY FIBER   Dietary fiber is defined as the collection of all dietary constituents that are not digested by the endogenous enzymes of mammals.[88] Fiber is composed of structural plant carbohydrates plus lignin; major fiber components in pets' diets include cellulose, hemicellulose, lignin, pectin, gums, and mucilages. The benefits of dietary fiber for gastrointestinal health and in the treatment and management of gastrointestinal disease in dogs and cats are now well recognized. Historically, the perceived benefits of fiber were limited to its physical effects on the gastrointestinal tract and distinctions were not always made between different fiber types. Fiber was not considered to be essential for the diets of dogs and cats. However, in the past 10 to 15 years, in vitro and in vivo studies have shown that different types of fiber have varying effects on the function and health of the gastrointestinal tract. Today, it is well known that the type of fiber included in diets for pets with gastrointestinal disease is as important as the level of fiber. The classification, characteristics, and functions of dietary fiber are discussed extensively in Chapters 2 and 10 (p. 14 and pp. 77-78).

With respect to gastrointestinal health, important fiber considerations are the degree to which a fiber type is fermented by intestinal bacteria and the amount and type of byproducts that are produced.[89-91] Both dogs and cats have active colonic bacteria and are capable of fermenting dietary fiber.[92-94] The amount of fermentation depends upon the amount of time the fiber is present in the tract, the composition of the diet, and the type of fiber that is present. For example, cellulose, gum karaya, and xanthan gum are almost nonfermentable in the intestine of the dog and cat.[92,94] In contrast, pectin and guar gum are rapidly fermented by canine and feline colonic microbes, while beet pulp and rice bran are moderately fermentable sources of fiber (Tables 35-1 and 35-2).

The most important end products of fiber fermentation are the SCFAs. These compounds, primarily acetic, butyric, and propionic acids, comprise a preferred energy source for colonocytes, which derive more than 70% of their energy requirement from luminally derived SCFAs.[95,96] Colonic cell proliferation is enhanced in the presence of SCFAs, probably as a result of increased availability of this energy source.[97] This is an important effect because epithelial cells of the gastrointestinal tract have high energy needs and a rapid turnover, with the average cell being replaced every 3 days. For example, dogs that consumed diets containing fermentable fiber had increased colon weights, mucosal surface area, and mucosal hypertrophy when compared with dogs

TABLE 35-1 FERMENTATION INDEX OF FIBER SOURCES FOR DOGS

FIBER SOURCE	FERMENTATION INDEX*
Cellulose	0.2
Oat fiber	0.4
Gum karaya	0.6
Peanut hulls	0.9
Xanthan gum	1.0
Gum arabic	1.0
Gum talha	1.3
Psyllium gum	1.4
Soy hulls	1.4
Rice bran	1.8
Beet pulp	2.5
Carob bean gum	3.4
Citrus pulp	3.4
Locust bean gum	5.3
Fructooligosaccharides	5.7
Citrus pectin	5.9
Guar gum	7.3
Lactulose	8.3

Adapted from Sunvold GD, Fahey GC Jr, Merchen NR, and others: Dietary fiber for dogs. IV. In vitro fermentation of selected fiber sources by dog fecal inoculum and in vivo digestion and metabolism of fiber-supplemented diets, *J Anim Sci* 73:1099–1109, 1995.
*Total 24-hour short-chain fatty acid production (mmol/g of substrate organic matter).

TABLE 35-2 FERMENTATION INDEX OF FIBER SOURCES FOR CATS

FIBER SOURCE	FERMENTATION INDEX*
Cellulose	0.1
Xanthan gum	0.5
Gum karaya	0.9
Gum arabic	1.3
Gum talha	1.8
Beet pulp	2.0
Rice bran	2.1
Carob bean gum	3.3
Sugar cane residue	3.4
Fructooligosaccharides	4.3
Locust bean gum	4.8
Guar gum	5.1
Citrus pectin	5.5

Adapted from Sunvold GD, Fahey GC Jr, Merchen NR, and others: Dietary fiber for cats: in vitro fermentation of selected fiber sources by cat fecal inoculum and in vivo utilization of diets containing selected fiber sources and their blends, *J Anim Sci* 73:2329–2339, 1995.
*Total 24-hour short-chain fatty acid production (mmol/g of substrate organic matter).

fed a diet containing nonfermentable fiber.[98,99] These changes appear to be due to a greater ratio of mucosal surface area to colonic mass and therefore are indicative of increased absorptive potential.[100]

The production of SCFAs from dietary fiber in the gastrointestinal tract has several other beneficial effects. SCFAs affect gut motility by increasing peristaltic contractions in the distal portion of the small intestine while possibly inhibiting colonic contractions.[101,102] It is postulated that the cumulative results of these two effects may prevent excessive fermentation in the small intestine while potentiating the absorption of SCFAs in the large intestine. Colonic blood flow increases in the presence of SCFAs.[103] This may occur due to a relaxation of resistance arteries in the colon or simply in response to increased metabolic activity of the colonocytes. Finally, the presence of SCFAs aids in the prevention of diarrhea by enhancing sodium absorption, maintaining normal intestinal electrolyte and fluid balance, promoting the growth of beneficial indigenous microflora, and inhibiting the proliferation of pathogenic microbes.[104,105]

When treating intestinal disease, the effect that SCFAs may have upon intestinal bacterial populations is an important consideration because bacterial and pathogen overgrowth is frequently seen as either the primary disease or as a consequence of other forms of intestinal disease (see pp. 455-457). An important function of indigenous bacterial populations in the intestine is to help prevent overgrowth of pathogenic bacteria, thus maintaining a healthy and balanced microbiota. Bacteria exert this effect by their patterns of SCFA production and through direct inhibition of the growth of other microbial species.[106,107] Beneficial bacteria such as *Bifidobacterium* and lactobacilli also aid in the digestion and absorption of food, provide a source of vitamins to the host animal, and stimulate gastrointestinal immune function (see pp. 467-470). Conversely, proliferation of harmful bacterial species causes or exacerbates intestinal disease through the production of toxins, carcinogens, or putrefactive substances. Both the relative abilities of beneficial and pathogenic bacteria to use fiber (carbohydrates) as a substrate, as well as the amount and pattern of SCFAs that are produced, must be considered in the selection of a fiber source.

There is also some evidence suggesting that IBD symptoms and intestinal healing following surgery may be positively influenced by fermentable fiber and SCFA production. The provision of specific bowel nutrients, including SCFAs, has been shown to protect intestinal tissue and promote restoration of normal intestinal function. For example, ulcerative colitis in humans is characterized by diminished rates of oxidation of butyrate in the large intestine.[108] Providing a supplemental source of butyrate to the colon has been shown to reduce the inflammatory response in patients with this disease.[109] A study with rats examined the effects of feeding diets with or without fermentable fiber after colonic anastomoses. During healing, the fiber-containing diet conferred a trophic effect on the surgical site, improving both wound strength and rate of healing.[110]

While some SCFA production is desirable because of their beneficial effects, more is not necessarily better. As stated previously, fiber types differ in the degree to which they are fermented by intestinal bacteria. Minimal fermentation and production of SCFAs occurs when fibers with low fermentability are fed. These include cellulose, peanut hulls, methylcellulose, and locust bean gum. Conversely, maximal production occurs when fermentable fiber mixtures containing pectin or guar gum are fed.[92-94] By comparison, fibers that are moderately fermentable include beet pulp, inulin, rice bran, and gum arabic. Rapid fermentation and the production of large amounts of SCFAs in the intestinal tract of both dogs and cats can cause the production of loose stools or diarrhea and excess gas, and may interfere with nutrient digestion and absorption.[111,112] Benefits are maximized by feeding optimal amounts of moderately fermentable fiber sources that provide optimal levels of SCFAs and at the same time have a nonfermentable component to provide bulk and contribute to normal peristalsis.

Both dogs and cats have active colonic bacteria and are capable of fermenting dietary fiber. The most important end products of fiber fermentation are the short-chain fatty acids (SCFAs), compounds that have several gastrointestinal benefits. SCFAs provide energy for colonocytes, promote normal peristalsis, increase blood flow to the large intestine, aid in electrolyte and fluid balance, and promote balanced intestinal microbial populations.

PREBIOTICS Prebiotics are nondigestible food ingredients that beneficially affect the host animal by influencing the growth and activity of selective bacterial colonies in the large intestine.[113] Most prebiotics are short-chain carbohydrates that are classified with fiber because they are plant derived, are not digested by mammalian enzymes, and are selectively fermented by certain intestinal microbes. Examples of prebiotics include inulin, galactooligosaccharides, lactulose, fructooligosaccharides (FOS) and mannanoligosaccharides (MOS).[113] FOS and MOS are highly fermentable prebiotics that have been studied for inclusion in pet foods. FOS contain fructose as their primary carbohydrate unit and are found naturally in a variety of fruits, vegetables, and grains. Concentrated sources of FOS include soybean hulls, psyllium, chicory, and sugar beet root (after pulp processing). FOS are also produced commercially through fermentation by *Aspergillus niger* (Figure 35-3).[114] MOS are related prebiotics that are comprised predominantly of mannose units and found naturally in yeast cells.

Although FOS and MOS both can function as prebiotics, the mechanism through which they affect the growth of intestinal microbes differs. FOS are selectively metabolized by certain beneficial bacterial species in the gastrointestinal tract.[115,116] For example, most *Bifidobacterium, Lactobacillus,* and *Bacteroides* species utilize FOS as an energy source as well as they do glucose. Conversely, harmful bacteria such as *Eubacterium, Salmonella,* and *Clostridium* species either do not metabolize FOS or metabolize them less efficiently than glucose.[2,117] Providing FOS in the diet supports the growth of health-promoting species, in particular *Bifidobacterium* and lactobacilli, and limit the growth of less beneficial or pathogenic species. In contrast to FOS, MOS functions as a prebiotic by preventing harmful gastrointestinal bacteria from attaching to the host's intestinal wall and colonizing. Certain species of pathogenic bacteria bind to mannose residues on the surface of intestinal cells, allowing colonization and preventing excretion. The presence of MOS in the large intestine competitively inhibits this attachment and promotes the fecal excretion of pathogenic bacterial species.

Early studies with human subjects found that the consumption of dietary FOS helped to prevent infection with *Clostridium* species and *Escherichia coli* and supported the growth of *Bifidobacterium*

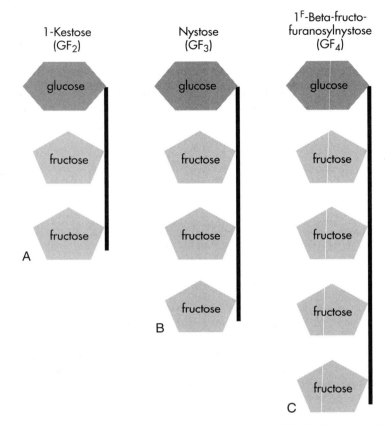

Figure 35-3 Common fructooligosaccharides. **A,** 1-Kestose (GF$_2$). **B,** Nystose (GF$_3$). **C,** 1^F-Beta-fructofuranosylnystose (GF$_4$).
(From NAVC: *New discoveries in canine gastrointestinal disease,* Dayton, Ohio, 1996, The Iams Company.)

populations.[117,118] Similarly, in vitro and in vivo studies have shown that FOS and lactosucrose (a functional trisaccharide that is highly fermentable) effectively alter the intestinal microbe populations in dogs and cats by increasing concentrations of lactobacilli and decreasing the concentration of *C. perfringens* (Figures 35-4 and 35-5).[119-121] Supplementation with MOS has been reported to significantly decrease total aerobe numbers and lactobacilli numbers in adult dogs.[122] A larger study found that feeding a commercial adult maintenance dry dog food that included two levels of supplemental FOS significantly decreased fecal *E. coli* concentrations when fed at both levels, and significantly decreased fecal concentrations of *Bacteroides* and eubacteria when fed at the higher level.[123] Including FOS also significantly increased fecal concentrations of lactobacilli, when fed at the lower level. No effects were found on

fecal counts of *C. perfringens* in this study. There is also some evidence that supplementation with prebiotics may positively influence immunoglobulin production by lactating female dogs and subsequently improve the immune health of their puppies.[124]

It should be noted that the microbial population responses that dogs have shown to prebiotics has not been consistent, and these effects appear to be influenced by numerous factors. A small pilot study showed that feeding a high protein food that contained a poor-quality protein source to dogs promoted the proliferation of *Clostridium* species in the large intestine, while feeding the same diet with a lower proportion of protein increased intestinal *Bifidobacteria* species.[125] Most significantly, adding a prebiotic (inulin from chicory) to the food further increased beneficial species when the lower protein food was fed, but only to a relatively small

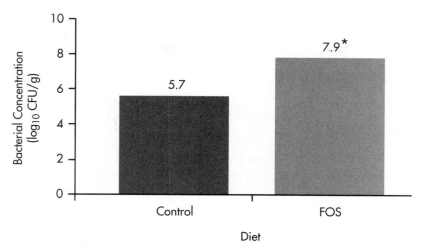

Figure 35-4   Effect of dietary fructooligosaccharides *(FOS)* on the concentration of lactobacilli in the feline large intestine. *, *P* < .05.
(From Sparkes AH, Papasouliotis K, Sunvold G, and others: The effect of dietary supplementation with fructo-oligosaccharides on the fecal flora of healthy cats, *Am J Vet Res* 59:436–440, 1998.)

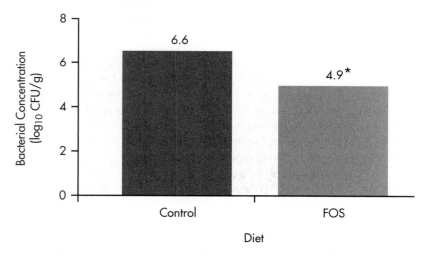

Figure 35-5   Effect of dietary fructooligosaccharides *(FOS)* on the concentration of *Clostridium perfringens* in the feline large intestine. *, *P* < .10.
(From Sparkes AH, Papasouliotis K, Sunvold G, and others: The effect of dietary supplementation with fructo-oligosaccharides on the fecal flora of healthy cats, *Am J Vet Res* 59:436–440, 1998.)

degree. Similarly, another study reported that feeding healthy dogs a dry food containing 1% supplemental FOS for 3 weeks significantly increased the number of both *Bifidobacteria* and *Clostridia* in fecal samples.[126] The researchers suggested that the base diet's level of fermentable fiber influenced the dogs' responses to FOS in this study. Finally, it has also been noted that the normal microbiota of dogs varies dramatically among dogs and can be affected by age, breed, and health status. These factors may subsequently influence an individual animal's response to prebiotic supplementation.[127]

Prebiotic supplementation may have a role in the treatment of SIBO or pathogen overgrowth in dogs. When dogs with SIBO were fed a diet containing 1% FOS for 45 days, significantly fewer aerobic and facultative anaerobic bacteria were found in both intestinal fluid and mucosal samples when compared with the samples of control dogs.[128] Another study found that Beagles fed diets containing either cellulose (nonfermentable fiber) or a combination of beet pulp and FOS had similar fecal bacterial densities, but those fed the FOS-containing diet had lower numbers of enterobacteria and clostridia and higher numbers of lactobacilli and streptococci, compared with those in dogs fed the nonfermentable fiber.[129] The dogs fed the FOS-containing food also had increased small intestinal mucosal weight and absorptive surface area and higher nutrient transport rates per unit of intestine. There is also clinical evidence of beneficial effects of FOS when included in the diets of dogs being treated for SIBO.[130] When dogs with suspected SIBO were treated with either antibiotic therapy for 30 days or were fed an FOS-containing diet for 60 days, fecal volume and fecal consistency normalized in both groups during treatment. Dogs treated with the antibiotic showed rapid improvement, but also quickly deteriorated following withdrawal of antibiotic therapy. Conversely, dogs fed the FOS-containing food experienced a gradual improvement in fecal consistency and volume, and normalization of these measures was maintained by dietary therapy throughout the study period.

When SIBO or pathogen overgrowth occur, the bacterial populations in the small intestine can be altered either by using antimicrobial drugs or by changing the diet to increase beneficial bacteria and inhibit the growth of undesirable species. While antibiotics are often effective in the treatment and management of SIBO, the risk of selectively killing the wrong populations exists, and this may result in exacerbation of SIBO. In addition, long-term use is usually required and may be associated with adverse side effects. Therefore dietary treatment, if effective, is more appealing to most pet owners. Providing a food that includes a prebiotic such as FOS may affect small intestinal bacterial populations in dogs with SIBO/ARD, and may provide an adjunctive therapy for treating SIBO/ARD-associated diarrhea.

Prebiotics are nondigestible food ingredients that beneficially affect the host animal by influencing the growth and activity of beneficial species of bacteria in the large intestine. Common examples are fructooligosaccharides, mannanoligosaccharides, inulin, and lactulose. Because

prebiotics help to support bifidobacteria and lactobacilli populations while reducing bacterial pathogens, these compounds can play a role in the management of SIBO/ARD and pathogen overgrowth.

FIBER/PREBIOTIC RECOMMENDATIONS

Current data suggest that appropriate levels of moderately fermentable fiber should be included in the elimination diet that is typically used to treat IBD in dogs and cats (see pp. 465-467). Although highly digestible diets that are very low in fiber have traditionally been used, it now appears that diets formulated to manage intestinal disease should contain between 3% and 7%, but not more than 10%, fiber (on a DMB).[131] A balance of fermentable and nonfermentable fiber sources should be fed to supply SCFAs and promote motility, respectively.[2] Both beet pulp and rice bran are moderately fermentable fibers and are appropriate for inclusion in gastrointestinal diets for dogs and cats. In addition, FOS and MOS are prebiotics that can provide SCFAs and be used to beneficially alter bacterial populations and numbers in pets with SIBO and pathogen overgrowth. The nutritional objective when selecting dietary fibers should be to select those that predispose to the colonization of beneficial indigenous microflora and promote sufficient SCFA production for intestinal epithelial health.

PROBIOTICS

Probiotics are live microorganisms that, when ingested, exert beneficial health effects that extend beyond their nutritional value.[132] These organisms are select strains of the same beneficial bacterial species that are specifically supported by prebiotics. While prebiotics function to alter gastrointestinal microbiota by providing substrate for selective microbes, probiotics can alter the gastrointestinal flora by supplying a direct source of beneficial microbes. A *synbiotic* is a preparation that includes both a probiotic and a prebiotic. Including a prebiotic that is a preferred substrate for the probiotic with the probiotic product can enhance its viability and proliferation in the host gastrointestinal tract. A potential synbiotic approach that may be effective for supporting companion animal gastrointestinal health or managing intestinal disease is to feed a pet food that includes a prebiotic along with a complementary probiotic supplement.

Historically, humans have consumed probiotics in the form of cultured yogurt, buttermilk, sauerkraut, and cheeses. However, in recent years, various types of probiotic supplements that are marketed for human and for pet use have become commercially available. Similar to human products, dog and cat probiotics are available in a variety of forms, including tablets and capsules, pastes, and liquids, and can also be directly incorporated into foods.[133] A wide variety of bacterial species and strains are also used in probiotics. The species that is used will directly affect the type of benefit that the supplement may have, as will dosage concentration and microbial viability. For example, preparations that provide too low a concentration or that do not adequately survive destruction by gastric acids and digestive enzymes may not allow sufficient colonization in the gastrointestinal tract to confer a health benefit.[134]

Gastrointestinal benefits that probiotics may provide to dogs and cats include the maintenance of balanced and healthy intestinal microbial populations; prevention of stress-induced, infectious, or antibiotic-associated diarrhea; and possibly management of SIBO and IBDs. Although their mechanisms of action are not completely understood, probiotics of varying species and strains can modify intestinal pH, enhance the local immune system, and inhibit the growth of intestinal pathogens. Pathogen proliferation is reduced through competition for nutrients and mucosal attachment sites and, for some probiotics, the production of inhibitory substances. Immune functions of probiotics include a direct effect upon gut-associated lymphoid tissue (GALT) as well as lesser-understood effects upon circulating immunoglobulins.[135]

Research studies have demonstrated that probiotics can survive passage through the stomach and small intestine of the dog and cat and are capable of effectively modifying the microbial environment of the large intestine. Two studies with healthy dogs and cats reported that supplementation with a strain of *Lactobacillus acidophilus* led to increased fecal numbers of *L. acidophilus* (a beneficial gut microbe), concomitantly with decreased numbers of *Clostridium* spp. and *Enterococcus* spp., suggesting an altered intestinal microbial balance.[136,137] Fecal pH also decreased in cats fed the probiotic, which indicates a colonic environment that was conducive to lactic acid bacterial species. Similarly, when healthy adult dogs were fed a strain of *Bifidobacterium*

animalis, fecal concentrations of clostridial pathogens decreased, and the pathogen *Clostridium difficile* decreased dramatically (Figure 35-6).[138] Immunological benefits were reported in studies of a strain of *Enterococcus faecium* that increased populations of certain serum immunoglobulins in puppies and kittens, and enhanced vaccination response in puppies.[135,139]

Probiotics may also be beneficial for the treatment or management of pets with gastrointestinal disease. When cats and kittens with chronic diarrhea were supplemented with a strain of *E. faecium*, significant improvements were observed, fecal bifidobacteria increased, and fecal *C. perfringens* decreased.[140,141] In another study, cats infected with campylobacteria showed a reduction in microbial shedding of this enteric pathogen when they were fed a diet containing a probiotic strain of *L. acidophilus*.[142] Similar results have been reported in dogs. When a group of dogs with IBDs were fed a combination of three lactobacilli species, probiotic supplementation positively affected the in vitro production of regulatory and proinflammatory cytokines from isolated duodenal tissue.[143] Other data show that young adult dogs supplemented with a strain of bifidobacteria prior to and during transition to a kennel environment had better stool scores during the transition and were less likely to experience loose stools or diarrhea

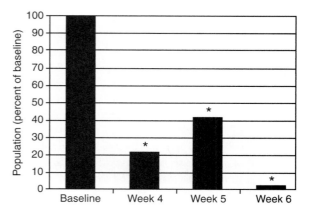

Figure 35-6   Effect of the probiotic *Bifidobacterium animalis* AHC7 supplementation on *Clostridium difficile* population in canine feces. *, Statistically significant difference from baseline, $P < .05$.

(From *Bifidobacterium animalis* AHC7 promotes gastrointestinal health in adult dogs, *Iams Company Abstract*, 2009.)

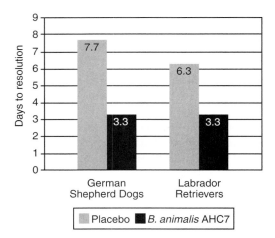

Figure 35-7   Days to diarrhea resolution in Labrador Retrievers and German Shepherd Dogs presented to a veterinary clinic for diarrhea.

(From Kelley RL, Kiely B, O'Mahony B, and others: Clinical benefits of probiotic canine-derived *Bifidobacterium animalis* strain AHC7 in dogs with acute idiopathic diarrhea, *Vet Ther* 10[3]:121–130, 2009.)

than were dogs that had not been supplemented.[144] When the same probiotic was fed to dogs presented to a veterinary clinic with diarrhea, the supplemented dogs experienced fewer number of days to resolution compared with dogs that were not supplemented (Figure 35-7).[145] Together, these studies suggest a role for probiotics in the treatment and management of gastrointestinal disorders in dogs and cats.

Probiotics are live microorganisms that, when ingested, provide beneficial health effects to the host animal by altering the gastrointestinal flora. Gastrointestinal benefits to dogs and cats include the maintenance of balanced and healthy intestinal microbial populations, prevention and management of diarrhea, and possibly management of small intestinal bacterial overgrowth and inflammatory bowel disorders.

Diet Digestibility

A final consideration when selecting a diet for pets with gastrointestinal disease is digestibility. Pet foods formulated for the management of gastrointestinal disease should always contain high-quality ingredients and be highly digestible. When nutrients are efficiently digested and absorbed in the proximal small intestine, the remainder of the bowel is allowed to rest and the delivery of undigested nutrients to the large intestine is minimized. This limits the risk of gaseousness and osmotic diarrhea in the large intestine due to malabsorption. Highly digestible protein sources are less antigenic because little dietary protein is absorbed intact into the mucosa (see Chapter 31, pp. 399-402). Diets that require minimal digestion also reduce gastric, pancreatic, biliary, and intestinal secretions and contribute to reduced total bacterial counts in the intestine. Gastrointestinal diets should have digestibility coefficients of 90% or greater (dry-matter [DM] digestibility) (Box 35-2).

References

1. Guilford WG: New ideas for the dietary management of gastrointestinal tract disease, *J Small Anim Pract* 35:620–624, 1994.

2. Reinhart GA, Sunvold GD: The role of diet in the treatment of gastrointestinal disease in dogs. In *Proc NAVC*, Orlando, Fla, 1996, pp 23–28.

3. Williams DA: Malabsorption, small intestinal bacterial overgrowth, and protein-losing enteropathy. In Guilford WG, Center SA, Strombeck DR, and others, editors: *Small animal gastroenterology*, ed 3, Philadelphia, 1996, Saunders.

4. Westermarck E, Skrzypczak T, Harmonien J: Tylosin-responsive chronic diarrhea in dogs, *J Vet Intern Med* 19:177–186, 2005.

5. Rutgers HC, Batt RM, Kelly DF: Lymphocytic-plasmacytic enteritis associated with bacterial overgrowth in a dog, *J Am Vet Med Assoc* 192:1739–1742, 1988.

6. Fogle JE, Bissett SA: Mucosal immunity and chronic idiopathic enteropathies in dogs, *Compend Contin Educ Pract Vet* 29:290–302, 2007.

7. Batt RM, Barnes A, Rutgers HC, Carter SD: Relative IgA deficiency and small intestinal bacterial overgrowth in German Shepherd Dogs, *Res Vet Sci* 50:106–111, 1991.

8. Littler RM, Batt RM, Lloyd DH: Total and relative deficiency of gut mucosal IgA in German Shepherd Dogs demonstrated by faecal analysis, *Vet Rec* 158:334–341, 2006.

9. German AJ, Day MJ, Ruaux CG: Comparison of direct and indirect tests for small intestinal bacterial overgrowth and antibiotic-responsive diarrhea in dogs, *J Vet Intern Med* 17:33–43, 2003.

10. Johnston KL: Small intestinal bacterial overgrowth, *Vet Clin North Am Small Anim Pract* 29:523–551, 1999.

11. Gruffy DD, Jones TJ, Papasouliotis K, and others: The uniqueness of the feline gut and its practical implications. In *Proceedings of the gastrointestinal health symposium: a pre-conference symposium*, 1997, World Veterinary Conference, pp 31–35.

12. Williams DA: Clinical diagnosis of canine small intestinal disease. In Reinhart GA, Carey DP, editors: *Recent advances in canine and feline nutrition, Iams nutrition symposium proceedings,* vol 2, Wilmington, Ohio, 1998, Orange Frazer Press.

13. Melgarejo T, Williams DA, O'Connell NC, Setchell KDR: Serum unconjugated bile acids as a test for intestinal bacterial overgrowth in dogs, *Dig Dis Sci* 45:407–414, 2000.

14. Melgarejo T, Williams DA, Setchell KD, and others: Serum total unconjugated bile acids (TUBA) in dogs with small intestinal bacterial overgrowth, *J Vet Intern Med* 11:114, 1997.

15. Johnston L, Lamport A, Batt RM: Unexpected bacterial flora in the proximal small intestine of normal cats, *Vet Rec* 132:362–363, 1993.

16. Rutgers HC, Batt RM, Elwood CM, and others: Small intestinal bacterial overgrowth in dogs with chronic intestinal disease, *J Am Vet Med Assoc* 206:187–193, 1995.

17. Balish E, Cleven D, Brown J, and others: Nose, throat, and fecal flora of Beagle dogs housed in locked or open environments, *Appl Environ Micro* 34:207, 1977.

18. Terada A, Hara H, Kato S, and others: Effects of lactosucrose (4-beta-D-galactosylsucrose) on fecal flora and fecal putrefactive product of cats, *J Vet Med Sci* 55:291–295, 1993.

19. Batt R, Rutgers H, Sancak A: Enteric bacteria: friend or foe? *J Small Anim Pract* 37:261–267, 1996.

20. Guarner F, Malagelada JR: Gut flora in health and disease, *Lancet* 361:512–519, 2003.

21. Macfarlane S, Macfarlane GT: Bacterial diversity in the large intestine, *Adv Appl Microbiol* 54:261–289, 2004.

22. Twedt DC: *Clostridium perfringens* associated diarrhea in dogs. In *Proc 11th Ann Conf Vet Intern Med Forum*, 1993, pp 121–125.

23. Scherk M: Inflammatory bowel disease and pancreatitis in cats. In *Proc WSAVA*, 2003, pp 25–31.

24. Watson P: Pancreatitis in the dog: dealing with a spectrum of disease, *In Pract* 26:64–77, 2004.

25. Xenoulis PG, Suchodolski JS, Steiner JM: Chronic pancreatitis in dogs and cats, *Compend Contin Educ Pract Vet* 30:166–181, 2008.

26. Steiner JM, Williams DA: Feline exocrine pancreatic disorders, *Vet Clin North Am Small Anim Pract* 29:551–575, 1999.

27. Newman S, Steiner J, Woosley K: Localization of pancreatic inflammation and necrosis in dogs, *J Vet Intern Med* 18:488–493, 2004.

28. DeCock HEV, Forman MA, Farver TB: Prevalence and histopathologic characteristics of pancreatitis in cats, *Vet Pathol* 44:39–49, 2007.

29. Cook AK, Breitschwerdt EB, Levine JF: Risk factors associated with acute pancreatitis in dogs: 101 cases (1985-1990), *J Am Vet Med Assoc* 203:673–679, 1993.

30. Lem KY, Fosgate GT, Norby B, Steiner JM: Associations between dietary factors and pancreatitis in dogs, *J Am Vet Med Assoc* 233:1425–1431, 2008.

31. Weiss DJ, Gagne JM, Armstrong PJ: Relationship between inflammatory hepatic disease and inflammatory bowel disease, pancreatitis, and nephritis in cats, *J Am Vet Med Assoc* 209:1114–1116, 1996.

32. Bishop MA, Steiner JM, Moore LE: Evaluation of the cationic trypsinogen gene for potential mutations in Miniature Schnauzers with pancreatitis, *Can J Vet Res* 68:315–318, 2004.

33. Batchelor DJ, Noble PJM, Taylor RH, and others: Prognostic factors in canine exocrine pancreatic insufficiency: prolonged survival is likely if clinical remission is achieved, *J Vet Intern Med* 21:54–60, 2007.

34. Wiberg ME: Pancreatic acinar atrophy in German Shepherd Dogs and Rough-Coated Collies: etiopathogenesis, diagnosis and treatment: a review, *Vet Q* 26:61–75, 2004.

35. Batchelor DJ, Noble PJM, Cripps PJ, and others: Breed associations for canine exocrine pancreatic insufficiency, *J Vet Intern Med* 21:207–214, 2007.

36. Brenner K, Harkin KR, Andrews GA, Kennedy G: Juvenile pancreatic atrophy in Greyhounds: 12 cases (1995-2000), *J Vet Intern Med* 23:67–71, 2009.

37. Batt RM: Exocrine pancreatic insufficiency, *Vet Clin North Am Small Anim Pract* 23:595–608, 1993.

38. Williams DA, Batt RM, McLean L: Bacterial overgrowth in the duodenum of dogs with exocrine pancreatic insufficiency, *J Am Vet Med Assoc* 191:201–206, 1987.

39. Steiner JM, Wilson BG, Williams DA: Development and analytical validation of a radioimmunoassay for the measurement of feline pancreatic lipase immunoreactivity in serum, *Can J Vet Res* 68:309–314, 2004.

40. Steiner JM, Teague SR, Williams DA: Development and analytic validation of an enzyme-linked immunosorbent assay for the measurement of canine pancreatic lipase immunoreactivity in serum, *Can J Vet Res* 67:175–182, 2003.

41. Williams DA, Batt RM: Sensitivity and specificity of radioimmunoassay of serum trypsin-like immunoreactivity for the diagnosis of canine exocrine pancreatic insufficiency, *J Am Vet Med Assoc* 192:195–201, 1988.

42. Steiner JM, Williams DA: Validation of a radioimmunoassay for feline trypsin-like immunoreactivity (fTLI) and serum cobalamin and folate concentrations in cats with exocrine pancreatic insufficiency (EPI), *J Vet Intern Med* 9:193, 1995.

43. Simpson JW: Diet and large intestinal disease in dogs and cats, *J Nutr* 128:2717S–2722S, 1998.

44. Richter KP: Lymphocytic-plasmacytic enterocolitis in dogs, *Sem Vet Med Surg Small Anim* 7:134–144, 1992.

45. Leib MS: Irritable bowel syndrome in dogs—fact or fiction? In *Proc NAVC*, 2009, pp 13–16.

46. Magne ML: Pathophysiology of inflammatory bowel disease, *Sem Vet Med Surg Small Anim* 7:112–116, 1992.

47. Johnson SE: Canine eosinophilic gastroenterocolitis, *Sem Vet Med Surg Small Anim* 7:145–152, 1992.

48. Breitschwerdt EB: Immunoproliferative enteropathy of Basenjis, *Sem Vet Med Surg Small Anim* 7:153–161, 1992.

49. Van Kruiningen HJ, Ryan MJ, Shindel NM: The classification of feline colitis, *J Comp Pathol* 93:275–294, 1983.

50. Dimski DS: Therapy for inflammatory bowel disease. In Kirk RW, Bonagura JD: *Kirk's current veterinary therapy XII*, Philadelphia, 1995, Saunders.

51. Tams TR: Chronic feline inflammatory bowel disorders. II. Feline eosinophilic enteritis and lymphosarcoma, *Compend Contin Educ Pract Vet* 8:464–471, 1986.

52. Jergens AE: Optimizing IBD therapy in dogs and cats: evidence-based observations. In *Proc AAHA Conf*, 2009, pp 207–210.

53. Leib M: Treatment of chronic idiopathic large-bowel diarrhea in dogs with a highly digestible diet and soluble fiber: a retrospective review of 37 cases, *J Vet Intern Med* 14:27–32, 2000.

54. Brockman DJ, Washabau RJ, Drobatz KJ: Canine gastric dilation/volvulus syndrome in a veterinary critical care unit: 2965 cases (1986-1992), *J Am Vet Med Assoc* 207:460–464, 1995.

55. Glickman LT, Glickman NW, Perez CM, and others: Analysis of risk factors for gastric dilatation and dilatation-volvulus in dogs, *J Am Vet Med Assoc* 204:1465–1471, 1994.

56. Bredal WP, Eggertsdottir AV, Austefjord O: Acute gastric dilatation in cats: a case series, *Acta Vet Scand* 37:445–451, 1996.

57. Glickman LT, Lantz GC, Schellengerg DB, and others: A prospective study of survival and recurrence following acute gastric dilatation-volvulus syndrome in 136 dogs, *J Am Vet Med Assoc* 34:253–259, 1998.

58. Brourman JD, Schertel ER, Allen DA, and others: Factors associated with perioperative mortality in dogs with surgically managed gastric dilatation-volvulus: 137 cases (1988-1993), *J Am Vet Med Assoc* 208:1855–1858, 1996.

59. Glickman L, Emerick T, Glickman N, and others: Radiological assessment of the relationship between thoracic conformation and the risk of gastric dilatation-volvulus in dogs, *Vet Radiol Ultrasound* 37:174–180, 1996.

60. Schellenberg D, Yi Q, Glickman N, and others: Influence of thoracic conformation and genetics on the risk of gastric dilatation-volvulus in Irish Setter dogs, *J Am Anim Hosp Assoc* 34:64–73, 1998.

61. Schaible RH, Ziech J, Glickman NW, and others: Predisposition to gastric dilatation-volvulus in relation to genetics of thoracic conformation in Irish Setters, *J Am Anim Hosp Assoc* 33:379–383, 1997.

62. Glickman LT, Glickman NW, Schellenberg DB, and others: Multiple risk factors for the gastric dilatation-volvulus syndrome in dogs: a practitioner/owner case-control study, *J Am Anim Hosp Assoc* 33:197–204, 1997.

63. Elwood CM: Risk factors for gastric dilatation in Irish Setter dogs, *J Small Anim Pract* 39:185–190, 1998.

64. Van Kruiningen HJ, Wojan LD, Stake PE, and others: The influence of diet and feeding frequency on gastric function in the dog, *J Am Anim Hosp Assoc* 23:145–153, 1987.

65. Ragjavan M, Glickman N, McCabe G: Diet-related risk factors for gastric dilatation-volvulus in dogs of high-risk breeds, *J Am Anim Hosp Assoc* 40:192–193, 2004.

66. Burrows CF, Bright RM, Spencer CP: Influence of dietary composition on gastric emptying and motility in dogs: potential involvement in acute gastric dilatation, *Am J Vet Res* 46:2609–2612, 1985.

67. Cott B, Shelton M, DeYoung DW: Preliminary report on a GDV questionnaire, *Purebred Dogs: Am Kennel Gaz* 92:76–77, 1975.

68. Caywood D, Teague HD, Jackson DA: Gastric gas analysis in the canine gastric dilatation-volvulus syndrome, *J Am Anim Hosp Assoc* 13:459–462, 1977.

69. Rogolsky B, Van Kruiningen HJ: Short-chain fatty acids and bacterial fermentation in the normal canine stomach and in acute gastric dilatation, *J Am Anim Hosp Assoc* 14:504–515, 1978.

70. Batt RM: Diagnosis and management of malabsorption in dogs, *J Small Anim Pract* 33:161–166, 1992.

71. Fossum T: Protein-losing enteropathy, *Sem Vet Med Surg Small Anim* 4:219–225, 1989.

72. Guilford WG: Effect of diet on inflammatory bowel diseases, *Vet Clin Nutr* 4:58–61, 1997.

73. Cummings JH, Antoine JM, Azpiroz F: Gut health and immunity, *Eur J Nutr* 43:118–173, 2004.

74. Jergens AE: Optimizing IBD treatment in dogs and cats, *Vet Clin North Am Small Anim Pract* 29:501–521, 1999.

75. Simpson JW: Management of colonic disease in the dog, *Waltham Focus* 5:17–22, 1995.

76. Nelson RW, Stookey LJ, Kazacos E: Nutritional management of idiopathic chronic colitis in the dog, *J Vet Intern Med* 2:133–137, 1988.

77. Sturgess K: Diagnosis and management of idiopathic inflammatory bowel disease in dogs and cats, *In Pract* 27:293–301, 2005.

78. Batt RM, Carter MW, McLean L: Wheat-sensitive enteropathy in Irish Setter dogs: possible age-related brush border abnormalities, *Res Vet Sci* 39:80–83, 1985.

79. Hall EJ, Batt RM: Development of wheat-sensitive enteropathy in Irish Setters: biochemical changes, *Am J Vet Res* 51:983–989, 1990.

80. Washabau RJ, Strombeck DR, Buffington CA, and others: Evaluation of intestinal carbohydrate malabsorption in the dog by pulmonary hydrogen gas excretion, *Am J Vet Res* 47:1402–1405, 1986.

81. Reinhart GA: New concepts in managing common pet allergies. In *Proc Conv Can Vet Med Assoc*, 1995, pp 9–14.

82. Reinhart GA, Sunvold GD: Practical applications of omega-3 and fermentable fiber in gastrointestinal patients. In *Proceedings of the gastrointestinal health symposium: a pre-conference symposium*, 1997, World Veterinary Congress.

83. Vilaseca J, Salas A. Guarner F, and others: Dietary fish oil reduces progression of chronic inflammatory lesions in a rat model of granulomatous colitis, *Gut* 31:539–544, 1990.

84. Rampton DS, Collins CE: Review article: thromboxanes in inflammatory bowel disease-pathogenic and therapeutic implications, *Ailment Pharmacol Ther* 7:357–367, 1993.

85. Aslan AC, Triadafilopoulos G: Fish oil fatty acid: supplementation in active ulcerative colitis; a double blind controlled, cross-over study, *Am J Gastroenterol* 87:432, 1992.

86. Hillier K, Jewel R, Forrell L, and others: Incorporation of fatty acids from fish oil and olive oil into colonic mucosal lipids and effects upon eicosanoid synthesis in inflammatory bowel disease, *Gut* 32:1151, 1991.

87. Stenson WF, Cort D, Rodgers J, and others: Dietary supplementation with fish oil in ulcerative colitis, *Ann Intern Med* 116: 609–614, 1998.

88. Eastwood M, Kritchevsky D: Dietary fiber: how did we get where we are? *Annu Rev Nutr* 25:1–8, 2005.

89. Reinhart GA, Moxley RA, Clemens ET: Source of dietary fiber and its effects on colonic microstructure, function and histopathology of Beagle dogs, *J Nutr* 24:2701S–2703S, 1994.

90. Clemens ET: Dietary fiber and colonic morphology. In Carey DP, Norton SA, Bolser SM, editors: *Recent advances in canine and feline nutritional research, Proceedings of the Iams international nutrition symposium*, Wilmington, Ohio, 1996, Orange Frazer Press.

91. Murdoch DB: Large intestinal disease. In Thomas DA, Simpson JW, Hall EJ, editors: *Manual of canine and feline gastroenterology*, Quedgeley, Gloucester, UK, 1996, British Small Animal Veterinary Association.

92. Sunvold GD, Fahey GC Jr, Merchen NR, and others: Dietary fiber for dogs. IV. In vitro fermentation of selected fiber sources by dog fecal inoculum and in vivo digestion and metabolism of fiber-supplemented diets, *J Anim Sci* 73:1099–1109, 1995.

93. Sunvold GD, Fahey GC Jr, Merchen NR, and others: Dietary fiber for cats: in vitro fermentation of selected fiber sources by cat fecal inoculum and in vivo utilization of diets containing selected fiber sources and their blends, *J Anim Sci* 73:2329–2339, 1995.

94. Sunvold GD, Titgemeyer EC, Bourquin LD, and others: Fermentability of selected fibrous substrates by cat fecal microflora, *J Nutr* 124(Suppl):2721S–2722S, 1994.

95. Bergman EN: Energy contributions of volatile fatty acids from the gastrointestinal tract in various species, *Physiol Rev* 70:567–590, 1990.

96. Hague S, Singh B, Parskeva C: Butyrate acts as a survival factor for colonic epithelial cells: further fuel for the in vivo versus in vitro debate, *Gastroenterology* 112:1036–1040, 1997.

97. Sakata T: Stimulatory effect of short-chain fatty acids on epithelial cell proliferation in the rat intestine: a possible explanation for trophic effect of fermentable fibre, gut microbes and luminal trophic factors, *Br J Nutr* 58:95–103, 1987.

98. Hallman JE, Moxley RA, Reinhart GA, and others: Cellulose, beet pulp and pectin/gum arabic effects on canine colonic microstructure and histopathology, *Vet Clin Nutr* 2:137–142, 1995.

99. Hallman JE, Reinhart GA, Wallace EA, and others: Colonic mucosal tissue energetics and electrolyte transport in dogs fed cellulose, beet pulp or pectin/gum arabic as their primary fiber source, *Nutr Res* 16:303–313, 1996.

100. Kripke S, Fox A, Berman J, and others: Stimulation of dietary fiber and its effect on colonic growth with intracolonic infusion of short chain fatty acids, *JPEN* 13:109–116, 1988.

101. Kamath PS, Hoepfner MT, Phillips SF: Short-chain fatty acids stimulate motility of the canine ileum, *Am J Physiol* 253: G427–G433, 1987.

102. Cherbut C: Effects of short-chain fatty acids on gastrointestinal motility. In Cummins JH, Rombear JL, Sakata T, editors: *Physiological and clinical aspects of short-chain fatty acids*, Cambridge, UK, 1995, Cambridge University Press.

103. Kvietys PR, Granger DN: Effect of volatile fatty acids on blood flow and oxygen uptake by the dog colon, *Gastroenterology* 80:962–969, 1981.

104. Roediger WEW, Rae DA: Trophic effect of short-chain fatty acids on mucosal handling of ions by the defunctioned colon, *Br J Surg* 69:23–25, 1982.

105. Kerley MS, Sunvold GD: Favorably modifying gut flora with a novel fiber (FOS). In *Proceedings of the gastrointestinal health symposium: a pre-conference symposium*, 1997, World Veterinary Congress.

106. Blomberg L, Henriksson A, Conway PL: Inhibition of adhesion of *Escherichia coli* K88 to piglet ileal mucus by *Lactobacillus* spp, *Appl Environ Micro* 59:34–39, 1993.

107. Kerley MS, Sunvold GD: Physiological response to short-chain fatty acid production in the intestine. In Carey DP, Norton SA, Bolser SM, editors: *Recent advances in canine and feline nutritional research, Proceedings of the Iams international nutrition symposium*, Wilmington, Ohio, 1996, Orange Frazer Press.

108. Chapman MAS, Grahn MF, Boyle MA, and others: Butyrate oxidation is impaired in the colonic mucosa of suffers of quiescent ulcerative colitis, *Gut* 35:73, 1994.

109. Scheppach WH, Sommer T, Kirchner GM, and others: Effect of butyrate enemas on the colonic mucosa in distal ulcerative colitis, *Gastroenterology* 103:51–56, 1992.

110. Rolandelli RH, Koruda MJ, Settle G, and others: The effect of enteral feedings supplemented with pectin on the healing of colonic anastomoses in the rat, *Surgery* 99:703, 1986.

111. Silvio J, Harmon DL, Gross KL, McLeod KR: Influence of fiber fermentability on nutrient digestion in the dog, *Nutrition* 16: 289–295, 2000.

112. Howard MD, Sunvold GD, Reinhart GA, and others: Effect of fermentable fiber consumption by the dog on nitrogen balance and fecal microbial nitrogen excretion, *FASEB J* 10:A257, 1996.

113. Macfarlane S, Macfarlane GT, Cummings JH: Review article: prebiotics in the gastrointestinal tract, *Aliment Pharmacol* 24: 701–714, 2006.

114. Brown DH: Applications of fructooligosaccharides in human foods. In Carey DP, Norton SA, Bolser SM, editors: *Recent advances in canine and feline nutritional research, Proceedings of the Iams international nutrition symposium*, Wilmington, Ohio, 1996, Orange Frazer Press.

115. Mitsuoka T, Hidaka H, Eida T: Effect of fructooligosaccharides on intestinal microflora, *Die Nahrung* 31:427–436, 1987.

116. Okazaki M, Fujikawa S, Matumoto N: Effect of xyloogliosaccharide on the growth of bifidobacteria, *Bifidobacteria Microflora* 9:77–86, 1990.

117. Hidaka H, Hirayaa M, Tokunaga T, and others: The effects of indigestible fructooligosaccharides on intestinal microflora and various physiological functions on human health. In Furda I, editor: *New developments in dietary fiber*, New York, 1990, Plenum Press.

118. Hidaka H, Eida T, Takizawa T, and others: Effects of fructooligosaccharides on intestinal flora and human health, *Bifidobacteria Microflora* 10:37–50, 1986.

119. Terada A, Hara H, Oishi T, and others: Effect of dietary lactosucrose on fecal flora and fecal metabolites of dogs, *Micro Ecol Health Dis* 5:87–92, 1992.

120. Gruffydd-Jones TJ, Papasouliotis K, Sparkes AH: Characterization of the intestinal flora of the cat and its potential for modification. In Reinhart GA, Carey DP, editors: *Recent advances in canine and feline nutrition, Iams nutrition symposium proceedings,* vol 2, Wilmington, Ohio, 1998, Orange Frazer Press.

121. Sparkes AH, Papasouliotis K, Sunvold G, and others: The effect of dietary supplementation with fructo-oligosaccharides on the fecal flora of healthy cats, *Am J Vet Res* 59:436–440, 1998.

122. Swanson KS, Grieshop CM, Flickinger EA, and others: Supplemental fructooligosaccharides and mannanoligosaccharides influence immune function, ileal and total tract nutrient digestibilities, microbial populations and concentrations of protein catabolites in the large bowel of dogs, *J Nutr* 132:980–989, 2002.

123. Unpublished study: Data on file at Procter and Gamble Pet Health and Nutrition Center, Lewisburg, Ohio, 2009.

124. Adogony V, Respondek F, Biourge V, and others: Effects of dietary FOS on immunoglobulins in colostrum and milk of bitches, *J Anim Physiol Anim Nutr* 91:169–174, 2007.

125. Zentek J, Marquart B, Pietrzak T, and others: Dietary effects on bifidobacteria and *Clostridium perfringens* in the canine intestine, *J Anim Physiol Anim Nutr* 87:397–407, 2003.

126. Beynen AC, Baas JC, Hoekemiejer PE, and others: Faecal bacterial profile, nitrogen excretion and mineral absorption in healthy dogs fed supplemental oligofructose, *J Anim Physiol Anim Nutr* 86:298–305, 2002.

127. Willard MD, Simpson RB, Cohen ND, Clancy JS: Effects of dietary fructooligosaccharides on selected bacterial populations in feces of dogs, *Am J Vet Res* 61:820–825, 2000.

128. Willard MD, Simpson RB, Delles EK, and others: Effects of dietary supplementation of fructo-oligosaccharides on small intestinal bacterial overgrowth in dogs, *Am J Vet Res* 55:654–659, 1992.

129. Buddington RK, Buddington KK, Sunvold GD: The influence of fermentable fiber on the small intestine of the dog: intestinal dimensions and transport of glucose and proline, *Am J Vet Res* 60:354–358, 1999.

130. Ruaux CG, Tetrick MA, Steniner JM, Williams DA: Fecal consistency and volume in dogs with suspected small intestinal bacterial overgrowth receiving broad spectrum antibiotic therapy or dietary fructo-oligosaccharide supplementation. In *Proc ACVIM Abst*, 2004, p 151.

131. Sunvold GD, Reinhart GA: Maintaining gastrointestinal health via colonic fermentation. In *Proc World Small Anim Vet Assoc*, 1997, pp 7–12.

132. Floch MH, Walker WA, Guandalini S: Recommendation for probiotic use—2008, *J Clin Gastroenterol* 42:S104–S108, 2008.

133. Weese JS, Arroyo L: Bacteriological evaluation of dog and cat diets that claim to contain probiotics, *Can Vet J* 44:212–215, 2003.

134. Weese JS, Anderson RE: Preliminary evaluation of *Lactobacillus rhamnosus* strain GG, a potential probiotic in dogs, *Can Vet J* 43:771–774, 2002.

135. Benyacoub J, Czarnecki-Maulden GL, Cavadini C, and others: Supplementation of food with *Enterococcus faecium* (SF68) stimulates immune functions in young dogs, *J Nutr* 133:1158–1162, 2003.

136. Baillon MA, Marshall-Jones ZV, Butterwick RF: Effects of probiotic *Lactobacillus acidophilus* strain DSM13241 in healthy adult dogs, *Am J Vet Res* 65:338–343, 2004.

137. Marshall-Jones ZV, Baillon MA, Croft JM, Butterwick RE: Effects of *Lactobacillus acidophilus* DSM13241 as a probiotic in healthy adult cats, *Am J Vet Res* 67:1005–1012, 2006.

138. Unpublished study: Data on file at Procter and Gamble Pet Health and Nutrition Center, Lewisburg, Ohio, 2009.

139. Veir JK, Knorr R, Cavadini C, and others: Effect of supplementation with *Enterococcus faecium* (SF68) on immune functions in cats, *Vet Ther* 8:229–238, 2007.

140. Czarnecki-Maulden GL, Cavadini C, Mrkvicka J: Effect of *E. faecum* SF68 on chronic, intractable diarrhea in adult cats. In *Nestle-Purina petcare brochure: role of probiotics in GI tract health*, 2007, pp 13–14.

141. Czarnecki-Maulden GL, Cavadini C, Mrkvicka J: *E. faecum* SF68 helps minimize naturally occurring diarrhea in kittens. In *Nestle-Purina petcare brochure: role of probiotics in GI tract health*, 2007, pp 14–15.

142. Baillon ML, Butterwick RF: The efficacy of a probiotic strain, *Lactobacillus acidophilus* DSM13241, in the recovery of cats from clinical *Campylobacter* infection. In *Proc ACVIM Forum*, 2003.

143. Sauter SN, Allenspach K, Gaschen F: Cytokine expression in an ex vivo culture system of duodenal samples from dogs with chronic enteropathies: modulation by probiotic bacteria, *Domest Anim Endocrinol* 29:605–622, 2005.

144. Unpublished study: Data on file at Procter and Gamble Pet Health and Nutrition Center, Lewisburg, Ohio, 2009.

145. Kelley RL, Kiely B, O'Mahony B, and others: Clinical benefits of probiotic canine-derived *Bifidobacterium animalis* strain AHC7 in dogs with acute idiopathic diarrhea, *Vet Ther* 10(3):121–130, 2009.

36

Nutritional Care of Cancer Patients

Because of increased knowledge and improvements in pet health care and nutrition in recent years, many companion animals are now living well into old age. As a result, cancer has become a relatively common disease in dogs and cats, occurring most frequently in pets who are older than 5 years.[1,2] In addition, because of improved methods of treatment, many pets with neoplastic disease achieve full remission and experience improved quality of life and survival times. Providing dogs and cats with optimal nutrition during the early stages of disease and throughout treatment and remission is an important component of care. Many cancer patients experience significant alterations in food intake, nutrient metabolism, and energy requirements. Research has shown that nutritional therapy is a key component in reducing the effects of these changes. In recent years, nutritional interventions that may also control or reduce malignant disease in pets have received attention. This chapter reviews the metabolic and physical changes associated with cancer cachexia, the nutrient and energy needs of pets with cancer, and current nutritional approaches to managing these patients.

CANCER CACHEXIA

Cancer cachexia is a frequently observed syndrome in human cancer patients characterized by progressive losses in body weight and lean tissue that cannot be completely accounted for by reduced food intake.[3] Clinical signs of weight loss and anorexia, along with cachexia's characteristic metabolic abnormalities, are also reported in dogs and cats with a wide variety of malignancies.[4] A principal underlying cause of cancer cachexia is tumor-induced alterations in the body's metabolism of carbohydrate, protein, and fat. Over time, these metabolic changes lead to anorexia, fatigue, weight loss, impaired immune function, and malnutrition. Cancer cachexia significantly affects a patient's quality of life, ability to withstand chemotherapy or radiation treatment, and survival time.[5] Furthermore, the metabolic changes of cachexia appear to occur in many patients

before clinical signs are observed.[6] This underscores the importance of early nutritional intervention when treating dogs and cats with cancer.

Although limited data are available, there is some evidence that the incidence of cancer cachexia differs between dogs and cats. Two pilot studies examined body weight and body condition status in dogs and cats that were diagnosed with a variety of types of cancer.[7,8] Severe weight loss and muscle wasting was frequently observed in cats with cancer, but was much less common in dogs. However, these results are controversial because other researchers report that dogs with cancer can exhibit the tumor-associated metabolic changes that contribute to cachexia while not showing clinical signs.[6] Although not studied in dogs, the presence of cancer cachexia in cats was found to be a significant negative prognostic factor for cancer survival, just as it is in human subjects.[8] The reason that dogs may not be as susceptible to clinically evident cachexia is not completely understood, and may be related to the dog's relatively lower dietary protein needs compared with the cat, the types of cancers that have been studied, and species differences in disease progression.

While cachexia is an important paraneoplastic syndrome, it is not the only cause of decreased food intake and loss of body condition in pets with cancer. Tumor-bearing animals may lose weight because of the presence of tumors or as a result of treatment-induced side effects. In some cases, such as oropharyngeal, gastric, or small-bowel tumors, the physical presence of a tumor can interfere with nutrient intake or assimilation. Surgical procedures, chemotherapy, and radiation therapy may also negatively affect nutrient intake and metabolism. Certain chemotherapies may alter smell and taste perceptions, resulting in decreased food intake or changes in food preferences.[9,10] Anorexia, vomiting, and diarrhea are also potential side effects of chemotherapy and radiation therapy. All of these effects must be addressed when assessing nutritional status and developing a dietary management protocol for pets with cancer.

Cancer cachexia is characterized by progressive losses in body weight and lean tissue that cannot be completely accounted for by reduced food intake. A principal underlying cause is tumor-induced alterations in the body's metabolism of carbohydrate, protein, and fat. Cancer cachexia significantly affects a patient's quality of life, ability to withstand chemotherapy or radiation treatment, and survival time. In addition, pets with cancer may lose weight because of the presence of tumors or as a result of treatment-induced side effects.

Phases of Cachexia

Three phases of cachexia have been identified in human subjects; it is presumed that the syndrome follows a similar pattern in dogs and cats. During the first phase, the patient does not exhibit clinical signs, but biochemical changes are evident. These include elevated blood lactate and insulin levels (peripheral insulin resistance) and alterations in amino acid and lipid profiles.[11] Dogs with lymphoma have significantly higher serum lactate and insulin concentrations following intravenous dextrose infusion, compared with levels in healthy dogs.[12] These changes occur even in dogs that are not showing clinical signs of cachexia. Clinical signs develop during the second stage. The patient begins to show anorexia, weight loss, and depression and has an increased risk of experiencing detrimental side effects of cancer therapy. The third and final stage is characterized by marked losses of body fat and protein stores, severe debilitation, weakness, and biochemical evidence of negative nitrogen balance. If left untreated, cancer cachexia can be the ultimate cause of death. Indirect calorimetry studies with rats have found that the three phases usually coincide with normal, increased, and decreased energy requirements, respectively.[13]

Alterations in Carbohydrate Metabolism

The biochemical alterations of cancer cachexia involve the metabolism of carbohydrate, protein, and lipids, which in turn affect basal metabolic rate. Together, this collection of biochemical changes leads to inefficient energy utilization by the host animal and enhanced energy use by the tumor. Alterations in carbohydrate metabolism are dramatic and are at least partially related to the metabolic needs of the tumor. Tumor cells preferentially metabolize glucose through anaerobic glycolysis for energy, and most are incapable of obtaining significant amounts of energy from either aerobic glycolysis or fat oxidation.[12,14] As a result, as a tumor grows, it uses the host's supply of glucose for energy, generating large amounts of lactate, the end product of anaerobic glycolysis. The host animal's hepatocytes convert this excess lactate to glucose via the Cori cycle, resulting in a shift in glucose metabolism from energy-producing oxidative pathways to energy-requiring gluconeogenic pathways. The end result is a gain of energy by the tumor and a net energy loss for the host. This alteration in carbohydrate metabolism occurs as early as the preclinical stage of cancer cachexia. Therefore nutritional intervention that is aimed at shifting metabolism to benefit the host over the tumor should begin as soon as a diagnosis is made.

In addition to elevated serum lactate, other biochemical abnormalities that occur in response to changes in carbohydrate use in tumor-bearing animals include altered serum insulin and glucagon secretion patterns, increased rate of gluconeogenesis and glucose turnover, and insulin resistance.[15-17] Although the majority of studies have been conducted with human cancer patients or laboratory animal models, there is evidence that these changes also occur in dogs (and presumably cats). Dogs with lymphoma, a common form of cancer in many breeds, show altered responses to glucose tolerance tests, and many develop insulin resistance.[12,18] These changes occur before and after the development of clinical signs and continue after remission is achieved.[18] It is hypothesized that insulin resistance in dogs with lymphoma is due to a post-receptor defect resulting in glucose intolerance. Regardless of the underlying cause, the prevalence of glucose intolerance and insulin insensitivity mandate the need to limit and carefully select the type of carbohydrate included in foods for pets with cancer.

Tumor cells preferentially metabolize glucose for energy, using the host's glucose and generating large amounts of lactate. Ultimately, the result is a gain of energy by the tumor and a net energy loss for the host. Tumor-bearing animals also have an increased incidence of insulin insensitivity and glucose intolerance.

Alterations in Protein Metabolism

Because both the tumor and the host have obligatory protein requirements, negative nitrogen balance is common in cancer patients.[19] Growing tumors require amino acids for protein synthesis and will also use host gluconeogenic amino acids for the production of glucose. Because tumors often have a high metabolic rate, this significantly affects host protein stores and can result in abnormal serum amino acid profiles.[20] The host experiences an increased rate of whole body protein turnover, characterized by a decreased rate of protein synthesis in skeletal muscle and an increased rate of synthesis in the liver.[21,22] In human cancer patients the shift in protein synthesis from muscle to liver is referred to as the acute-phase reactant response, and its onset is a negative prognostic factor for survival. If not corrected, this protein imbalance eventually leads to increased loss of skeletal muscle (muscle wasting), hypoalbuminemia, compromised immunity, impaired gastrointestinal function, and delayed wound healing.

Studies of human cancer patients have shown that serum levels of the gluconeogenic amino acids alanine, glutamic acid, aspartic acid, and glycine generally decrease, while concentrations of the branch-chain amino acids (BCAAs) (leucine, isoleucine, and valine) are normal or increased.[20,23] This shift reflects the increased proteolysis of skeletal muscle as the three BCAAs make up approximately ⅓ of skeletal muscle protein. Studies of dogs with cancer have also found changes in serum amino acid profiles. A group of 32 dogs with a variety of cancers had decreased serum levels of glycine, glutamine, valine, cystine, and arginine and elevated levels of isoleucine and phenylalanine, compared with values that were reported in the group of healthy control dogs.[24,25]

Although the biochemical pathways are complex and are not completely understood, the primary underlying cause of skeletal muscle protein breakdown in cancer patients appears to be the up-regulation of the ubiquitin-proteasome proteolytic pathway.[26,27]

Activation of this pathway is responsible for the muscle wasting that is seen in a variety of disease and trauma states, including diabetes, hyperthyroidism, and in response to fasting, sepsis, and burns. With cancer, several tumor-derived factors and cytokines have been identified that influence this proteolytic pathway. These include proteolysis induction factor, tumor necrosis factor-alpha, and interleukin-1-beta.

Alterations in Lipid Metabolism

Loss of body fat accounts for the majority of the weight lost by humans and animals with cancer cachexia.[28] Although reduced food intake is a significant contributor to this loss, humans and animals with cancer also experience decreased lipogenesis and increased lipolysis. This metabolic shift is a result of decreased lipoprotein lipase activity and appears to also be influenced by several specific tumor-derived cytokines.[29,30] The result is elevated serum concentrations of free fatty acids (FFAs), very–low-density lipoproteins (VLDLs), triglycerides, acetoacetate, and beta-hydroxybutyrate.[31,32] In human patients with cancer, altered lipid profiles have been associated with immunosuppression and decreased survival time.[33] Similarly, dogs with untreated lymphoma had significantly elevated concentrations of serum triglycerides, FFAs, and VLDLs when compared with healthy controls.[24,34] Although serum cholesterol concentration increased in response to chemotherapy, other lipid parameters did not normalize during treatment or when the dogs attained remission.

Changes in Energy Requirements

As discussed previously, tumors obtain energy primarily through the anaerobic metabolism of glucose, resulting in the production of lactate. The host must then recycle this lactate through the Cori cycle, which leads to a net loss of energy. Additional energy costs to animals with cancer may include cytokine-induced increases in glucose recycling, protein degradation, and energy expenditure.[35,36] Therefore, at least theoretically, energy expenditure in cancer patients is expected to increase. However, studies using indirect calorimetry to measure energy expenditure in tumor-bearing subjects have reported varying results.[13,37-39] Some investigators have reported increased energy expenditure in humans and animals with neoplastic disease. Conversely, others have found normal or reduced energy needs. These discrepancies are probably a result of several factors. Because cancer cachexia develops in stages and biochemical alterations typically precede clinical signs, animals that are in the preclinical stage of cachexia are expected to have normal energy requirements. Conversely, individuals with active, untreated cachexia may have elevated energy expenditure, while those in the final stages may be hypometabolic. Additional factors that significantly affect energy needs include the type and size of tumor and the patient's phase of treatment, severity of clinical signs, and level of activity.

Several studies using indirect calorimetry have been conducted to determine whether there are significant changes in resting energy expenditure (REE) in dogs with cancer.[40-42] In one study, 22 dogs with naturally occurring lymphoblastic lymphoma were fed isocaloric amounts of either a high-carbohydrate or a high-fat diet before and during chemotherapy.[41] The initial REE values in dogs with lymphoma before treatment were significantly lower than those of healthy control dogs. After 6 weeks of chemotherapy, REE values decreased further in the dogs with lymphoma, even after remission was achieved in the majority of dogs. Although there were no significant differences in mean REE between the two diet groups, the dogs fed the high-fat diet maintained slightly higher energy expenditures than those fed the high-carbohydrate diet. An important consideration in this study is the fact that the healthy control animals were slightly younger than the dogs with cancer (mean ages of 5.4 versus 7 years, respectively). Although slight, this age difference may account for the lower initial mean REE in dogs with lymphoma. However, it would not account for the further decreases seen during treatment and remission. A possible explanation for these decreases may be that the dogs with lymphoma were in the first silent phase of cancer cachexia at the start of the study. This was followed by a reduction in metastatically active tumor tissue in response to treatment or possibly in response to a decrease in host metabolism caused by a loss of lean body tissue. A common side effect of chemotherapy is decreased energy intake, which could lead to a loss of lean body tissue and a decreased metabolic rate.

A second study examined the effects of surgical excision of various types of tumors on energy expenditure in dogs.[42] Removal of tumors did not significantly affect REE, regardless of tumor type. In addition, the energy expenditure of tumor-bearing dogs prior to surgery was not significantly greater or less than that of a control group of healthy dogs. In contrast to the previously described study of dogs with lymphoma, this study indicated that REE and energy needs of dogs with other types of cancer are not significantly different from healthy dogs of the same age.

Although studies of the energy requirements of dogs with cancer are limited (no studies have been published for cats), results thus far indicate that the energy needs of cancer patients do not significantly increase, and they may decrease slightly with some types of cancer. In addition, removal of the cancer through surgery or chemotherapy does not appear to appreciably affect energy needs. These data do not support the standard tenet that patients with neoplastic disease have increased energy requirements. Rather, it seems that the energy needs of dogs and cats with cancer must be addressed on an individual basis and may vary with the type of cancer, stage of the disease, and method of treatment.

DIETARY MANAGEMENT OF CANCER PATIENTS

The metabolic changes associated with cancer occur before clinical signs are seen, emphasizing the importance of early nutritional intervention. Because many dogs and cats with cancer have decreased food intakes, a major goal of nutritional therapy is to select a food that is highly palatable and energy dense. The food's nutrient profile should be tailored to address the metabolic alterations of cancer cachexia, maintain normal body condition, and prevent weight loss. Provision of an appropriate diet with select nutrients may reverse some of the deleterious effects of neoplastic disease, improve the pet's ability to tolerate chemotherapy or radiation treatment, and enhance overall quality of life. Specific dietary recommendations should consider the stage of disease, energy needs, current and past nutritional status, and ability or willingness to eat.

Diet Characteristics

Current data indicate that food selected for cancer patients should take advantage of the differences in metabolic needs between the host animal and the tumor.

The food's caloric distribution should emphasize calories originating from fat and protein, rather than from carbohydrate, because fatty acids and amino acids are not the preferred fuel source for most tumors. A diet that contains reduced carbohydrate and elevated protein and fat may supply a readily available source of energy, meet the host's protein needs, and limit the supply of carbohydrate to tumor cells.[28,43] Human cancer patients with cachexia have shown improvements in body weight, adipose stores, energy and nitrogen balance, and ability to metabolize glucose when dietary fat is increased.[44,45] Similarly, dogs with lymphoma fed a high-fat diet had lower mean lactate and insulin levels after remission when compared with dogs fed isocaloric amounts of a high-carbohydrate diet.[41] A food that contains 50% to 60% of total calories from fat, 30% to 50% of calories from protein, and the remaining portion of calories from soluble carbohydrate is recommended for dogs and cats with cancer.[46] In addition to shifting metabolism away from carbohydrate and toward fat, another benefit of feeding a high-fat diet to cancer patients is the increased energy density and palatability of these foods.

The type of fat that is included in foods for pets with cancer is also an important consideration. In recent years, the importance of omega-3 fatty acids for human and pet cancer patients and the effects of this class of fatty acids on tumor development and metastasis have been studied. (A complete review of these fatty acids and their use in pet foods is included on pp. 387-395.) The antiinflammatory effects of omega-3 fatty acids on multiple systems of the body suggest a role in treating cancer patients. There is an increasing body of evidence showing that omega-3 fatty acids, particularly eicosapentaenoic acid (EPA) and docosahexaenoic acid (DHA), limit tumor growth.[47-50] Studies using animal models have shown that supplementation with EPA and DHA helps to prevent cachexia and metastatic disease.[51] There is also indirect evidence that omega-3 fatty acids may be metabolically helpful in preventing the recurrence of cancer after remission has been achieved.[52] Although the underlying mechanism is not completely understood, the effect appears to be related to incorporation of long-chain omega-3 fatty acids into tumor cell membranes. This alters membrane fluidity and permeability, potentially increasing tumor cell susceptibility to both chemotherapeutic agents and to the host's own immune system. Increasing cell membrane

omega-3 fatty acids also shifts prostaglandin synthesis away from prostaglandin E_2 (PGE$_2$) and toward PGE$_1$. Cyclooxygenase metabolites such as PGE$_2$ play a role in the progression of several forms of cancer, and blocking their production can inhibit tumor growth.[53]

Results of trials with human cancer patients have reported clinical benefits of omega-3 fatty acid supplementation. When 85 subjects with upper gastrointestinal cancers were fed either an omega-3 fatty acid and arginine supplement or a placebo, those receiving the supplement had improved nitrogen intake and balance, an increased rate of wound healing, reduced incidence of complications, and shortened hospitalization time when compared with patients receiving the placebo.[47] While the design of this study confounded fatty acid and arginine effects, the results suggest a benefit of omega-3 fatty acids for human cancer patients. Similar results were reported when cancer patients were supplemented with omega-3 fatty acids, arginine, and ribonucleic acid (RNA).[54]

Although a limited number of clinical studies have been conducted, current research indicates that companion animals with cancer may also benefit from omega-3 fatty acids. When dogs with lymphoma were fed a food supplemented with EPA, DHA, and arginine, supplemented dogs had lower plasma lactate responses to glucose tolerance tests and increased disease-free intervals and survival times when compared with dogs that were not supplemented.[55] Similar to the previous study with human subjects, the design of this study prevented any conclusions about a singular effect of omega-3 fatty acids because arginine was included in the supplement. A subsequent study fed the same therapeutic food to dogs that had nasal tumors and were receiving radiation therapy.[56] Dogs fed the therapeutic food had higher serum concentrations of EPA, DHA, and arginine when compared with serum concentrations in the control group of dogs. Increases in serum EPA and DHA were positively correlated with reduced tissue concentrations of proinflammatory agents and decreased tissue damage, and improved owner-reported performance in response to radiation treatment. Effects of fatty acids alone (in the absence of arginine) on canine cancer cell lines have also been reported.[57] In vitro studies have shown that supplementation with EPA, gamma-linolenic, and conjugated linoleic acid inhibited proliferation of bladder, osteosarcoma, prostatic, and bladder cell lines. EPA had the most potent effect, and these effects were enhanced when EPA was used in conjunction with the other fatty acids. Finally, although one mechanism of action of omega-3 fatty acids that has been postulated is augmentation of the effects of chemotherapy or radiation treatment, a recent study found that supplementation with omega-3 fatty acids in dogs with lymphoma did not significantly affect the pharmokinetics of doxorubicin.[58]

Pet foods formulated for cancer patients should also contain slightly higher concentrations of protein than the levels needed for adult maintenance. Providing optimal levels of high-quality protein contributes to a positive nitrogen balance in the face of potentially increased requirements during active neoplastic disease. Losses of lean body tissue can occur during cancer cachexia and as a result of anorexia or decreased food intake. The food should contain between 30% and 50% of calories from protein, with the higher end of this range appropriate for cats.[59] Because tumor cells preferentially use gluconeogenic amino acids for energy, a food that is specifically enriched with certain amino acids may be beneficial. For example, although arginine can exert metabolic effects that are both proneoplastic and antineoplastic, supplemental arginine has been shown to inhibit tumor growth and metastasis and may enhance survival time in dogs with cancer.[55,60,61] A diet that contains increased BCAAs may also be beneficial. Although no studies have yet have been conducted with canine or feline patients, human cancer patients with cancer cachexia who received supplemental BCAAs reported a benefit to quality of life and showed improvements in nitrogen balance.[62] In addition, in vitro work with several types of canine cancer cells showed that supplementation with BCAA did not increase cancer cell proliferation, and increasing leucine appeared to inhibit cancer cell growth.[63] However, the ability of BCAAs to preserve lean body tissue in people or animals with cancer cachexia has not yet been demonstrated. Therefore additional studies that examine the metabolic and clinical effects of including BCAAs in diets for dogs with cancer are needed before recommendations can be made.

Antioxidant nutrients have been identified as having potential roles in both the prevention and treatment cancer. In the body, antioxidants function to sequester reactive oxygen species (ROS) that are generated during aerobic metabolism, thus preventing or reducing oxidative stress. Oxidative stress leads to cellular and deoxyribonucleic acid (DNA) damage and the production of inflammatory mediators, and is thought to be a risk factor for the development and progression of certain types of cancer.[64] For this reason, the antioxidant nutrients have been studied for their efficacy in cancer prevention and treatment. Similar to some human cancer patients, metabolic markers of oxidative stress have been reported to increase in dogs with lymphoma and mammary carcinoma.[65,66] It is theorized that providing supplemental antioxidants may reduce clinical signs associated with these metabolic changes and may also be helpful in reducing the adverse effects of chemotherapy and radiation therapy. There is in vitro evidence with cancer cells and in vivo work with laboratory animals suggesting that beta-carotene, lutein, and other carotenoids may inhibit tumor cell growth.[67-69] However, not all studies have shown a benefit, and clinical trials, especially with dog and cat cancer patients, have not been reported. In addition, one argument against the use of supplemental antioxidants during cancer treatment is that the presence of increased antioxidants in tissues may interfere with the antitumor effects of radiation and some chemotherapies, and may counteract some of the cellular benefits of omega-3 fatty acids.[64,70,71] Because individual antioxidant nutrients have different properties and cellular effects, controlled clinical studies are needed to fully elucidate potential benefits of the various antioxidant nutrients for dogs and cats with cancer.

Diets for pets with cancer should be formulated to account for the metabolic changes associated with neoplastic disease. A diet that is nutrient dense, highly digestible, high in fat and protein, and low in carbohydrate is appropriate. Increasing omega-3 fatty acids, particularly eicosapentaenoic acid and docosahexaenoic acid, may also be beneficial.

Calculating Energy Needs

The energy needs of companion animals with cancer can be affected by the type of tumor and the animal's stage of disease, willingness to eat, and activity level.

Adjustments in energy needs should be made for cancer patients who are clinically ill or experiencing severe side effects from treatment. Because ill animals are often kept in thermoneutral environments, have decreased food intakes, and are inactive, the formulas used to determine normal maintenance energy requirements for dogs and cats will not usually provide accurate estimates for some cancer patients. Conversely, an animal's resting energy requirement (RER) reflects the energy needed during a resting, postabsorptive state in a thermoneutral environment. Formulas for RER may therefore provide a better estimate of energy needs in cancer patients. An additional "illness factor" can be added to this estimate based upon the pet's degree of illness and metabolic state. For dogs, an estimate of RER can be made using the formula RER (kilocalories [kcal]/day) = 70 × (body weight$_{[kg]}$)$^{0.75}$.[72-74] An estimate for cats can be calculated using the formula RER (kcal/day) = 40 × (body weight$_{kg}$). The RER estimates may need to be adjusted to account for additional energy needs for the demands of underlying disease. For dogs with cancer, a factor of 1.25 to 2 has been recommended, while 1.25 to 1.5 has been suggested for cats.

METHODS OF FEEDING

Feeding ill patients can be achieved through delivery of nutrients enterally (into the intestinal tract) or parenterally (intravenously). Enteral feeding always should be the delivery method of choice, provided the pet has a functional gastrointestinal tract. Compared with parenteral methods, enteral feeding prevents mucosal atrophy and bacterial overgrowth, presents less risk to the patient, and is more convenient and affordable for clients. Parenteral nutrition is only suggested when the gastrointestinal tract cannot be used and when there is an anticipated need for long-term intravenous feeding.

Oral feeding of a canned or dry ration should be the first choice for cancer patients. Many dogs and cats with cancer are capable of consuming, digesting, and assimilating food but are reluctant to eat an adequate volume of food. Decreased intake or anorexia occurs as a result of the metabolic or physiological effects of disease or in response to surgery, chemotherapy, or radiation therapy. Some pets can be encouraged to eat by offering small meals or hand-feeding, warming the food to body temperature, adding warm water to enhance the aroma and

texture, or changing the type of food that is offered. Metoclopramide is often given to ameliorate nausea associated with chemotherapy, and it may stimulate eating. Similarly, chemical appetite stimulants such as benzodiazepine derivatives or antiserotonin agents may be helpful in getting reluctant pets to eat. However, these drugs can have variable responses and may not be appropriate for some cancer patients because of physiological contraindications and potential side effects.

When a patient is unwilling or unable to consume food orally, a feeding tube can be used. Nasoesophageal tubes provide short-term feeding to patients with normal gastrointestinal function, but they are not appropriate for animals with severe esophageal or gastric disease. Other types of enteral feeding routes are esophagostomy tubes, gastrostomy tubes, and jejunostomy tubes. An esophagostomy tube delivers nutrients into the distal esophagus, a gastrostomy tube delivers nutrients directly into the stomach, and a jejunostomy tube bypasses the entire upper gastrointestinal tract and delivers nutrients to the small intestine. All three of these tubes require surgical placement and can be left in position for extended periods of time. However, while bolus (meal) feeding can be used with nasoesophageal, esophagostomy, and gastrostomy tubes, a constant rate of infusion must be used with a jejunostomy tube. More complete discussions of the use, placement, and management of enteral feeding tubes are beyond the scope of this chapter and can be found in other veterinary publications.[72]

The formula selected for tube feeding should have the same characteristics as the food that would be used for oral feeding. An energy- and nutrient-dense formula minimizes the volume that must be fed. Providing a high proportion (50% or more) of calories as fat also helps delay gastric emptying and prevent diarrhea. The formula should include a partially soluble fiber source that helps slow gastric emptying and supports normal gastrointestinal tract function.[11] A formula that is too nutrient dense may induce vomiting or osmotic diarrhea, especially if a large volume is administered at one time. Therefore a balancing act between providing adequate nutrients, calories, and fluid and preventing nausea or diarrhea is often required when tube-feeding cancer patients. A blenderized canned cat or dog food works well with gastrostomy tubes, while liquid commercial veterinary products for dogs and cats can be used with nasogastric and jejunostomy tubes. The pet's total daily requirements should be administered in at least five to eight small-bolus feedings per day, except when jejunostomy feeding is used. If diarrhea occurs, reduction of the rate of feeding, feeding smaller increments, or decreasing the total amount of formula administered may help the intestinal tract to adapt.

Parenteral nutrition is the only option for nutritional support in cancer patients that cannot tolerate enteral feeding, usually because of a nonfunctional or severely diseased gastrointestinal tract.[72,75] Regardless of the underlying disease being treated, parenteral nutrition is generally not considered for veterinary patients unless the patient is expected to require support for several days and the gastrointestinal tract is expected to heal given a sufficient period of rest. The long-term benefits of parenteral nutrition are often questionable because this route of delivery is associated with mucosal atrophy and increased medical risks such as sepsis and metabolic anomalies. Parenteral nutrition may also be cost prohibitive for many clients. When it is used, a parenteral formula for dog and cats with cancer should contain a limited amount of dextrose and 60% to 70% of calories as fat. Avoiding glucose- or lactate-containing solutions is especially important, given the metabolic changes associated with cancer.[76] As with enteral feeding, the goal is to provide the host with a readily available energy source while limiting the energy available to the tumor.

CONCLUSION

The primary challenge when feeding cancer patients is to provide adequate calories, essential nutrients, and fluids in the face of the decreased food intake and metabolic alterations that are often associated with neoplastic disease. Although more clinical trials are needed with dogs and cats with different types of cancer, current research supports the use of foods that contain increased amounts of fat and protein, reduced carbohydrate, and elevated levels of omega-3 fatty acids.

References

1. Patronek GJ, Waters DJ, Glickman LT: Comparative longevity of pet dogs and humans: implications for gerontology research, *J Gerontol* 52A:B171–B178, 1997.

2. Waters DJ, Jeffreys AB: Critical issues in aging and cancer: implications for effective cancer prevention. In *Proc NAVC*, 2006, pp 16–21.

3. Tisdale MJ: Cancer anorexia and cachexia, *Nutr* 17:438–442, 2003.

4. Ogilvie GK: Paraneoplastic syndromes. In Ettinger S, Feldman E: *Textbook of veterinary internal medicine*, ed 4, Philadelphia, 1999, Saunders.

5. Crow SE, Oliver J: Cancer cachexia, *Compend Contin Educ Pract Vet* 43:2004–2012, 1979.

6. Vail DM, Ogilvie GK, Wheeler SL: Metabolic alterations in patients with cancer cachexia, *Compend Contin Educ Pract Vet* 12: 381–387, 1990.

7. Michel KE, Sorenmo K, Shofer FS: Evaluation of body condition and weight loss in dogs presented to a veterinary oncology service, *J Vet Intern Med* 18:692–695, 2004.

8. Baez JL, Michel KE, Sorenmo K, Shofer FS: A prospective investigation of the prevalence and prognostic significance of weight loss and changes in body condition in feline cancer patients, *J Feline Med* 9:411–417, 2007.

9. Kokal WA: The impact of antitumor therapy on nutrition, *Cancer* 55:273–278, 1985.

10. Trant AS, Serin J, Douglass HO: Is taste related to anorexia in cancer patients? *Am J Clin Nutr* 36:45–58, 1982.

11. Ogilvie GK: Interventional nutrition for the cancer patient, *Clin Tech Small Anim Pract* 13:224–231, 1998.

12. Vail DM, Ogilvie GK, Wheeler SL, and others: Alterations in carbohydrate metabolism in canine lymphoma, *J Vet Intern Med* 4:8–11, 1990.

13. Zyliez S, Schwantje O, Wagener DJT, and others: Metabolic response to enteral food to different phases of cancer cachexia in rats, *Oncology* 47:87–91, 1990.

14. Hansell DT, Davies JWL, Barns J, and others: The oxidation of body fuel stores in cancer patients, *Ann Surg* 204:637–642, 1986.

15. Burt ME, Lowry SF, Gorschboth C, and others: Metabolic alterations in a noncachectic animal tumor system, *Cancer* 47:2138–2146, 1981.

16. Norton JA, Maher M, Wesley R, and others: Glucose intolerance in sarcoma patients, *Cancer* 55:3022–3027, 1984.

17. Inculet RI, Peacock JL, Gorschboth CM, Norton JA: Gluconeogenesis in the tumor-influenced rat hepatocyte: importance of tumor burden, lactate, insulin and glucagon, *J Natl Cancer Inst* 79:1039–1046, 1987.

18. Ogilvie GK, Walters LM, Salman MD, and others: Treatment of dogs with lymphoma with adriamycin and a diet high in carbohydrate or high in fat, *Am J Vet Res* 8:95–104, 1994.

19. Kurzer M, Meguid MM: Cancer and protein metabolism, *Surg Clin North Am* 66:969–1001, 1986.

20. Landel AM, Hammong WG, Meguid MM: Aspects of amino acid and protein metabolism in cancer-bearing states, *Cancer* 55:230–237, 1985.

21. Norton JA: The influence of tumor-bearing on protein metabolism in the rat, *J Surg Res* 30:456–462, 1981.

22. Norton JA, Stein TP, Brennan MF: Whole body protein synthesis and turnover in normal and malnourished patients with and without known cancer, *Ann Surg* 194:123–128, 1981.

23. Warren RS, Jeemvanandam M, Brennan MF: Protein synthesis in the tumor-influenced hepatocyte, *Surgery* 98:275–281, 1985.

24. Ogilvie GK, Vail DM, Wheeler SL, and others: Alterations in fat and protein metabolism in dogs with cancer. In *Proc Vet Cancer Soc*, Estes Park, Colo, 1988.

25. Ogilvie GK, Walters LM, Salman MD: Alterations in select aspects of carbohydrate, lipid and amino acid metabolism in dogs with non-hematopoietic malignancies, *Am J Vet Res* 8:62–66, 1994.

26. Baracos VE: Regulation of skeletal-muscle-protein turnover in cancer-associated cachexia, *Nutrition* 16:1015–1018, 2000.

27. Laxarus DD, Destree AT, Mazzola LM, and others: A new model of cancer-cachexia: contribution of the ubiquitin-proteosome pathway, *Am J Physiol* 277:E332–E341, 1999.

28. Ogilvie GK, Vail DM: Nutrition and cancer: recent developments, *Vet Clin North Am Small Anim Pract* 20:969–985, 1990.

29. McAndrew PF: Fat metabolism and cancer, *Surg Clin North Am* 66:1003–1012, 1986.

30. Davenport DJ: Use of nutraceuticals in cancer therapy, *Proc NAVC* 20:777–780, 2006.

31. Alexopoulos CG, Blatsios B, Avgerinos A: Serum lipids and lipoprotein disorders in cancer patients, *Cancer* 60:3065–3070, 1987.

32. Alexander HR: Substrate alterations in a sarcoma-bearing rat model: effect of tumor growth and resection, *J Surg Res* 48:471–475, 1990.

33. Kern KA, Norton JA: Cancer cachexia, *J Parenteral Nutr* 12:286–298, 1988.

34. Ford RB, Babineau C, Ogilvie GK, and others: Serum lipid profiles in dogs with lymphoma. In *Proc Vet Canc Soc*, Raleigh, NC, 1989.

35. Del Ray A, Besedovsky H: Interleukin 1 affects glucose homeostasis, *Am J Physiol* 253:R794–R798, 1987.

36. Beutler B, Cerami A: Cachectic tumor necrosis factor: an endogenous mediator of shock and inflammation, *Immunol Res* 5:281–293, 1986.

37. Arbeit JM: Resting energy expenditure in controls and cancer patients with localized and diffuse diseases, *Ann Surg* 199:292–298, 1984.

38. Dempsey DT, Knox LS, Mullen JL, and others: Energy expenditure in malnourished patients with colorectal cancer, *Arch Surg* 121:789–795, 1986.

39. Hansell DT, Davies JWL, Durns HJG: The relationship between resting energy expenditure and weight loss in benign and malignant disease, *Ann Surg* 203:240–245, 1986.

40. Ogilvie GK: Energy metabolism in diseased and critically ill dogs: new horizons, *Vet Clin Nutr* 4:138–142, 1997.

41. Ogilvie GK, Walters LM, Fettman MJ, and others: Energy expenditure in dogs with lymphoma fed two specialized diets, *Cancer* 71:3146–3152, 1993.

42. Ogilvie GK, Salman MD, Fettman MJ, and others: Resting energy expenditure in dogs with nonhematopoietic malignancies before and after excision of tumors, *Am J Vet Res* 57:1463–1467, 1996.

43. Rossi-Fanelli F, Cascino A, Muscaritoli M: Abnormal substrate metabolism and nutritional strategies in cancer management, *JPEN* 15:680–683, 1991.

44. Dempsey DT, Mullen JL: Macronutrient requirements in the malnourished cancer patient, *Ann Surg* 55:290–294, 1985.

45. Shein PS: The oxidation of body fuel stores in cancer patients, *Ann Surg* 204:637–642, 1986.

46. Mauldin GE: Feeding the cancer patient. In Carey DP, Norton SA, Bolser SM, editors: *Recent advances in canine and feline nutritional research, Proceedings of the Iams international nutrition symposium*, Wilmington, Ohio, 1996, Orange Frazer Press.

47. Lowell JA, Parnes HL, Blackburn GL: Dietary immunomodulation: beneficial effects on carcinogenesis and tumor growth, *Crit Care Med* 18:S145–S148, 1990.

48. Ramesh G, Das UN, Koratkar R, and others: Effect of essential fatty acids on tumor cells, *Nutrition* 8:343–347, 1992.

49. Begin ME, Ellis G, Das UN, and others: Differential killing of human carcinoma cells supplemented with n-3 and n-6 polyunsaturated fatty acids, *J Natl Cancer Inst* 77:2053–2057, 1986.

50. Plumb JA, Luo W, Kerr DJ: Effect of polyunsaturated fatty acids on the drug sensitivity of human tumor cell lines resistant to either cisplastin or doxorubicin, *Br J Cancer* 67:728–733, 1993.

51. Tisdale MJ, Brennan RA, Fearon KC: Reduction of weight loss and tumor size in a cachexia model by a high fat diet, *Br J Cancer* 56:39–43, 1987.

52. Roush GC, Pero RW, Powell J, and others: Modulation of the cancer susceptibility measure, adenosine diphosphate ribosyl transferase (ADPRT), by differences in n-3 and n-6 fatty acids, *Nutr Cancer* 16:197–207, 1991.

53. Mohammed SI, Khan KNM, Sellers RS, and others: Expression of cyclooxygenase-1 and -2 in naturally-occurring canine cancer, *Prostaglandins Leukot Essent Fatty Acids* 70:479–483, 2004.

54. Daly JM, Lieberman M, Goldfine J, and others: Enteral nutrition with supplemental arginine, RNA, and omega-3 fatty acids: a prospective clinical trial, *Proc Am Con Parenteral Enteral Nut JPEN* 15:19S, 1991.

55. Olgivie GK, Fettman MJ, Mallincfrodt CH, and others: Effect of fish oil, arginine, and doxorubicin chemotherapy on remission and survival time for dogs with lymphoma, *Cancer* 88:1916–1928, 2000.

56. Anderson CR, Ogilvie GK, LaRue SM, and others: Effect of fish oil and arginine on acute effects of radiation injury in dogs with neoplasia: a double-blind study. In *Proc Vet Cancer Soc*, Chicago, 1997.

57. Knapp DW, Mohammet SI, Hayek MG: Fatty acid regulation of cancer cell growth. In *NAVC Proc*, 2004, pp 22–26.

58. Selting KA, Ogilvie GK, Gustafson DL, and others: Evaluation of the effects of dietary n-3 fatty acid supplementation on the pharmokinetics of doxorubicin in dogs with lymphoma, *Am J Vet Res* 67:145–151, 2006.

59. Donahue S: Nutritional support of hospitalized patients, *Vet Clin North Am Small Anim Pract* 19:475–495, 1989.

60. Tachibana K, Mukai K, Hirauka I, and others: Evaluation of the effect of arginine enriched amino acid solution on tumor growth, *JPEN* 9:428–434, 1985.

61. Barbul A, Isto DA, Wasserkrug HL, and others: Arginine stimulates lymphocyte immune response in healthy human beings, *Surgery* 90:244–251, 1981.

62. Cangiano C, Laviano A, Meguid MM, and others: Effects of administration of oral branched-chain amino acids on anorexia and caloric intake in cancer patients, *J Natl Cancer Inst* 88:550–552, 1996.

63. Wakshlag JJ, Kallfelz FA, Wakshlag RR, Davenport GM: The effects of branched-chain amino acids on canine neoplastic cell proliferation and death, *J Nutr* 136:2007S–2010S, 2006.

64. Freeman LM: Antioxidants in cancer treatment: helpful or harmful? *Compend Contin Educ Pract Vet* 31:154–158, 2009.

65. Szczubial M, Kankofer M, Lopuszynski W: Oxidative stress parameters in bitches with mammary gland tumours, *J Vet Med Physiol Pathol Clin Med* 51:336–340, 2004.

66. Winter JL, Barber L, Griessmar PC: Antioxidant status and biomarkers of oxidative stress in canine lymphoma, *J Vet Intern Med* 23:311–316, 2009.

67. Palozza P, Serini S, Di Nicuolo F, Calviello G: Modulation of apoptotic signaling by carotenoids in cancer cells, *Arch Biochem Biophys* 430:105–109, 2004.

68. Prakash P, Russell RM, Krinsky NI: In vitro inhibition of proliferation of estrogen-dependent and estrogen-independent human breast cancer cells treated with carotenoids and retinoids, *J Nutr* 131:1574–1580, 2001.

69. Chew BP, Park JS, Wong MW, Wong TS: A comparison of the anti-cancer activities of dietary beta-carotene, canthaxanthin and astaxanthin in mice in vivo, *Anticancer Res* 19:1849–1853, 1999.

70. Block KI, Koch AC, Mead MN: Impact of antioxidants supplementation on chemotherapeutic efficacy: a systematic review of the evidence from randomized controlled trials, *Cancer Treat Rev* 33:407–418, 2007.

71. Moss RW: Do antioxidants interfere with radiation therapy for cancer? *Integr Cancer Ther* 6:281–293, 2007.

72. Chan DL, Freeman LM: Nutrition in critical illness, *Vet Clin North Am Small Anim Pract* 36:1125–1241, 2006.

73. Buffington CAT: Enteral nutritional support, *Vet Clin Nutr* 3:10–13, 1996.

74. Reinhart GA, Hayek MG: Nutritional support in the critical care patient. In *Proc XXI Cong World Small Anim Vet Assoc*, 1996, pp 66–68.

75. Lippert AC, Fulton RB, Parr AM: A retrospective study of the use of total parenteral nutrition in dogs and cats, *J Vet Intern Med* 7:52–64, 1993.

76. Vail DM, Ogilvie GK, Fettman MJ, and others: Exacerbation of hyperlactatemia by infusion of lactated Ringer's solution in dogs with lymphoma, *J Vet Intern Med* 4:228, 1990.

37

Nutrition and Mobility

It has been reported that almost one fourth of dogs visiting veterinary practices are diagnosed with musculoskeletal disorders.[1] Of these cases, 70% involved mobility or lameness issues of the appendicular skeleton. The incidence in dogs that are less than 1 year of age is about 22%, and more than 90% of these cases are thought to be influenced by nutritional factors.[2] Developmental skeletal diseases are most prevalent in the large and giant breeds, and their onset is usually associated with periods of rapid growth. The most common of these disorders are canine hip dysplasia (CHD), several forms of osteochondrosis, hypertrophic osteodystrophy (HOD) (also called *metaphyseal osteopathy*), and panosteitis. Congenital disorders that affect mobility include medial patellar luxation and Legg-Calvé-Perthes disease. Other causes of lameness and impaired mobility include ruptured cruciate, infectious arthritis, and rheumatoid arthritis. Finally, osteoarthritis (OA) is a common disorder in middle-aged and older pets and eventually develops with almost all forms of musculoskeletal disease. Free-choice feeding of diets that are nutrient- and energy-dense or supplementation with certain nutrients during growth are important factors in the etiology of developmental skeletal disease. In addition, nutritional management, along with antiinflammatory and pain medication, plays a critical role in alleviating clinical signs and supporting joint heath in pets affected with OA.

GENERAL CONSIDERATIONS

The musculoskeletal system is composed primarily of muscle, ligaments, tendons, cartilage, and bone. It provides structural support for multiple organ and metabolic functions as well as locomotion, mastication, and respiration. Because the musculoskeletal system is integrated with the cardiovascular, respiratory, neurologic, hemolymphatic, digestive, and endocrine systems, primary disorders of any of these interrelated systems can directly affect the musculoskeletal system. Therefore, when evaluating any lameness issue, other body functions and systems should also be considered.

Musculoskeletal dysfunction of the appendicular skeleton can involve one or more limbs. There can be muscle, tendon, joint, or bone involvement in one or more limbs. There may be swelling, pain, weakness, or atrophy present in muscles or tendons. Similarly, evaluation of affected joints may reveal swelling, heat, pain, crepitation, luxation or subluxation, and either increased or decreased range of motion. The bone itself may be involved. Fractures, bony enlargement, abnormal conformation, growth disturbances, and increased or decreased density seen on radiographs are all indictors that a bone may be the primary source of lameness. In all cases, a thorough veterinary examination and medical history are necessary for diagnosis of musculoskeletal disease.

DEVELOPMENTAL SKELETAL DISORDERS

Canine Hip Dysplasia

CHD is a biomechanical disease of the coxofemoral joint, characterized by incongruity between surfaces of the head of the femur and the acetabulum. Over time, this subluxation causes remodeling of the joint, typified by shallowing of the acetabulum, flattening of the femoral head, and development of OA. The degree of subluxation and joint laxity determines the degree of femoral head remodeling and development of degenerative joint disease over the dog's lifetime (Figure 37-1).[3] Together, joint laxity (which becomes evident after 2 months of age) and OA, which can become evident as early as 4 months of age or be delayed for years, determine the severity of the disease in an individual. Affected dogs range from being asymptomatic throughout life to being severely crippled at a young age.

CHD is the most frequently encountered orthopedic disease in veterinary medicine. It has a multifactorial etiology, involving both a strong genetic component and a number of potential environmental factors.[4] Although all dogs are susceptible, breeds that have an increased

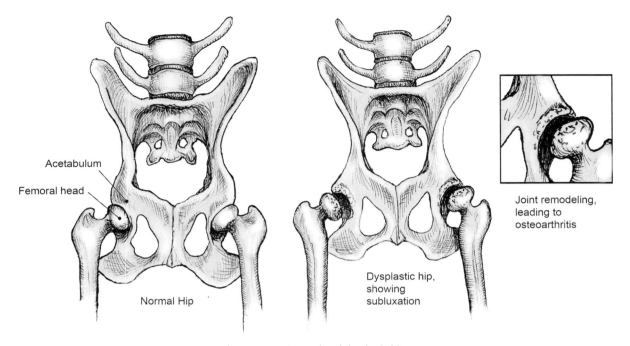

Acetabulum

Femoral head

Normal Hip

Dysplastic hip,
showing
subluxation

Joint remodeling,
leading to
osteoarthritis

Figure 37-1   Normal and dysplastic hips.

risk of developing CHD include the Bulldog, Pug, Saint Bernard, Clumber Spaniel, Boykin Spaniel, and Bloodhound.[5] The prevalence of CHD in some breeds may be higher than 70%.[6] Of the environmental influences, diet and growth rate are believed to be most important. A dog's rate of growth during the period from 3 months to 8 months of age is critical in the development of CHD (Figure 37-2). Dogs demonstrating a high rate of growth and excessive weight gain during this period have a higher frequency and more severe degenerative changes than do dogs growing at rates equal to or below their breed standard.[7] Additionally, excessive external muscular forces acting on the hip joint from strenuous or excessive exercise during periods of growth may prevent the femoral head from remaining in close contact with the acetabulum during development.

Dogs with severe hip dysplasia may show clinical signs of the disease when they are less than a year of age, but signs more typically appear in middle-aged dogs. Depending on the degree of CHD, obvious signs of OA may not be observed until the dog is middle aged or older because the hip joint develops more articular cartilage abnormalities as animals age. Clinically, dogs with hip dysplasia have difficulty rising from a lying or sitting position especially after exercise. They may move both legs together when running or loping and appear to "bunny-hop." There may be pain associated with palpation of the joint on physical examination or even a notable laxity within the joint. If chronic, there may also be atrophy or muscle wasting of the pelvic and hind-limb muscles.

Canine hip dysplasia (CHD) is a developmental skeletal disease characterized by incongruity between surfaces of the head of the femur and the acetabulum. Over time, this subluxation causes remodeling of the joint and development of osteoarthritis. Large and giant breeds are more susceptible to CHD, and risk is increased if a dog experiences a high rate of growth and excessive weight gain during development.

Osteochondrosis

Osteochondrosis is characterized by a focal disruption in endochondral ossification, which causes impaired maturation of epiphyseal cartilage.[8] It can occur in

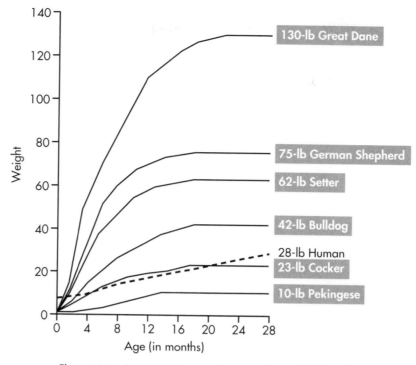

Figure 37-2   Representative growth curves of several dog breeds.

both the physis and epiphysis of growth cartilage and at multiple points throughout the skeleton. In growing dogs, osteochondrosis of the articular epiphyseal cartilage most commonly occurs in the shoulder, stifle, hock, and elbow. Clinical signs include pain, lameness, and occasionally swelling around the affected joint. One or multiple joints may be affected, and signs typically appear when dogs are between 5 and 9 months of age. Subsequent to the development of osteochondrosis, acute inflammatory joint disease or OA develops when the cartilage joint surface is disrupted. A common manifestation of osteochondrosis is osteochondritis dissecans. This occurs when a segment of articular (joint) cartilage is separated from the underlying bone and subchondral bone is exposed to synovial fluid. If this piece of cartilage breaks off into the joint, it is commonly referred to as a "joint mouse" and typically requires surgical removal. As with CHD, the etiology of osteochondrosis appears to be multifactorial. Identified risk factors include age, sex, breed, rapid growth rate, and excessive weight gain, and possibly nutrient excesses

(particularly of calcium).[9,10] Breeds that demonstrate the highest incidence of this disorder include the Bernese Mountain Dog, Great Dane, Labrador Retriever, Golden Retriever, Newfoundland, and Rottweiler.[11,12]

Hypertrophic Osteodystrophy

HOD occurs primarily in the large and giant breeds of dogs and is characterized by excessive bone deposition and retarded bone resorption. Breeds showing a high incidence include Great Danes, Saint Bernards, Boxers, Chesapeake Bay Retrievers, Irish Setters, German Shepherd Dogs, and Labrador Retrievers.[12] The distal ulna, radius, and tibia are most commonly affected. Radiographically, an irregular, translucent zone initially appears in the metaphysis and is separated from the growth plate by an excessively dense band of bone. As the disease progresses, additional bone is deposited outside of the periosteum, and soft-tissue swelling and subperiosteal hemorrhages develop around affected metaphyseal areas. Signs include acute pain and swelling, lameness, intermittent pyrexia, and occasional anorexia. The observed swelling is due to both fibrous thickening of the periosteum and the deposition of new periosteal bone. HOD primarily affects dogs that are growing rapidly, and the initial signs are typically seen when dogs are between 3 months and 6 months of age.

Panosteitis

Panosteitis is a common cause of lameness in young, large-breed dogs and is typically diagnosed when dogs are between 5 and 12 months of age. Males are more frequently affected than females, and Great Pyrenees, German Shepherd Dogs, Mastiffs, and Basset Hounds are at increased risk.[12] Panosteitis is characterized by generalized inflammation of the long bones, specifically the humerus, radius, ulna, femur, and tibia.[13] In more than half of the reported cases, the disorder moves from leg to leg, eventually affecting almost all of the long bones. Affected dogs show a sudden onset of moderate to severe lameness, with no history of injury or trauma. A defining characteristic of panosteitis is its tendency to shift, moving from one limb to another over a period of several months or more. Because of this, panosteitis is often erroneously referred to as "growing pains" in young dogs, as it is often seen during periods of rapid growth. Affected puppies may show a loss of appetite and transient fever during acute episodes. Although dogs may show extreme lameness and pain upon palpation of the affected limbs, panosteitis is a self-limiting disorder in the vast majority of dogs. Still, this disorder can be very concerning to owners because some dogs show intermittent lameness for up to 18 months or more.

Nutritional Factors Influencing Developmental Skeletal Diseases

Most forms of developmental skeletal disease are influenced by genetics and are considered to be polygenetic diseases. However, heredity cannot fully explain their occurrence, and phenotypic expression depends upon a variety of environmental influences. For example, although a limited number of breeds have been studied, heritability coefficients for CHD are estimated to be between 0.1 and 0.4.[14-16] This means that 60% or more of the factors that influence the phenotypic expression of CHD are environmental in nature. Although it is difficult to identify all of the external components involved in these disorders, nutrition and rate of growth play an important role. A number of nutrients have been examined, including energy, protein, vitamin C, fat, carbohydrate, and calcium. The data indicate that the most important nutritional factors in the development of skeletal disease in dogs are excess caloric intake and excessive intake of calcium during growth.

EXCESS CALORIC INTAKE Excess energy intake during growth commonly occurs as a result of feeding a high-quality, growth diet to a young dog on a free-choice basis or feeding excess quantities of food on a portion-controlled basis. Some owners believe that puppies should be kept "plump" in appearance, and that a rotund puppy is a healthy puppy. However, when puppies are fed excessive amounts of a balanced diet, growth rate is maximized before excess weight in the form of fat is gained. As a result, a growing dog that appears to be slightly overweight is usually growing at a maximal rate. Studies with dogs, humans, and other species have shown that the consumption of excess calories resulting in a maximal or an above-average growth rate is not compatible with optimal and healthy skeletal development.[17,18]

The first study to demonstrate the relationship between overnutrition, rapid growth, and developmental skeletal disease was conducted with growing Great Danes.[19] Two groups of growing puppies were fed a highly palatable, energy-dense food throughout growth. The first group was fed free-choice, and the second group was fed amounts of food that were restricted to two thirds of the intake of the first group. The dogs that were fed free-choice grew significantly faster than did the dogs fed restricted amounts of food, and bone tissue was significantly affected by the rapid growth rate. A variety of skeletal abnormalities were observed in the dogs that were fed free-choice, including enlargement of the costochondral junctions and the epiphyseal-metaphyseal regions of long bones, hyperextension of the carpus, and sinking of the metacarpophalangeal and metatarsophalangeal joints. These changes were associated with pain and varying degrees of lameness. It was concluded that generalized overnutrition, in the form of excess energy, protein, calcium, and phosphorus, caused increased growth rate in these dogs that contributed to abnormal skeletal development.

Subsequently, other studies were conducted with growing dogs of several large breeds, including German Shepherd Dogs, Golden Retrievers, and Labrador Retrievers. In one study, a group of puppies that had high parental frequencies of CHD were examined. The incidence and severity of dysplasia was greater in puppies that had rapid growth rates as a result of increased caloric intake, when compared with puppies that were fed restricted amounts of food.[20] Similarly, when a group of puppies was hand-reared at a reduced rate of growth, they developed a very low incidence of hip dysplasia.[21,22] In contrast, a control group that was fed to allow a much higher growth rate showed a very high incidence of hip dysplasia.

A well-controlled longitudinal study with a group of 48 Labrador Retrievers found that dogs fed 25% less food than dogs fed free-choice, starting after weaning and continuing throughout life, had significantly less hip joint laxity at 30 weeks of age and a significantly lower incidence of CHD.[18,23] Of the dogs in the free-choice group, 16 of 24 developed CHD by 2 years of age, compared with 7 of the 24 dogs in the limited-feeding group. OA was observed in the hips of 7 of the 24 free-choice dogs by the time they were 1 year old, while none of the limited-feeding dogs showed OA at 1 year.[24] By 5 years of age, 12 of the 23 remaining free-choice dogs (52%) and only 3 of the 23 limited-feeding dogs (13%) had radiographic signs of hip OA, and the degree of OA was more severe in free-choice dogs than in the restricted-feeding dogs. Additional evaluations showed that arthritic changes to hips and shoulders increased linearly (rather than bimodally) throughout life, and these changes were more frequent, occurred earlier, and were more severe in dogs fed free-choice compared with dogs fed restricted amounts of food.[25,26] Finally, the dogs fed free-choice weighed more and had higher body condition score values during growth and throughout life; a significant and positive correlation was found between body weight and the presence and severity of OA.[24]

The skeletal system of dogs is most susceptible to physical and metabolic stressors during the first 12 months of life. It is theorized that abnormal skeletal development during periods of rapid growth results from overloading the growing skeleton with prematurely increased muscle mass and body weight.[27] This theory is supported by the fact that rapidly growing male dogs of the large and giant breeds are more frequently affected than are smaller females.[28] There also appears to be a correlation between increasing body size and the occurrence of the lesions associated with osteochondrosis.[29] A comparison between the bones of large and small breeds of dogs during periods of rapid growth shows that the bones of large breeds are relatively less dense than are the bones of small breeds at similar stages of development. Bones of large breeds have a thinner cortex, larger medullary cavity, and a less dense spongiosa.[29,30] It is possible that the bones of large dogs during growth are not as strong as those of smaller dogs during the same period. This may be the basis for the genetic predispositions toward skeletal abnormalities in the large and giant breeds. Recent evidence suggests that mechanical stress on the joints caused by excessive weight during growth and throughout life also contributes to the development of OA.[24]

In addition to weight-related mechanical stressors, overnutrition has direct effects that negatively influence skeletal development. Studies with Great Danes have shown that overnutrition stimulates accelerated skeletal growth.[29] Great Dane puppies were fed a diet formulated for growth from weaning to 6 months of age. Puppies in one group were fed free-choice (ad libitum), and puppies in the second group were restricted to 70% to 80% of the amount consumed by the first group. As in previous studies, dogs fed ad libitum weighed significantly more than the restricted group at 6 months of age. Bone measurement data showed that accelerated skeletal growth, in the form of increased size and volume of bone, contributed significantly to the increased weight. The male dogs that experienced overnutrition also showed an increased rate of bone remodeling, resulting in enlarged bones with relatively low densities and low resistance to the greater weight they were required to bear. It appears that if a large dog is allowed to attain its maximal growth rate by consuming excess amounts of a balanced diet, the accelerated growth rate creates a rapidly growing skeleton that is less strong and less able to withstand the biomechanical stresses of the greater muscle mass and body weight that are put on it. Not only do these dogs weigh more, but their bones are less able to handle the added weight. The end result is the development of aberrations in ossification, damage to developing cartilage and growth plates, and premature closure of growth plates. Most often this manifests as osteochondrosis, but these changes may also be involved in the onset of several other developmental skeletal diseases.

Excess energy intake during growth is a significant risk factor for developmental skeletal disease in dogs. This most commonly occurs as a result of feeding a high-quality, growth diet to a young dog on a free-choice basis or feeding excess quantities of food on a portion-controlled basis. The resulting rapid growth rate is not compatible with healthy skeletal development because of mechanical stresses placed on developing bones and changes in bone growth.

Feeding for Optimal Growth Rate

The final skeletal height of a dog is strongly influenced by genetics. Providing adequate, but not excessive, amounts of a balanced diet enables an animal to achieve its potential size but at a slower rate than if excess food is provided. Feeding an energy-dense, nutrient-balanced food at a level that promotes a high rate of growth decreases the time it takes the dog to attain adult size and can contribute to abnormal skeletal development. Conversely, feeding restricted amounts of a balanced food, to achieve a slower growth rate, results in an animal of the same size, but at a later point in time. Allowing the skeleton to develop slowly, and feeding to maintain a lean body condition, eliminates the biomechanical stresses of excess weight and the changes in bone development that are associated with rapid growth and overweight body conditions.

The best way to attain a moderate growth rate is to strictly monitor body weight during growth and to feed to attain a lean body condition (Box 37-1; see Chapter 28, Figure 28-2, p. 324). The chief contributor to rapid growth and weight gain is dietary energy. Because fat is much more energy dense than protein or carbohydrate, high-fat diets contribute significantly to excess energy intake. Several commercial dog foods are specifically formulated for large-breed puppies. These foods contain slightly lower fat and energy than typical puppy foods and have a protein concentration that is balanced to maintain an appropriate protein-to-energy ratio. Although dietary protein was once identified as a potential contributor to skeletal abnormalities, studies have

shown that dietary protein level is not a risk factor for the development of skeletal disorders in growing dogs.[31] A general recommendation is to select a food that has a moderately reduced energy content (between 3.5 and 3.8 kilocalories [kcal]/gram [g] of dry food) compared with typical puppy foods, and between 12% and 16% fat. The food should contain a minimum of 22% high-quality protein, with an optimum level of between 26% and 28% (23% to 26% of calories).[32] Calcium levels should be between 0.8% and 1.2% (see pp. 499-500).

Large- and giant-breed dogs should always be fed on a portion-controlled basis during growth. Free-choice feeding is not recommended because it increases the risk of overconsumption and is not conducive to monitoring daily intake and controlling rate of growth. In addition, ad libitum feeding appears to affect several of the hormonal regulatory systems of growth.[33] Circulating levels of insulin-like growth factor-1, thyroxine (T_4), and triiodothyronine (T_3) were found to be higher in growing dogs that were fed ad libitum when compared with levels in dogs that were fed on a portion-controlled basis. It is possible that ad libitum feeding promotes the metabolic processes that support rapid growth rate. Portion-controlled feeding allows the owner to feed an amount of food that maintains optimum growth rate

---

BOX 37-1 PRACTICAL FEEDING TIPS: FEEDING GROWING DOGS TO DECREASE THE RISK OF DEVELOPMENTAL SKELETAL DISEASE

Select a complete and balanced dog food that has been formulated for growth in large and giant breeds.

Feed this food throughout the first 1 to 2 years of life.

Use a portion-controlled feeding regimen and carefully measure the amount of food that is fed each day.

Provide an amount of food that will support an average rate of growth for a dog's breed.

Provide an amount of food that will maintain a lean body condition throughout growth.

Strictly monitor weight gain and body condition until the dog reaches maturity.

Do not supplement the diet with minerals, vitamins, or additional foods.

and body condition and to gradually adjust the dog's intake as energy needs change during growth.

The amount to feed can be estimated from guidelines provided on the food's package and then adjusted to attain ideal body condition (see Chapter 28, Figure 28-2, p. 324). Because growing large- and giant-breed dogs have very steep growth curves, their intake requirements can change dramatically over short periods of time. Therefore puppies should be weighed and evaluated at least once every 2 weeks. Young puppies should be fed three to four meals per day until they are 4 months old and two meals per day thereafter. A well-formulated, breed-size–specific growth diet should be fed throughout the dog's growth period. For large and giant breeds, this corresponds to the first 12 to 24 months of life, depending upon the dog's breed and adult size.

The best way to attain a moderate growth rate is to strictly monitor dogs' body weight during growth and to feed to attain a lean body condition. A growth food that contains slightly reduced fat and energy should be selected for large- and giant-breed puppies. Feeding on a portion-controlled basis is also recommended because this allows the owner to feed an amount of food that maintains optimum growth rate and body condition and to gradually adjust the dog's intake as energy needs change.

Excess Calcium Intake and Skeletal Disease

Calcium is a nutrient that is commonly supplemented to the diets of dogs and, less commonly, to the diets of cats. The reason most often cited for calcium supplementation relates to its essential role in normal skeletal growth and development. Supplements such as dicalcium phosphate and bone meal are added to a growing dog's diet during growth spurts or when problems such as hyperextension of the carpus or sinking of the metacarpophalangeal joints occur. Some breeders encourage all of their puppy buyers to routinely supplement their puppy's diet with calcium during the entire first year of life as a prophylactic measure. Some believe that calcium supplementation is not only necessary for proper bone development but that it also prevents the development of certain skeletal disorders. Regardless of the good intentions, there are potential risks when excessively high levels of calcium are either included in the diet itself or added to an adequate and balanced diet.

Research has shown that normal growth in puppies can be supported by a calcium intake of 0.37% available calcium or 0.6% total calcium.[34] The Association of American Feed Control Officials' (AAFCO's) *Nutrient Profiles* for dog foods sets minimum levels for calcium of 0.8% for growth and reproduction and 0.5% for adult maintenance. The profile also mandates a maximum level of 2.5% calcium in all dog foods. This maximum level was included because published data show that excess calcium during growth may contribute to abnormal skeletal development and increase a dog's risk of skeletal disease.

A series of studies were conducted in the 1980s to determine the effect of varying levels of dietary calcium upon the occurrence of developmental skeletal disease in growing Great Danes.[35,36] An experimental diet was formulated that met the recommendations of the 1974 National Research Council's (NRC's) *Nutrient Requirements for Dogs*. Both the control group and the experimental group of dogs received this food throughout growth. In addition, the experimental group received calcium carbonate supplementation to achieve a level of 3.3% in the diet, three times the amount recommended by the NRC at that time.[37,38] Dogs that were fed excessive calcium during growth developed chronic hypercalcemia and hypophosphatemia. Skeletal differences between the control and experimental dogs included a higher percentage of total bone volume, retarded bone maturation, retarded bone remodeling, and a decreased number of osteoclasts (bone resorption cells) in the dogs receiving calcium supplementation. This group also showed a higher incidence and severity of cartilage irregularities associated with osteochondrosis at the distal and proximal humeral cartilages. Clinically, calcium-supplemented dogs exhibited retained cartilage cones, severe lateral deviation of the feet, and radius curvus syndrome.

When plasma calcium levels increase, the hormone calcitonin is secreted from the thyroid gland. Calcitonin functions to lower plasma calcium to normal levels; it exerts this effect by decreasing the activity of osteoclasts, which leads to decreased bone resorption and slowed cartilage maturation.[19,35] This is a normal hormonal response to both eating and calcium influx, and calcitonin functions along with parathyroid hormone (PTH) to closely regulate calcium homeostasis. However, the chronic elevation of calcitonin suppresses bone resorption for an abnormal period of time, resulting in a gradual thickening and increased density of cortical bone. For example, when growing Beagles were supplemented with 2.3 g of calcium per day for 2 months, the thyroid glands of supplemented dogs contained significantly increased proportions of calcitonin-producing C cells and decreased proportions of thyroid follicles, when compared with those of the control dogs.[39] High dietary calcium intake caused thyroid C-cell hyperplasia, which would suggest the occurrence of chronic hypercalcitoninism in these dogs. Additionally, electron microscopy of the thyroid C cells of dogs fed excess calories, protein, and calcium showed that these cells were releasing larger amounts of calcitonin than were the C cells of dogs fed restricted diets. In growing dogs, these changes interfere with normal bone remodeling and development. The deposition of excessive subperiosteal bone that results may cause the clinical signs of HOD and Wobbler syndrome, and the chronic effects of calcitonin on cartilage maturation may result in the eventual detachment of the articular cartilage that is seen in osteochondrosis.

A more recent study, again with Great Danes, fed the same diets described previously plus a third experimental diet that contained additional phosphorus to provide a balanced calcium-to-phosphorus ratio.[40] Puppies in this study were fed the high calcium diets during the period of most rapid growth, between 6 and 17 weeks of age. At 17 weeks, all of the puppies were switched to the control diet, which contained normal calcium and phosphorus levels (1.04% and 0.82%, respectively). Puppies fed the high calcium-only diet developed hypercalcemia and hypophosphatemia that persisted throughout the experimental diet feeding period. Puppies fed the food containing elevated calcium and phosphorus had normal serum calcium values during this period and slightly lowered plasma phosphorus levels. Although both groups of puppies that were fed excessive calcium showed skeletal disturbances during the feeding period, changes were more severe in puppies fed excessive calcium without phosphorus. This difference was attributed to the hypercalcemia and subsequent reduction in PTH secretion,

leading to hypophosphatemia. This study also found that normalizing dietary calcium levels after 17 weeks of age corrected some skeletal abnormalities, but joint changes that were consistent with osteochondrosis still developed in the puppies that were fed the diet containing high calcium without added phosphorus.

To further examine the effects of elevated calcium when a normal calcium to phosphorus ratio is maintained, Great Dane puppies were fed diets containing three levels of calcium (0.48%, 0.8%, and 2.7%).[41] Each diet contained sufficient phosphorus to provide a consistent calcium-to-phosphorus ratio of 1.2:1.0. To control for other factors that can affect skeletal development, the experimental diets had reduced caloric density and contained 26% protein and 14% fat. Puppies were assigned to the three diets at the age of weaning, and they were fed the experimental diets for 18 months. Even when balanced with phosphorus, increasing dietary calcium had a rapid and direct effect on the amount of mineral deposited in maturing bones. Bone mineral content and bone density were positively correlated with dietary calcium and phosphorus beginning almost immediately after weaning and continuing until the dogs were 6 months old. Six of the 15 dogs that were fed the highest level of calcium (2.7%) showed clinical signs of lameness during the first 6 months of the study, and three of these dogs showed clinical signs of HOD. After 6 months, the bone density differences seen between the high-, medium-, and low-calcium groups gradually diminished and were not apparent by the time that the dogs were 12 months old (Table 37-1). Similar to the results of Schoenmakers et al.,[40] dogs fed high amounts of calcium that were balanced with

TABLE 37-1 BONE MINERAL CONTENT OF GREAT DANES FED THREE DIFFERENT LEVELS OF DIETARY CALCIUM

AGE (MONTHS)	LOW CALCIUM (G)	MODERATE CALCIUM (G)	HIGH CALCIUM (G)
2	77.55[b]	83.27[b]	110.38[a]
6	905.06[b]	1066.63[c]	1201.87[c]
12	1768.64[b]	1916.68[a,b]	2072.70[a]
14	2031.21	2069.72	2132.20

[a,b,c], Values within a row with different superscripts differ (P<0.05).

phosphorus did not develop hypercalcemia. Conversely, dogs fed the highest calcium diet had low total and ionized serum calcium values when they were between 4 and 7 months of age. This decrease was not observed in dogs fed the low- and medium-level calcium diets. It is likely that these values are a result of increased deposition of circulating calcium into developing bone, possibly in response to chronically increased calcitonin levels. The normalization of bone composition between the three groups after 6 months of age may reflect the natural maturation of the dogs' regulatory mechanisms that control calcium absorption and excretion (see below).

The influence that excess calcium intake has upon skeletal development in growing dogs appears to be due, at least in part , to the inability of young dogs to regulate calcium and absorption and excretion. Dietary calcium is absorbed across the intestinal epithelium through either active transport or passive diffusion. The active transport mechanism is saturable, is carrier mediated, and depends on the animal's vitamin D status. The second mechanism is a nonsaturable, diffusional transfer that is directly dependent on the concentration of available calcium in the intestinal lumen. Passive diffusion is the predominant pathway for calcium absorption in neonates and young animals.[42] As an animal matures, active transport of calcium becomes more prominent and calcium absorption becomes more tightly controlled. For example, puppies of weaning age absorb at least 50% of dietary calcium, regardless of the quantity that is ingested.[43] In contrast, the percentage of calcium that adults absorb from their diet varies between 10% and 90%, depending on the composition of the food, the calcium content of the diet, and the physiological state of the animal.[44]

For example, a study with growing dogs (Great Danes) reported that 45% of dietary calcium was absorbed when a normal level of calcium was fed (1.1% of the diet's dry matter [DM]).[45] This percentage increased to 80% when the level of calcium was decreased to 0.55%. Conversely, when the calcium level was increased to 3.3%, 45% of the calcium was still absorbed. As a result, calcium balance was significantly more positive in the dogs fed a high level of the mineral when compared with the balance in the dogs that were fed either normal or low concentrations. The mineral content of cortical and cancellous bone was greater in the high-calcium dogs, and there was decreased bone

turnover and remodeling of the skeleton. As dogs age and reach maturity, they appear to be able to adapt to high calcium intakes by decreasing the proportion that is absorbed. Because young dogs have reduced ability to regulate calcium absorption and also have rapidly developing and changing skeletons, they are especially susceptible to the adverse effects of high dietary calcium.

The large and giant breeds of dogs are especially susceptible to the pathological effects of excess calcium consumption, presumably because of their rapid growth rate, heavier weights, and larger overall size.[29] However, while studies with Great Danes have consistently shown a detrimental response to calcium excess, relatively few other large or giant breeds have been studied, and not all large-breed dogs that are fed foods containing high levels of calcium develop skeletal abnormalities.[46] For example, studies of a large cross-breed dog called the Foxhound-Boxer-Ingelheim Labrador (FBI) reported that FBIs fed excessive calcium during growth had lower calcium retention when compared with Beagle puppies fed the same diet, and the FBIs showed no indications of skeletal disease.[47] Conversely, subclinical skeletal abnormalities have been reported in some smaller breeds fed excess calcium during growth, such as Beagles, but not in others, such as Miniature Poodles.[48,49] These results suggest that dog breeds may differ in their degree of susceptibility to the detrimental effects of calcium excess on skeletal development. Factors that may be important include genetic influences on a dog's structure and conformation, body composition, growth rate, and possibly calcium metabolism and homeostatic mechanisms.

Dietary Calcium Recommendations (Large and Giant Breeds)

It appears that the mechanisms of calcium homeostasis that prevent puppies from absorbing excess amounts of calcium are not fully functional prior to 6 months of age. Therefore the safety margins for optimal calcium and phosphorus intake early in life are relatively narrow, especially for large- and giant-breed dogs. The food that is fed to puppies from weaning and throughout growth should contain adequate but not excessive calcium. A calcium level slightly lower than 1% appears to be beneficial for large-breed puppies. While 0.4% is too low, a level of 0.8% is optimal. Because changes in mineral composition in response to dietary calcium are present as early as 2 months of age, and skeletal problems can be present by 5 to 6 months, the large-breed growth diet should be introduced at weaning.

Some breeders continue to suggest feeding an adult maintenance rather than a commercial puppy food to large- and giant-breed puppies. However, because some maintenance diets are substantially lower in energy density than growth diets, the dog must be fed a higher volume of the maintenance diet to meet its energy needs. If the calcium level in the adult diet is similar to that in the puppy food (e.g., 1.1% or more), then the total calcium the puppy consumes when fed the maintenance diet will actually be greater.[50] Likewise, if a growing dog is fed an appropriate amount of a high-quality pet food formulated for growth, supplementation with calcium is unnecessary and contraindicated. If a pet owner is feeding the pet a food that appears to contain inadequate or unavailable levels of calcium, switching the dog to a high-quality commercial diet is safer than attempting to correct the imbalance in the poor diet through supplementation.

Foods that are fed to puppies from weaning and throughout growth should contain adequate but not excessive calcium. A calcium level slightly lower than 1% is recommended for large-breed puppies, with 0.8% optimal. An adult maintenance food should not be fed because puppies may still be at risk of consuming too much calcium. Likewise, supplementation with calcium is unnecessary and contraindicated.

CONGENITAL AND MEDICAL MOBILITY DISORDERS

Congenital Medial Patellar Luxation

Congenital medial patellar luxation is an orthopedic condition characterized by hypermobile patellas. It can affect dogs (both large and small breeds) and cats, and occurs unilaterally or bilaterally. The Orthopedic Foundation for Animals (OFA) reports an incidence rate of more than 40% in Pomeranians and about 25% in Cocker Spaniels.[5] Patellar luxation is classified into four grades, depending on the degree to which the patella slips from its seat in the trochlear sulcus to a medial joint location. The least severe grade (1) occurs when the patella slips from its normal location slightly or rarely, and the most severe grade (4) occurs when there is complete and permanent luxation of the patella from the trochlear sulcus. The cause of congenital medial patellar luxation is unknown; however, it presumably has a genetic component because it occurs more frequently in certain familial lines of purebred dogs.

Legg-Calvé-Perthes Disease

Legg-Calvé-Perthes disease (LCPD) is a disorder that occurs most frequently in small and miniature breeds of dogs. The syndrome is characterized by the interruption of the blood supply to the femoral epiphysis and eventual death of the osteocytes in the affected area. While the body attempts to repair the lesions, portions of the femoral head may collapse, causing articular surface incongruities and OA. Although the etiology is unknown, factors such as genetics, cytotoxic factors, fat embolization of the epiphyseal vessels, and decreased epiphyseal blood flow secondary to increased intraarticular pressure may contribute to the development of LCPD.

LCPD may develop unilaterally or bilaterally, and signs typically develop when dogs are between 4 and 11 months of age. Pain and lameness develop, along with eventual pelvic muscle atrophy. Many affected dogs are painful on palpation and manipulation of the hip joint and crepitation may be noted. Radiographs are the best way to confirm a diagnosis of LCPD.

Cranial Cruciate Ligament Rupture

Cranial cruciate ligament rupture is one of the most frequently observed injuries in the dog and is also occasionally seen in the cat. The ligament may be partially or completely ruptured. Meniscal damage may or may not occur with cruciate rupture. In all cases, affected animals can develop degenerative joint changes within a few weeks of the initial injury, and severe OA changes can be seen within a few months postinjury.[51] Although any dog may rupture the cruciate, this injury is commonly seen in middle-aged and inactive dogs that are overweight. Active, athletic animals also can rupture the cruciate, and usually this occurs during an athletic activity that causes overextension of the joint. Clinical signs include non–weight-bearing lameness that may partially resolve over time. However, OA changes develop rapidly with this injury, leading to chronic lameness and impaired mobility.

Infectious Arthritis

Infectious arthritis is an arthritic disorder that results from the introduction of an infectious agent to one or more joints. There are numerous underlying causes of infectious arthritis, but all result in the invasion of infectious agents into one or more joint capsules. The joint inflammation that occurs may be mild or severe and can lead to necrosis of the synovial membrane in the joint and production of a fibrinopurulent exudate. Joint motion is eventually reduced and either fibrous or bony ankylosis may be a final outcome of uncontrolled infectious arthritic. Clinical signs include lameness and pain in one or more joints, usually associated with joint effusion or swelling. When systemic infection is present, the animal may also show additional signs of depression, fever, anorexia, and lymphadenopathy. Chronic cases lead to severe OA or bony ankylosis.

Rheumatoid Arthritis

Rheumatoid arthritis is a chronic, progressive, immune-mediated disease that can affect many joints. Middle-age or senior dogs and small breeds are most often affected. Initially clinical signs include joint pain and effusion, shifting leg lameness, fever, anorexia, and depression. As the disease progresses, there may be crepitation upon palpation of affected joints and increased joint laxity. Similar to human patients, some dogs develop luxation or angular deformities of the areas affecting the bones. Although the etiology of rheumatoid arthritis is not completely understood, it appears to be immunologic in nature. Immunoglobulin G (IgG), IgM, and IgA antibodies (rheumatoid factors) are produced and form immune complexes with altered IgG. This leads to joint inflammation with intraarticular and synovial membrane infiltration by plasma cells, lymphocytes, and polymorphonuclear neutrophils (PMNs). The result is cartilage and subchondral bone destruction by enzymatic activity combined with natural weight-bearing forces. The supporting structures in the joint then break down and the joint can luxate or subluxate.

OSTEOARTHRITIS— A COLLECTIVE SYNDROME

Regardless of the primary cause of lameness or altered mobility (developmental, metabolic, genetic, or traumatic), the usual end result involves OA as the animal ages. OA (also called *degenerative joint disease*) is a chronic, progressive disease characterized by articular cartilage destruction, thickening of subchondral bone and osteophyte formation. In some, but not all, cases, inflammation of the synovial membrane and joint effusion develops. The incidence of OA has been estimated to be as high as 20% in dogs more than 1 year of age, and risk increases as animals become middle aged and older.[52,53] Clinical signs vary from mild pain, with no changes in mobility, to severe pain and functional disability. Affected animals develop lameness, joint heat or swelling, pain and stiffness following exercise, decreased range of motion, and muscle atrophy.

Understanding the Articular Surface of Joints and OA Development

The skeleton is an important structural component of the body, keeping all the organs safe and organized as well as providing a means for the animal to move and function properly. The joints between bones act as shock absorbers, protecting the surface of the bones and allowing flexibility and range of motion. Cells lining the joint capsule produce the synovial fluid. Synovial fluid lubricates the articular surfaces of the joints, prevents contact of the surfaces, supplies nutrients to the cells of the articular cartilage, and removes any waste products produced within the joint. The presence of synovial fluid within joints contributes to an almost friction-free, wear-resistant articulating surface that allows bones to function together without damage.

Proteoglycan and collagen are two extracellular components, found within the articular cartilage, that contribute to health of the joint's articulating surface. Proteoglycan is a large molecule composed of multiple glycosaminoglycan (GAG) chains that include hyaluranan, chondroitin sulfate, dermatan sulfate, heparin sulfate, and keratin sulfate. Collagen is a structural protein composed of a triple helix of polypeptide alpha-chains. These two joint components work together; proteoglycans provide a high hydration capacity to the cartilage and collagen fibers that contribute to tensile strength.

Mature articular cartilage is organized in several distinct zones. Superficial or articular surface includes chondrocytes and collagen and a relatively small number of proteoglycans. Deeper cartilage layers (i.e., closer to the bone) are composed of less collagen and more proteoglycans. As an animal ages, normal physiological changes include a decrease in collagen and GAG content (especially chondroitin sulfate) and a reduction in joint hydration.[54,55] The size of the proteoglycans also decreases. These age-related changes result in less capability to withstand the forces associated with normal joint function.[56]

In addition to the effects of aging, trauma and injury also cause physiological change to joints. Three general types of joint injury are microdamage or blunt trauma, chondral fractures, and osteochondral fractures.[57] Microdamage can be caused by repetitive blunt trauma to the joint or a single traumatic impact. It is characterized by a loss of matrix components (primarily proteoglycans) without chondrocyte damage. The chondrocytes may be capable of repairing the damage by restoring lost proteoglycans and matrix components, if the traumatic event is acute. If blunt trauma continues (for example, when a dog jumps on an injured joint), joint damage may become irreversible.[57] Chondral fractures occur when there is superficial damage to the articular surface without damage to the subchondral plate. Chondrocytes in the injured area proliferate and synthesize more extracellular matrix protein. However, because chondrocytes cannot migrate from one area to another, complete repair does not occur if damage is extensive.[58] Osteochondral fracture is a full-thickness defect, involving damage through the cartilage to the bone, leading to severe chondrocyte loss and bone marrow cell involvement. Because vascular tissue is involved, this type of injury invokes a full inflammatory response. Fibroblasts differentiate into chondrocytes in an attempt to repair the tissue, resulting in structurally abnormal articular cartilage.[57,58] Repaired tissue will have lower proteoglycan content and altered forms of collagen. The long-term end result is compromised joint function.

Dogs with OA also have abnormalities with chondrocyte function. Normally chondrocytes produce proteoglycans, collagen, fibronectin, and other components to maintain joint integrity and health. When lameness, disease, or chronic injury disrupts the homeostasis of the joint, the articular cartilage undergoes progressive degeneration. Initially there is increased synthesis of the extracellular matrix. However, the new proteoglycans are not of the same composition as those found in non-injured joints. For example, proteoglycans produced in OA joints contain lower levels of keratin sulfate, and the ratio of chondroitin-4-sulfate to chondroitin-6-sulfate is increased.[59,60] Proteoglycan and collagen breakdown (degeneration) also occurs, as a result of increased activity of the matrix metalloproteinases (MMP) and other proteases.[61,62] Other peptides and fibronectin components stimulate chondrocytes and synovial cells to release arachidonic acid metabolites such as prostaglandin E_2 (PGE_2), leukotriene B_4, and thromboxane, causing increased inflammation of the joint capsule lining.[62]

Over time, chondrocyte necrosis becomes evident, the synthesis of the extracellular matrix decreases, and degradative activity continues. The joint's collagen network becomes disorganized. Functional proteoglycans are removed from the extracellular matrix, which decreases the water content of the cartilage, and thus the flexibility and resilience of the joint becomes compromised. Chondrocytes are gradually exposed to more damage and trauma from the normal mechanical stresses of walking and movement, accelerating the osteoarthritic process.[61]

The goal in treating mobility and lameness disorders is to reduce pain and inflammation, prevent or slow further degeneration of affected joints, and support or restore function. Surgical treatment is often the primary recommendation for some types of mobility disorder, such as cranial cruciate ligament rupture or with certain cases of hip dysplasia. For others, medical management provides the primary or adjunctive therapy and is used to alleviate pain and decrease long-term negative effects of OA. Medical management of OA is an integrative approach that includes nutritional management and weight control, as well as pharmacological and exercise/activity management.

Nutritional Management

Because of potential side effects from nonsteroidal anti-inflammatory drugs (NSAIDs) and glucocorticoids, many pet owners and veterinarians have been looking to alternative or adjunctive methods for supporting joint health. Including nutrients that help to protect joint health in a pet's diet can lower the need for the use of NSAIDs. Additionally certain supplements may have beneficial effects on pets with OA, reduce the amount of NSAIDs needed, and have positive effects on joint repair and health.[63]

FATTY ACID SUPPLEMENTATION As discussed in other chapters, certain eicosanoids that are produced from omega-6 fatty acids (such as PGE_2, leukotriene B_4, leukotriene C_4, and thromboxane A_2) are local proinflammatory chemical mediators. Conversely, eicosanoids that are produced from omega-3 fatty acids, in particular eicosapentaenoic acid (EPA), are less inflammatory. Eicosanoid production in tissues can be altered by adjusting the fatty acids in the diet. For example, feeding dogs foods that contained increased omega-3 fatty acids and an adjusted ratio of 5:1 to 10:1 led to increased production of omega-3 (less-inflammatory) eicosanoids.[64]

There is evidence in human subjects that providing omega-3 fatty acids in the diet can ameliorate clinical signs of joint inflammation. For example, patients with rheumatoid arthritis whose diet was supplemented with fish oil and evening primrose oil experienced reduced inflammation and decreased pain medication dosages.[65-67] In dogs, there is evidence that increasing omega-3 fatty acids in the diet of dogs with ruptured cranial cruciate ligaments may benefit joint health by altering synovial fluid MMP levels.[68] Additional studies are needed to examine the long-term benefits of omega-3 fatty acids for pets with OA and their potential to allow reduced dosages of antiinflammatory medications.

GLYCOSAMINOGLYCANS As discussed previously (pp. 501-502), GAGs are part of the proteoglycans that form cross-linkages with collagen within cartilage and other connective tissues. The GAGs that have relevance to connective tissue and joints are chondroitin-4-sulfate, chondroitin-6-sulfate, keratin sulfate, dermatan sulfate, and nonsulfated hyaluronic acid. Hyaluronic acid promotes healthy synovial fluid viscosity and lubricates the synovial membranes in joints. Along with the other GAGs, hyaluronic acid provides elasticity, flexibility, and tensile strength to articular cartilage and tendons. The GAGs have antiinflammatory effects on connective tissues and act directly in the structural repair of joint tissue. Additionally, they provide chondrocytes with

increased availability of chondroitin sulfate and hyaluronic acid precursors. An injectable, partially synthetic polysulfated GAG product has been approved by the Food and Drug Administration (FDA) for the use in dogs and horses suffering from noninfectious degenerative joint disease. In addition, oral nutraceuticals of chondroitin sulfate are available. These products may help to reduce inflammation and pain, normalize synovial fluid viscosity, and promote repair of joint cartilage by retarding degradation caused by increased activity of joint proteolytic enzymes. For example, human subjects with OA in one or both knee joints showed improved mobility and a reduction in clinical signs when supplemented with 1200 milligrams (mg) of chondroitin sulfate per day.[69]

GLUCOSAMINE Glucosamine compounds are amino sugars produced from glucose and the amino acid glutamine and are a primary component of the GAGs and proteoglycans found in the extracellular matrix of joints. As nutraceuticals, these compounds may function to protect and regenerate connective tissue and cartilage in joints affected with OA. For example, in vitro studies with chondrocytes report that glucosamine has a stimulatory effect on cells by increasing the production of collagen and proteoglycans.[70] Both glucosamine sulfate and glucosamine HCl (a salt of D-glucosamine) have joint activity, but most studies have focused on glucosamine sulfate because the body eventually converts D-glucosamine into glucosamine sulfate. For example, a study with Beagles reported that supplementation with a combination of glucosamine, chondroitin sulfate, and ascorbate increased biosynthetic activity in cartilage segments by 50% and decreased proteolytic degradation by 59%.[48]

Glucosamine products are commonly used for many joint, cartilage, or disc-degenerating conditions such as hip dysplasia, spondylosis, OA, osteochondritis, and other nonspecific joint injuries or ailments. The benefits appear to be protective and restorative, which leads to less discomfort and inflammation, thus promoting more mobility. Many veterinary practitioners recommend nutraceuticals with a combination of both glucosamine and chondroitin sulfate. To date, there have not been any studies demonstrating safety concerns about these products. However, one study of joint effects in Beagles supplemented with 1600 mg sodium chondroitin sulfate and 2000 mg glucosamine hydrochloride per day reported statistically significant, but clinically unimportant, changes in hemoglobin, hematocrit, white blood cell count, segmented neutrophils, and red blood cell count following 30 days of supplementation.[71] No changes were noted in any bleeding or clotting parameters.

Chondroitin sulfate and glucosamine may help to reduce inflammation and pain, normalize synovial fluid viscosity, and promote repair of joint cartilage in joints affected by osteoarthritis. Long-term benefits appear to be protective and restorative, contributing to reduced discomfort and inflammation and promoting increased mobility. Many veterinary practitioners recommend nutraceuticals that include a combination of glucosamine and chondroitin sulfate.

Weight Control for Mobility Management

Regardless of the underlying initial cause of OA, disease progression will be worsened in the presence of an overweight or obese condition (see Chapter 28 for a complete discussion of obesity). For example, human subjects who are moderately or severely overweight are 3.5 times more likely to develop OA than those who are at their ideal weight. Moreover, moderate weight loss can significantly decrease risk of OA development in human patients.[72,73] Another study with human subjects reported that weight loss led to complete relief of pain in one or more joints in 90% of affected patients.[74] A study with dogs examined the effects on weight loss in dogs with CHD. Dogs that achieved an 11% to 18% body-weight reduction were significantly less lame when lameness scores following weight loss were compared with scores at the start of the study period (Figure 37-3).[75] Another study reported that dogs fed a restricted diet throughout life had significantly less severity of OA lesions in the shoulder as adults when compared with dogs that were fed ad libitum.[76]

Because of the relationship between overweight conditions and OA, some veterinary orthopedic specialists no longer recommend total hip replacements in obese dogs.[77] Instead overweight dogs are started on a weight-reduction program with the goal of reducing body fat to 20% to 25% of body weight. During the weight-loss program, antiinflammatory medications

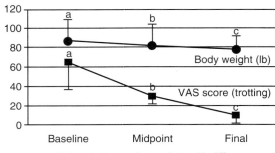

Values between time points with different letters differ significantly $P<0.05$

Figure 37-3   Change in body weight and Visual Analog Scale (*VAS*) lameness ratings during weight loss in dogs.
(From Impellizeri JA, Tetrick MA, Muir P: Effect of weight reduction on clinical signs of lameness in dogs with hip osteoarthritis, *J Am Vet Med Assoc* 216:1089–1091, 2000.)

and nutritional joint supplements are used, as needed, to control pain and discomfort. A substantial number of owners report that their dog's mobility and comfort improved enough with weight loss and moderate exercise to prevent the need for a surgical intervention.[77] Guidelines for weight-loss and weight-control programs for pets with OA are the same as those for other pets and are discussed in detail in Chapter 28 (pp. 326-335).

Osteoarthritis (OA) progression and symptoms are worsened when pets are overweight or obese. Reducing body weight can delay the onset of OA and in affected animals helps to reduce pain, increase mobility, and allow decreased dependency on antiinflammatory medications.

Pharmacological Management

NSAIDs or corticosteroids are frequently included in treatment protocols for traumatic or degenerative joint conditions. Both function by decreasing the production of proinflammatory arachidonic acid metabolites that are released during cellular membrane damage.[78] Both of these drug categories directly inhibit cyclooxygenase enzymes that produce eicosanoids such as leukotrienes, thromboxanes, prostaglandins, and prostacyclins.[79]

Of the two categories, most veterinary practitioners today include NSAIDs as part of their treatment protocols because of the many options that are available and because of fewer long-term side effects when compared with corticosteroids. Different NSAIDs block various parts of the arachidonic cascade, and, as a result, one product may work better than another for different patients or different types of mobility disorders. This allows veterinarians to select a specific drug that may work best with a particular patient. Generally, although NSAIDs have fewer detrimental long-term effects than corticosteroids, these drugs may still be associated with vomiting, diarrhea, anorexia, lethargy, and gastroduodenal ulceration.

Exercise/Activity Management

Historically, humans diagnosed with OA were advised to live a sedentary life of inactivity and to not partake in physical exercise. However, with a quieter lifestyle, muscle atrophy and overall loss of muscle mass occurs, which can eventually increase stress on joints. It has been determined in humans with OA that moderate exercise is important for maintaining muscle strength, stamina, and range of motion within joints. Sustaining some type of active lifestyle can also allow reduced dependency on medications.[80,81] Studies with animals have demonstrated similar results.[82] Today, exercise and activity management is an important aspect of therapy with companion animals with OA.

Each animal's past activity history should be assessed because those having an inactive lifestyle should not be forced into an exercise program that is beyond their capabilities. Two aspects should be considered when determining the type of exercise program to initiate with the animal. First, the type of exercise should be considered. Exercise that involves low-impact or non–weight-bearing activities is recommended for OA patients. In humans, low-impact activities such as walking or bicycling have been considered beneficial.[81,83] When dealing with dogs, walking (on a leash or on a controlled animal treadmill) is considered a low-impact activity, while swimming is considered an ideal non–weight-bearing exercise. Both these activities reduce load on OA joints while maintaining, and in some cases building, muscle mass and strength, resulting in less discomfort and pressure on damaged cartilage.

Although most clients may not have access to a swimming area for their pets, there are many animal physical therapy facilities available now across the United States that provide low-impact physical programs for animals. These facilities offer a controlled, professionally supervised environment where underwater treadmills or small pools are used. Dogs initially may swim for only 1 to 3 minutes for 3 or more days a week, gradually increasing duration as stamina improves.[77] It is important for pet owners to understand that high-impact activities such as trotting, running, jumping, and climbing over rough terrains will overstress joints with OA by causing more inflammation, damage, and subsequently pain (Figure 37-4).

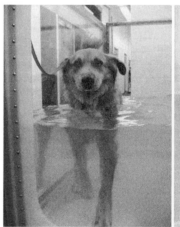
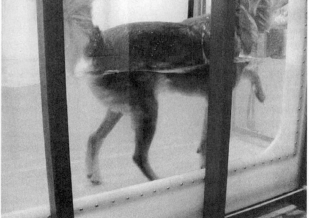

Figure 37-4   Dog exercising on an underwater treadmill.
(From Millis DL: Physical therapy for dogs with joint disease. In *Clinical perspectives on canine joint disease*, Proc NAVC, 2001, p 24.)

A second aspect of designing an exercise program is the length of time to commit to the activity. Animals with a sedentary lifestyle should initially limit exercise to a short 5- to 15-minute walk, several days a week. If the owner notices their pet has more joint stiffness after starting an exercise program, the duration of each session should be reduced. As the pet develops more muscle mass, strength, and stamina, the duration of each walk or bout of exercise can be gradually increased. Animals that already have a fully active lifestyle such as hunting, sled-racing, or agility dogs should have their type of exercise program changed to a low-impact activity such as walking, but the time spent doing so may be more substantial to keep the muscle mass and strength they already have.

Regular exercise is an important component of treatment for pets with osteoarthritis (OA). Recommended activities include regular walking, swimming, or water therapy. High-impact activities such as trotting, running, jumping, and climbing over rough terrains will overstress joints with OA, so these activities should be limited or avoided.

Determining response to nutritional and pharmacological interventions in pets with OA can be challenging, because most studies rely on the pet owners' perception of how well their dogs are responding. A more analytical approach to determine results may be an option in the future. For example, a recent study found that assessing multiple gene products from cartilage biopsy samples from dogs with OA provided a direct measure of existing chondrocyte metabolism and may be useful as a measure of cartilage health and response to OA treatments.[84]

References

1. Johnson JA, Austin C, Breuer GJ: Incidence of canine appendicular musculoskeletal disorders in 16 veterinary teaching hospitals from 1980-1989, *J Vet Comp Orthop Trauma* 7:56–69, 1994.

2. Richardson DC, Zentek J: Nutrition and osteochondrosis, *Vet Clin North Am Small Anim Pract* 28:115–135, 1998.

3. Smith GK, LaFond E, Heyman SJ: Biomechanical characterization of passive laxity of the hip joint in dogs, *Am J Vet Res* 58:1078–1082, 1997.

4. Richardson DC, Toll PWL: Relationship of nutrition to developmental skeletal disease in young dogs, *Vet Clin Nutr* 4:6–13, 1997.

5. Orthopedic Foundation for Animals (OFA): Website. http://www.offa.org. Accessed September 28, 2009.

6. Paster ER, LaFond E, Biery DN, and others: Estimates of prevalence of hip dysplasia in Golden Retrievers and Rottweilers and the influence of bias on published prevalence figures, *J Am Vet Med Assoc* 226:387–392, 2005.

7. Kasstrom H: Nutrition, weight gain and development of hip dysplasia, *Acta Radiol* 334(Suppl):135–179, 1975.

8. Ythehus B, Carlson CS, Ekman S: Etiology and pathogenesis of osteochondrosis, *Vet Pathol* 44:429–448, 2007.

9. Slater MR, Scarlett JM, Kaderly RE, and others: Breed, gender, and age risk factors for canine osteochondritis dissecans, *J Vet Comp Orthop Trauma* 4:100–106, 1991.

10. Slater MR, Scarlett JM, Donoughue S, and others: Diet and exercise as potential risk factors for osteochondritis dissecans in dogs, *Am J Vet Res* 53:2119–2124, 1992.

11. Coopman F, Verhoeven G, Saunders J, and others: Prevalence of hip dysplasia, elbow dysplasia and humeral head osteochondrosis in dog breeds in Belgium, *Vet Rec* 163:654–658, 2008.

12. LaFond E, Breur GJ, Austin CC: Breed susceptibility for developmental orthopedic diseases in dogs, *J Am Anim Hosp Assoc* 38:467–477, 2002.

13. Trostel CT, Pool RR, McLaughlin RM: Canine lameness caused by developmental orthopedic diseases: panosteitis, Legg-Calvé-Perthes disease and hypertrophic osteodystrophy, *Compend Contin Educ Pract Vet* 25:282–293, 2003.

14. Van Hagen MAE, Ducro BJ, van de Broek J, Knol BW: Incidence, risk factors, and heritability estimates of hind limb lameness caused by hip dysplasia in a birth cohort of Boxers, *Am J Vet Res* 66:307–312, 2005.

15. Dietschi E, Schawalder P, Gaillard C: Estimation of genetic parameters for canine hip dysplasia in the Swiss Newfoundland population, *J Anim Breed Gen* 120:150–161, 2003.

16. Engler J, Hamann H, Distl O: Estimation of genetic parameters for radiographic signs of hip dysplasia in Labrador Retrievers, *Berliner Munchen Tier Wochen* 121:359–364, 2008.

17. Dluzniewska KA, Obtulowicz A, Koltek K: On the relationship between diet, rate of growth and skeletal deformities in school children, *Folia Med Craco* 7:115–126, 1965.

18. Kealy RD, Olsson SE, Monti KL, and others: Effects of limited food consumption on the incidence of hip dysplasia in growing dogs, *J Am Vet Med Assoc* 201:857–863, 1992.

19. Hedhammer A, Wu F, Krook L, and others: Overnutrition and skeletal disease—an experimental study in growing Great Dane dogs, *Cornell Vet* 64(Suppl 5):1–159, 1974.

20. Kasstrom H: Nutrition, weight gain and development of hip dysplasia, *Acta Radiol* 334(Suppl):135–179, 1975.

21. Lust G, Geary JC, Sheffy BE: Development of hip dysplasia in dogs, *Am J Vet Res* 34:87–91, 1973.

22. Lust G, Rendano VT, Summers BA: Canine hip dysplasia: concepts and diagnosis, *J Vet Med Assoc* 187:638–640, 1985.

23. Kealy RD, Lawler DF, Ballam JM, and others: Five-year longitudinal study on limited food consumption and development of osteoarthritis in coxofemoral joints of dogs, *J Am Vet Med Assoc* 210:222–225, 1997.

24. Kealy RD, Lawler DF, Ballam JM: Evaluation of the effect of limited food consumption on radiographic evidence of osteoarthritis in dogs, *J Am Vet Med Assoc* 217:1678–1680, 2000.

25. Smith GK, Paster ER, Powers MY, and others: Lifelong diet restriction and radiographic evidence of osteoarthritis of the hip joint in dogs, *J Am Vet Med Assoc* 229:690–693, 2006.

26. Runge JJ, Biery DN, Lawler DF, and others: The effects of lifetime food restriction on the development of osteoarthritis in the canine shoulder, *Vet Surg* 37:102–107, 2008.

27. Olsson SE, Reiland S: The nature of osteochondrosis in animals, *Acta Radiol Scand* 358(Suppl):299–306, 1978.

28. Trangerud C, Grondalen A, Indrebo A, and others: A longitudinal study on growth and growth variables in dogs of four large breeds raised in domestic environments, *J Anim Sci* 85:76–83, 2007.

29. Dammrich K: Relationship between nutrition and bone growth in large and giant dogs, *J Nutr* 121:S114–S121, 1991.

30. Crenshaw TD, Budde RQ, Lauten SD, and others: Nutritional effects on bone strength in the growing canine. In Reinhart GA, Carey DP, editors: *Recent advances in canine and feline nutrition, Iams nutrition symposium proceedings,* vol 2, Wilmington, Ohio, 1998, Orange Frazer Press.

31. Nap RC, Hazewinkel HAW, Vorrhout G, and others: The influence of the dietary protein content on growth in giant breed dogs, *J Vet Comp Orthop Trauma* 6:1–8, 1993.

32. Lepine AJ: Nutritional management of the large breed puppy. In Reinhart GA, Carey DP, editors: *Recent advances in canine and feline nutrition, Iams nutrition symposium proceedings,* vol 2, Wilmington, Ohio, 1998, Orange Frazer Press.

33. Blum JW, Zentek J, Meyer H: Untersuchngen einer unterschiedlichen Energiveeersorgung auf die Wachstumsintensitat und Skelettentwicklung bei wachsenden Doggen, *J Vet Med* 39:568–574, 1992.

34. Association of American Feed Control Officials (AAFCO): Pet food regulations. In *AAFCO official publication*, Atlanta, 2008, AAFCO.

35. Hazewinkel HAW, Goedegebuure SA, Poulos PW, and others: Influences of chronic calcium excess on the skeletal development of growing Great Danes, *J Am Anim Hosp Assoc* 21:377–391, 1985.

36. Goedegebuure SA, Hazewinkel HAW: Morphological findings in young dogs chronically fed a diet containing excess calcium, *Vet Pathol* 23:594–605, 1986.

37. National Research Council (National Academy of Sciences): *Nutrient requirements of dogs*, Washington, DC, 1974, National Academy Press.

38. National Research Council (National Academy of Sciences): *Nutrient requirements of dogs*, Washington, DC, 1985, National Academy Press.

39. Stephens LC, Norrdin RW, Benjamin SA: Effects of calcium supplementation and sunlight exposure on growing Beagle dogs, *Am J Vet Res* 466:2037–2042, 1985.

40. Schoenmakers I, Hazewinkel HAW, Voorhout G, and others: Effect of diets with different calcium and phosphorus contents on the skeletal development and blood chemistry of growing Great Danes, *Vet Rec* 147:652–660, 2000.

41. Lauten SD, Cox NR, Brawner WR, and others: Influence of dietary calcium and phosphorus content in a fixed ratio on growth and development in Great Danes, *Am J Vet Res* 63:1036–1047, 2002.

42. Allen LH: Calcium bioavailability and absorption: a review, *Am J Clin Nutr* 35:783–808, 1982.

43. Tryfonidou MA, Van den Broek J, van den Brom WE, Hazewinkel HAW: Intestinal calcium absorption in growing dogs is influenced by calcium intake and age but not by growth rate, *J Nutr* 132:3363–3368, 2002.

44. Hedhammer A, Krook L, Schrijver HF, and others: Calcium balance in the dog. In Anderson RS, editor: *Nutrition of the dog and cat*, Oxford, England, 1980, Pergamon Press.

45. Hazewinkel HAW, Brom WE, van den Klooster AT, and others: Calcium metabolism in Great Dane dogs fed diets with various calcium and phosphorus levels, *J Nutr* 121:S99–S106, 1991.

46. Dobenecker B, Keinzle E, Koslin R, Matis U: Mal- and overnutrition in puppies with and without disorders of skeletal development, *J Anim Phys Anim Nutr* 80:76–81, 1998.

47. Dobenecker B: Apparent calcium absorption in growing dogs of two different sizes, *J Nutr* 134:2151S–2153S, 2004.

48. Dobenecker B, Kasbeitzer N, Flinspach S, and others: Calcium-excess causes subclinical changes of bone growth in Beagles but not in Foxhound-crossbred dogs, as measured in X-rays, *J Anim Physiol Anim Nutr* 90:394–401, 2006.

49. Nap RC, Hazewinkel HAW, van den Brom WI: ^{45}Ca kinetics in growing Miniature Poodles challenged by four different dietary levels of Ca, *J Nutr* 123:1826–1833, 1993.

50. Kuhlman G, Boourge V: Nutrition of the large and giant breed dog with emphasis on skeletal development, *Vet Clin Nutr* 4:89–95, 1997.

51. Brinker WO, Piermattei DL, Flo GL: *Handbook of small animal orthopedics and fracture treatment*, Philadelphia, 1983, Saunders.

52. Johnston SA: Osteoarthritis: joint anatomy, physiology, and pathobiology, *Vet Clin North Am Small Anim Pract* 27:699–723, 1997.

53. Egenvall A, Bonnett BN, Olson P, Hadhammar S: Gender, age and breed pattern of diagnoses for veterinary care in insured dogs in Sweden during 1996, *Vet Rec* 146:551–557, 2000.

54. Nakano T, Aherne FX, Thompson JR: Changes in swine knee articular cartilage during growth, *Can J Anim Sci* 59:167–179, 1979.

55. Venn MF: Variation of chemical composition with age in human femoral head cartilage, *Ann Rheum Dis* 37:168–174, 1978.

56. Lepine AJ: A morphologic and physiologic review of articular cartilage. In *Proc Vet Orthoped Soc*, 2000, pp 6–13.

57. Frenkel SR, DiCesare PE: Degradation and repair of articular cartilage, *Front Biosci* 4:671–685, 1999.

58. Buckwalter JA, Rosenberg LC, Hunziker EB: Articular cartilage composition structure response to injury and methods of facilitating repair. In *Articular cartilage and knee joint function, Bristol-Myers/Zimmer orthopaedic symposium*, New York, 1988, Raven Press, pp 19–56.

59. Poole AR: An introduction to the pathophysiology of osteoarthritis, *Front Biosci* 4:662–670, 1999.

60. Dijkgraaf LC, De Bont LG, Boering G, Liem RS: The structure, biochemistry, and metabolism of osteoarthritis cartilage: a review of the literature, *J Oral Maxillofac Surg* 53:1182–1192, 1995.

61. Malemud CJ, Goldberg VM: Future directions for research and treatment of osteoarthritis, *Front Biosci* 4:762–771, 1999.

62. Muir H: Cartilage structure and metabolism and basic changes in degenerative joint disease, *Aust N Z J Med* 8:1–5, 1978.

63. Sanderson RO, Beata C, Flipo RM, and others: Systematic review of the management of canine osteoarthritis, *Vet Rec* 164:418–424, 2009.

64. Vaughn DM, Reinhart GA, Lauten DS, and others: Evaluation of effects of dietary n-6 to n-3 fatty acid ratios on leukotriene B synthesis in dog skin and neutrophils, *Vet Dermatol* 5:163–173, 1994.

65. Belch JJF, Ansell D, Madhok R, and others: Effects of altering dietary essential fatty acids on requirements for non-steroidal anti-inflammatory drugs in patients with rheumatoid arthritis: a double blind placebo controlled study, *Ann Rheum Dis* 47:96–104, 1988.

66. Lau CD, Morley KD, Belch JJF: Effects of fish oil supplementation on non-steroidal anti-inflammatory drug requirement in patients with mild rheumatoid arthritis—a double blind placebo controlled study, *Br J Rheumatol* 32:982–989, 1993.

67. Geusens P, Wouters C, Nijs J, and others: Long-term effects of omega-3 fatty acid supplementation on active rheumatoid arthritis—a 12-month double blind, controlled study, *Arthritis Rheum* 37:824–829, 1994.

68. Hansen RA, Harris MA, Pulhar GE, and others: Fish oil decreases matrix metalloproteinases in knee synovia of dogs with inflammatory joint disease, *J Nutr Biochem* 19:101–108, 2008.

69. Bourgeois P, Chales G, Dehais J, and others: Efficacy and tolerability of chondroitin sulfate 1200 mg/day vs chondroitin sulfate 3 × 400 mg/day vs placebo, *Osteoarthritis Cartilage* 6(Suppl A):25–30, 1998.

70. Anderson MA: Oral chondroprotective agents. Part I. Common compounds, *Compendium* 21:601–609, 1999.

71. McNamara PS, Barr SC, Erb HN: Hematological, hemostatic and biochemical effects in dogs receiving an oral chondroprotective agent for thirty days, *Am J Vet Res* 57:1390–1394, 1996.

72. Felson DT, Zhang Y, Anthony JM, and others: Weight loss reduces the risk for symptomatic knee osteoarthritis in women. The Framingham Study, *Ann Intern Med* 116:535–539, 1992.

73. Schrager M: Slimming down reduces arthritis risk, *Phys Sports Med* 23:22, 1995.

74. McGoey BV, Beitel M, Saplys RJ: Effect of weight loss on musculoskeletal pain in the morbidly obese, *J Bone Joint Surg* 72-B:323, 1990.

75. Impellizeri JA, Tetrick MA, Muir P: Effect of weight reduction on clinical signs of lameness in dogs with hip osteoarthritis, *J Am Vet Med Assoc* 216:1089–1091, 2000.

76. Runge JJ, Beiry DN, Lawler DF, and others: The effects of lifetime food restriction on the development of osteoarthritis in the canine shoulder, *Vet Surg* 37:102–107, 2008.

77. Millis DL: Physical therapy for dogs with joint disease. In *Proc NAVC*, 2001, pp 22–27.

78. Johnston SA, Fox SM: Mechanism of action of anti-inflammatory medications used for the treatment of osteoarthritis, *J Am Vet Med Assoc* 210:1486–1492, 1997.

79. Hayek MG, Lepine AJ, Sunvold GD, Reinhart GA: Nutritional management of joint problems in dogs. In *Proc Vet Orthoped Soc*, 2000, pp 18–23.

80. Kovar PA, Allegrante JP, MacKenzie CR, and others: Supervised fitness walking in patients with osteoarthritis of the knee. A randomized, controlled trial, *Ann Intern Med* 116:529–534, 1992.

81. Røgind H, Bibow-Neilsen B, Jensen B, and others: The effects of a physical training program on patients with osteoarthritis of the knees, *Arch Phys Med Rehabil* 79:1421–1427, 1998.

82. Otternes IG, Eskra JD, Bliven ML, and others: Exercise protects against articular cartilage degeneration in the hamster, *Arthritis Rheum* 41:2068–2076, 1998.

83. Mangione KK, McCully K, Gloviak A, and others: The effects of high-intensity and low-intensity cycle ergometry in older adults with knee osteoarthritis,, *J Gerontol A Biol Sci Med Sci* 54:184–190, 1999.

84. Matyas JR, Huang D, Chung M, Adams ME: Regional quantification of cartilage type II collagen and aggrecan messenger RNA in joints with early experimental osteoarthritis, *Arthritis Rheum* 46:1536–1543, 2002.

38

Nutrition and the Heart

The heart provides several basic functions in the body. It provides a transport mechanism for oxygen and nutrients to other organs and body systems. It also helps transport carbon dioxide and other metabolic wastes to excretory organs. Hormones and other enzymes are moved from one organ to another by the heart to provide for basic functions of the reproductive and thyroid systems. In addition, the heart helps with thermoregulation, keeping the body at a consistent and ideal temperature.

There are several requirements for normal cardiac function. First, there needs to be adaptable coronary circulation. The vessels that supply oxygen and nutrients to the heart must be functional and capable of adapting to meet increased demands when needed. There also must be a flexible response by myocardial contractile cells so that when the animal needs additional cardiac output during stress or exercise, the cells of the heart can provide for a higher heart rate and cardiac output. The valves of the heart must function normally and maintain healthy blood flow. Finally, normal peripheral vascular response is needed to maintain normal blood pressure under a variety of physiological states.

When any of these functions is impaired, the heart begins to undergo a state of imbalance, eventually resulting in congestive heart failure (CHF). Clinically, animals with heart disease may show signs of syncope, coughing or respiratory difficulty, exercise intolerance, and cyanosis. Additional signs include cardiac murmurs, rhythm disturbances, cardiac enlargement, and/or excessively weak or strong arterial pulses.

TYPE AND INCIDENCE

Heart disease is one of the most commonly diagnosed diseases of dogs in the United States and Europe.[1] In dogs, heart disease can be either congenital or acquired. Common congenital heart conditions include aortic stenosis (AS), patent ductus arteriosis (PDA), ventricular septal defect (VSD), and pulmonic stenosis (PS).

Some of these conditions appear to have a hereditary component and are found more frequently in certain breeds or lines of purebred dogs. Acquired heart disease is more common than congenital disease in dogs and cats. However, companion animals rarely suffer from atherosclerosis and coronary disease.[2] The most common form of acquired heart disease in dogs is chronic valvular disease. There are many different types of valvular diseases; chronic mitral insufficiency, tricuspid insufficiency, mitral stenosis, aortic insufficiency, pulmonic insufficiency, and bacterial endocarditis are the most common forms that are diagnosed in dogs. Of these, chronic mitral insufficiency is the most common and is typically observed in middle- to older-age dogs. It also appears more often in certain breeds such as the Cavalier King Charles Spaniel, Dachshund, Miniature and Toy Poodles, Chihuahuas, and many of the Terrier breeds.[3] In chronic mitral insufficiency, there is retrograde flow of blood from the left ventricle to the left atrium during ventricular systole or contraction. This results in reduced flow to the peripheral circulation, an increased backflow to the atrium, and blood volume overload in the heart. Dogs with this heart problem usually eventually develop CHF.

Acquired heart disease is more common than congenital heart disease in dogs and cats. However, companion animals rarely suffer from atherosclerosis and coronary disease. Chronic mitral insufficiency is one of the most common heart problems in dogs and is seen in middle- to older-age dogs. It occurs more often in Cavalier King Charles Spaniels, Dachshunds, Miniature and Toy Poodles, Chihuahuas, and some Terrier breeds.

Another common heart problem in dogs is dilated cardiomyopathy (DCM). This disease typically occurs in dogs that are middle-aged to older; however, some breeds have been reported to develop it early in life. For example, Portuguese Water Dogs can develop DCM and show clinical signs of CHF as young as 2 to 3 months of age.[4] There also appears to be a genetic predisposition in several large- and giant-breed dogs. Irish Wolfhounds, Great Danes, Saint Bernards, Newfoundlands, Doberman Pinschers, and Boxers are breeds that show an increased incidence of DCM.[5,6] Over half of all Dobermans and one third of Boxers are estimated to develop the disease in their lifetime.[5,6] Although they are not considered a large- or giant-breed dog, Cocker Spaniels also have a tendency to develop a form of DCM that previously was considered only a feline cause of cardiomyopathy; DCM in Cocker Spaniels can be caused by a taurine deficiency.

DCM is a primary myocardial disease characterized by cardiac chamber enlargement, arrhythmias, and diminished cardiac contractility. Eventually these dogs show signs of CHF, if not managed properly. Clinically, these dogs can show signs of weakness, collapse, lethargy, abdominal distention, tachycardia, tachypnea, dyspnea, coughing, syncopy, weight loss, anorexia, and sudden death. Two multibreed studies done on dogs with DCM demonstrated survival after 1 year of being diagnosed with DCM at only 17.5% and 37.5%, respectively, with the median survival times of only 27 and 65 days, respectively.[7,8]

In cats, DCM used to be the most common type of heart disease. However, in the late 1980s Pion et al.[9] reported an association with DCM and taurine deficiency in cats. Fortunately, it was found that administration of taurine to cats' diets could reverse the myocardial changes seen.[9] Since that finding was demonstrated, commercial cat food manufacturers have increased the amount of taurine in their products, and there has been a dramatic reduction in the incidence of feline DCM. Although it is possible to still see a case of DCM in cats fed a poor-quality homemade, vegetarian, or unbalanced diet, most cases of feline DCM are seen as a taurine-independent variant of DCM, or seen as end-stage hypertrophic cardiomyopathy (HCM).[10]

Currently in cats, the most common heart disease is HCM. Its incidence appears to be increasing. A recent publication reported 21% of overtly healthy cats had heart murmurs, and 86% of these cats, when evaluated using echocardiography, had structural cardiac disease, primarily HCM.[11] This is in comparison to studies conducted in the 1970s and 1980s where only 1.6% of all cats referred to a veterinary hospital were reported to have HCM.[12] Although most cats listed to be at risk for this condition include domestic long- and short-haired cats, in purebred lines, Maine Coon cats seem to have a heritable or familial tendency toward the disease.[13]

Cats with HCM have a symmetrical or asymmetrical hypertrophy of the left ventricular wall, papillary muscles, and septum restricting the size of the left ventricular lumen. The myocardial cells are enlarged, and the left ventricular filling is impaired from reduced left ventricular compliance. There often is a secondary left atrial enlargement present. If there is atrial enlargement, arrhythmias may be more commonly detected. Cat with HCM usually develop CHF and arterial thromboembolism (ATE) with ATE reportedly developing in up to 48% of affected cats.[12,14-17] Clinically, cats with HCM demonstrated signs of weakness, labored breathing, lethargy, syncope, arrhythmias, and hindlimb pain or paralysis if ATE was present. Cats with HCM have a mean survival time of less than 2 years.[14]

The most common heart disease in cats is hypertrophic cardiomyopathy (HCM). Cats with HCM usually develop congestive heart failure and approximately half will develop arterial thromboembolism (ATE). Clinically, cats with HCM demonstrated signs of weakness, labored breathing, lethargy, syncope, arrhythmias, and hindlimb pain or paralysis if ATE was present.

CARDIAC CACHEXIA

Cardiac cachexia is defined as muscle wasting and weight loss that commonly occurs in humans, dogs, and cats with cardiac disease. For example, one study reported that more than 50% of dogs with DCM showed some degree of cardiac cachexia.[18] Similar to cancer cachexia, the weight loss that occurs with cardiac cachexia includes a substantial and unusually high loss of lean body tissue. Although many veterinarians consider cachexia to be an end-stage development in animals with CHF, it can occur in early stages of CHF.[19] Similar to cancer cachexia, the metabolic changes may precede obvious physical changes. The loss of lean body mass can affect many different systems and is associated with shortened survival time. As muscle tissue is metabolized, the animal experiences muscle wasting, a loss of strength, and eventually compromised immune function. For example, dogs with cardiac cachexia have lower CD4+ lymphocytes and are at increased risk for anemia.[20]

Anorexia is a very common problem in pets with CHF and contributes to the onset of cardiac cachexia. It has been reported to occur in up to 84% of dogs with CHF and in at least 38% of cats with cardiac disease.[21-23] Reduced appetite may be secondary due to the fatigue and respiratory dyspnea commonly seen with CHF, but it can also be due to side effects of medications or feeding a new food that may be less palatable.[24] An increase in energy requirements is also a factor that needs to be evaluated when considering the loss of lean body mass. In humans, it has been documented that some may need up to a 30% increase in overall energy requirements when diagnosed with CHF.[25] This increase in energy requirements may be due to tachycardia or tachypnea.[10] Therefore dogs and cats may also benefit from increasing the total energy in their diet. Metabolic alterations may also contribute to the loss of lean body mass. Cytokine elevation, tumor necrosis factor, and interleukin-1 occur in patients with CHF.[24] These inflammatory mediators can increase energy requirements, increase breakdown of lean body mass, and directly cause anorexia.[24] Interestingly, in 68% of dogs with CHF, anorexia was a contributing factor for owners opting to euthanize their pets.[21] Therefore controlling, or at least addressing, the issue of cardiac cachexia and anorexia nutritionally is important to prolong survival time in dogs and cats with CHF.

Cardiac cachexia and anorexia are common in pets with congestive heart failure (CHF). The resultant loss of lean body mass can affect many different systems and is associated with shortened survival time. Decreased interest in food may be secondary to fatigue and respiratory dyspnea, but may also be due to side effects of medications or feeding a new food that is less palatable. Therefore nutritional management of cardiac cachexia and anorexia is important to prolong survival time and improve the quality of life for pets with CHF.

TREATMENT PROTOCOLS

Medical treatment goals for cats with HCM are those that include reducing heart rate, management of CHF when present, and either treating or preventing ATE. Common medications to achieve this include diltiazem, beta-blockers, furosemide, and angiotensin-converting enzyme (ACE) inhibitors. To prevent or treat ATE, aspirin, warfarin, dalteparin or enoxaparin, and clopidigrel are common options. Dogs with DCM are often prescribed medications such as ACE inhibitors, beta-blockers, pimobendan, digoxin, antiarrhythmics, and diuretics such as furosemide.

NUTRITION AND CARDIAC DISEASE

In addition to medical therapy, nutritional modification is an important component of treatment protocols for dogs and cats with CHF. Nutritional modification can support a good quality of life, and, in some cases, may ameliorate some of the clinical effects of heart disease.

In many cases, preventing or reversing anorexia is part of nutritional treatment. Because some medications given to heart patients can cause anorexia as a side effect, reducing the dose or altering the number of doses per day may be helpful. Food palatability is an important consideration. Many therapeutic foods are available in both a canned and dry form, so switching between the two may be beneficial. Warming the food in a microwave (either canned foods or wetted dry foods) and offering small, frequent meals throughout the day can also help with acceptance. Additionally, adding small amounts of certain flavor enhancers such as honey, yogurt, or diluted tuna juice may improve acceptance of the food.

Specific Nutritional Modifications in Managing Cardiovascular Disease

A variety of nutritional modifications may help to slow progression of cardiac disease and improve the quality of life in animals with cardiovascular disease. Specific nutrients of interest include sodium, taurine, carnitine, fatty acids, antioxidants, and protein.

SODIUM Animals with cardiovascular disease have impaired ability to excrete sodium in the urine because of decreased cardiac output.[26] Therefore dietary salt restriction is typically recommended as an aid to control fluid accumulation. The degree of sodium restriction should be dependent on the stage of heart failure and is directed at controlling sodium-responsive clinical signs. Restricting sodium too extensively, especially in asymptomatic dogs, may lead to increased blood pressure via an activated renin-angiotensin-aldosterone system.[27] Although this may not have negative long-term effects, early neuroendrocrine activation may not be desirable.[28] Therefore a food containing maintenance levels of sodium can be fed to pets with early-stage cardiovascular disease (sodium <0.40% dry matter). High-salt table scraps or treats should be avoided. For example, a study showed that dogs with cardiac disease but without CHF were able to maintain both sodium and potassium levels when fed either a low- or a high-sodium diet.[29] Another study reported that a low-sodium diet fed to dogs with asymptomatic cardiac disease had no beneficial effect on cardiac size or function but, rather, led to increased aldosterone concentration and heart rate.[28]

The stage of heart disease at which to institute sodium restriction in dogs and cats is still unclear. A general recommendation is to reduce sodium to less than 0.30% of dry matter when clinical signs appear.[10] This can be accomplished by feeding a pet food that is formulated for senior pets because many of these products contain slightly reduced sodium. Foods should be evaluated individually, or the pet food company should be contacted to ensure that an adequate product is selected. As CHF becomes more severe, veterinary diets specifically formulated for heart patients should be considered because these products are more restricted in sodium. It is also important to assess the food's palatability because low-sodium foods may not be well accepted by pets with congestive heart disease (CHD).

The sodium content of treats and human foods that may be used to administer medications is also an important consideration. Because pets with CHD often show a reduced interest in food, some owners use dog treats, hot dogs, cheese, peanut butter, or lunch meats to administer pills. All of these foods are high in sodium and so are contraindicated. In one study, although owners reported that they were aware of the importance of sodium, they often failed to consider the type of treats they were using to administer medications.[30] In fact, 92% of the dogs studied were fed high-sodium treats or table scraps. In another study, 62% of pet owners used high-sodium human or pet foods for pill administration.[31] High-sodium foods should be avoided when giving medications to all pets with CHD, regardless of the stage of disease. Other "human" treats that should be avoided include canned fish, margarine or butter, canned vegetables, potato chips, pretzels, pop corn, and other salty snacks. Dog treats and snacks that are specifically formulated to be low in sodium are acceptable, but other over-the-counter pet treats should not be fed.

The degree of sodium restriction for pets with heart disease is directed toward controlling sodium-responsive clinical signs. Foods containing maintenance levels of sodium can be fed to pets with early-stage cardiovascular disease. High-salt table scraps or treats should always be avoided. It is generally recommended to reduce sodium to <0.30% of dry matter when clinical signs appear. As congestive heart failure becomes more severe, veterinary diets specifically formulated for heart patients should be considered.

TAURINE Taurine is a sulfur-containing amino acid. As discussed in Chapters 4 and 12 (pp. 22 and 97-100), taurine is found in high concentrations in the myocardium, skeletal muscle, central nervous system, and platelets, and is important for normal heart function.[32] Although the exact mechanisms through which taurine affects heart function are not completely understood, taurine modulates cellular calcium concentrations and availability in heart muscle, directly affects contractile proteins, and serves as a natural antagonist of angiotension II.[32-35] Additionally, taurine may protect the heart by inactivating free radicals and changing cellular osmolality.[36]

Taurine is an essential amino acid for the cat, and a deficiency can cause DCM. Until the late 1980s, DCM was one of the most common heart conditions diagnosed in cats. In 1987, an association between clinical cases of DCM in cats and taurine levels in pet food was found; taurine supplementation completely reverses the condition (see Chapter 12, pp. 97-100 for a complete discussion).[9] Commercial pet food companies that increased the concentration of taurine have further supplemented taurine levels in feline diets, and thus there has been a dramatic reduction in cases of DCM in cats. Occasionally a few cases of DCM are reported in cats, but these cases are usually not a result of a taurine-deficient diet. Rather, these cases may represent a taurine-independent variant of DCM in cats or are associated with end-stage HCM.[10]

In the dog, taurine is currently classified as a conditionally essential amino acid (see Chapter 12, pp. 99-100 for a complete discussion). Dogs of some breeds that are diagnosed with DCM have been found to have low plasma taurine concentrations.[37-40] Affected breeds include the American Cocker Spaniel, Golden Retriever, Labrador Retriever, Saint Bernard, Newfoundland, and English Setter. Although the underlying causes are not known, it appears that some breeds (or lines) have a naturally occurring higher requirement for taurine or a breed-specific metabolic abnormality that affects taurine need.[41-43] Taurine deficiency has also been associated with lamb meal and rice diets, soybean-based diets, and high-fiber diets (see Chapter 12, pp. 97-100 for a complete discussion).[39,40,41,44-48] Any factor that results in increased colonic bacteria populations leads to increased taurine loss in the feces and thus an increased dietary requirement for this nutrient.[44,49] Taurine is found naturally in animal-based proteins; so, providing diets that include a sufficient level of high-quality animal proteins ensures adequate taurine intake.

Blood and plasma taurine levels are measured in dogs with DCM; levels of blood and plasma taurine together more accurately reflect skeletal and cardiac muscle taurine levels than either test alone.[35] If circulating taurine is low, supplementation of taurine is warranted. Even if the concentration is within the normal reference range, supplementing taurine for dogs with DCM, especially those breeds that are predisposed to taurine deficiency, may be beneficial.[35,40,42,44] The recommended dose of taurine is 500 to 1000 milligrams (mg) given three times daily to small dogs under 25 kilograms (kg), and 1 to 2 grams (g) given two or three times daily to larger dogs (25 to 40 kg).[35] Clinical improvement is often rapid, but changes to echocardiograms may not be reflected for up to 2 to 4 months, or even longer.[35]

L-CARNITINE   L-carnitine is a vitamin-like, water-soluble molecule synthesized by the body from lysine and methionine. It is concentrated in skeletal and cardiac muscle and is necessary for fatty acid metabolism and energy production.[50] Carnitine is especially important for cardiac tissue because the heart obtains approximately 60% of its total energy from oxidation of long-chain fatty acids.[51] Carnitine functions in the transport of long-chain fatty acids into cellular mitochondria, where beta-oxidation takes place.[52,53] Carnitine also plays a role in detoxification of the mitochondria by helping to remove accumulating short- and medium-chain fatty acids.[35]

Carnitine deficiency will cause primary myocardial disease and has been reported in many species. In humans, primary L-carnitine deficiency has been shown to occur as a result of genetic defects that affect the synthesis, transport, intestinal absorption, or excessive degradation of carnitine.[54] Secondary carnitine deficiency is seen in vegetarians, infants fed formulas not supplemented with carnitine, and in patients undergoing long-term parenteral nutrition.[54] In dogs the incidence is not known; however, carnitine deficiency has been recognized in a family of Boxers with DCM.[55] Other cases of carnitine deficiency and DCM in dogs have also been reported.[38,56-59]

Myopathic carnitine deficiency is characterized by low concentration of carnitine in the myocardium; it is estimated to occur in 17% to 60% of cases of canine DCM.[35] However, it is unknown if carnitine deficiency is a cause of DCM in dogs or if it is a secondary effect. Myocardial cells of dogs with DCM are damaged, which may lead to secondary loss of carnitine from heart tissue. Conversely, onset of carnitine deficiency prior to development of DCM was reported in three dogs, which suggests that carnitine deficiency can lead to DCM.[35] Although a causal relationship has not been proven, some veterinary cardiologists recommend carnitine supplementation for dogs with DCM (50 to 100 mg/kg three times daily).[19] If a carnitine deficiency is suspected, supplementation may improve survival time and quality of life.[58] Similar to taurine supplementation, clinical response to carnitine supplementation may be rapid while echocardial changes may take 2 to 4 months to be evident.

FATTY ACIDS   Supplementation with omega-3 polyunsaturated fatty acids may be beneficial to dogs with CHF and cardiovascular disease. Specifically, dogs with CHF have been shown to have plasma fatty acid abnormalities, including decreased concentration of eicosapentaenoic acid (EPA) and docosahexaenoic acid (DHA) when compared with normal dogs.[18] In a study of dogs with DCM, fish oil supplementation at a dose of 25 mg/kg EPA and 18 mg/kg DHA was administered and resulted in normalization of plasma fatty acid profiles.[18] Fatty acids in the supplemented form of fish oils can also have antiarrhythmic effects.[60-62] In humans, dietary supplementation with fish oils was associated with a reduction of more than 70% of ventricular premature contractions ccurring in a 24-hour period in 44% of the patients.[63] Similarly, a study of Boxers diagnosed with right ventricular cardiomyopathy reported that supplementation with fish oil significantly reduced arrhythmias and may be helpful in treating this condition in this breed.[61]

When cardiac cachexia is present, increasing the proportion of omega-3 fatty acids in the food may beneficially modulate cytokine production. Reduction of cytokines is correlated to improved survival time in dogs with CHF.[18] Supplementing with fish oils that are high in omega-3 fatty acids can decrease cytokine production in dogs with CHF, improve cardiac cachexia, and in some cases help with palatability issues leading to an increase in food intake.[18] Overall, acknowledging and addressing the issue of cardiac cachexia in dogs and cats is critical in prolonging survival times and modulating the long-term effects seen with CHF.

ANTIOXIDANTS   Reactive oxygen species (ROS) are a byproduct of oxygen metabolism and can be damaging to normal tissues and cell growth. Dogs with CHF experience increased oxidant "stress" as a result of abnormal myocardial function and have a reduced concentration of naturally occurring lipid-soluble antioxidants.[64,65] Supplementation with vitamin C and vitamin E increases plasma concentrations of these antioxidants and reduces plasma F2-alpha–isoprostanes, a marker for oxidative stress.[28] Other antioxidants such as coenzyme Q10 have been helpful in humans with DCM. Some veterinary clinicians have had some apparent success with this antioxidant, although clinical studies on dogs have not yet been published.[19] Supplementation with various antioxidants may be beneficial to animals with DCM and other cardiovascular conditions based on the information that is currently available.

HIGH-QUALITY PROTEIN   High-quality protein has been discussed in other areas of this chapter when considering nutritional modification in treating the cardiac patient. For example, it is important in providing the proper amino acids for taurine production and to prevent muscle wasting or loss of lean body mass. In the 1960s some authors recommended protein restriction for dogs with CHF to prevent "metabolic stress" on the liver caused by excessive dietary protein.[66] However, there are no known published studies to support this theory in dogs and cats, and this practice may actually be detrimental to these patients by predisposing them to a more substantial loss in lean body mass. Because cardiac cachexia is so common in animals with CHF, protein restriction should be limited to only those with concurrent and severe renal disease.[64] In fact, when choosing a diet for heart patients, protein-restricted foods that are formulated for kidney disease should not be used unless serum levels such as blood urea nitrogen and creatinine warrant this.

Other Nutritional Considerations— Obesity

Overweight conditions can exacerbate heart disease because obesity is associated with elevated cardiac output, increased plasma and extracellular fluid volume, increased neurohumoral activation, reductions in urinary sodium and water excretion, elevated blood pressure, increased heart rate, abnormal systolic and diastolic ventricular function, and exercise intolerance.[67] Therefore weight reduction in animals with cardiac disease may be beneficial. In fact, in one study it was demonstrated that weight reduction in obese dogs with pulmonary disease resulted in improved pulmonary function.[68] Therefore a gradual weight reduction in animals with cardiac problems may be helpful, although consideration as to the type of diet is important. Diets geared toward adipose tissue loss rather than protein or amino acid loss are needed to minimize any concurrent or future cardiac cachexia that may occur.

CONCLUSION

When treating dogs and cats with cardiovascular disease, nutritional modification should be considered a primary part of the treatment protocol. Proper nutrition not only helps prolong survival time and enhance the quality of life, but may help reduce the amount of certain medication needed, such as diuretics to reduce the load on the heart and other organs.

References

1. Buchanan JW: Prevalance of cardiovascular disorder. In Fox PR, Sisson D, Moise NS, editors: *Textbook of canine and feline cardiology*, ed 2, Philadelphia, 1999, Saunders, pp 457–470.

2. Fox PR: Pathology of the cardiovascular system. In Fox PR, editor: *Canine and feline cardiology*, New York, 1988, Churchill Livingstone, pp 637–657.

3. Häggström J, Kvart C, Pedersen HD: Acquired valvular heart disease. In Ettinger SJ, Feldman EC, editors: *Textbook of veterinary internal medicine*, ed 6, St Louis, 2005, Saunders.

4. Alroy J, Rush J, Freeman L, and others: Inherited infantile dilated cardiomyopathy in dogs: genetic, clinical, biochemical and morphologic findings, *Am J Med Genet* 95:57–66, 2000.

5. Calvert CA, Jacobs GJ, Smith DD, and others: Association between results of ambulatory electrocardiography and development of cardiomyopathy during long-term follow-up of Doberman Pinschers, *J Am Vet Med Assoc* 216:34–39, 2000.

6. Meurs KM, Spier AW, Wright NA, and others: Comparison of in-hospital versus 24-hour ambulatory electrocardiography for detection of ventricular premature complexes in mature Boxers, *J Am Vet Med Assoc* 218:222–224, 2001.

7. Tidholm A, Svensson H, Sylven C: Survival and prognostic factors in 189 dogs with dilated cardiomyopathy, *J Am Anim Hosp Assoc* 33:364–368, 1997.

8. Monnet E, Orton EC, Salam M, and others: Idiopathic dilated cardiomyopathy in dogs: survival and prognostic indicators, *Vet Intern Med* 9:12–17, 1995.

9. Pion PD, Kittleson MD, Rogers QR, and others: Myocardial failure in cats associated with low plasma taurine: a reversible cardiomyopathy, *Science* 237:764–768, 1987.

10. Freeman LM, Rush JE: Nutrition and cardiomyopathy: lesions from spontaneous animal models, *Curr Heart Failure Rep* 4:84–90, 2007.

11. Cote E, Manning AM, Emerson D, and others: Assessment of the prevalence of heart murmurs in overtly healthy cats, *J Am Vet Med Assoc* 225:384–388, 2004.

12. Atkins CD, Gallo AM, Kurzman ID, Cowen P: Risk factors, clinical signs, and survival in cats with a clinical diagnosis of idiopathic hypertrophic cardiomyopathy: 74 cases (1985-1989), *J Am Vet Med Assoc* 201:613–618, 1992.

13. Meurs KM, Sanchez X, David RM, and others: A cardiac myosin binding protein C mutation in the Maine Coon cat with familial hypertrophic cardiomyopathy, *Hum Mol Genet* 14:3587–3593, 2005.

14. Rush JE, Freeman LM, Fenollosa N, Brown DJ: Population and survival characteristics of cats with hypertrophic cardiomyopathy: 260 cases (1990-1999), *J Am Vet Med Assoc* 220:202–207, 2002.

15. Kittleson MD: Feline myocardial disease. In Ettinger SJ, Feldman EC, editors: *Textbook of veterinary internal medicine*, ed 6, St Louis, 2005, Saunders.

16. Kittleson MD, Meurs KM, Munro MJ, and others: Familial hypertrophic cardiomyopathy in Main Coon cats: an animal model of human disease, *Circulation* 99:3172–3180, 1999.

17. Baty CJ: Feline hypertrophic cardiomyopathy: an update, *Vet Clin Small Anim* 34:1227–1234, 2004.

18. Freeman LM, Rush JE, Kehayias JJ, and others: Nutritional alternations and the effect of fish oil supplementation in dogs with heart failure, *J Vet Intern Med* 12:440–448, 1998.

19. Freeman LM: Interventional nutrition for cardiac disease, *Clin Tech Small Anim Pract* 13:232–237, 1998.

20. Freeman LM, Rush JE: Relationship between cachexia and lymphocyte subpopulations and hematologic parameters in dogs with spontaneously-occurring congestive heart failure. In *Proceedings of the third cachexia conference*, vol 82, Rome, Italy, December 8-10, 2005.

21. Mallery KF, Freeman LM, Harpster NK, and others: Factors contributing to the decisions for euthanasia in dogs with congestive heart failure, *J Am Vet Med Assoc* 214:1201–1204, 1999.

22. Freeman LM, Rush JE, Cahalane AK, and others: Dietary patterns in dogs with cardiac disease, *J Am Vet Med Assoc* 223:1301–1305, 2003.

23. Torin DS, Freeman LM, Rush JE: Dietary patterns of cats with cardiac disease, *J Am Vet Med Assoc* 230:862–867, 2007.

24. Freeman LM, Roubenoff R: The nutrition implications of cardiac cachexia, *Nutr Rev* 52:340–347, 1994.

25. Poehlman ET, Scheffers, Gottieb SS, and others: Increased resting metabolic rates in patients with congestive heart failure, *Ann Intern Med* 121:860–862, 1994.

26. Boegehold MA, Kotchen TA: Relative contributions of dietary Na+ and Cl– to salt-sensitive hypertension, *Hypertension* 14:579–583, 1989.

27. Pedersen HD: Effects of mild mitral valve insufficiency, sodium intake, and place of blood sampling on the rennin-angiotensin system in dogs, *Acta Vet Scand* 37:109–118, 1996.

28. Freeman LM, Rush JE, Markwell PJ: Effects of dietary modification in dogs with early chronic valvular disease, *J Vet Intern Med* 20:1116–1126, 2006.

29. Pensinger R: Dietary control of sodium intake in spontaneous congestive heart failure in dogs, *Vet Med* 59:752–784, 1964.

30. Freeman LM, Rush JE, Cahalane AK, and others: Evaluation of dietary patterns in dogs with cardiac disease, *J Am Vet Med Assoc* 223:1301–1305, 2003.

31. Freeman LM, Rush JE, Cahalane AK, Markwell PJ: Dietary patterns of dogs with cardiac disease, *J Nutr* 132:1632S–1633S, 2002.

32. Tenaglia A, Cody R: Evidence for a taurine-deficient cardiomyopathy, *Am J Cardiol* 62:136–139, 1998.

33. Huxtable RJ, Chubb J, Asari J: Physiological and experimental regulation of taurine content in the heart, *Fed Proc* 39:2685–2690, 1980.

34. Schaffer SW, Kramer J, Chovan JP: Regulation of calcium homeostasis in the heart by taurine, *Fed Proc* 39:2691–2694, 1980.

35. Sanderson SL: Taurine and carnitine in canine cardiomyopathy, *Vet Clin Small Anim* 36:1325–1343, 2006.

36. Huxtable RJ: Physilogical actions of taurine, *Physiol Rev* 72:101–163, 1992.

37. Kramer GA, Kittleson MD, Fox PR: Plasma taurine concentrations in normal dogs and in dogs with heart disease, *J Vet Intern Med* 9:253–258, 1995.

38. Kittleson MD, Keene B, Pion PD, and others: Results of the multicenter Spaniel trial (MUST), *J Vet Intern Med* 11:204–211, 1997.

39. Freeman LM, Rush JE, Brown DJ, and others: Relationship between circulating and dietary taurine concentrations in dogs with dilated cardiomyopathy, *Vet Ther* 2:370–378, 2001.

40. Fascetti AJ, Reed JR, Roger QR, and others: Taurine deficiency in dogs with dilated cardiomyopathy: 12 cases (1997-2001), *J Am Vet Med Assoc* 223:1137–1141, 2003.

41. Backus RC, Ko KS, Fascetti AJ: Low plasma taurine concentration in Newfoundland dogs is associated with low plasma methionine and cysteine concentrations and low taurine synthesis, *J Nutr* 136:2525–2533, 2006.

42. Sanderson SL, Gross KL, Ogburn PN, and others: Effects of dietary fat and L-carnitine on plasma and whole blood taurine concentrations and cardiac function in healthy dogs fed protein-restricted diets, *Am J Vet Res* 62:1616–1623, 2001.

43. Pion PD, Sanderson SL, Kittleson MD: The effectiveness of taurine and levocarnitine in dogs with heart disease, *Vet Clin North Am Small Anim Pract* 28:1495–1514, 1998.

44. Delaney SJ, Kass PH, Rogers QR, Fascetti AJ: Plasma and whole blood taurine in normal dogs of varying size fed commercially prepared food, *J Anim Physiol Anim Nutr* 87:236–244, 2003.

45. Spitze AR, Wong DL, Rogers QR, Fascetti AJ: Taurine concentrations in animal feed ingredients; cooking influences taurine content, *J Anim Physiol Anim Nutr* 87:251–261, 2003.

46. Torres Cl, Backus RC, Fascetti AJ, Rogers QR: Taurine status in normal dogs fed a commercial diet associated with taurine deficiency and dilated cardiomyopathy, *J Anim Physiol Anim Nutr* 87:359–372, 2003.

47. Backus RC, Cohen G, Pion PD, and others: Taurine deficiency in Newfoundlands fed commercially available complete and balanced diets, *J Am Vet Med Assoc* 223:1130–1136, 2003.

48. Belanger MC, Quellet M, Queney G, and others: Taurine-deficient dilated cardiomyopathy in a family of Golden Retrievers, *J Am Anim Hosp Assoc* 41:284–291, 2005.

49. Stratton-Phelps M, Backus RB, Rogers QR, and others: Dietary rice bran decreases plasma and whole-blood taurine in cats, *J Nutr* 132:1745S–1747S, 2002.

50. Rebouche CJ, Engel AG: Kinetic compartmental analysis of carnitine metabolism in the dog, *Arch Biochem Biophys* 220:60–70, 1983.

51. Neely JR, Morgan HA: Relationship between carbohydrate metabolism and energy balance of heart muscle, *Annu Rev Physiol* 36:413–459, 1974.

52. Stumpt DA, Parker WD Jr, Angelini C: Carnitine deficiency, organic acidemias, and Reye's syndrome, *Neurology* 35:1041–1045, 1985.

53. Gilbert EF: Carnitine deficiency, *Pathology* 17:161–169, 1985.

54. Paulson DJ: Carnitine deficiency-induced cardiomyopathy, *Mol Cell Biochem* 180:33–41, 1998.

55. Keene BW: L-carnitine deficiency in canine dilated cardiomyopathy. In Kirk RW, Bonagura JD, editors: *Current veterinary therapy XI*, Philadelphia, 1992, Saunders.

56. Sanderson S, Osborne C, Ogburn P, and others: Canine cystinuria associated with carnitinuria and carnitine deficiency (abstract), *J Vet Intern Med* 9:212, 1995.

57. McEntee K, Clercx C, Snaps F, and others: Clinical, electrocardiographic and echocardiographic improvements after L-carnitine supplementation in a cardiomyopathic Labrador, *Canine Pract* 20:12–15, 1995.

58. Keene BW, Panciera DP, Atkins CE, and others: Myocardial L-carnitine deficiency in a family of dogs with cardiomyopathy, *J Am Vet Med Assoc* 198:647–650, 1991.

59. Costa ND, Labuc RH: Case report: efficacy of oral carnitine therapy for dilated cardiomyopathy in Boxer dogs, *J Nutr* 124:2687S–2692S, 1995.

60. Endres S, Ghorbani R, Kelley VE, and others: The effect of dietary supplementation with n-3 polyunsaturated fatty acids on the synthesis of interleukin-1 and tumor necrosis factor by mononuclear cells, *N Engl J Med* 320:265–271, 1989.

61. Smith CE, Freeman LM, Rush JE, and others: Omega-3 fatty acids in Boxer dogs with arrhythmogenic right ventricular cardiomyopathy, *J Vet Intern Med* 21:265–273, 2007.

62. Kang JX, Leaf A: Antiarrhythmic effects of polyunsaturated fatty acids: recent studies, *Circulation* 94:1774–1780, 1996.

63. Sellmayer A, Witzgall H, Lorenz RL, and others: Effects of dietary fish oil on ventricular premature complexes, *Am J Cardiol* 76:974–977, 1995.

64. Freeman LM, Brown DJ, Rush JE: Assessment of degree of oxidative stress and antioxidant concentrations in dogs with idiopathic dilated cardiomyopathy, *J Am Vet Med Assoc* 215:644–646, 1999.

65. Freeman LM, Rush JE, Milbury PE, Blumber JB: Antioxidant status and biomarkers of oxidative stress in dogs with congestive heart failure, *J Vet Intern Med* 19:537–541, 2005.

66. Pensinger RR: Nutritional management of heart disease. In Kirk RW, editor: *Current veterinary therapy III*, Philadelphia, 1968, Saunders, pp 229–232.

67. Alexander JK: The heart and obesity. In Hurst JW, editor: *The heart*, ed 6, New York, 1986, McGraw-Hill, p 1452.

68. Brinson JJ, McKiernan BC: Respiratory function in obese dogs with chronic respiratory disease and their response to treatment, *J Vet Intern Med* 12:209, 1998.

Appendix 1 Estimated Metabolizable Energy Requirements of Adult Dogs

WEIGHT (LB)	WEIGHT (KG)	INACTIVE (KCAL/DAY)[*]	ACTIVE (KCAL/DAY)[*]
2	0.91	88.37	120.92
4	1.82	148.61	203.37
6	2.72	201.43	275.64
8	3.63	249.94	342.02
10	4.54	295.47	404.33
12	5.45	338.77	463.58
14	6.36	380.29	520.39
16	7.26	420.34	575.21
18	8.17	459.17	628.33
20	9.08	496.92	680.00
25	11.35	587.45	803.88
30	13.62	673.53	921.67
35	15.89	756.08	1034.63
40	18.16	835.72	1143.62
45	20.43	912.90	1249.24
50	22.70	987.97	1351.96
55	24.97	1061.18	1452.14
60	27.24	1132.74	1550.06
65	29.51	1202.82	1645.96
70	31.78	1271.57	1740.04
75	34.05	1339.10	1832.45
80	36.32	1405.51	1923.33
85	38.59	1470.89	2012.79
90	40.86	1535.31	2100.96
95	43.13	1598.85	2187.90
100	45.40	1661.56	2273.71
105	47.67	1723.48	2358.45
110	49.94	1784.68	2442.19
115	52.21	1845.18	2524.98
120	54.48	1905.03	2606.88
125	56.75	1964.26	2687.93
130	59.02	2022.89	2768.17
135	61.29	2080.97	2847.64
140	63.56	2138.51	2926.38
145	65.83	2195.54	3004.42
150	68.10	2252.08	3081.79

*Inactive adult dogs: metabolizable energy requirement = $95 \times (W_{kg})^{0.75}$. Active adult dogs: metabolizable energy requirement = $30 \times (W_{kg})^{0.75}$.

Appendix 2 Estimated Metabolizable Energy Requirements of Adult Cats

Weight (lb)	Weight (kg)	Lean adult (kcal/day)[*]	Overweight adult (kcal/day)[*]
2	0.91	93.74	125.08
3	1.36	123.00	147.10
4	1.82	149.14	165.04
5	2.27	173.20	180.45
6	2.72	195.70	194.10
7	3.18	216.99	206.45
8	3.63	237.30	217.77
9	4.09	256.79	228.28
10	4.54	275.57	238.10
12	5.45	311.37	256.12
14	6.36	345.25	272.41
16	7.26	377.56	287.35
18	8.17	408.56	301.21
20	9.08	438.45	314.18
22	9.99	467.36	326.39
24	10.90	495.41	337.95
26	11.80	522.71	348.94

[*]Lean adult cats: metabolizable energy requirement $= 100 \times (W_{kg})^{0.67}$. Overweight adult cats: metabolizable energy requirement $= 130 \times (W_{kg})^{0.40}$.

Appendix 3

Standard Weights for American Kennel Club Dog Breeds (lb)

Group 1—sporting

BREED	MALE	FEMALE
Brittany	35-40	30-40
Pointer	55-75	45-64
German Shorthaired Pointer	55-70	45-60
German Wirehaired Pointer	60-75	50-65
Chesapeake Bay Retriever	65-80	55-70
Curly-Coated Retriever	65-70	65-70
Flat-Coated Retriever	50-65	45-60
Golden Retriever	65-75	55-65
Labrador Retriever	65-80	55-70
English Setter	60-75	55-65
Gordon Setter	55-80	45-70
Irish Setter	~70	~60
American Water Spaniel	28-45	25-40
Clumber Spaniel	70-85	55-70
Cocker Spaniel	25-30	20-25
English Cocker Spaniel	28-34	26-32
English Springer Spaniel	49-54	40-45
Field Spaniel	35-50	35-50
Irish Water Spaniel	55-65	45-58
Sussex Spaniel	35-45	35-45
Welsh Springer Spaniel	35-45	30-40
Vizsla	45-55	40-50
Weimaraner	60-75	55-70
Wirehaired Pointing Griffon	55-65	50-60

Group 2—hound

BREED	MALE	FEMALE
Afghan Hound	~60	~50
Basenji	~24	~22
Basset Hound	65-75	50-65
Beagle, 13″	13-18	13-16
Beagle, 15″	17-22	15-20
Black and Tan Coonhound	70-85	55-70
Bloodhound	90-110	80-100
Borzoi	75-105	70-90
Dachshund, Miniature	~10	~10
Dachshund, Standard	16-22	16-22
American Foxhound	65-75	55-65
English Foxhound	65-75	50-70
Greyhound	65-70	60-65

Continued

Group 2—hound, cont'd

BREED	MALE	FEMALE
Harrier	40-50	35-45
Ibizan Hound	~50	~45
Irish Wolfhound	~120	~105
Norwegian Elkhound	~55	~48
Otter Hound	75-115	65-100
Petit Basset Griffon Vendeen	40-45	40-45
Pharaoh Hound	55-70	50-65
Rhodesian Ridgeback	~75	~65
Saluki	50-70	45-65
Scottish Deerhound	85-110	75-95
Whippet	20-28	18-23

Group 3—working

BREED	MALE	FEMALE
Akita	70-85	65-75
Alaskan Malamute	85-95	75-85
Bernese Mountain Dog	75-90	65-80
Boxer	55-70	50-60
Bullmastiff	110-130	100-120
Doberman Pinscher	65-80	55-70
Giant Schnauzer	70-85	60-75
Great Dane	120-180	100-130
Great Pyrenees	100-125	85-115
Komondor	100-130	80-110
Kuvasz	100-115	70-90
Mastiff	75-190	160-180
Newfoundland	130-150	100-120
Portuguese Water Dog	42-60	35-50
Rottweiler	80-95	70-85
Saint Bernard	130-180	120-160
Samoyed	50-65	45-60
Siberian Husky	45-60	35-50
Standard Schnauzer	30-40	25-35

Group 4—terrier

BREED	MALE	FEMALE
Airedale Terrier	45-60	40-55
American Staffordshire Terrier	45-55	40-50
Australian Terrier	12-14	12-14
Bedlington Terrier	17-23	17-23
Border Terrier	13-15	11-14
Bull Terrier	52-62	45-55
Cairn Terrier	~14	~13
Dandie Dinmont Terrier	13-24	18-24
Fox Terrier, Smooth	17-19	15-17
Fox Terrier, Wire	17-19	15-17
Irish Terrier	~27	~25

Group 4—terrier, cont'd

BREED	MALE	FEMALE
Kerry Blue Terrier	33-40	30-38
Lakeland Terrier	~17	~17
Manchester Terrier, Standard	12-22	12-22
Miniature Bull Terrier	15-20	15-20
Miniature Schnauzer	16-18	12-16
Norfolk Terrier	11-12	11-12
Norwich Terrier	11-12	11-12
Scottish Terrier	19-22	18-21
Sealyham Terrier	23-24	21-23
Skye Terrier	25-30	20-25
Soft-Coated Wheaten Terrier	35-40	30-35
Staffordshire Bull Terrier	28-28	24-34
Welsh Terrier	18-22	16-18
West Highland White Terrier	12-14	11-13

Group 5—toy

BREED	MALE	FEMALE
Affenpinscher	7-8	7-8
Brussels Griffon	10-12	8-10
Chihuahua	2-7	2-7
English Toy Spaniel	8-14	8-14
Italian Greyhound	8-15	8-15
Japanese Chin	14-20	14-20
Maltese	4-6	4-6
Manchester Terrier	7-12	7-11
Miniature Pinscher	10-12	9-11
Papillon	8-10	7-9
Pekingese	10-14	10-14
Pomeranian	4-8	4-7
Toy Poodle	7-10	7-10
Pug	14-18	14-18
Shih Tzu	12-17	10-15
Silky Terrier	8-10	8-10
Yorkshire Terrier	5-8	4-6

Group 6—nonsporting

BREED	MALE	FEMALE
Bichon Frise	9-12	9-12
Boston Terrier	15-24	15-24
Bulldog	45-55	40-50
Chinese Shar-Pei	45-55	35-45
Chow Chow	45-60	40-50
Dalmatian	50-65	45-55
Finnish Spitz	25-35	25-30
French Bulldog	20-28	20-28
Keeshond	40-50	40-50
Lhasa Apso	13-15	13-15
Poodle, Standard	50-60	45-55

Continued

Group 6—nonsporting, cont'd

BREED	MALE	FEMALE
Poodle, Miniature	17-20	15-20
Schipperke	12-18	12-16
Tibetan Spaniel	9-15	9-15
Tibetan Terrier	18-30	18-30

Group 7—herding

BREED	MALE	FEMALE
Australian Cattle Dog	35-45	35-45
Australian Shepherd	45-65	45-65
Bearded Collie	55-65	50-60
Belgian Malinois	60-70	43-55
Belgian Sheepdog	60-70	43-55
Belgian Tervuren	60-70	43-55
Bouvier des Flanders	70-90	70-90
Briard	65-75	60-70
Collie	65-75	50-65
German Shepherd Dog	75-90	65-80
Old English Sheepdog	60-70	60-70
Puli	29-33	29-33
Shetland Sheepdog	16-22	14-18
Welsh Corgi, Cardigan	30-38	25-34
Welsh Corgi, Pembroke	27-30	25-28

Glossary

acanthosis nigricans diffuse hyperplasia of the spinous layer of the skin, with gray, brown, or black pigmentation.

accretion growth by addition of material.

acrodermatitis severe skin lesions.

adipocyte hyperplasia an increase in the number of fat cells, occurring normally during certain developmental periods such as early growth and, occasionally, puberty.

adipocyte specialized cells that store large amounts of triglyceride.

alopecia the absence of hair from the skin areas where it is normally present.

anabolism any process by which organisms convert substances into other components of the organism's chemical architecture.

anorexia lack or loss of the appetite for food.

arrhythmia lacking a steady rhythm.

articular cartilage cartilage covering the articular surfaces of the bones, forming a synovial joint.

ascites effusion and accumulation of serous fluid in the abdominal cavity.

ataxia failure of muscular coordination; irregularity of muscular action.

azotemia an excess of urea or other nitrogenous compounds in the blood.

bone meal the dried, ground, and sterilized product from undecomposed bones.

BUN blood urea nitrogen.

byproduct secondary products in addition to the principal product; the parts that are left after the economically valuable pieces are harvested.

calculolytic pertaining to the destruction or decomposition of a calculus.

calorie the amount of heat energy that is necessary to raise the temperature of 1 gram of water from 14.5° C to 15.5° C. Because the calorie is such a small unit of measure, the kilocalorie, equal to 1000 calories, is most often used in the science of animal nutrition.

cardiomyopathy deterioration of the function of the myocardium (heart muscle) for any reason.

carnivorous eating or subsisting on primarily animal material.

carpus the joint between the paw and the forelimb (the wrist in humans).

cation an ion carrying a positive charge owing to a deficiency of electrons; in an electrochemical cell, cations migrate toward the cathode.

cellulose an unbranched, long-chain polysaccharide that is a component of dietary fiber; forms the skeleton of most plant structures and plant cells.

chondrodysplasia an inherited disease characterized by abnormal growth at the ends of bones.

chylomicron a class of lipoproteins responsible for the transport of exogenous cholesterol and triglycerides from the small intestine to tissues after meals.

colostrum the first product of the mammary gland following parturition.

coprophagy the ingestion of dung or feces.

corn gluten meal the dried residue from corn after the removal of the larger part of the starch and germ and the separation of the bran.

costochondral pertaining to a rib and its cartilage.

creatinine the end product of creatine metabolism, found in muscle and blood and excreted in the urine.

crepitation dry, crackling sound like that of grating the ends of a fractured bone.

crystalluria excretion of crystals in the urine, in some cases producing urinary tract irritation.

cyanosis a bluish discoloration of the skin and mucous membranes as a result of excessive concentration of reduced hemoglobin in the blood.

cystitis inflammation of the urinary bladder.

cystocentesis perforation or tapping, as with an aspirator, trocar, or needle, to remove urinary bladder contents.

demodicosis skin disease caused by the mange mite *Demodex canis* in dogs.

deoxyribonucleic acid (DNA) a nucleic acid that constitutes the genetic material of all cellular organisms.

dietary thermogenesis also called the *specific dynamic action of food*; the energy needed by the body to digest, absorb, and assimilate nutrients.

duodenum the first or proximal portion of the small intestine extending from the pylorus to the jejunum.

dyspnea difficult or labored respiration.

dystocia abnormal labor or birth.

echocardiography noninvasive diagnostic procedure that uses ultrasound to study the structure and function of the heart.

eicosanoids biologically active substances that are metabolites of 20-carbon fatty acids; includes prostaglandins, leukotrienes, prostacyclins, and thromboxanes.

emesis the reflex act of ejecting the contents of the stomach through the mouth; vomiting.

endocarditis inflammation of the endocardium and heart valves.

endogenous developing or originating within the organism or arising from causes within the organism.

energy density for a pet food, refers to the number of calories provided by the food in a given weight or volume. In the United States, it is expressed as kilocalories of metabolizable energy per kilogram or pound of diet; in Europe, kilojoule per kilogram is used.

energy imbalance occurs when an animal's daily energy consumption is either greater or less than its daily requirement, leading to changes in growth rate, body weight, and body composition.

enterohepatic pertaining to the intestine (entero) and the liver (hepatic).

epiphysis the expanded articular end of a long bone, developed from a secondary ossification center.

erythropoiesis the production of erythrocytes (red blood cells).

essential nutrients nutrients that cannot be synthesized by the body at a rate adequate to meet body needs and that must be supplied in the diet.

estrus the recurrent, restricted period of sexual receptivity in female mammals.

exogenous developing or originating outside the organism.

extravasation a discharge or escape, as of blood from a vessel into the tissues.

germ as in wheat germ, the plant embryo found in seeds and frequently separated from the bran (outer coat of a seed) and starch endosperm during milling.

glomerulosclerosis fibrosis and scarring that result in senescence of the renal glomeruli.

gluconeogenesis the formation of glucose from molecules that are not carbohydrates, as from amino acids, lactate, and the glycerol portion of fats.

gluten the tough, thick, proteinaceous substance that remains when the flour, wheat, or other grain is washed to remove the starch.

glycosuria the excretion of an abnormal concentration of glucose in the urine.

grain the seed from cereal plants (e.g., wheat, rice, barley, oats).

Heinz bodies coccoid inclusion bodies resulting from oxidative injury to and precipitation of hemoglobin, seen in the presence of certain abnormal hemoglobins and erythrocytes with enzyme deficiencies.

hematocrit the ratio of the total red cell volume to the total blood volume.

hemicellulose a heterogeneous group of branched-chain polysaccharides that, together with pectin, forms the matrix of plant cells within which cellulose fibers are enmeshed.

hemolytic anemia anemia as a result of intravascular fragmentation of red blood cells.

hepatic lipidosis an abnormal accumulation of fats and fat-like substances in the liver.

hepatomegaly enlargement of the liver.

hepatopathy disease or disorder of the liver.

homeostasis the maintenance of stability in the body's internal environment, achieved by a system of control mechanisms activated by negative feedback.

hydrolysis the splitting of a compound into fragments by the addition of water. The hydroxyl group is incorporated in one fragment and the hydrogen atom in the other.

hydroxyapatite an inorganic compound, found in the matrix of bone and the teeth, that is composed of calcium, phosphorous, hydrogen, and oxygen and provides rigidity.

hypercalcemia increased calcium concentration in the blood.

hyperkeratosis thickening of the stratum corneum (outer layer of skin), often associated with qualitative abnormality of the keratin.

hyperlipidemia a general term for elevated concentrations of triglyceride and/or cholesterol in the plasma of fasted animals.

hyperphagia ingestion of a greater than optimal quantity of food.

hyperplasia increase in cell number.

hypertrophy increase in cell size.

hypophosphatemia decreased phosphorous concentration in the blood.

hypothalamus gland located in the brain that exerts control over the function of a portion of the pituitary gland. Its nuclei comprise part of the mechanism that activates, controls, and integrates the peripheral autonomic mechanisms, which include a general regulation of water balance, body temperature, sleep, and food intake.

iatrogenic any adverse condition occurring as the result of treatment, especially infections acquired during the course of treatment.

icterus jaundice.

idiopathic self-originated or of unknown causation.

inappetence lack of appetite.

indole a compound that is produced by the decomposition of tryptophan in the intestine; it is partly responsible for the peculiar odor of the feces.

jejunum the portion of the small intestine that extends from the duodenum to the ileum.

keratin scleroprotein that is the principal constituent of epidermis, hair, nails, horny tissues, and the organic matrix of the enamel of teeth.

keratinization the development of or conversion into the structural protein keratin.

kilojoule the amount of mechanical energy that is required for a force of 1 newton to move a weight of 1 kilogram a distance of 1 meter. To convert kilocalories to kilojoule, the number of kilocalories is multiplied by 4.184.

lactic acid an end product of glycolysis that provides energy anaerobically in skeletal muscle during heavy exercise. It can be oxidized aerobically in the heart for energy production or can be converted back to glucose (gluconeogenesis) in the liver.

leukotriene one of a group of biologically active compounds formed from 20-carbon fatty acids that function as regulators of allergic and inflammatory reactions.

ligand a molecule that binds to another molecule; commonly refers to a small molecule that binds specifically to a larger molecule.

lipemia retinalis a milky appearance of the veins and arteries of the retina, occurring as a result of hyperlipidemia.

lipidosis a term for several of the lysosomal storage diseases in which there is an abnormal accumulation of lipids in the reticuloendothelial cells. Also called *lipid storage disease.*

lipogenesis the formation of fat; the transformation of non-fat food materials into body fat.

lipoid granuloma a small, nodular, delimited aggregation of lipid cells; a xanthoma.

lumen the cavity or channel within a tube or tubular organ (e.g., the intestine).

lymphadenopathy chronic abnormal enlargement of the lymph nodes (usually associated with disease).

meal an ingredient that has been ground or otherwise reduced in particle size.

meat and bone meal the same as meat meal, except that meat and bone meal can contain a great deal more bone (raising the ash content and lowering the protein quality).

meat byproducts the nonrendered, clean parts, other than meat, derived from slaughtered mammals; include, but are not limited to, lungs, spleen, kidneys, brain, liver, blood, bone, and stomach/intestine, without their contents.

meat meal the rendered product from mammal tissues exclusive of blood, hair, hoof, horn, hide trimmings, manure, stomach, and rumen contents, except in such amounts as may occur unavoidably in good processing practices.

meniscus the disk of cartilage that serves as a cushion between the ends of bones that meet at a joint.

metabolism the sum of all the physical and chemical processes by which living, organized substance is produced and maintained (anabolism); also the transformation by which energy is made available for the uses of the organism (catabolism).

metabolizable energy (ME) the amount of energy that is ultimately available to the tissues of the body after losses in the feces and urine have been subtracted from the gross energy of food. It is the value that is most often used to express the energy content of pet food ingredients and commercial diets.

metaphysis the wider part at the extremity of the shaft of a long bone, adjacent to the epiphyseal disk. During development it contains the growth zone and consists of spongy bone; in the adult it is continuous with the epiphysis.

methemoglobinemia the presence of methemoglobin in the blood, resulting in cyanosis.

necrosis cell and tissue death.

neoplasia the progressive multiplication of cells under conditions that would not elicit or would cause cessation of multiplication of normal cells; may be malignant or benign.

nephrosclerosis sclerosis (invasion of connective tissue at the expense of active tissue) of the kidney.

neuropathies general term denoting functional disturbances and/or pathological changes in the peripheral nervous system.

nonessential nutrients nutrients that can be synthesized by the body at a level sufficient to meet body needs; can be obtained either through de novo synthesis or from the diet.

nutraceutical a food or naturally occurring food supplement thought to have a beneficial effect on human or animal health.

omnivorous subsisting on both plants and animals.

os penis a heterotopic bone developed in the fibrous septum between the corpora cavernosa and above the urethra, forming the skeleton of the penis.

osmosis the passage of pure solvent from a solution of lesser to one of greater solute concentration when the two solutions are separated by a membrane that selectively prevents the passage of solute molecules but is permeable to the solvent.

ossification the process of creating bone; that is, of transforming cartilage (or fibrous tissue) into bone.

osteochondrosis a disease of the growth or ossification centers of bones that begins as a degeneration or necrosis, followed by regeneration or recalcification.

osteocyte a mature bone cell of adult bone that is isolated in a lacuna of the bone substance.

parakeratosis retention of nuclei in the cells of the stratum corneum of the epidermis, as in psoriasis.

parturition the act or process of giving birth.

pearled barley dehulled barley grain.

periosteum a specialized connective tissue covering all bones of the body and possessing bone-forming potentialities.

peristalsis rhythmic movements produced by the functioning longitudinal and circular muscle fibers of the small intestine to propel food forward.

phylogeny the evolutionary history of a group of organisms.

polydipsia chronic excessive thirst.

polyphagia excessive eating.

polyuria the passage of a large volume of urine in a given period of time.

postprandial occurring after a meal.

poultry byproduct meal ground, rendered, clean parts of the carcasses of slaughtered poultry such as necks, feet, undeveloped eggs, and intestines, exclusive of feathers except in such amounts as might occur unavoidably in good processing practices.

poultry byproducts nonrendered, clean parts of carcasses of slaughtered poultry such as heads, feet, and viscera free from fecal content and foreign matter except in such trace amounts as might occur unavoidably in good processing practices.

poultry meal (also includes chicken meal if the origin is strictly chicken) the dry rendered product from a combination of clean flesh and skin, with or without the accompanying bone, derived from the parts of whole carcasses of poultry exclusive of feathers, heads, feet, and entrails.

prepuce a covering fold of skin over the penis.

proprioception perception/awareness of position provided by sensory nerve terminals that give information concerning movements and position of the body.

prostacyclin a prostaglandin synthesized by endothelial cells lining the cardiovascular system; a physiological antagonist of thromboxane.

prostaglandins any of a group of components derived from unsaturated 20-carbon fatty acids, primarily arachidonic acid.

proteoglycan group of polysaccharide-protein conjugates present in connective tissue and cartilage; form the ground substance in the extracellular matrix of connective tissue and also have lubricant and support functions.

pruritus descriptive of any of various conditions marked by itching.

purulent consisting of or containing pus.

pylorus the distal opening of the stomach surrounded by a strong band of circular muscle through which the stomach contents are emptied into the duodenum.

pyoderma any purulent skin disease.

pyrexia a fever or febrile condition; abnormal elevation of body temperature.

senescence the process or condition of growing old, especially the condition resulting from the transitions and accumulations of the deleterious aging processes.

skatole a crystalline amine with a strong characteristic odor, found in feces; produced by the decomposition of proteins in the intestine and directly from the amino acid tryptophan by decarboxylation.

stenosis narrowing or stricture of a duct or canal.

struvite a urinary calculus composed of magnesium ammonium phosphate.

subluxation an incomplete or partial dislocation; in the case of canine hip dysplasia, the head of the femur partially dislodges from the cup (acetabulum) of the pelvic bone.

suppuration the formation of pus.

syncopy sudden, usually temporary, loss of consciousness generally caused by insufficient oxygen in the brain; fainting.

tachycardia abnormally rapid heartbeat.

tachypnea increased rate of breathing.

taurine a beta-amino acid that contains a sulfonic group rather than a carboxylic group and so cannot form a peptide bond. It is an essential amino acid for cats, but not for dogs.

theobromine a methylxanthine contained in chocolate; has physiological properties similar to those of caffeine.

thermogenesis the production of heat by physiological processes.

thromboembolism occlusion of a blood vessel by an embolus that has broken away from a thrombus (clot).

thromboxane an extremely potent inducer of platelet aggregation and platelet-release reactions; also a vasoconstrictor; it is a physiological antagonist of prostacyclin.

urethritis inflammation of the urethra.

urolithiasis the disease condition associated with the presence of urinary calculi or stones.

villi multitudinous, threadlike projections that cover the surface of the mucosa of the small intestine and serve as the sites of absorption (by active transport and diffusion) of fluids and nutrients.

vulva the region of the external genital organs of the female.

xanthoma a tumor composed of lipid-laden foam cells.

Index

Page numbers followed by f, t, or b indicate figures, tables, or boxes, respectively.